$120.00

AF768329

CLINICAL NEUROSURGERY

CONGRESS OF NEUROLOGICAL SURGEONS
1951
ERUDITIO OBSERVANTIA SOCIETAS

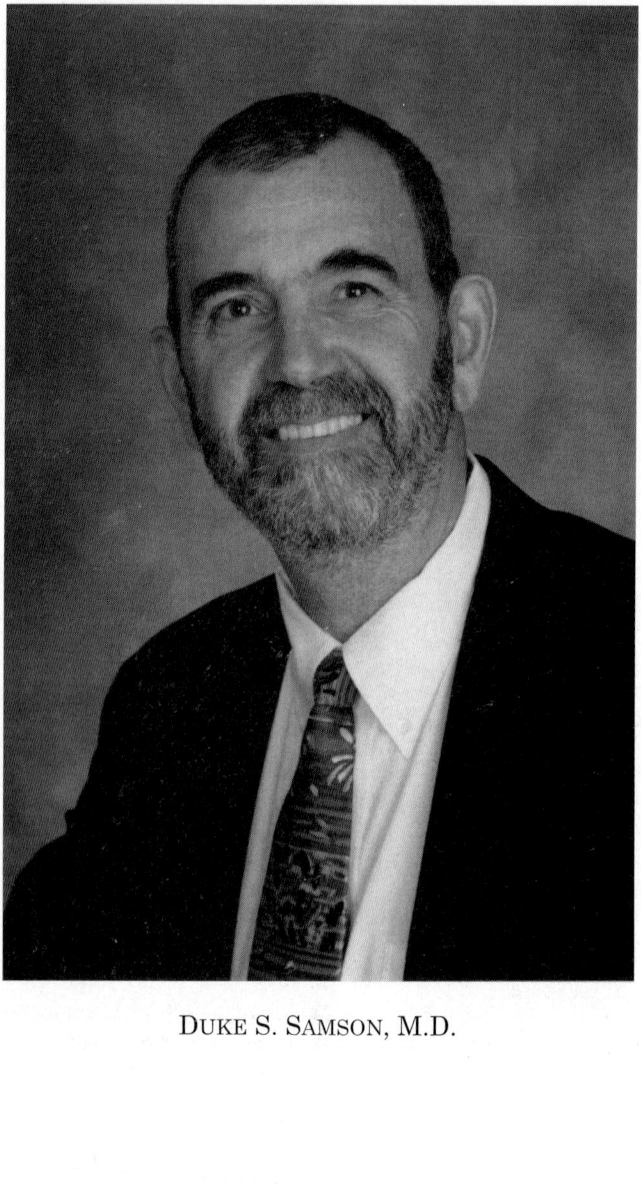

Duke S. Samson, M.D.

CLINICAL NEUROSURGERY

Volume 47

Proceedings

OF THE

CONGRESS OF NEUROLOGICAL SURGEONS

Boston, Massachusetts
1999

LIPPINCOTT WILLIAMS & WILKINS
A **Wolters Kluwer** Company
Philadelphia • Baltimore • New York • London
Buenos Aires • Hong Kong • Sydney • Tokyo

LIPPINCOTT
WILLIAMS
& WILKINS

Accurate indications, adverse reactions, and dosage schedules for drugs are provided in this book, but it possible that they may change. The reader is urged to review the package information data of the manufacturers of the medications mentioned.

Printed in the United State of America
(ISBN 0-7817-3034-1)

Preface

The 49th Annual Meeting of the Congress of Neurological Surgeons was held at the John B. Hynes Veterans Convention Center in Boston Massachusetts from October 30 to November 4, 1999. Volume 47 of *Clinical Neurosurgery* represents the official compendium of the platform presentations from that meeting, and I am privileged to be its Editor-in-Chief for the next three years.

The Annual Meeting Chairman, Dr. Issam A. Awad, and the Scientific Program Chairman, Dr. Vincent C. Traynelis, organized and led an outstanding meeting. Our Honored Guest, Dr. Duke S. Samson, offered thoughtful and instructive contributions throughout the meeting. The Presidential Address by Dr. Hunt Batjer provided an intriguing historic perspective on the challenges faced by neurosurgeons and an inspiring call to action for all of our members.

Splendid New England fall weather attended this event in the beautiful and historic city of Boston. As always, members of the Congress were treated to an excellent scientific and social program. All participants of the multiple meeting committees should be congratulated on their fine work. In particular, I wish to thank the contributors to *Clinical Neurosurgery* for their cooperation and timeliness in submitting their manuscripts and to my Associate Editors for their diligent editing of these manuscripts. I would like to express my gratitude, as well, to Vicki Vaughn at Lippincott Williams & Wilkins who ushered this project through to fruition. And, finally, I would like to acknowledge the efforts of my dedicated secretary, Brenda Gropman, for her superb assistance. I look forward to seeing you all once again at our 50th anniversary meeting and celebration in San Antonio, Texas, September 23–28, 2000.

MATTHEW A. HOWARD III, M.D.
Editor

J. PAUL ELLIOTT, M.D.
Associate Editor

MICHAEL M. HAGLUND, M.D., PH.D., MPH
Associate Editor

GUY M. MCKHANN II, M.D.
Associate Editor

Honored Guests

1952—Professor Herbert Olivecrona, Stockholm, Sweden
1953—Sir Geoffrey Jefferson, Manchester, England
1954—Dr. Kenneth G. McKenzie, Toronto, Canada
1955—Dr. Carl W. Rand, Los Angeles, California
1956—Dr. Wilder G. Penfield, Montreal, Canada
1957—Dr. Francis C. Grant, Philadelphia, Pennsylvania
1958—Dr. A. Earl Walker, Baltimore, Maryland
1959—Dr. William J. German, New Haven, Connecticut
1960—Dr. Paul C. Bucy, Chicago, Illinois
1961—Professor Eduard A. V. Busch, Copenhagen, Denmark
1962—Dr. Bronson S. Ray, New York, New York
1963—Dr. James L. Poppen, Boston, Massachusetts
1964—Dr. Edgar A. Kahn, Ann Arbor, Michigan
1965—Dr. James C. White, Boston, Massachusetts
1966—Dr. Hugh A. Kravenbühl, Zurich, Switzerland
1967—Dr. W. James Gardner, Cleveland, Ohio
1968—Professor Normal M. Dott, Edinburgh, Scotland
1969—Dr. Wallace B. Hamby, Cleveland, Ohio
1970—Dr. Barnes Woodhall, Durham, North Carolina
1971—Dr. Elisha S. Gurdjian, Detroit, Michigan
1972—Dr. Francis Murphey, Memphis, Tennessee
1973—Dr. Henry G. Schwartz, St. Louis, Missouri
1974—Dr. Guy L. Odom, Durham, North Carolina
1975—Dr. William A. Sweet, Boston, Massachusetts
1976—Dr. Lyle A. French, Minneapolis, Minnesota
1977—Dr. Richard C. Schneider, Ann Arbor, Michigan
1978—Dr. Charles G. Drake, London, Ontario, Canada
1979—Dr. Frank H. Mayfield, Cincinnati, Ohio
1980—Dr. Eben Alexander, Jr., Winston-Salem, North Carolina
1981—Dr. J. Garber Galbraith, Birmingham, Alabama
1982—Dr. Keiji Sano, Tokyo, Japan
1983—Dr. C. Miller Fisher, Boston, Massachusetts
1984—Dr. Hugo V. Rizzoli, Washington, DC
Dr. Walter E. Dandy (posthumously), Baltimore, Maryland
1985—Dr. Sidney Goldring, St. Louis, Missouri
1986—Dr. M. Gazi Yasargil, Zurich, Switzerland
1987—Dr. Thomas W. Langiftt, Philadelphia, Pennsylvania

1988—Professor Lindsay Symon, London, England
1989—Dr. Thoralf M. Sundt, Jr., Rochester, Minnesota
1990—Dr. Charles Byron Wilson, San Francisco, California
1991—Dr. Bennett M. Stein, New York, New York
1992—Dr. Robert G. Ojemann, Boston, Massachusetts
1993—Dr. Albert L. Rhoton, Jr., Gainesville, Florida
1994—Dr. Robert F. Spetzler, Phoenix, Arizona
1995—Dr. John A. Jane, Charlottesville, Virginia
1996—Dr. Peter J. Jannetta, Pittsburgh, Pennsylvania
1997—Dr. Nicholas T. Zervas, Boston, Massachusetts
1998—Dr. John M. Tew
1999—Dr. Duke S. Samson

Officers of the Congress of Neurological Surgeons 1999

H. HUNT BATJER, M.D.
President

DANIEL L. BARROW, M.D.
President-Elect

PAUL C. MCCORMICK
Vice-President

MARK N. HADLEY
Secretary

STEPHEN M. PAPADOPOULOS, M.D.
Treasurer

EXECUTIVE COMMITTEE

PAUL C. MCCORMICK
Vice-President

MARK N. HADLEY
Secretary

STEPHEN M. PAPADOPOULOS, M.D.
Treasurer

EXECUTIVE COMMITTEE

ISSAM A. AWAD, M.D.
JAMES R. BEAN, M.D.
PAUL J. CAMARATA, M.D.
MARK H. CAMEL, M.D.
RICHARD G. ELLENBOGEN, M.D.
DOUGLAS S. KONDZIOLKA, M.D.
MICHAEL L. LEVY, M.D.
CHRISTOPHER M. LOFTUS, M.D.
JOEL D. MACDONALD, M.D.
TIMOTHY B. MAPTSONE, M.D.
STANLEY B. MARTIN, M.D.
NELSON M. OYESIKU, M.D.
JOSEPH M. PIEPMEIER, M.D.
GERALD E. RODTS, JR., M.D.
WARREN R. SELMAN, M.D.
VINCENT TRAYNELIS, M.D.

Editors-in-Chief
Clinical Neurosurgery

Volume	*Date*	*Editor-in-Chief*
1	1953	Raymond K. Thompson, M.D.
2	1954	Raymond K. Thompson, M.D. & Ira J. Jackson, M.D.
3	1955	Raymond K. Thompson, M.D. & Ira J. Jackson, M.D.
4	1956	Ira J. Jackson, M.D.
5	1957	Robert G. Fisher, M.D.
6	1958	Robert G. Fisher, M.D.
7	1959	Robert G. Fisher, M.D.
8	1960	William H. Mosberg, Jr., M.D.
9	1961	William H. Mosberg, Jr., M.D.
10	1962	William H. Mosberg, Jr., M.D.
11	1963	John Shillito, Jr., M.D., & William H. Mosberg, Jr., M.D.
12	1964	John Shillito, Jr., M.D.
13	1965	John Shillito, Jr., M.D.
14	1966	Robert G. Ojemann, M.D. & John Shillito, Jr., M.D.
15	1967	Robert G. Ojemann, M.D.
16	1968	Robert G. Ojemann, M.D.
17	1969	Robert G. Ojemann, M.D.
18	1970	George T. Tindall, M.D.
19	1971	George T. Tindall, M.D.
20	1972	Robert H. Wilkins, M.D.
21	1973	Robert H. Wilkins, M.D.
22	1974	Robert H. Wilkins, M.D.
23	1975	Ellis B. Keener, M.D.
24	1976	Ellis B. Keener, M.D.
25	1977	Ellis B. Keener, M.D.
26	1978	Peter W. Carmel, M.D.
27	1979	Peter W. Carmel, M.D.
28	1980	Peter W. Carmel, M.D.
29	1981	Martin H. Weiss, M.D.
30	1982	Martin H. Weiss, M.D.
31	1983	Martin H. Weiss, M.D.
32	1984	John R. Little, M.D.
33	1985	John R. Little, M.D.
34	1986	John R. Little, M.D.
35	1987	Peter McL. Black, M.D., Ph.D.
36	1988	Peter McL. Black, M.D., Ph.D.
37	1989	Peter McL. Black, M.D., Ph.D.
38	1990	Warren R. Selman, M.D.
39	1991	Warren R. Selman, M.D.

40	1992	Warren R. Selman, M.D.
41	1993	Christopher M. Loftus, M.D.
42	1994	Christopher M. Loftus, M.D.
43	1995	Christopher M. Loftus, M.D.
44	1996	M. Sean Grady, M.D.
45	1997	M. Sean Grady, M.D.
46	1998	M. Sean Grady, M.D.
47	1999	Matthew A. Howard III, M.D.

CONGRESS OF NEUROLOGICAL SURGEONS

1951

ERUDITIO OBSERVANTIA SOCIETAS

Contributors

P. David Adelson, M.D., Associate Professor of Neurosurgery, Children's Hospital of Pittsburgh and the University of Pittsburgh, Pittsburgh, Pennsylvania (Chapter 17)

E. Alexander III, M.D., Director of Section on Stereotactic and Functional Neurosurgery, Department of Neurosurgery, Brigham and Women's Hospital, Boston, Massachusetts (Chapter 13)

Alessandra Alfieri, M.D., Center for Minimally Invasive Innovative Microneurosurgery, Department of Neurological Surgery, University of Pittsburgh School of Medicine, Pittsburgh, Pennsylvania (Chapter 5)

Issam A. Awad, M.D., M.Sc., F.A.C.S., The Nixdorff-German Professor, Department of Neurosurgery, Yale University School of Medicine, New Haven, Connecticut (Chapter 11)

Koang Hum Bak, M.D., Ph.D., Department of Neurosurgery, The Cleveland Clinic Foundation, Cleveland, Ohio (Chapter 33)

Daniel L. Barrow, M.D., MBNA/Bowman Profess and Chairman, Department of Neurosurgery, Emory University School of Medicine, Atlanta, Georgia (Chapter 9)

H. Hunt Batjer, M.D., Michael J. Marchese Professor and Chair, Department of Neurological Surgery, Northwestern University Medical Center, Chicago, Illinois (Chapter 1)

Craig Baumgartner, P.A.-C, M.B.A., Department of Neurological Surgery, Evanston Hospital, Evanston, Illinois (Chapter 6)

Edward C. Benzel, M.D., F.A.C.S., Department of Neurosurgery, The Cleveland Clinic Foundation, Cleveland, Ohio (Chapter 33)

Peter M. Black, M.D., Ph.D., Neurosurgeon-in-Chief, Brigham and Women's and Children's Hospital, Boston, Massachusetts (Chapter 2)

Harsimran S. Brara, M.D., Department of Neurosurgery, University of Florida School of Medicine, Gainesville, Florida (Chapter 30)

Benjamin S. Carson, Sr., M.D., Professor and Director, Pediatric Neurosurgery, The Johns Hopkins Medical Institutions, Baltimore, Maryland (Chapter 21)

C. Michael Cawley, M.D., Assistant Professor, Department of Neurosurgery, Emory University School of Medicine, Atlanta, Georgia (Chapter 28)

Ivan Ciric, M.D., Professor of Neurological Surgery, Northwestern University Medical School; Bennett-Tarkington Chair in Neurosurgery, Evanston Hospital, Evanston, Illinois (Chapter 6)

Michael L. Cunningham, M.D., Ph.D., Chief, Craniofacial Service, Seattle Children's and Regional Medical Center; Assistant Professor, Department of Pediatrics, University of Washington School of Medicine, Seattle, Washington (Chapter 16)

Moise Danielpour, M.D., Department of Neurological Surgery, University of California, San Francisco, California (Chapter 22)

Catherine Daumas-DuPont, M.D., Department of Neurological Surgery, Centre Hospital Paris, France (Chapter 7)

Paul W. Detwiler, M.D., Chief Resident, Division of Neurological Surgery, Barrow Neurological Institute, Phoenix, Arizona (Chapter 37)

Curtis A. Dickman, M.D., Director of Spinal Research, Associate Chief of Spinal Neurosurgery, Division of Neurological Surgery, Barrow Neurological Institute, Phoenix, Arizona (Chapter 28)

James M. Drake, Division of Neurosurgery, University of Toronto, Toronto, Ontario, Canada (Chapter 18)

Gary Duckwiler, M.D., Associate-Professor, Department of Radiological Sciences, University of California, Los Angeles, California (Chapter 12)

Richard G. Ellenbogen, M.D., Chief, Division of Pediatric Neurological Surgery, Seattle Children's Hospital and Regional Medical Center; Associate Professor of Neurosurgery, University of Washington School of Medicine, Seattle, Washington (Chapter 16)

Lisa A. Ferrara, M.S., Department of Neurosurgery, The Cleveland Clinic Foundation, Cleveland, Ohio (Chapter 33)

Richard G. Fessler, M.D., Ph.D., Department of Neurosurgery, University of Florida, Gainesville, Florida (Chapter 30)

R. M. Friedlander, M.D., Department of Neurosurgery, Brigham and Women's Hospital, Boston, Massachusetts (Chapter 13)

Sydney C. Gary, M.D. Section of Neurobiology, Yale University, New Haven, Connecticut (Chapter 4)

Y. Pierre Gobin, M.D., Assistant Professor, Department of Radiological Sciences, University of California, Los Angeles, California (Chapter 12)

Joseph S. Gruss, M.D., Chief, Division of Plastic and Reconstructive Surgery, Seattle Children's Hospital and Regional Medical Center; Associate Professor of Neurosurgery, University of Washington School of Medicine, Seattle, Washington (Chapter 16)

Mark N. Hadley, M.D., Department of Neurological Surgery, University of Alabama, Birhingham, Alabama (Chapter 27)

Regis W. Haid, Jr., M.D., Department of Neurosurgery, The Emory Clinic, Atlanta, Georgia (Chapters 29, 32)

Susan Hockfield, Ph.D. Section of Neurobiology, Yale University, New Haven, Connecticut (Chapter 4)

Daniel Huddle, D.O., Assistant Professor of Diagnostic Radiology and Neurosurgery, The Neurovascular Surgery Program, Yale University School of Medicine, New Haven, Connecticut (Chapter 11)

Hae-Dong Jho, M.D., Ph.D., Director, Minimally Invasive Innovative Mirconeurosurgery, Department of Neurological Surgery, University of Pittsburgh School of Medicine, Pittsburgh, Pennsylvania (Chapter 5)

Iain Kalfas, M.D., F.A.C.S., Department of Neurosurgery, The Cleveland Clinic Foundation, Cleveland, Ohio (Chapter 33)

William Kerr, Jr., M.D., Department of Neurological Surgery, Evanston Hospital, Evanston, Illinois (Chapter 6)

J.R.W. Kestle, FRCSC, Division of Neurosurgery, Primary Children's Medical Center, Salt Lake City, Utah (Chapter 18)

Frank LaMarca, M.D., Department of Neurological Surgery, Evanston Hospital, Evanston, Illinois (Chapter 6)

Jorge J. Lastra, M.D., Department of Neurosurgery, The Cleveland Clinic Foundation, Cleveland, Ohio (Chapter 33)

Sunghoon Lee, M.D., Resident in Neurosurgery, The Neurovascular Surgery Program, Yale University School of Medicine, New Haven, Connecticut (Chapter 11)

Paul M. Lin, M.D., Emeritus Clinical Professor, Department of Neurosurgery, Temple University Health Sciences Center, Philadelphia, Pennsylvania (Chapter 26)

Mark E. Linskey, M.D., Associate Professor, Neurosurgery, University of Arkansas for Medical Sciences; Co-Director, Arkansas Cancer Research Center Neuro-oncology Program; Co-Director, University of Arkansas for Medical Sciences Gamma Knife Center; Director, Arkansas Cancer Research Center Brain Tumor Research Laboratory, Little Rock, Arkansas (Chapter 3)

J. S. Loeffler, Department of Neurosurgery, Brigham and Women's Hospital, Boston, Massachusetts (Chapter 13)

Christopher M. Loftus, M.D., F.A.C.S., Esther and Ted Greenberg Professor and Chairman, Department of Neurosurgery, University of Oklahoma College of Medicine, Oklahoma City, Oklahoma (Chapter 4)

Todd G. Mainprize, M.D., Resident, Division of Neurosurgery, University of Toronto, Toronto, Ontario, Canada (Chapter 15)

Mark R. McLaughlin, M.D., Department of Neurosurgery, Emory University School of Medicine, Atlanta, Georgia (Chapter 29, 32)

David Mclone, M.D., Ph.D., Department of Neurosurgery, Children's Memorial Hospital, Chicago, Illinois (Chapter 19)

Yuichi Murayama, M.D., Division of Interventional Neuroradiology and Leo G. Rigler Radiological Research Center, University of California School of Medicine. Los Angeles, California (Chapter 12)

Maureen O'Donnell, M.D., MSc., FRCPC, Assistant Professor, Department of Pediatrics, Children's and Women's Health Center of British Columbia and University of British Columbia, Vancouver, British Columbia, Canada (Chapter 24)

T. C. Origitano, M.D., Ph.D, F.A.C.S., Department of Neurological Surgery, Loyola University Medical Center, Maywood, Illinois (Chapter 10)

In-Sung Park, M.D., Ph.D., Department of Neurological Surgery, Center for Minimally Invasive Innovative Microneurosurgery, University of Pittsburgh School of Medicine, Pittsburgh, Pennsylvania (Chapter 5)

T. S. Park, M.D., Shi H. Huang Professor of Neurosurgery, Washington University School of Medicine, St. Louis, Missouri (Chapter 23)

Warwick J. Peacock, Department of Neurological Surgery, University of California, San Francisco, California (Chapter 22)

Debi Pierce, B.S., Department of Neurological Surgery, Evanston Hospital, Evanston, Illinois (Chapter 6)

Randall W. Porter, M.D., Division of Neurological Surgery, Barrow Neurological Institute, St. Joseph's Hospital and Medical Center, Phoenix, Arizona (Chapter 28)

Gregory J. Pryzbylski, M.D., Director of Neurotrauma, Assistant Professor, Department of Neurosurgery, Jefferson Medical College, Philadelphia, Pennsylvania (Chapter 25)

Charles J. Riedel, M.D., Assistant Professor, Neurological Surgery, Neurological Institute. Columbia University, New York Presbyterian Hospital, New York, New York (Chapter 31)

Gerald E. Rodts, Jr., M.D., Department of Neurosurgery, Emory University School of Medicine, Atlanta, Georgia (Chapters 29, 32)

Sami Rosenblatt, M.D., Department of Neurological Surgery, Evanston Hospital, Evanston, Illinois (Chapter 6)

James T. Rutka, M.D., Ph.D. FRCS, Professor and Chairman, Neurosurgery, Director, The Arthur and Sonia Labatt Brain Tumor Research Centre, Dan Family Chair in Neurosurgery, The Hospital for Sick Children, University for Sick Children, Toronto, Ontario, Canada (Chapter 15)

Duke S. Samson, M.D., Professor and Chairman, Department of Neurosurgery, University of Texas Health Sciences Center, Dallas, Texas (Chapter 8)

R. Michael Scott, M.D., Professor of Surgery, Harvard Medical School; Director, Pediatric Neurosurgery, The Children's Hospital, Boston, Massachusetts (Chapter 20)

Paul Steinbok, M.B.B.S., B.Sc., FRCSC, Head, Division of Pediatric Neurosurgery, British Columbia's Children's Hospital; Professor, Department of Surgery, University of British Columbia, Vancouver, British Columbia, Canada (Chapter 24)

Philip E. Stieg, Ph.D., M.D., Associate Chief, Section on Cerebrovascular Neurosurgery, Brigham and Women's Hospital, Boston, Massachusetts (Chapter 13)

Brian R. Subach, M.D., Department of Neurosurgery, Emory University School of Medicine, Atlanta, Georgia (Chapters 29, 32)

Michael D. Taylor, M.D., Resident, Division of Neurosurgery, University of Toronto, Toronto, Ontario, Canada (Chapter 15)

S. Tuli, M.D., Division of Neurosurgery, The Hospital for Sick Children, Toronto, Ontario, Canada (Chapter 18)

Fernando Vinuela, M.D. Professor and Director, Interventional Neuroradiology Division, University of California School of Medicine, Los Angeles, California (Chapter 12)

Jonathan Zhang, M.D., Department of Neurosurgery, Emory University School of Medicine, Atlanta, Georgia (Chapter 32)

Biography Duke S. Samson, M.D.

Duke Samson was born in Odessa, Texas in January 1943. Following graduation from Odessa High School in 1961, he attended Stanford University, where he majored in psychology and played intercollegiate football and rugby. He graduated from Washington University Medical School in 1969 and completed a surgical internship at Duke University Medical Center. His neurosurgical residency at the University of Texas Southwestern Medical School was highlighted by a fellowship with Professor Gerard Guiot in Paris and Professor M. G. Yasargil in Zurich. Dr. Samson entered the United States Army Medical Corps in 1975, serving both at Clark Air Force Base in the Republic of the Philippines and Walter Reed Army Medical Center. In 1977 he joined the faculty at Southwestern, focusing his clinical and investigative interests on vascular diseases of the nervous system. Dr. Samson was promoted to Professor of Surgery in 1984 and assumed the chairmanship of the division of neurological surgery the following year. In 1987, neurosurgery at Southwestern achieved departmental status and he accepted the W. Kemp Clark Chair, established in honor of the divisions chairman. On sabbatical leave from the chairmanship in 1998, Dr. Samson was named Director of the Mobility Foundation, a multi-disciplinary center dedicated to clinical research in cerebrovascular diseases and spinal cord injury. He currently holds both the Kimberly-Clark Distinguished Chair and the Lois and Darwin Smith Distinguished Chair in Neurological Surgery.

Duke and his wife, Dr. Patricia Bergen, who is a member of the Department of General Surgery at Southwestern, are proud parents of Lorne Daniel, age nine, and Gabriel Stanford, age seven.

Bibliography of Duke S. Samson, M.D.

JOURNAL PUBLICATIONS

1. Samson DS, Clark WK. Current review of brain abscess. *Amer J Med* 54;201–210, 1973.
2. Samson DS, Hodosh RM, Clark WK. Surgical management of unruptured asymptomatic aneurysm. *J Neurosurg* 46:731–734, 1977.
3. Samson DS, Watts C, Clark WK. Cerebral revascularization for transient ischemic attacks. *Neurology* 27:767–771, 1977.
4. Samson DS, Hodosh RM, Clark WK. Microsurgical evaluation of the pterional approach to aneurysms of the distal basilar circulation. *Neurosurg* 3(2):135–141, 1978.
5. Samson DS, Boone SC. Extracranial-Intracranial (EC-IC) arterial bypass: Past performance and current concepts. *Neurosurgery* 3(1):79–86, 1978.
6. Boone SC, Samson DS. Observations on Moya-Moya Disease: A case treated with superficial temporal middle cerebral artery anastomosis. *Surg Neurol* 19:189–193, 1978.
7. Samson DS, Hodosh RM. Microsurgical treatment of transient cerebral ischemia: Preliminary studies in 50 cases. *JAMA* 241(4):376–378, 1979.
8. Boone SC, Samson DS. Technical Notes: Salvage of a nonfunctional superficial temporal-middle cerebral artery anastomosis. *Neurosurgery* Vol. 4, No. 3:254, 1979.
9. Samson DS, Hodosh RM, Reid WR, Beyer CW, Clark WK. Risk of intracranial aneurysm surgery in the good grade patient—early versus later operation. *Neurosurgery* 5:422–426, 1979.
10. Stewart RM, Samson DS, Diehl J, Inton R. Ditmore QM. Unruptured cerebral aneurysms presenting as recurrent transient neurological deficits. *Neurology* 30(1):47–51, 1980.
11. Ditmore QM, Samson DS, Beyer CW. Traumatic middle cerebral artery aneurysm: case report. *Neurosurgery* 6(3):293–296, 1980.
12. Samson DS, Neuwelt EA, Beyer CW, Ditmore QM. Failure of extracranial-intracranial arterial bypass in acute middle cerebral artery occlusion: a case report. *Neurosurgery* 6(2):185–188, 1980.
13. Gewertz BL, Samson DS, Ditmore QM, Bone GE. Management of penetrating injuries of the internal carotid artery at the base of the

skull utilizing extracranial-intracranial bypass. *J. Trauma* 20(5):65–369, 1980.
14. Samson DS, Ditmore QM, Beyer CW. Intra-arterial use of isobutyl-2-cyanoacrylate in the treatment of intracranial arteriovenous malformations. *Neurosurgery* 8(1):43–51, 1981.
15. Samson DS, Ditmore QM, Beyer CW. Intravascular use of isobutyl-2-Cyanoacrylate in the treatment of carotid cavernous fistulae. *Neurosurgery* 8(1):52–55, 1981.
16. Samson DS, Gewertz B, Beyer CW, Hodosh RM. Saphenous vein bypass in microsurgical treatment of cerebral ischemia. *Arch Surg* 116:1578–1582, 1981.
17. Samson DS, Beyer CW. Furosemide in the intraoperative reduction of intracranial pressure in the subarachnoid hemoorhage patient. *Neurosurgery* 10(2):167–169, 1982.
18. Samson DS. Cervical carotid injuries. *Clinical Neurosurgery* 29:647–656, 1982.
19. Samson DS. Surgical treatment of intracranial arteriovenous malformations. *Texas Medicine,* February 1983, 52–59. "Recipient of the Harriet Cunnhingam Citation for Meritorious Scientific Writing."
20. Samson DS, Batjer HH. Intraoperative Aneurysm Rupture. To be published in the Proceedings of the Second International Symposium of Cerebral Aneurysm Surgery in the Acute Stage-Graz, Austria, September, 1984.
21. Rosenstein J, Batjer HH, Samson DS. Use of the extracranial-intracranial arterial bypass in the management of refractory vasospasm, a case report. *Neurosurgery* 17:474–479, 1985.
22. Samson DS, Batjer HH. Arteriovenous malformations of the cerebellar vermis. *Neurosurgery* 16:341–349, 1985.
23. Dohrmann PJ, Batjer HH, Samson D, Suss RA. Recurrent subarachnoid hemorrhage complicating a traumatic carotid-cavernous fistula. *Neurosurgery* 17:480–483, 1985.
24. Close LG, Mickey BE, Samson DS, Anderson RG, Schaefer SD. Resection of upper aerodigestive tract tumors involving the middle cranial fossa. *Laryngoscope* 95(8):908–914, 1985.
25. Batjer HH, Samson DS. Arteriovenous malformations of the posterior fossa: clinical presentation, diagnostic evaluation, and surgical treatment. *J Neurosurgery* 64:849–856, 1986.
26. Batjer HH, Samson DS. Arteriovenous malformations of the posterior fossa: clinical presentation, diagnostic evaluation and surgical treatment. *Neurosurgical Review* 9:287–296, 1986.
27. Batjer HH, Suss R, Samson DS. Intracranial arteriovenous malformations associated with aneurysms. *Neurosurgery* 18:29–35, 1986.

28. Batjer HH, Samson DS. Intraoperative aneurysmal rupture: incidence, outcome, and suggestions for surgical management. *Neurosurgery* 18:701–707, 1986.
29. Batjer HH, Mickey BM, Samson DS. Potential roles for early revascularization in acute cerebral ischemia. *Neurosurgery* 18:283–291, 1986.
30. Batjer HH, Samson DS. The use of extracranial-intracranial arterial bypass in the management of symptomatic vasospasm. *Neurosurgery* 19:235–246, 1986.
31. Batjer HH, Mickey BM, Samson DS. Enlargement and rupture of distal basilar aneurysm following iatrogenic carotid occlusion. *Neurosurgery* 20:624–628, 1987.
32. Batjer HH, Samson DS. Surgical approaches to trigonal arteriovenous malformations. *J. Neurosurgery* 67:511–517, 1987.
33. Batjer HH, Devous MD, Meyer YJ, Purdy PD, Samson DS. Cerebrovascular hemodynamics in arteriovenous malformation complicated by normal perfusion pressure breakthrough. *Neurosurgery* 22:503–509, 1988.
34. Batjer HH, Devous MD, Purdy PD, Mickey BM, Bonte FJ, Samson DS. Improvement in regional cerebral blood flow and cerebral vasoreactivity following extracranial-intracranial bypass. *Neurosurgery* 22:913–919, 1988.
35. Paine JT, Batjer HH, Samson DS. Intraoperative ventricular puncture. *Neurosurgery* 22:1107–1109, 1988.
36. Batjer HH, Purdy PD, Neiman M, Samson DS. Subtemporal transdural use of detachable balloons for traumatic carotid cavernous fistulae. *Neurosurgery* 22:290–296, 1988.
37. Batjer HH, Frankfurt AI, Purdy PD, Smith SS, Samson DS. Use of etomidate, temporary arterial occlusion, and intraoperative angiography in large and giant cerebral aneurysm surgery. *J Neurosurgery* 68:234–240, 1988.
38. Batjer HH, Samson DS. Causes of morbidity and mortality from surgery of aneurysms of the distal basilar artery. *Neurosurgery* 25:904–916, 1989.
39. Batjer HH, Purdy PD, Giller CA, Samson DS. Evidence of redistribution of cerebral blood flow during treatment for intracranial arteriovenous malformation. *Neurosurgery* 26:599–605, 1989.
40. Purdy P, Devous M, White C, Batjer HH, Samson DS, Brewer K, Hodges K. Reversible middle cerebral artery embolization in dogs without intracranial surgery. *Stroke* 20:1368–1376, 1989.
41. Megison P, Batjer H, Purdy P, Samson DS. Spontaneous resolution of arteriovenous malformation without hemorrhage: A case report. *Am J Neuroradiology* 10:204, 1989.

42. Purdy PD, Devous MD Sr, Batjer HH, White CL III, Meyer Y, Samson DS. The microfibrillar collagen model of canine cerebral infarction. *Stroke* 20:1361–1367, 1989.
43. Giller CA, Stieg P, Batjer HH, Samson DS, Purdy PD. Transcranial Doppler ultrasound as a guide to graded therapeutic carotid artery occlusion. *Neurosurgery* 26:307–311, 1990.
44. Purdy PD, White CL III, Batjer HH, Brewer K, Hodges K, Samson DS. Intracarotid hydroxyethyl methacrylate solution causing stroke in dogs. *J. Neurosurgery* 73:756–759, 1990.
45. Batjer HH, Samson DS. Management of intraoperative aneurysm rupture. *Clin Neurosurg* 36:275–288, 1990.
46. Batjer HH, Samson DS. Retrograde suction decompression of giant paraclinoidal aneurysms: Technical note. *J Neurosurg* 73:305–306, 1990.
47. Purdy PD, Samson DS, Batjer HH, Risser RC. Preoperative embolization of cerebral arteriovenous malformations with polyvinyl alcohol particles: Experience in 51 adults. *Am J Neuroradiology* 11:501–510, 1990.
48. Batjer HH, Samson DS. Causes of morbidity and mortality from surgery of aneurysms of the distal basiler artery. *Stroke* 21:693, 1990.
49. Purdy PD, Batjer HH, Samson DS, Risser RC, Bowman GW. Intraarterial sodium amytal administration of guide preoperative embolization of cerebral arteriovenous malformations. *J Neurosurg Anesthesiol* 3(2):103–106, 1991.
50. Batjer HH, Samson DS. Emergent aneurysm surgery without cerebral angiography for the comatose patient. *Neurosurgery,* 28:283–287, 1991.
51. Purdy PD, Batjer HH, Samson DS. Management of hemorrhagic complications from preoperative embolization of arteriovenous malformations. *J Neurosurg* 74:205–211, 1991.
52. Giller CA, Mathews D, Purdy P, Kopitnik TA, Batjer HH, Samson DS. The transcranial Doppler appearance of acute carotid artery occlusion. *Ann Neurol* 31:101–103, 1992.
53. Purdy PD, Batjer HH, Risser RC, Samson D. Arteriovenous malformations of the brain: choosing embolic materials to enhance safety and ease of excision. *J Neurosurg* 77:217–222, 1992.
54. Eckard DA, Purdy PD, Girson MS, Samson D, Kopitnik T, Batjer HH. Intraarterial papaverine for relief of catheter-induced intracranial vasospasm. *American Journal of Roentgenology* 158:883–884, 1992.
55. Batjer HH, Samson DS. Reoperation for aneurysms and vascular malformations. *Clin Neurosurg* 39:140–147, 1992.
56. Samson D. Aneurysm perspective. *Clin Neurosurg.* 40:124–136, 1993.

57. Kopitnik TA, Samson DS. Management of subarachnoid hemorrhage. *J Neurol Neurosurg Psychiatry* 56(9):947–959, 1993.
58. Samson DS, Batjer HH, Bowman G, Mootz L, Krippner WJ, Meyer YJ, Allen BC. A Clinical Study of the parameters and effects of temporary arterial occlusion in the management of intracranial aneurysms. *Neurosurgery* 34(1):22–28; discussion 28–29, 1994.
59. Batjer HH, Kopitnik TA, Giller CA, Samson DS. Surgery for paraclinoidal carotid artery aneurysms. *J Neurosurg* 80(4):650–658, 1994.
60. Kopitnik TA, Batjer HH, Samson DS. Combined transsylvian-subtemporal exposure of cerebral aneurysms involving the basilar apex. *Microsurgery* 15(8):534–540, 1994.
61. Batjer HH, Kopitnik, TA Jr, Giller CA, Samson DS. Surgical management of proximal carotid artery aneurysms (Review) (19 refs). *Clin Neurosurgery* 41:21–38, 1994.
62. Samson D, Steiner L, Stein BM, Debrun G. What is your general approach to the management of brain stem AVMs? *Surg Neurol* 44(2):107–108, 1995.
63. Vardiman AB, Kopitnik TA, Purdy PD, Batjer HH, Samson DS. Treatment of traumatic arterial vasospasm with intra-arterial papaverine infusion. *Am J Neuroradiol* 16(2):319–321, 1995.
64. Horowitz M, Purdy P, Unwin H, Carstens G 3rd, Greenlee R, Hise J, Kopitnik T, Batjer H, Rollins N, Samson D. Treatment of dural sinus thrombosis using selective catheterization and urokinase. *Ann Neurol* 38(1):58–67, 1995.
65. Horowitz M, Fichtel F, Samson D, Purdy P. Intracavernous carotid artery aneusysms: the possible importance of angiographic dural waisting. A case report. *Surg Neurol* 46(6):549–552, 1996.
66. Horowitz M, Samson D, Purdy P. Does electrothrombosis occur immediately after embolization of aneurysm with Guglielimi detachable coils? *AJNR Am J Neuroradiol* 18(3):520–513, 1997.
67. Fleckenstein JL, Purdy PD, Mendelsohn DB, Chason DP, Ginsburg MI, Samson DS. Aneurysm clip testing for ferromagnetic properties; clip variability issues. *Radiology* 202(3):640–642, 1997.
68. Samson D. The future of aneurysm surgery (letter; comment). *Surg Neurol* 49(6):582–583, 1998.
69. Giller CA, Wills MJ, Giller AM, Samson. Distribution of hematocrit values after aneurysmal subarachnoid hemorrhage. *J Neuroimaging* 8:169–170, 1998.
70. Horowitz M, Kopitnik T, Landreneau F, Krummerman J, Batjer HH, Thomas G, Samson, D. Posteroinferior cerebellar artery aneurysms: surgical results for 38 patients. *Neurosurgery* 43(5):1026–1032, 1998.

71. Horowitz MB, Kopitnik TA, Landreneau F, Ramnani DM, Rushing EJ, George E, Purdy PP, Samson, Duke. Multidisciplinary approach to traumatic intracranial aneurysms secondary to shotgun and handgun wounds. *Surg Neurol* 51(1):31–41; discussion 41–42, 1999.
72. Samson D, Batjer HH, Kopitnik TA Jr. Current results of the surgical management of aneurysms of the basilar apex. *Neurosurgery* 44(4)697–702; discussion 702–704, 1999.
73. Horowitz M, Purdy P, Kopitnik T, Dutton K, Samson D. Aneurysm retreatment after Guglielmi detachable coil and nondetachable coil embolizaton: report of nine cases and review of the literature. *Neurosurgery* 44(4):712–719; discussion 719–720, 1999.
74. White JA, Horowitz MB, Samson D. Dural waisting as a sign of subarachnoid extension of cavernous carotid aneusysms: a follow-up case report. *Surg Neurol* 52(6):607–609; discussion 609–610, 1999.

BOOKS

1. Samson DS, Batjer HH. *Intracranial Aneurysm Surgery: Techniques.* Futura Publishing Company, Mount Kisco, New York, 1990.

BOOK CHAPTERS

1. Samson DS, Clark WK. Therapy of brain abscess. *Current Therapy,* ed. Conn HF., pp. 634, WB Saunders, Philadelphia, 1975.
2. Samson DS, Hodosh RM, Clark WK. Treatment of spontaneous subarachnoid hemorrhage. *The Treatment of Neurologic Diseases,* ed. R. Rosenberg, pp. 117–142, Spectrum Publications, Jamaica, New York, 1978.
3. Samson DS, Beyer CW, Mayhood MA. Serum and CSF brain-specific isoenzyme profiles in experimental cerebral ischemia and infarction. *Proceedings of The Fourth International Symposium of Microsurgical Anastomoses for Cerebral Ischemia.* Springer-Verlag, New York, 1978.
4. Samson DS, Hodosh RM, Beyer CW. Timing of aneurysm surgery as a function of clinical grade. *Subarachnoid Hemorrhage and Cerebral Vasospasm,* ed. Wilkins RH, pp. 463–466, Williams and Wilkins, 1979.
5. Samson DS, Beyer DW. Thiopental coma in the treatment of cerebral ischemia/infarction. *Subarachnoid Hemorrhage and Cerebral Vasospasm,* ed. Wilkins RH, pp. 634–636, Williams and Wilkins, 1979.
6. Samson DS, Gewertz BL, Beyer CW, Hodosh RM. Use the saphe-

nous vein interposition grafts in the treatment of cerebral ischemia. *Microsurgical Anastomoses in Cerebral Ischemia,* ed. Kletter G, Springer-Verlag, Munich, 1981.

7. Samson DS. Current management of carotid artery injuries. *Clinical Neurosurgery,* Williams and Wilkins, 1981.
8. Samson DS, Mickey BM. Tissue adhesives in neurosurgery. *Clinical Neurosurgery,* Williams and Wilkins, pp. 429–444, 1981.
9. Samson DS, Gewertz B. Saphenous vein grafts to the middle cerebral artery. *Stroke and the Extracranial Vessels,* ed. Robert R. Smith, Raven Press, New York, 1984.
10. Samson DS, Batjer HH. Intraoperative aneurysmal rupture, in Auer LM (ed): *Proceedings of the Second International Symposium—Cerebral Aneurysm Surgery in the Acute Stage,* Graz, Austria, 1984.
11. Samson DS, Batjer HH. Intraoperative aneurysmal rupture, in Auer LM (ed). *Timing of Aneurysm Surgery.* Berlin, New York, Walter de Gruyter, 1985, pp 313–321.
12. Samson DS. The Fronto-Temporal or Pterional Approach to Aneurysms of the Basilar Artery. *Textbook of Cerebrovascular Surgery,* eds. Fein J, Flamm E, Springer-Verlag, New York, 1985.
13. Samson DS, Batjer HH. Intraoperative aneurysmal rupture—incidence, outcome and surgical management, in Kikuchi H, Fukushina T, Watanabe K (eds). *Intracranial Aneurysms—Surgical Timing and Techniques.* Japan, Nishimura Co., 1986, pp. 123–131.
14. Batjer HH, Samson DS. Surgery of Arteriovenous Malformations, in Dudley H, Carter DC, Russel RCG. (eds): *Operative Surgery* 4th edition. London, Butterworth, 1989, pp 219–230.
15. Batjer HH, Samson DS. Intraoperative Aneurysmal Rupture, in Wilkins RH, Rengachary SS (eds): *Neurosurgery Update,* McGraw-Hill Book Company, 1991, pp 100–105.
16. Samson DS, Batjer HH. Preoperative evaluation of the risk/benefit ratio for arteriovenous malformations of the brain, in Wilkins RH, Rengachary SS (eds): *Neurosurgery Update* II, McGraw-Hill Book Company, 1991 pp 129–133.
17. Batjer HH, Samson DS. Arteriovenous malformations, in Little JR, Awad IA (eds): *Reoperative Neurosurgery.* Baltimore, Williams and Wilkins, 1992 pp 219–237.
18. Samson DS, Batjer HH. Intracerebral hematomas secondary to ruptured aneurysms and intracranial vascular malformations, In Kaufman HH (ed): *Intracerebral Hematomas:* New York, Raven Press, 1992, pp 75–84.

19. Batjer HH, Samson DS. Basilar apex aneurysms, in Apuzzo MLJ (ed): *Brain Surgery—Complication Avoidance and Management.* New York, Churchill Livingstone, 1993 Vol. 1, pp 1040–1083.
20. Batjer HH, Samson DS. Distal anterior cerebral artery aneurysm, in Rengachary SS, Wilkins RH (eds): *Neurosurgical Operative Atlas,* Vol. 2, No. 2, Baltimore, Williams and Wilkins, pp 119–132.
21. Batjer HH, Samson DS. Basilar bifurcation aneurysm, in Rengachary SS, Wilkins RH (eds): *Neurosurgical Operative Atlas.* Baltimore, Williams and Wilkins, (in press).
22. Samson DS, Batjer HH. Lobar Arteriovenous Malformations, in Apuzzo MLJ (ed): *Brain Surgery—Complication Avoidance and Management.* New York, Churchill-Livingstone, 1993.
23. Batjer HH, Kopitnik TA, Purdy PD, Samson DS. Giant cerebral aneurysms, in Awad IA (ed): *Current Management of Cerebral Aneurysms* (in press)
24. Batjer HH, Kopitnik TA, Purdy PD, Samson DS. Aneurysm surgery: Vertebral and Pica, in Carter LP, Spetzler RF (eds): *Neurovascular Surgery.* New York, McGraw-Hill 1995.
25. Samson D, Batjer H. Posterior fossa arteriovenous malformations, in Carter LP, Spetzler RF (eds): *Neurovascular Surgery.* New York, McGraw-Hill 1995.
26. Batjer HH, Samson DS. Limits of temporary arterial occlusion, in Da Pian R (ed): *New Trends in Management of Cerebro—vascular Malformations.* Wien, New York, Springer-Verlag, 1994.
27. Batjer HH, Samson DS, Purdy PD. Clinical evaluation of cerebral perfusion in AVM patients, in da Pian R (ed): *New Trends in Maangement of Cerebrovascular Malformations.* Wien, New York, Springer-Verlag, 1994.
28. Purdy PD, Batjer HH, Kopitnik TA, Risser R, Samson DS. Use of ethanol in preoperative AVM embolization, in Da Pian R (ed): *New Trends Management of Cerebrovascular Malformations.* Wien, New York, Springer-Verlag, 1994.
29. Purdy PD, Batjer HH, Kopitnik TA, Samson DS. The team approach to combined embolization and resection of arteriovenous malformations in Da Pian R (ed): *New Trends Management of Cerbrovascular Malformations.* Wien, New York, Springer-Verlag, 1994.
30. Batjer HH, Samson DS. Basilar bifurcation aneurysm. In Tindall GT, Cooper PR, Barrow DL (eds): *The Practice of Neurosurgery.* Baltimore, Williams and Wilkins (in press).
31. Samson D, Batjer H. The transsylvian approach to basiler aneurysms, in Da Pian R (ed): *New Trends in Management of Cere-*

brovascular Malformations. Wien, New York, Springer-Verlag, 1996.

32. Samson D, Batjer H, Purdy P. The surgery of posterior fossa arteriovenous malformations, in Da Pian R (ed): *New Trends in Management of Cerebrovascular Malformations.* Wien, New York, Springer-Verlag, 1996.
33. Samson DS. Surgery for unruptured intracranial aneurysms. In: Wilkins RH, Rengachary SS, eds. *Neurosurgery.* 2nd ed. New York: McGraw Hill, 1996.
34. Samson DS. Uses of extracranial-intracranial arterial bypass in current practice. In: Tindall GT, Cooper OR, Barrow DL, eds. *The Practice of Neurosurgery.* Baltimore: Williams & Wilkins, 1994 (in press)
35. Dexter MA, Samson DS. Vertebral artery reconstruction for vertebrobasilar insufficiency. In: Ernst CB, Stanley JC (eds.), *Current Therapy in Vascular Surgery.* Mosby, Philadelphia, 1998 (in press).
36. Dexter MA, Samson DS, Batjer HH, Kopitnik TA, Horowitz MB. Surgical treatment of basilar apex aneurysms. In: Batjer HH, Loftus CM (eds.), *Textbook of Neurological Surgery,* Lippincott-Raven, Philadelphia, submitted for publication, 1998 (in press).
37. Samson D. Developments in Surgery of Posterior Circulation Aneurysms. Matthew Howard, M. D. (ed): *CNS-Volume 47* Lippincott Williams & Wilkins. Baltimore, Maryland, 2000 (in press).

MISCELLANEOUS

1. Samson DS. Neurosurgical conflicts and concerns. *Basic Neuroradiology,* a symposium. University of Texas, October 21–23, 1977.

ABSTRACTS

1. Samson DS, Clark WK. Surgical treatment of brain abscess and subdural empyema. Annual Meeting, Southern Neurosurgical Society, Houston, Texas 1971.
2. Samson DS, Hodosh RM, Clark WK. Pediatric epidural hematoma. Annual Meeting American Association of Neurologic Surgeons, Atlanta, Georgia, April, 1974.
3. Samson DS, Watts C, Clark WK. Initial results in treatment of transient ischemic episodes with cerebral revascularization. Joint Meeting on Stroke and Cerebral Circulation, Dallas, Texas, February, 1976.
4. Samson DS, Hodosh RM, Clark WK. Surgical treatment of unruptured aneurysms. Annual Meeting of American Association of Neurological Surgeons, San Francisco, California, April, 1976.

5. Samson DS, Neilson KD, Clark WK. Transsphenoidal surgery of endocrine-active pituitary tumors. Annual Meeting American Medical Association, Dallas, Texas, July, 1976.
6. Samson DS, Watts C, Clark WK. Cerebro-revascularization in the treatment of transient cerebral ischemia. Annual Meeting of Congress of Neurological Surgery, New Orleans, Louisiana, October, 1976.
7. Samson DS, Watts C, Clark WK. Initial results of ED-IC bypass in treatment of transient ischemia. Annual Meeting of American Academy of Neurology, Atlanta, Georgia, April, 1977.
8. Samson DS, Hodosh RM, Clark WK. Microsurgical comparisons of two operative approaches to the distal basilar artery. Annual Meeting of Congress of Neurological Surgery, San Francisco, California, October, 1977.
9. Beyer CW, Samson DS, Mayhood MA. Brain isoenzyme elevations in an experimental stroke model. London, Ontario, Canada, September, 1978.
10. Stewart MR, Samson DS, Diehl JD. Neurologic deficits in patients with unruptured aneurysms. American Academy of Neurology Annual Meeting, 1979.
11. Samson DS. Early versus late aneurysm surgery in the good grade aneurysm patient. Second International Conference on Cerebral Vasospasm. July 6, 1979. Amsterdam, Holland.
12. Samson DS, Beyer DW. The use of thiopental barbiturate coma in the treatment of vasospasm induced cerebral ischemia/infarction. July 7, 1979. Amsterdam, Holland.
13. Samson DS, Ditmore QM, Gewertz GL, Bone GE. Management of penetrating injuries of the internal carotid artery at the base of the skull utilizing extracranial-intracranial bypass approach. The American Association for the Surgery of Trauma Annual Meeting, 1979.
14. Samson DS. Surgical therapy of non-bacterial CNS infection; Symposium on Infection of Central Nervous System. Annual Meeting American Association of Neurological Surgeons, Los Angeles, California, April 25, 1979.
15. Samson DS, Hodosh RM. The risk of intracranial aneurysm surgery in the good grade patient—early versus later operation. Annual Meeting, Congress of Neurological Surgery, Las Vegas, Nevada, October, 1979.
16. Samson DS. A current management of brain abscess. Annual Meeting, Congress of Neurological Surgery, Las Vegas, Nevada, October, 1979.
17. Beyer CW, Samson DS, Hodosh RM. Preoperative evaluation of cerebral autoregulation and systemic tolerance of induced hy-

potension. Annual Meeting of the American Academy of Neurological Surgery, Memphis, Tennessee, November, 1979.

18. Samson DS. The pterional approach of aneurysms of the distal basilar artery. Annual Meeting, American Association of Neurological Surgeons, New York, April 1980.
19. Mickey BM, Samson DS. Neurosurgical applications of the cyanoacrylate adhesives. Annual Meeting, Congress of Neurological Surgeons, Houston, Texas, October, 1980.
20. Mickey BM, Samson DS. Experimental adhesive properties of IBC in the subarachnoid space. Annual Meeting, American Association of Neurological Surgeons, Boston, MA, April, 1981.
21. Samson DS. Saphenous vein interposition grafts—an alternative in EC-IC bypass. Annual Meeting, American Association of Neurological Surgeons, Boston, Mass., April, 1981.
22. Samson DS. The Nipride challenge in cerebral vasospasm. Annual Meeting, Texas Medical Association, Dallas, Texas, May, 1981.
23. Samson DS. Intravascular use of Isobutyl-2-Cyanoacrylate. Annual Meeting, Texas Medical Association, Dallas, Texas, May, 1981.
24. Samson DS, Gewertz B, Beyer CW, Hodosh RM. The use of saphenous vein interposition grafts in the microsurgical treatment of cerebral ischemia. Annual Meeting, International Cardiovascular Society, Dallas, Texas, June, 1981.
25. Samson DS. Management of carotid artery injuries. Annual Meeting, Congress of Neurological Surgeons, Los Angeles, California, October, 1981.
26. Samson DS. Results with IBC embolization in the surgical treatment of arteriovenous malformations. Annual Meeting, American Association of Neurologic Surgeons, Honolulu, Hawaii, April, 1982.
27. Samson DS. Causes, cures, complications and intracranial aneurysm surgery. Annual Meeting, Congress of Neurological Surgeons, Toronto, Canada, October, 1982.
28. Samson DS, Batjer HH, Hodosh RM. Re-evaluation of saphenous vein interposition grafts in the treatment of cerebral ischemia: A five year experience. Annual Meeting, Congress of Neurological Surgeons, Chicago, Illinois, October, 1983.
29. Samson DS, Batjer HH. Arteriovenous malformations of the superior vermis and roof of the fourth ventricle: radio-graphic anatomy, surgical exposure and treatment. Annual Meeting, Congress of Neurological Surgeons, Chicago, Illinois, October, 1983.
30. Samson DS, Batjer HH. Carotid cavernous fistulae: Current treatment and complications. Annual Meeting, Congress of Neurological Surgeons, Chicago, Illinois, October, 1983.

31. Samson DS, Batjer HH. Intraoperative aneurysmal rupture. Presented at Second International Symposium—Cerebral Aneurysm Surgery in the Acute Stage. Graz, Austria, September, 1984.
32. Samson DS, Batjer HH. Mortality and morbidity in arteriovenous malformation surgery. Annual Meeting, Congress of Neurological Surgeons, New York, New York, September, 1984.
33. Batjer HH, Samson DS. Potential roles for early revascularization procedures in acute cerebral ischemia. Annual Meeting, American Heart Association, Miami, Florida, 1984. Abst. *Circulation* 70(4):II–135, 1984.
34. Bonte FJ, Devous MD, Samson DS, Batjer HH, Chehabi HH. Single-photon tomographic study of regional brain blood flow in patients with arteriorevnous malformations. Annual Meeting, The Radiological Society of North America, Nov, 1984.
35. Samson DS, Batjer HH. Arteriovenous malformations of the cerebellar hemispheres, tonsils, brainstem and cerebellar pontine angle. Presented at Annual Meeting, American Association of Neurological Surgeons, Atlanta, Georgia, April, 1985.
36. Batjer HH, Samson DS. The use of extracranial-intracranial arterial bypass in the management of symptomatic vasospasm. Presented at Annual Meeting, Congress of Neurological Surgeons, Honolulu, Hawaii, Sept. 29–Oct. 4, 1985.
37. Batjer H, Suss R, Samson DS. Intracranial arteriovenous malformations assoicated with aneurysm. Presented at Congress of Neurological Surgeons—Post Convention Meeting, Maui, Hawaii, October 5, 1985.
38. Batjer H, Devous M, Mickey BM, Chehabi HH, Bonte FJ, Samson DS. Cerebrovascular reactivity and ischemia associated with intracranial arteriovenous malformations. Presented at Annual Meeting, Congress of Neurological Surgeons, Honolulu, Hawaii, Sept. 29–Oct. 4, 1985.
39. Devous MD Sr, Batjer HH, White SR, Samson DS, Mickey BM, Bonte FJ. DSPECT determination of regional cerebral blood flow at rest and following Diamox induced vasodilation in patients with AVMs, *J Nucl Med* 27:733, 1986.
40. Batjer HH, Samson DS. Surgical approaches to trigonal arteriovenous malformations. Presented at Annual Meeting, American Assoc. of Neurological Surgeons, Denver, Colorado, April 13–17, 1986.
41. Samson DS, Batjer HH. Surgical Therapy of posterior fossa AVM's. Presented at Luncheon Seminar, Annual Meeting. Congress of Neurological Surgeons, New Orleans, La., September 14–18, 1986.
42. Devous MD Sr, Batjer HH, Mickey BM, Samson DS, Bonte FJ. Dy-

namic SPECT measurements of vasodilatory reserve in regions of cerebral steal in patients with arteriovenous malformations. *J Nucl Med* 28:591–592, 1987.
43. Devous MD Sr, Batjer HH, Mickey BM, Samson DS, White SR, Bonte FJ. Dynamic SPECT measurements of vasodilatory reserve in regions of cerebral steal in patients with arteriovenous malformation. *J Cereb Blood Flow Metab* 7 (Suppl 1):S200, 1987.
44. Bonte FJ, Devous MD Sr, Chehabi HH, Samson DS, Batjer HH, Mickey BM. Single-photon tomography study of regional cerebral blood flow in patients with transient ischemic attacks. *J Nucl Med* 28:633, 1987.
45. Batjer HH, Frankfurt AI, Purdy PD, Smith SS, Samson DS. Use of etomidate-induced EEG suppression, temporary arterial occlusion, and intraoperative angiography in the management of difficult large and giant cerebral aneurysms. Presented at Annual Meeting, American Assoc. of Neurological Surgeons, Dallas, Texas, May, 1987.
46. Batjer HH Devons MD Sr, Seibert GB, Samson DS. Intracranial arteriovenous malformation: Factors influencing hyperemic complications and outcome. Presented at the 50th annual meeting of American Academy of Neurological Surgery, Cincinnati, Ohio, September 15, 1988.
47. Purdy PD, Devous MD, White III CL, Samson DS, Batjer HH. Reversible middle cerebral artery embolization in dogs without intracranial surgery. Presented at the 13th International Joint Conference on Stroke and Cerebral Circulation, February 19, 1988, San Diego, Calfironia. Abstract in *Stroke* 19:137, 1988.
48. Devous MD, Purdy PD, Batjer HH, White CL, Samson DS. Relations among regional cerebral blood flow, neurological status, and histopathology in the avitene model of canine cerebral infarction. *J Cereb Blood Flow Metab* 9:S636, 1989.
49. Batjer HH, Purdy PD, Samson DS. Management of hemorrhagic complications of pre-operative embolization of arteriovenous malformations. Presented at Forty-third Annual Meeting of Neurosurgical Society of America, Pebble Beach, California, April 9, 1990.
50. Purdy PD, White CL III, Batjer HH, Brewer K, Hodges K, Samson D. Intracarotid hydroxyethyl methacrylate solution causes stroke in dogs. Presented at the 28th Annual Meeting of the American Society of Neuroradiology, Los Angeles, California, March 19–23, 1990.
51. Purdy, PD, Samson D, Batjer HH, Risser RC. Preoperative embolization of cerebral arteriovenous malformations with polyvinyl

alcohol particles: experience in 63 procedures. Presented at the 28th Annual Meeting of the American Society of Neuroradiology, Los Angeles, California, March 19–23, 1990.

52. D'Alise MD, Stanford GG, Bruce DA, Samson DS. The Parkland Rapid Exam (PRE): A New Scoring System for Neurological Injury in Trauma Triage. Presented at the 1995 Annual Meeting of the Southern Neurosurgucal Society, Dorado, Puerto Rico, April 5–9, 1995.

Contents

II

GENERAL SCIENTIFIC SESSION II
NEUROVASCULAR DECISION MAKING

III

GENERAL SCIENTIFIC SESSION III
PEDIATRIC UPDATE FOR THE GENERAL NEUROSURGEON

IV

GENERAL SCIENTIFIC SESSION IV
LUMBAR INTERBODY FUSIONS

CHAPTER

1

Presidential Address—The End of the Beginning (Again!)

H. HUNT BATJER, M.D.

Ladies and Gentlemen, Members, and Special Guests,

I am deeply honored to have had the opportunity to represent you as the President of The Congress of Neurological Surgeons (CNS). Working with past and current leadership of this organization has been one of the most extraordinary opportunities anyone could ever imagine. The energy and commitment of the CNS Executive Committee should make each of you proud and comfortable in the knowledge that our future as neurosurgeons is in great hands. But let me make one point clear—We need you to come forth and join in the effort. Too often we see the same names appearing again and again doing the work for our specialty. This problem follows logically from two principles taught to me by my father, Henry Batjer: 1) There is an unlimited amount of work to do but only a limited number of people willing to do it and 2) There appear to be two types of people in the world—those that are willing to work and those that are willing to let them!

Organized medicine and organized neurosurgery function as a meritocracy—step up to the plate and offer your talents. The service to your specialty and to our patients' health is an extraordinary high calling. Some of my most enjoyable times, have occurred while serving with this Executive Committee, such as last summer when two miserable specimens (Dr. Barrow and Mr. Willard) were humiliated on the golf course by two finely tuned athletic machines (Drs. Hadley and Batjer). In addition, this year, I had the opportunity to travel widely on behalf of this organization. I made two trips to Japan, one trip to Australia, and one trip to New Zealand, and attended an innumerable number of meetings in Washington and other North American cities.

I have truly enjoyed getting to know you and to understand the difficulties you face. I have learned that we face many of the same problems. The key in the future will be to attack them with the appropriate mix of national, state, and local strategies. I hope I have represented you well.

The CNS has grown remarkably in stature during its first 49 years of life. We have evolved a unique partnership with the American

Association of Neurological Surgeons. Our specialty interfaces with many outside entities, including all three branches of the Federal Government, State governments, regulatory bodies such as the FDA and HCFA, and other medical organizations. The "spokesperson" for our specialty comes in two forms: 1) Through the Joint AANS/CNS Officers under the signature of both Presidents and 2) Through the Washington Committee under the signature of Katie Orrico or its Chairman. This dynamic partnership affords bipartisan leadership and representation in all of our public interfaces and assures that your interests and those of your patients' will be well served.

I would like to especially thank and acknowledge several people:

1) My parents, Henry Batjer and Eleanor Stanlis. Without their presence, my course on this planet would have been problematic from the start! Their support and guidance over the years can never be repaid. I can only hope to do as well as a father and a professional.
2) The Batjer girls. Janet, Hannah, Devon, Hunter, and Ashley have spent much of this year alone. Their love and understanding have been the highest possible incentive to get home!
3) My colleagues at Northwestern. These fine people have absorbed substantial extra burdens during my absences this year and I will never forget their support.
4) Kemp Clark. Dr. Clark was the Chief of Neurosurgery at University of Texas Southwestern when I began my training on his service. His recruitment efforts, which included this year's Honored Guest, set the stage for the development of one of the truly outstanding programs in this country.
5) Charles Drake. I had the extreme pleasure of spending a clinical fellowship on Dr. Drake's service in London. I am sad for all of the young neurosurgeons who will not have the opportunity to listen to his wise and honest perspective. I will always miss the smell of his pipe tobacco and the sound of his grumblings in the back of the room as controversies were being discussed.
6) Duke Samson. Dr. Samson became my mentor during my internship and I continue learning from him to this day. He is a master surgeon and master surgical educator without peer. No one significantly influenced my life more than this year's CNS Honored Guest.

THE "M" WORD

I would like to use this brief time to put into perspective our current unique vantage point. We find ourselves at the simultaneous close of three critical periods of time: 1) The second millennium, 2) The 20th century, and 3) The decade of the 1990's.

In order to better understand our current position and opportunities, it is of interest to study each of these three remarkable epochs and analyze what features set the stage for success or failure. To do this, we must study the environment at the *beginning* not the end of each. As these three periods of time began, we must ask what was the relationship between *intellectual expansion, technology, and the political environment?* Were these factors acting synergistically or antagonistically?

I hope to provide a brief snapshot into the medical, surgical, and political environments of the beginning of each of these remarkable periods and contrast them with our current environment as it goes forward into the 21st century and third millennium. My focus, therefore, will be on *the beginning* of these epochs to better understand the issues of the day and hopefully demonstrate a repetitive cycle of problems that intermittently stifled growth, only to be overcome by an unrelenting force that pushed for new knowledge. I hope to share with you a reason for my own extreme enthusiasm for our future and explain why this moment in time is truly "The End of the Beginning."

TRANSITIONS

The athletes and former athletes among us know very well the meaning of a "transition game." This designation refers to the ability to rapidly switch from a defensive posture to an offensive attack. Through his extraordinary abilities, Michael Jordan created great awareness of how brief a transition game can be and how successful the outcome is if careful strategic planning and superior talent are brought to bear. As neurosurgeons, we deal daily with transitional moments in the operating room that could also be termed "turning the corner." As we perform the early phases of dissection of a complex large basilar artery aneurysm, the anatomy often looks as if it cannot be reconstructed meaningfully. However, as the masters have taught us, there are certain transitional strategies, which when implemented, seemingly make solutions appear before our eyes. In the case of the basilar aneurysm, it often occurs as we begin to mobilize the P1 segment origin and dissect the back wall. A similar circumstance occurs in the treatment of intracranial arteriovenous malformations. The initial dissection occurs in the subarachnoid space as we map out all of the afferent and efferent vasculature. This critical phase helps resolve the Gordian knot but must cease and transition into the subpial dissection at a moment intuitive to the experienced surgeon, as the battle will only be won in the brain. How to implement transitional thinking to economic and political upheaval and change is less intuitive to physicians.

As I review key historical moments, including the present in this perspective, we should examine the *transition strategies* applied by physicians, scientists, and surgeons to determine if they leverage their opportunities to maximize the future advances or fail to seize the moment. For most advances relevant to the surgical neurosciences, a synergy between intellectual exploration, technological advances, and political climate must be present. I will use these three yardsticks as we examine the previously mentioned points in time to illustrate why we are incredibly advantaged at this moment.

THE BEGINNING OF THE SECOND MILLENNIUM

The beginning of the second millennium in the year 1000 AD marked an optimistic emergence from the Dark Ages. The Dark Ages are classically described, as noted in Figure 1.1, as the period of time from the fall of Rome to the Goths in 476 AD to the year 1000. On the other hand, the Medieval world was still mired in the "age of faith," which extended from the fall of Rome to the fall of Constantinople in 1453 AD. An extraordinary heritage of neurosurgery had been developed through ancient civilizations in which Neolithic man had learned to perform surgery on the nervous system. Clear evidence of trephination can be found in pre-Columbian society in the former Mesopotamia, ancient Egypt, and ancient China. An extraordinary period of intellectual growth occurred in the final centuries before Christ. Roman and Greek societies fostered extraordinary inquiry and growth through the teachings of Pythagoras, Hippocrates, Socrates, Plato, and Aristotle. These intellectual developments, as related to medicine and surgery, continued through the teachings of Galen around 200 AD. Extraordinary deductive reasoning had been developed during the time of Hippocrates around 400 BC relating to trephinations for skull fractures, epilepsy, blindness, and headache (1, 5, 7). Remarkably, students were taught to avoid the temporal region for fear of damage "to the artery." Surgeons were taught to leave a small shell of bone to protect the dura, as the inevitable suppuration would naturally extrude this last bit of bone. Greek and Roman physicians were also taught not to remove bone over the cranial sutures due to adherence of the underlying dura. Among other technical problems, progress in neurological surgery was precluded by a lack of anesthesia and instrumentation.

In a very real sense, these remarkable societies were "The First Beginning" of neurosurgery. Unfortunately, progress ceased when the Roman Empire fell. This remarkable moment in time initiated what can be called the Neurosurgical Dark Ages. This era persisted for a variety of reasons through the Renaissance and into the 19th century. The fall

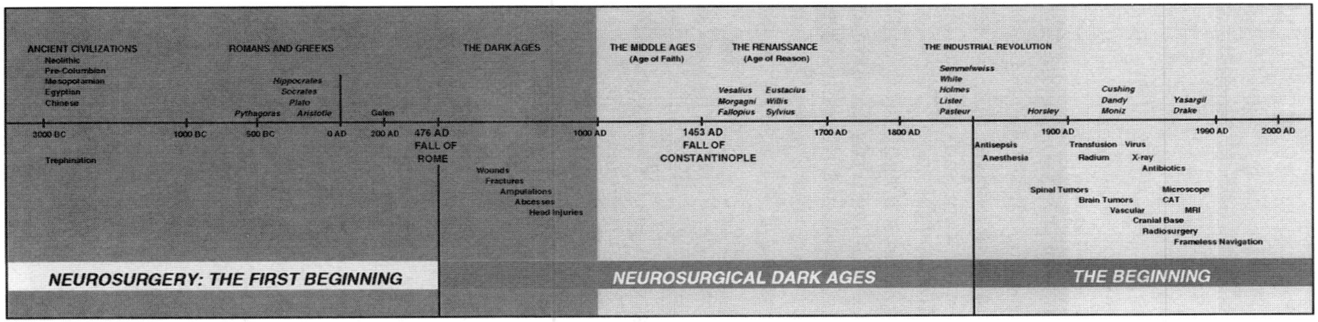

FIG. 1.1 Timetable reflecting societal progress with medical implications from the time of ancient civilizations to the present.

of the Roman Empire and the commencement of the Middle and Dark ages heralded an "Age of Faith" where man no longer learned by his own observations. Interest in the sciences declined as teachers focused on the magical and the unnatural phenomena. As Roman institutions fell, law and medicine were some of the first to go. Physicians and patients had to fend for themselves, and non-clerical physicians ceased to exist. As we approached the beginning of the Second Millennium, an interesting series of regulatory agencies were established such that physician's fees were very high and defined by ordinance. Punishment for malpractice was severe. Physicians' rights and penalties to be incurred were often defined by the social rank of their patients. Physicians were of very low status and not highly educated. Medical procedures largely consisted of exorcism and the internal and external application of plant substances.

As the Church became more established, it attempted to maintain a link with the intellectual past, and the conquerors gave deference to the church of Rome in the traditions of the culturally superior peoples they had conquered. This fortuitous event clearly rejuvenated the care of the sick but without the substantial scientific roots of the Roman and Greek past. For example, St. Benedict forbade the study of medicine (5). Physicians ultimately became an integral part of monastic life. Most of the well-developed surgical procedures of the past were abandoned and were replaced by cauterization techniques. Pharmacology abandoned all experimental aspects and regressed to herbalism and folk medicine. Medical procedures consisted of prayer, the laying on of hands, the use of holy oil, exorcism, and the use of sacred engravings. Surgical procedures were confined to the treatment of wounds, fractures, amputations, abscesses, and head injury. In general, the surgical principles dictated "cut it out or cut it off." These regressive medical times were partially explainable by increased reliance on the Church for teaching. The healing mission of Christ was felt to include "Miracle Cures" and people felt powerless to help themselves.

Western European peoples emerged from the Dark Ages with a spirit of optimism that belied the misery to come from war, plagues, and famine. Thus, one can perceive that at this moment in time, the beginning of the Second Millennium, there was *very little opportunity* for early progress, particularly in the surgical disciplines. Intellectual growth that had been such a fixture of Roman and Greek societies had stopped. Technology remained a substantial limitation and the political climate of the day favored mysticism over science.

THE BEGINNING OF THE 20TH CENTURY.

The beginning of the 20th century found a remarkably different world. The world of neurosurgery had clearly emerged from its own Dark Ages.

Remarkably, with one important exception the Renaissance did not impact our discipline in a favorable way. While the intellectual, academic, and artistic gifts of this remarkable era will be an integral part of life for civilized man as long as there are civilized people, the only major benefit to the neurosciences occurred in the 14th century when a ban on human dissection was eliminated. This single event prompted prolific anatomical studies by Vesalius, Fallopius, Eustacius, Willis, Sylvius, and Morgagni. Detailed information about the nervous system now emerged from the primitive understanding elucidated by Hippocrates.

Two other seminal events positioned physicians and surgeons optimally at the beginning of the 20th century: *antisepsis and anesthesia.* Previous surgical ventures were limited in scope due to the necessary brevity of the procedures (lack of anesthesia) and the inevitable suppuration. The remarkable work of Semmelweiss, Holmes, Lister, Pasteur, and others clearly launched the surgical world as we now know it. Just before the turn of the century, Victor Horsley removed the first intraspinal tumor. Educational programs in surgical disciplines were receiving significant attention as the 20th century began. There was increasing regulation and standardization of medical curricula as well as surgical training. Regarding surgery, however, these curricula focused largely on *duration* and *not content,* a circumstance that arguably exists today.

Therefore, remarkable scientific development had occurred and political structures were nurturing of the sciences and medicine. At the turn of the century, the only deficit was in technology, but this changed quickly. These ingredients, together with the training of intellectual horsepower stimulated by progress in the late 19th century, set the stage for a century of spectacular growth in the neurosciences. This synergy, unimpeded by minor technological problems and a rapid crescendo of decades of world conflict, resulted in a rapid crescendo of cascading events, such as the understanding of transfusions, identification of viruses, x-ray, radium, and ultimately antibiotics. In retrospect, it seems remarkable that the major red blood cell types were only reported in 1901 by Lance Steiner and routine testing before each transfusion commenced in 1908. In 1941, Florey and Chain clearly established the therapeutic value of Flemming's penicillin.

As one views the episode of growth beginning at the dawn of the 20th century in perspective, progress occurring over typical five-year intervals of time would have required centuries in ages past. In this "century of neurosurgery," Horsley's advances were rapidly followed by Cushing and Dandy, spurred on by the creation of angiography by Moniz in 1927 (6). The microsurgical era represented another technological advance capitalized upon by the genius of Yasargil and Drake in recognizing immediate applications. As the 1990s approached, refinements of the principle of electrosurgery (4) and spectacular new neuroimaging, including computed tomography (CT) scanning and magnetic resonance imaging (MRI), set the stage for an extraordinary optimistic decade.

THE BEGINNING OF THE 1990S

In spite of the apparent assets and synergies existing in 1990, political difficulties entered the equation. Cost for medical care were rising at an alarming rate, and in the United States, the presidential election of 1992 framed the debate of how to pay for health care. In 1990, the matrix of industries comprising health care consumed 14% of the gross domestic product and this was felt to be too much. These resources totaled $670 billion per year, which translated to $2,566 per citizen (2). While the Clinton administration proposal to restructure health care in the US failed, numerous forces were concurrently working toward cost containment. This resource-based methodology, utilized through the Health Care Financing Agency and remarkable expansion and penetration of managed care organizations of various types, dramatically reshaped surgical health care. Clearly, the targeted issues of these governmental and private agencies were "expensive technologies" and "expensive procedures." Remarkable arguments surfaced in the Medicare debate that clearly involved societal ethical mores. End of life issues were targeted as 30% of total Medicare budgeting that was consumed during the last year of life, with one-half of that sum used in the last 60 days of life. Hospice structures were developed in order to contain these costs and advance directives were strongly promoted. These initiatives were only marginally successful in curtailing costs. The consolidation of managed care enterprises as well as federally driven reductions in Medicare allocation to the surgical disciplines significantly interrupted an overall increase in health care expenditures for a relatively brief period of time. However, these initiatives did nothing to curb the bloated and growing administrative costs associated with health care, which now consume more than 20% of the health care dollar. The lack of synergy between intellectual development, technological development, and political climate limited the true neuroscience growth potential of the decade of the 1990s.

THE BEGINNING OF THE THIRD MILLENNIUM

So where do we find ourselves today? In the United States, health care represents one-seventh of the US economy and totals $1 trillion per year. Due to a variety of factors, 44 million Americans do not have health insurance coverage (often by the individual's choice). Hospitals are now being hit by the provisions of the Balanced Budget Act of 1997, and many of our greatest institutions are in immediate danger of insolvency. Graduate medical education may become a yearly federal budgetary football. Patients feel out of control and are striking back. Employers are unhappy about rising healthcare costs and their unhappy employees. Health maintenance organizations are being clobbered by increased liability from their unhappy clients, while escalating costs make them less attractive for employers. I can only imaging Marcus Welby studying the formula for Medicare Physician Reimbursement (Figure 1.2) How would Dr. Cushing react to the "bullet points" of Evaluation and Management documentation guidelines?

Our learned medical societies (including the CNS!) and our finest institutions have been thrown off course by these upheavals. Of necessity we have had to focus on the enormous threat to fiscal survival for physician practices and hospitals. Our academic centers have faced extraordinary risk through Physicians at Teaching Hospitals (PATH) audits in which the Office of Inspector General could arrive and confiscate ten of millions of dollars under the guise of "fraudulent billing based on ambiguous and unbelievably complex documentation guidelines. Our advocacy efforts have focused on how best to control loss, or worse, on how to control *rate* of loss! These multiple factors threaten the two most important facets of specialty care—Quality and Access.

RBRVS: Components

$$\text{Payment} = \text{CF} \times [\text{RVU}_{wk} \times \text{GPCI}_{wk}] + [\text{RVU}_{pe} \times \text{GPCI}_{pe}] + [\text{RVU}_{mp} \times \text{GPCI}_{mp}]$$

wk =	Work = 50%
pe =	Practice Expense = 46%
mp =	Malpractice = 4%
GPCI =	Geographic Practice Cost Index
CF =	Conversion Factor = $34.73 for 1999

FIG. 1.2 Resource-Based Methodology at its Finest!

Needless to say, resources have been redirected from research and technology into the defensive actions noted above. The direct result has been stagnation from an intellectual and technological standpoint during the 1990s.

So what is there to be happy about? In the words of Henry Batjer, "Things seem to get sonofabitcher all the time!" The beginning of the next century and the next millennium do not imply "the beginning of the end" for the neurosciences. History teaches us that progress and growth come in fits and starts, and require synergy of intellect, technology, and political structure for meaningful advances to be made. In perspective, we have been static for a trivial period of time.

We are now poised and optimally positioned for unbelievable forward advances, particularly in the arenas of neural-regeneration, tissue salvage, gene therapies, prevention, stem cell implantation, skeletal remodeling, and safer intracranial and spinal navigation with functional road mapping. We have exactly the right people in the right place at the right time. Neuroscientists among us, together with our colleagues from industry, have created extraordinary new tools. Our current societal and political environment is intolerant of mediocrity. We are at center stage.

HOW DO WE DO IT?

I am not the kind of guy who would rail about our problems and obliquely point to a bright future without some tangible suggestions.

Value What we Bring to the Table

Figure 1.3 illustrates a screw. This is a very good screw and sells for less than 25 cents at the local hardware store a short drive from all of our homes. Figure 1.4 illustrates another screw. This is also a very good screw and sells for nearly $1000. Our industrial partners have been remarkably successful in differentiating the product or service they bring to the market place in the eyes of the consumer. These differentiating characteristics have translated to increased value of that product or service. We have clearly failed to capitalize on the remarkable service we bring to the public, and we can no longer accept this. We deal with diseases of critical public health importance and we treat an organ that has extraordinary value to even the mystical societies at the first millennium. Let us take these assets to the market place.

Fiscal Responsibility

We must run our practices with a heightened sense of cost control, balancing true business principles with compassionate care. Medicine and neurosurgery are not classical businesses but without attention to

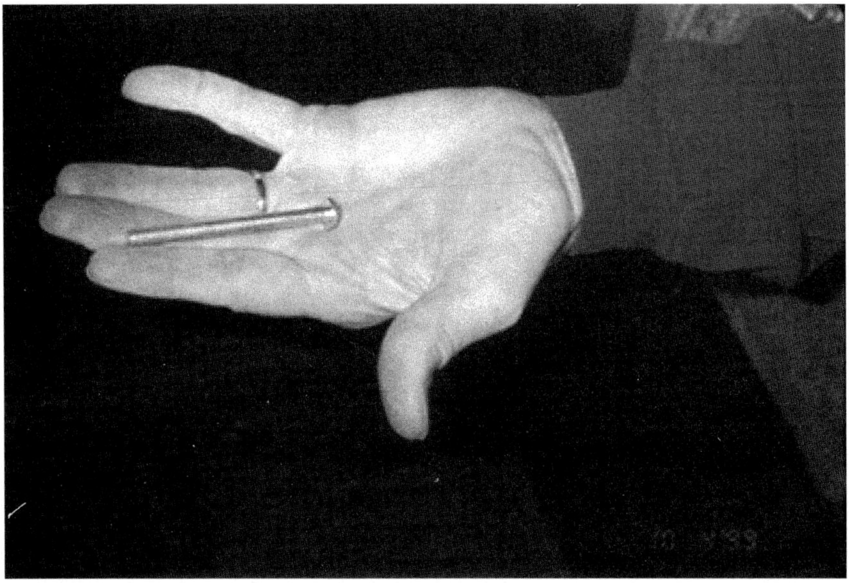

FIG. 1.3 "A screw"

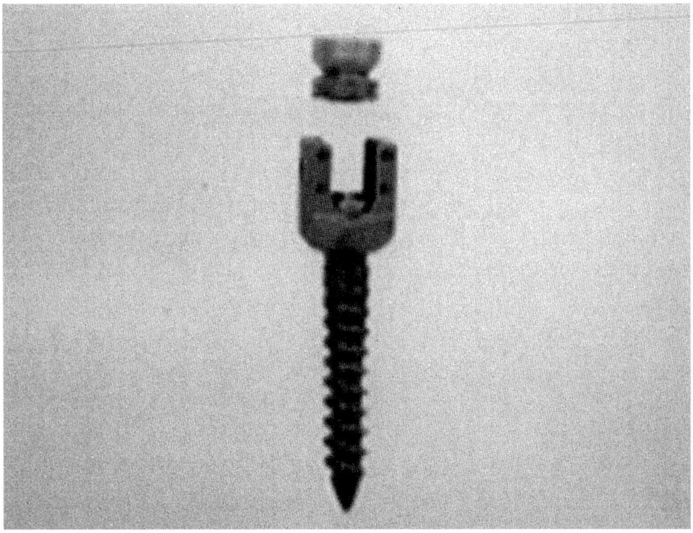

FIG. 1.4 "An instrument"

business principles, our practices will fail. No money, no mission. However, if we run our practices as true businesses, we violate the "The Oath of Hippocrates." If we ask ourselves at each patient encounter "Is this how I would treat one of my own family members?" the result will be *better access* and *better quality of care.*

Keep Your Eye on the Ball

We must navigate interesting, frustrating, and rapidly changing financial and political realities to ensure survival of our practices. Regardless of how well we navigate these uncertainties, if we fail to serve the public by advancing the science and practice of medicine with tangible benefits and minimizing human suffering, we will be viewed by history as failures (and we should be). Ladies and Gentlemen, here is *The Ball.* Let us check our report card. Figure 1.5 illustrates a glioblastoma multiforme in a 57-year-old man. How will this gentleman fare under my care compared to how he might have fared under Dr. Cushing's care in the 1930s? Figure 1.6 illustrates a large stroke, which represents the third leading cause of death in this country. How many victims of this disease are caught before irreversible damage is done? Do they recover quicker than they did in previous decades? Figure 1.7 illustrates a fatal hypertensive cerebral hemorrhage. Are we not able to measure and treat high blood pressure? Figure 1.8 represents a severe subarachnoid hemorrhage from a ruptured aneurysm. We have beautiful and sophisticated technology that allows precise and even perfect anatomical treatment for the offending lesion. It is difficult to feel terrifically satisfied knowing that only one-half of the victims of this disease recover their premorbid state and occupation. I find it fascinating that some of our clinical scholars and surgeons are at this moment teaching neurologists, primary care physicians, and neurosurgeons that we should not preemptively strike this disease, treat unruptured aneurysms, and *prevent* subarachnoid hemorrhage! I wish some of these therapeutic nihilists could get to know some of the families of the patients I treat. I wonder if these physicians are capable of "feeling their pain." Figure 1.9 shows a ruptured giant fusiform basilar trunk aneurysm in an 18-year-old girl. How do you feel about our strategic and technical solutions to this problem? (3) Figure 1.10 illustrates a brain injury from a gun shot wound. Figure 1.11 illustrates a thoracic spine fracture resulting in a paraplegia. I personally feel that the final two conditions are more sociological in nature than neurological. However, we as neurosurgeons have pivotal roles to play. The maximum advantage we can bring will be in the arena of prevention. How many of our members actually participate in their local chapters of Think First? We have documented evidence that getting the message to young children changes behaviors. This is our responsibility and we must get the message out. We must do better.

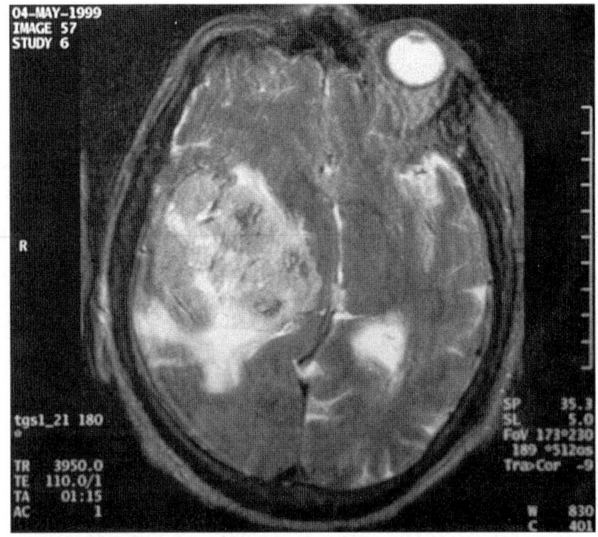

FIG. 1.5 Glioblastoma multiforme

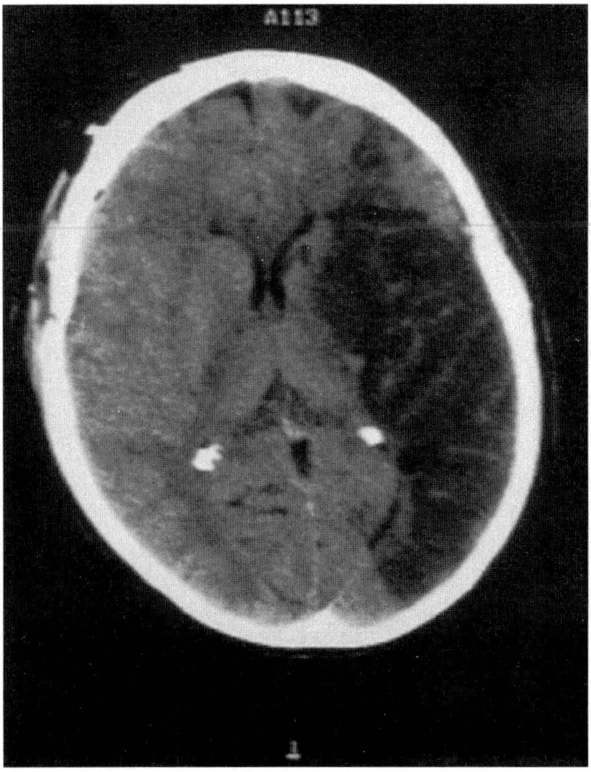

FIG. 1.6 Large dominant cerebral infarction

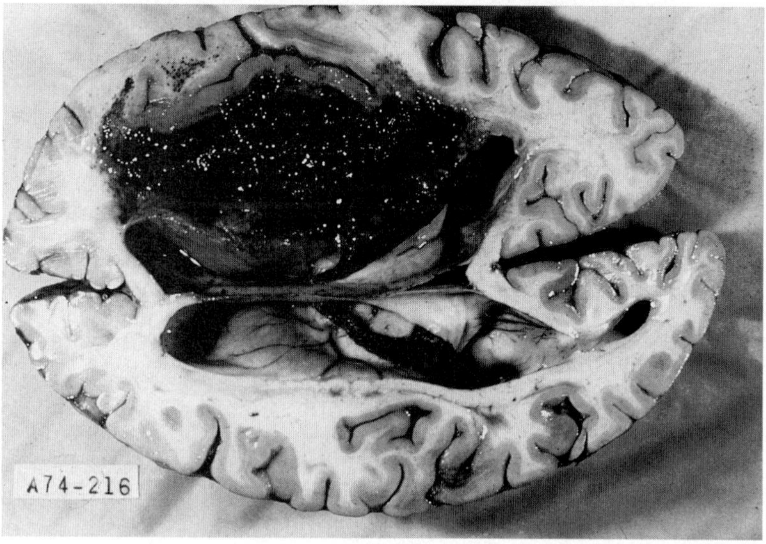

FIG. 1.7 Fatal Gangliar hypertension hemorrhage

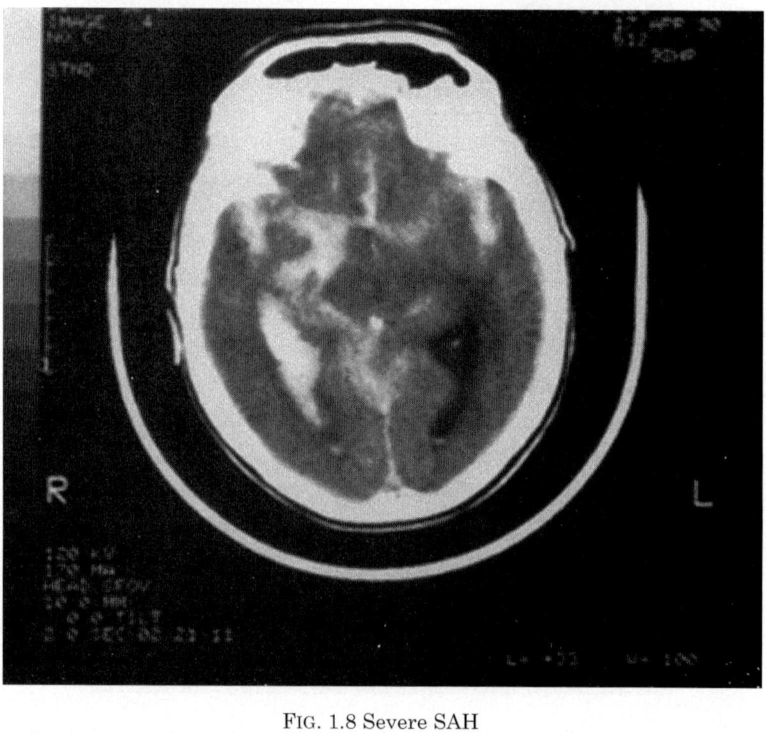

FIG. 1.8 Severe SAH

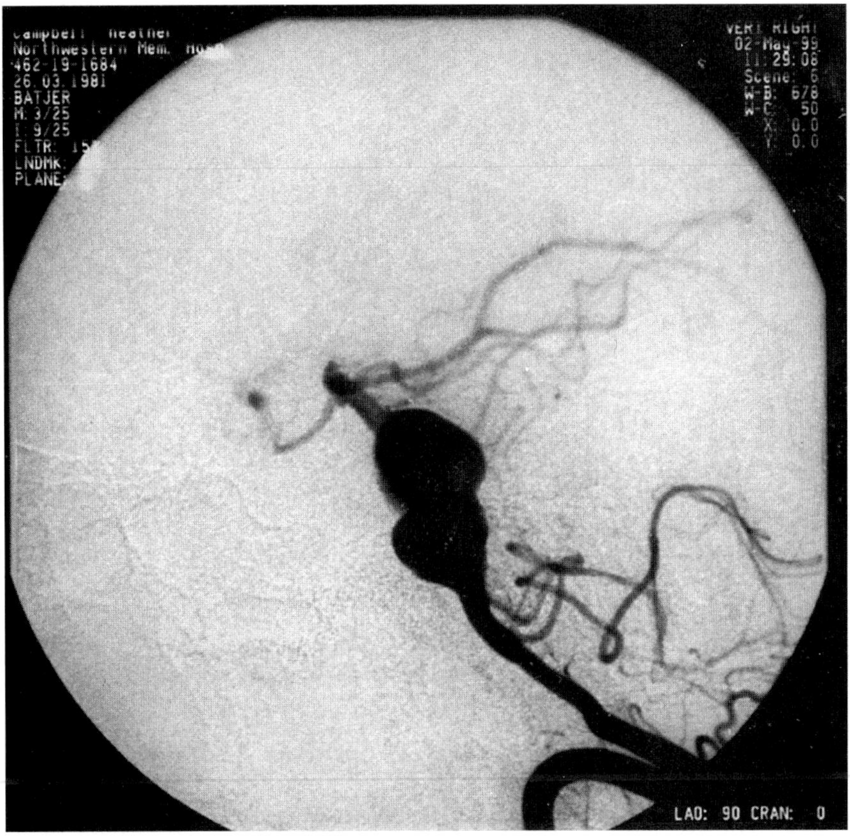

FIG. 1.9 Giant fusiform basilar trunk aneurysm

These cases recall a less than terrific coach I once had who stood before our high school basketball team and stated "Men, this is no time to rest on your laurels because you do not have any."

Invest in the Future

We must commit the necessary people, time, and resources to our key diseases. Our strongest weapon is the creativity of our young members. We must give them time and resources. This will cost money and we must *do it.*

Training Programs

In many ways, our training strategies do not differ substantively from our predecessors of the turn of the century. Our programs still focus on service rather than education and we have been unsuccessful in providing a critical outpatient experience while under pressure from hospitals

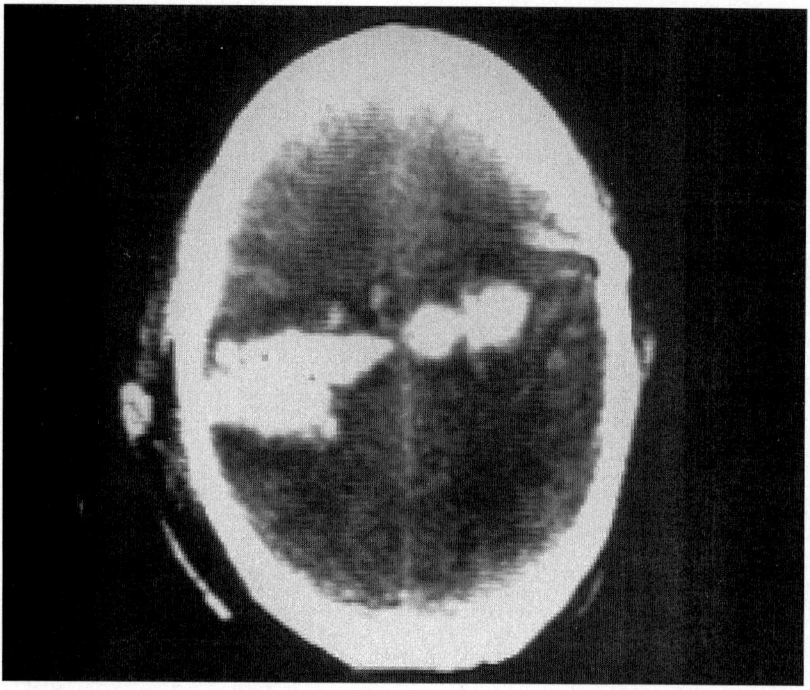

FIG. 1.10 GSW to the brain

and managed care organizations to minimize the days of hospital admissions. "The one size fits all" strategy is clearly anachronistic. We must critically rethink how we teach our young neurosurgeons knowing that we have a very finite resource that is increasingly under political pressure. In the next year, graduate medical education funding could become a line item on the federal budget subject to political whim. Let us go forward and alter our training methodology to optimally train our residents for the job they will in fact be doing, not the job their professors are doing. We need to strive for education, not indentured servitude.

Don't Wait

Do not wait to see how the next century and the next millennium will treat us. We will not get lucky. We must attack the future.

General Patton found himself positioned at precisely the right place at precisely the right time with precisely the right instrument. At this moment, we share many of those strategic advantages. We are poised for a true *Renaissance in Neuroscience* using the creative and intellectual horsepower that we have assembled which can harness and direct

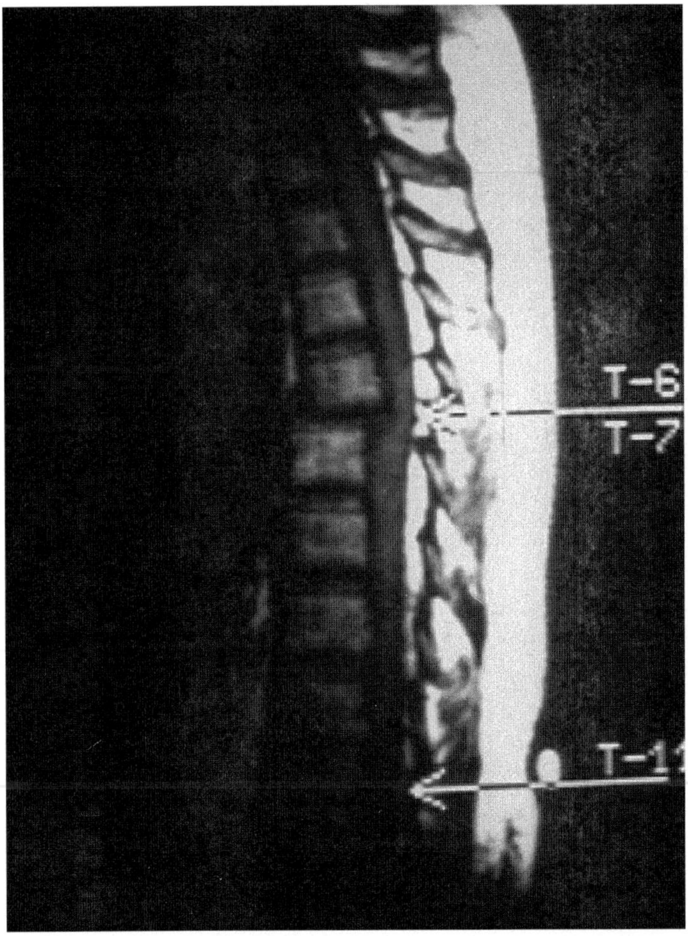

FIG. 1.11 Thoracic spine fracture, dislocation

the marvelous new technologies that have emerged. If we do this right, we will have launched a new golden age of better care, fewer diseases, and quicker and more complete recoveries. If we keep our eyes on "the ball" and focus on the long term goal of improving the public's health, we too will soar like eagles into an unimaginable future and be remembered as "the best there ever was" and "the best there ever will be."

REFERENCES

1. Adams F: *The genuine works of Hippocrates.* London: Printed for the Syndenham Society, Vol I, pp. 470–482, 1849.

2. Batjer HH: Cerebrovascular care in the next decade: Cost, prudence, progress, and rationing. In Batjer HH (ed): *Cerebrovascular Disease.* New York: Lippincott-Raven Publishers, 1978.
3. Batjer HH, Samson DS: Causes of morbidity and mortality form surgery of aneurysms of the distal basilar artery. **Neurosurgery** 25:904–916, 1989.
4. Cushing H, Bovie WT: Electro-surgery as an aid to the removal of intracranial tumors. **Surg Gynec Obst** 47:751–784, 1928.
5. Lyons AS, Petrucelli RJ: *Medicine-An Illustrated History.* New York: Harry N. Abrams, Inc. Publishers, 1978.
6. Moniz E: L'encephalographie arterielle, son importance dans la localization des tumeurs cerebrales. **Rev Neurol** 2:72–90, 1927.
7. Walker AE (ed). *A History of Neurological Surgery.* Baltimore: Williams and Wilkins Company, 1951.

I

General Scientific Session I Treatment of CNS Neoplasms and Aneurysms: The End of the Beginning

CHAPTER

2

Surgery for Cerebral Gliomas: Past, Present, and Future

PETER M. BLACK, M.D., PH.D.

ACKNOWLEDGMENT

I am indebted to Christopher Black for his help in preparation of this manuscript.

INTRODUCTION

Most neurosurgeons have a love-hate relationship with cerebral gliomas. On the one hand, these tumors tend to be infiltrative and ultimately incurable by surgery alone. On the other, they are common and sometimes complex to remove safely.

Even today there is controversy about how aggressive to be with surgery for gliomas (11, 26). However, increasing evidence suggests that both low- and high-grade gliomas are best treated with major resection. Removal of the imaged abnormality in low-grade gliomas appears to be an important component of long-term remission (9, 10, 15, 16, 21, 65, 81), and major resection makes quality of life and survival better for high-grade gliomas (2, 15, 34, 50, 51, 90).

The past, present, and future of cerebral glioma surgery involves both biology and technology. Figure 2.1 summarizes our progress. In the past, we have had modest technology and modest understanding of biology. At present, we have robust technology but modest understanding of glioma biology. In the future, I believe there will be both robust technology and biology and the increasing recognition of the molecular neurosurgeon as local oncologist.

THE PAST (1913–1967)—"THE BEGINNING"

The past era of cerebral glioma surgery was characterized by modest technology and biology. It is helpful to compare the work of Cushing with that of neurosurgeons today. Harvey Cushing, neurosurgeon of the century (16, 19, 28, 40, 65, 71), did most of his neurosurgery at the Peter Bent Brigham Hospital, one of the forerunners of the present

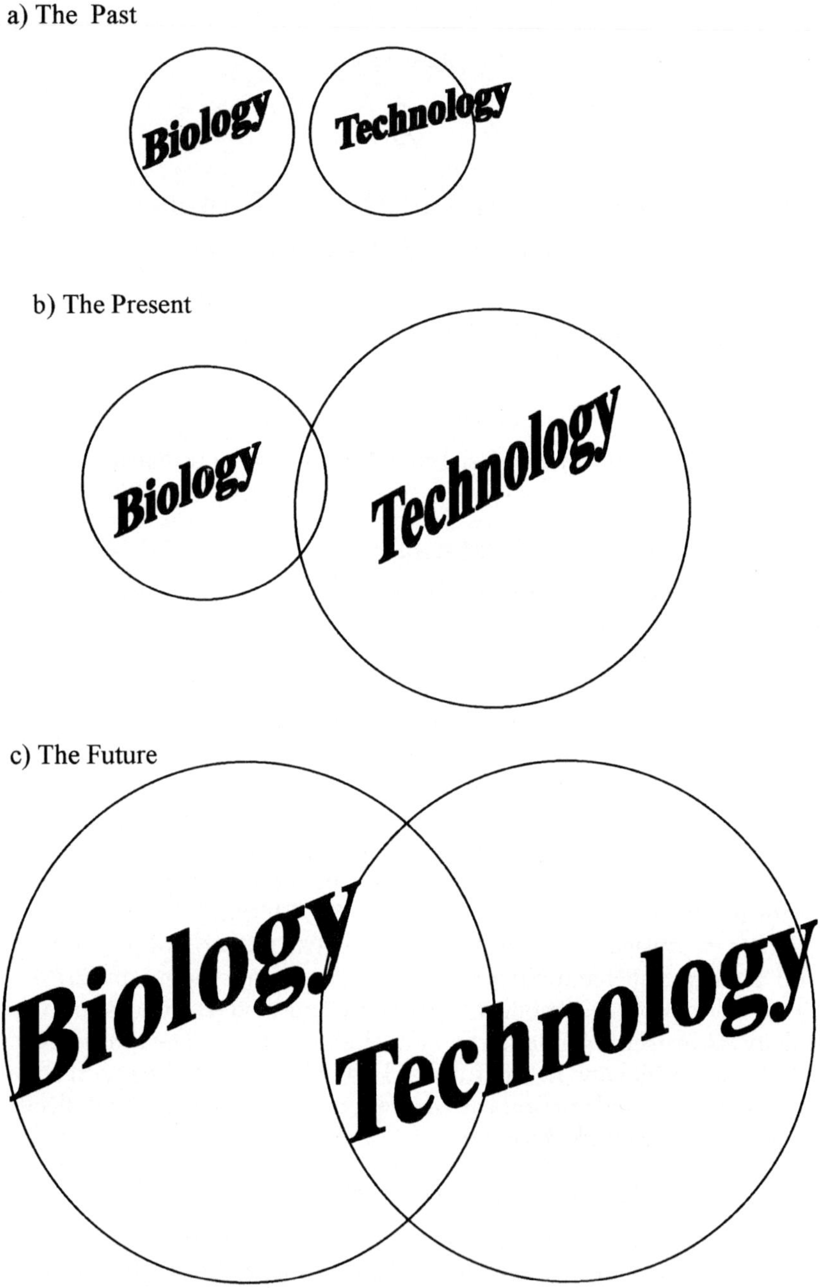

FIG. 2.1 Past, present, and future of cerebral glioma surgery
FIG. 2.1a: The past—modest biology, modest technology, little interaction
FIG. 2.1b: The present—modest biology, robust technology, modest interaction
FIG. 2.1c: The (hopeful) future—robust biology, robust technology, robust interaction

Brigham and Women's Hospital (13, 19). The Brigham and Women's Hospital was formed in 1987 by the union of the Peter Bent Brigham Hospital, the Boston Hospital for Women, the Boston Lying-in Hospital, and the Robert Breck Brigham Hospital (16, 76). In the period from 1913–1933, Cushing carried out more than 2000 operations for brain tumor (19). His surgical approaches and illustrations have been collected in a historical volume (17). The procedures and their outcomes have been summarized in his remarkable monograph "Intracranial tumors. Notes upon a series of 2000 verified cases with surgical-mortality percentages pertaining thereto" (36).

Technology

It is noteworthy that Cushing emphasized the importance of major resection for malignant gliomas and his techniques allowed this to be done in a way not achieved by lesser surgeons. In his summary of his experience he writes that: "The larger and more formidable the lesion appears to be, the more radical is the effort made to remove its major portion . . ."(36).

The concept that major surgery allows better surgical survival in malignant gliomas is an important concept even today; the neurosurgeon is well advised to remove the enhancing component completely or to leave such a lesion along and perform just a stereotactic biopsy (26). The result of partial resection is often malignant brain swelling of the rest of the tumor. Cushing also recognized that radiation therapy might be helpful in the management of gliomas (91).

It is remarkable how similar Cushing's series of tumors is to this author's series, as shown in Figure 2.2. Gliomas counted for essentially the same fraction of brain tumors in his time as they did in the years 1987–98. However, the morbidity and mortality have improved remarkably in the last 65 years. For Cushing, the mortality for 164 astrocytomas was 10.4% and for 208 glioblastomas was 24.2%. At present the surgical (30-day) mortality for 343 low-grade gliomas in the author's series was 0%, for 149 anaplastic astrocytomas 0%, and for 255 glioblastomas 0.4%.

A number of technological improvements helped to diminish mortality. The use of corticosteroids to control brain swelling, the understanding that as much as possible of a malignant tumor should be removed, improved neuroanesthesia, resident neurosurgeon coverage, and improved intensive care, including intracervical pressure (ICP) monitoring, were all important. For the surgery itself, electrocautery, developed by Cushing for its neurosurgical applications, and suction with a tradition sucker, were the main tools of the neurosurgeon's trade in his time. Angiography and ventriculography were the imaging modalities

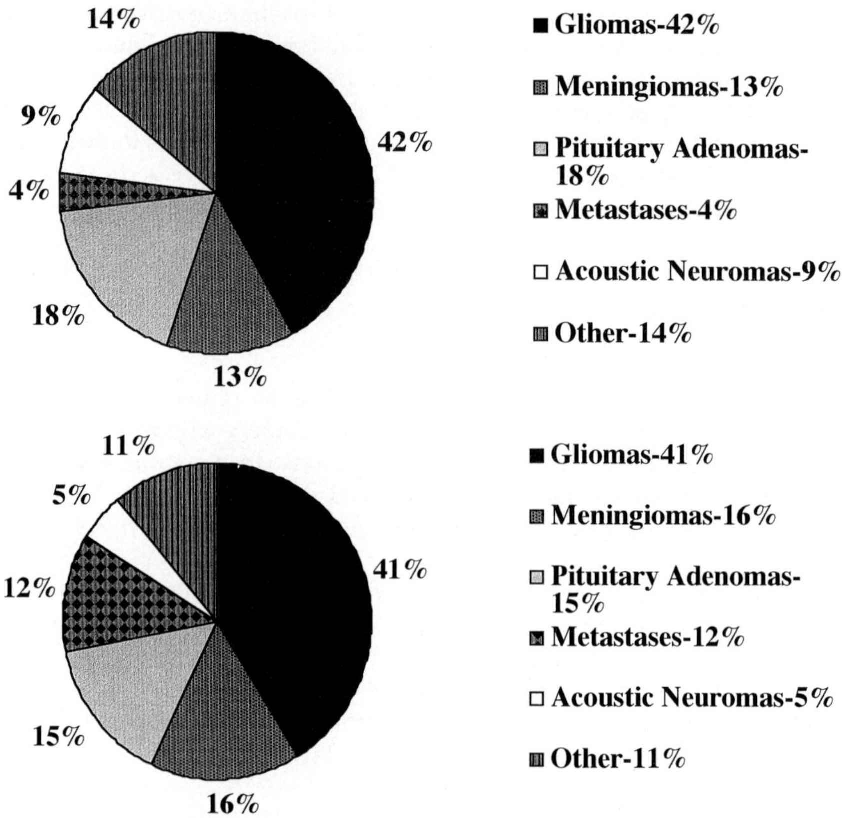

FIG. 2.2 Comparison of Harvey Cushing's and the author's total cases.
FIG. 2.2a: Harvey Cushing's 2000 total cases (1913–1933).
FIG. 2.2b: The author's 2489 cases from 1987 to 1999.

from the 30s to the 60s but could only establish shifts in brain structures: it was not possible to view the brain tumor itself. However, the beginnings of the techniques that would become critical to glioma surgery of the present time were being developed. The most important of these was stereotaxis, the concept of linking surgery to imaging. Early attempts included the Horsley and Clarke apparatus (53), the device developed by Spiegel and Wycis (97), and the Tailarach system. In a premonitory way these led to the image-guided surgery revolution.

Biology

During this time, understanding of brain tumor biology was developing slowly. Most work was done with cell culture, but the culture conditions markedly changed the nature of the findings. There were a few animal models of gliomas but they were not very good. There was debate about the classification of gliomas, and the uncertainty in this made the comparison of treatment modalities difficult. The understanding of glioma biology reflected the understanding of cancer biology in general, which was in a developmental stage. Moreover, there was little interaction between biology and surgery.

THE PRESENT (1967–1999)—"THE END OF THE BEGINNING"

The modern era in glioma neurosurgery is characterized by robust technology but modest biology (11, 23, 25).

Technology

The modern technological era in neurosurgery began with the introduction of the operating microscope into routine surgical use. Pioneered by Ted Kurze and Peardon Donaghy for neurosurgical application following the example of ear-nose-throat surgeons, the operating microscope was popularized by Yasargil and his followers until it revolutionized the practice of tumor neurosurgery (100, 103). The capacity to view cranial nerves, arteries, and other small structures allowed a precision in surgery that was new and exciting.

Although the operating microscope became an important part of neurosurgery for skull base, pituitary, intraventricular, and other tumors, it was not particularly helpful in glioma surgery. Some surgeons argued that it permitted the microscope establishment of the tumor margin, but for the majority of surgeons, loupe magnification was still used. There were, however, important adjuncts to microsurgery that set the tone for later development. These included skeletal fixation, bipolar cautery, power craniotomes, and the ultrasonic aspirator.

However, three technological capabilities *have* been particularly important in advancing the field of glioma surgery. These are: accurate imaging and localization of the tumor to be resected, a reliable navigation system for guidance of resection, and an understanding of eloquent areas to be avoided.

ACCURATE IMAGING AND LOCALIZATION OF THE TUMOR TO BE RESECTED

For gliomas, the most important development of the present era has been the advance in imaging. This allowed the recognition of tumor and its characteristics. With computed tomograph (CT) it was possible for the first time to view the blood-brain barrier breakdown caused by a tumor directly (27). With magnetic resonance imaging (MRI), this capability became even more robust, with an enhanced ability to establish increased water content of brain caused by permeable new blood vessels in the tumor. Much remains to be done in tumor imaging, however. Present techniques only allow demonstration of the blood-brain barrier breakdown around tumors; in the future, it may be possible to visualize the tumor cells themselves. Radioisotope-labeled molecules may be one way of imaging tumor directly that may be increasingly important in the future, as demonstrated by Kassis and colleagues (56).

A RELIABLE NAVIGATION SYSTEM FOR GUIDANCE OF RESECTION

As important as visualization of the tumor is the use of computing power to manipulate it. This occurred first with modern adaptation of previous stereotactic frames, the Brown-Roberts-Wells (BRW) and Leksell being the first widely used CT-compatible frames (5, 51, 66). These combined the power of visualization with the capacity to manipulate. The result was a revolution that is still with us.

Stereotactic biopsies could be done safely and accurately, which significantly improved the capacity to identify a bran mass. Improved target-centered frames were developed that allowed both biopsy and surgical resection of lesions (35). The concept that a lesion should be followed for months to see whether it progresses was modified; now, biopsies could be done early to establish the nature of the lesion. Craniiotomies could be done with computer-guided precision (35, 57, 78). Stereotactic radiosurgery and implantation of brachytherapy seeds could also be carried out (18, 69, 70, 95). Our experience with linac radiosurgery using the Radionics X-knife system in glioblastomas has shown a median survival of 18 months after diagnosis (95). This is at least as good as interstitial brachytherapy with high activity seeds (70) and illustrates the importance of local therapies. These modalities made a great difference in the management of glioblastomas, essentially doubling survival for patients who were eligible for them.

Framed systems were followed by frameless systems (6, 7). These provided the accuracy of framed units without the inconvenience of applying a base ring. They generally used a fiducial system with computer guided reconstruction of the brain and the lesion. They placed the power of computing in the hands of the surgeon, giving him or her the ability to work with MRI vision instead of physiological vision. They could be used to localize a tumor, identify its margins, and resect it safely. In a similar way to the use of the endoscope in general surgery, they markedly advanced the field.

At the Brigham and Women's Hospital, we have been able to use both a commercially available system of frameless stereotaxis—the Radionics OTS system—and our own system, the Brigham and Women's Hospital Surgical Navigator. We have carried out over 100 craniotomies with the Radionics OTS system. We have found it easy to use and accurate in its localization of lesions to within one centimeter. It has been most useful with CT imaging. This limits its use in low-grade gliomas, where the mass is best seen with MRI.

The surgical navigator has several differences from commercially available systems (60, 80). It uses skin-to-skin registration and therefore does not need fiducials. It has very powerful segmentation and three-dimensional reconstruction paradigms and can incorporate surface vessels into the registration. It also has the capacity to be interactive with the surgeon, allowing points from the operating field to be entered in the reconstructed scan.

The principles used in the BWH surgical navigator have recently been incorporated in the Visual Technologies, Inc., (VTI system). This may be the next generation of image-guided surgical systems. It uses electromagnetic guidance rather than direct line-of-site navigation, is readily used with MRI and the operating microscope, and has powerful reconstruction capacities.

The major problem, however, with all systems that use preoperatively acquired images is that volumes may shift during the surgery. First with the GE Signa SP scanning system and then with similar systems from other manufacturers, we have entered a new era of image guided surgery, as will be discussed.

AN UNDERSTANDING OF ELOQUENT AREAS

Techniques for identifying eloquent regions of the brain have become extremely important in glioma surgery. These include functional MRI, transcutaneous magnetic stimulation, and positron emission tomography (PET) scanning. PET can be coregistered with MRI and therefore, allow understanding of the area that is used in a particular function; however, its spatial resolution is not very satisfactory. Functional MRI is probably the most important future technique; it depends on blood flow changes and can represent the area involved quite accurately. It can also be superimposed on a three-dimensional rendering of the brain surface. Transcutaneous magnetic stimulation is particularly useful for motor mapping. In this, a strong magnetic field is passed across the intact skull and defines sites in which maximum movement occurs (45).

Perhaps the most effective technique, however, is one that has not changed significantly since Cushing's time—the mapping of the brain with direct cortical stimulation. It was shown in 1987 that the same techniques that had been used for epilepsy surgery could be applied to tumor surgery, and this has made a great difference in the approach to gliomas (24). With medazolam and fentanyl or propofol as the anesthetic agent, tumors in speech, motor, or sensory areas can be removed routinely. In 156 adult patients with these techniques, it was possible to divide patients into 81 who had no deficit preoperatively and 75 with a preoperative deficit (37, 38). In 81 patients without a deficit, only one patient had a new problem after brain mapping and resection of the lesion. In 75 patients who had a preoperative deficit in speech, movement, or sensation, there was an 8% incidence of postoperative difficulty. This tended to occur after the surgery was completed and in a delayed manner, making it difficult to predict. One of the conclusions from this paper is that it is better to operate on a patient when there is no preoperative deficit than waiting for a deficit to occur. We have now operated on more than 300 patients with these techniques and find them straightforward and important.

In children or in some adults, it may be difficult to do surgery under local anesthesia, although the procedure was tolerated well by 95% of patients in our previous series (38). An alternative is to use subdural grids and strips to map the brain at the bedside. On many occasions now this has been used with patients who have seizures, with the capacity to be certain about the localization of speech and motor areas. An example of this technique is a 14-year-old girl with seizures and an apparent low-grade glioma. It was possible to insert subdural grids and strips for phase III evaluation of her seizures and then map her cortex at the bedside to identify motor cortex definitively. The grids could be mapped onto the three-dimensional reconstruction of the motor cortex to allow precise correlation with the imaged abnormality. The oligodendroglioma could then be successfully removed.

An alternative to this is evoked potential recording demonstrating primary sensory cortex; from this, the motor cortex can be inferred. This technique has been used with only partial success because it is sometimes difficult to demonstrate phase reversal.

Another option is intraoperative mapping under general anesthesia using motor potentials. However, it may be difficult to establish the site of motor stimulation precisely with this technique (45).

Biology

An understanding of glioma biology must begin with classification, which is still based on morphological characteristics (42). The most recent glioma classification proposed by the World Health Organization is presented in Table 2.1. Low-grade gliomas are divided into several histopathological types, which include astrocytomas, gangliogliomas, dysembryoplastic neuroepithelial tumors, oligodendrogliomas, neurocytomas, mixed gliomas and gangliogliomas. The pathological criteria for these are variable from center to center and this must be kept in mind in evaluating these tumors. However, it appears that most of them do not extensively infiltrate the brain around the tumor. Malignant gliomas include glioblastomas, anaplastic astrocytomas, anaplastic oligodendrogliomas, and primitive neuroectodermal tumors. These tumors stimulate angiogenesis, divide rapidly, and invade the brain.

The attempt to derive new classification systems based on molecular and developmental understandings is a critically important part of present glioma biology. Whatever the classification system, however, the surgeon must recognize how an understanding of biology affects what he or she is doing. Two of the most important features of gliomas that limit effective treatment at present are invasion and heterogeneity. Invasion defeats the surgeon and heterogeneity defeats the oncologist.

Invasion has been studied by a number of investigators, many of them in neurosurgical laboratories. DeRidder et al. found that invasion was directly related to tumorigenicity (41). Pedersen et al. followed the migratory pattern of human glioma cells transplanted into the rat brain with a lacz marker, showing extensive invasion (86). Chicoine and Silbergeld showed patterns of invasion in animals (33) and then in patients' biopsied tissue at a distance from the enhancing tumor. At least four centimeters from the margin of the apparent glioma and in brain that appeared histologically normal, there were cells that were able to develop anchorage-independent growth in soft agar and had a malignant karyotype (96). Rosenblum et al. analyzed the pattern of invasion of malignant gliomas, showing that white matter tracts are the most common pathway used (88).

Invasion requires adhesion to the extracellular matrix (ECM), selective remodeling of the matrix, and cell movement (89). For adhesion to the ECM, cell membrane integrins allow attachment of cells to matrix proteins collagen, fibronectin, or laminin (89). Differential attachment occurs depending on the integrin array expressed. For example, laminin is deposited at the invading front of tumor cells. Increased expression of a laminin-associated integrin in these cells is also found.

Malignant glial cells also remodel the extracellular matrix by the secretion of proteases, which include serine proteases, metalloproteases, cysteine proteases, and aspartine proteases (59). There is an upregulation of metalloproteases in glioma cells and these cell lines secrete matrix metalloprotease-2. Cathepsin B is elevated in malignant gliomas and excreted into the extracellular space. Mikkelson et al. demonstrated that staining with cathepsin B correlates with degree of malig-

TABLE 2.1
WHO Histological Typing of CNS Tumors (from 64)

1 Tumors of Neuroepithelial Tissue
- 1.1 Astrocytic Tumors
  - 1.1.1 Astrocytoma
    - 1.1.1.1 Variants: Fibrillary
    - 1.1.1.2 Protoplasmic
    - 1.1.1.3 Gemistocytic
  - 1.1.2 Anaplastic (malignant) astrocytoma
  - 1.1.3 Glioblastoma
    - 1.1.3.1 Variants: Giant cell glioblastoma
    - 1.1.2.1 Gliosarcoma
  - 1.1.4 Pilocytic astrocytoma
  - 1.1.5 Pleomorphic xanthoastrocytoma
  - 1.1.6 Subependymal giant cell astrocytoma (Tuberous Sclerosis)
- 1.2 Oligodendroglial tumors
  - 1.2.1 Oligodendroglioma
  - 1.2.2 Anaplastic (malignant) oligodendroglioma
- 1.3 Ependymal tumors
  - 1.3.1 Ependymoma
    - 1.3.1.1 Variants: Cellular
    - 1.3.1.2 Papillary
    - 1.2.1.3 Clear cell
  - 1.3.2 Anaplastic (malignant) ependymoma
  - 1.3.3 Myxopapillary ependymoma
  - 1.3.4 Subependymoma
- 1.4 Mixed Gliomas
  - 1.4.1 Oligo-astrocytoma
  - 1.4.2 Anaplastic (malignant) oligo-astrocytoma
  - 1.4.3 Others
- 1.5 Choroid plexus tumors
  - 1.5.1 Choroid plexus papilloma
  - 1.5.2 Choroid plexus carcinoma
- 1.6 Neuroepithelial tumors of uncertain origin
  - 1.6.1 Astroblastoma
  - 1.6.2 Polar spongioblastoma
  - 1.6.3 Gliomatosis cerebri
- 1.7 Neuronal and mixed neuronal-glial tumors
  - 1.7.1 Gangliocytoma
  - 1.7.2 Dysplastic gangliocytoma of cerebellum (Lhermitte-Duclos)
  - 1.7.3 Desmoplastic infantile ganglioglioma
  - 1.7.4 Dysembryoplastic neuroepithelial tumor
  - 1.7.5 Ganglioglioma
  - 1.7.6 Anaplastic (malignant) ganglioglioma
  - 1.7.7 Central neurocytoma
  - 1.7.8 Paraganglioma of the filum terminale
  - 1.7.9 Olfactory neuroblastoma (Aesthesioneuroblastoma)
    - 1.7.9.1 Variant: (Olfactory neuroepithelioma

continued

TABLE 2.1
WHO Histological Typing of CNS Tumors (from 64)

1.8	Pineal parenchymal tumors
1.8.1	Pineocytoma
1.8.2	Pineoblastoma
1.8.3	Mixed/transitional pineal tumors
1.9	Embryonal tumors
1.9.1	Medulloepithelioma
1.9.2	Neuroblastoma
1.9.2.1	Variant: Ganglioneuroblastoma
1.9.3	Ependymoblastoma
1.9.4	Primitive neuroectodermal tumors (PNETS)
1.9.4.1	Medulloblastoma
1.9.4.1.1	Variants: Desmoplastic medulloblastoma
1.9.4.1.2	Medullomyoblastoma
1.9.4.1.3	Melanotic medulloblastoma

nancy in glioma cells (77). To change the matrix, glioma cells also secrete ECM components, such as glycoproteins and glycosaminoglycans. Among the glycoproteins, laminin, collagen, tenascin, and vitronectin are substrates for different integrin receptors that are permissive for migration. Among glycosaminoglycans, hyaluronate is produced in large amounts. CD 44, a hyaluronate receptor, is able to mediate and integrate the function of different cell-surface receptors, facilitating cell motility. Recent data suggest that it is expressed more in neoplastic cells than in normal cells and that its suppression decreases invasion of glioma cells.

The third feature of invasiveness is cell motility. Cells move by mechanisms that are very poorly understood but involve cytoskeleton and membrane changes, such as ruffling. The acquisition of the so-called migratory phenotype requires: 1) rearrangement of cellular receptors, such as integrins, that mediate response between ECM, components and the cytoskeleton, 2) ability of the cell to produce and secrete proteases, 3) modification of the ECM, and 4) secretion of motility factors such as autocrine motility factor, autotaxin, and glioma-derived motility factor.

Considerable controversy exists regarding the ability of glioma cells to penetrate the basement membrane, which would lead to the potential for systemic metastases (85). Functional basement membranes in the brain include the basement membrane of blood vessels, rich in collagen IV, and the glia limitans externa. Glioma cells adhere to the basement membrane of endothelial cells but usually fail to penetrate it; they are able to penetrate the glial part of the glial limitans and to invade the Virchow-Robin space but not the vascular basement membrane that remains intact.

Heterogeneity is a characteristic of glioma cells that makes it difficult to use any single chemotherapeutic agent (4). Sources of heterogeneity in malignant gliomas include polyclonality, differential expression of growth factors or their receptors, differential DNA repair capability, and differential antigen expression for immune response (68).

There is conflicting evidence for the clonality of gliomas (43). Some glioma subtypes that would seem to contain very different cell types are monoclonal. For example, Hakim et al. demonstrated that gangliogliomas, which have neuronal and glial cells, are monoclonal (47). Most malignant gliomas also appear to be monoclonal despite their various cell types. Bigner et al. (12) demonstrated that the genetic makeup of gliomas is heterogeneous using chromosomal analyses, and Shapiro et al. demonstrated multiple subpopulations in human malignant gliomas (94).

Malignant gliomas express both ligands and receptors for platelet-derived growth factor (PDGF) (46, 75), epidermal growth factor (EGF), and vascular endothelial growth factor (VEGF) (24). These may be very differently distributed within human gliomas. For example, Strommer et al. used immunohistochemistry with a monoclonal antibody to epidermal growth factor receptor (EGFR) in 57 human malignant gliomas to show that expression of EGFR was heterogeneous in the same tumor (99). Stavrou et al. similarly demonstrated the antigenic heterogeneity of human gliomas (98). Pederson et al. demonstrated major differences in response to a variety of growth factors (87). Darling et al. showed how important heterogeneity was for determining the response to cytotoxic drugs (39).

This biology has important implications for the neurosurgeon (101). For low-grade gliomas which do not invade extensively, it suggests that major surgical resection might be an important step toward long-term remission. This in turn makes the use of brain mapping and intraoperative guidance important. For malignant gliomas, biology means that extensive surgery, while helpful in relieving mass effect, cannot hope to be effective alone in long-term control. This does not, of course, mean that contemporary chemotherapy does achieve that control (19). Heterogeneity means that some clones may be resistant to whatever radiation or chemotherapy is used, allowing cells to recover and create new colonies (52).

THE FUTURE—2000 AND BEYOND—"THE BEGINNING OF THE END"

Part of the future for glioma surgery is with us already with advanced technology and advanced biology both likely to progress over the next generation, and with an increasing interaction between them.

Almost certainly the advanced technology will be based on imaging in better identification of tumor, better identification of functional brain, and ability to adapt to changes during resection. We will not discuss identification of tumor and functional brain here, as developments in these areas are likely to be natural outgrowths to present developments. What is important to recognize, however, is the significant advance likely in intraoperative imaging.

Technology

INTRAOPERATIVE MRI AND THE OPERATING ROOM OF THE FUTURE

The intraoperative MRI at Brigham and Women's Hospital is a collaborative project with General Electric Corporation (3, 20, 21, 55, 72, 73, 79, 93, 102). It is a MRI that can be used for intraoperative image guidance (3, 6, 13) (Fig. 2.3). The 0.5 Tesla superconducting "open configuration" magnet was designed with coils in two separate but communicating

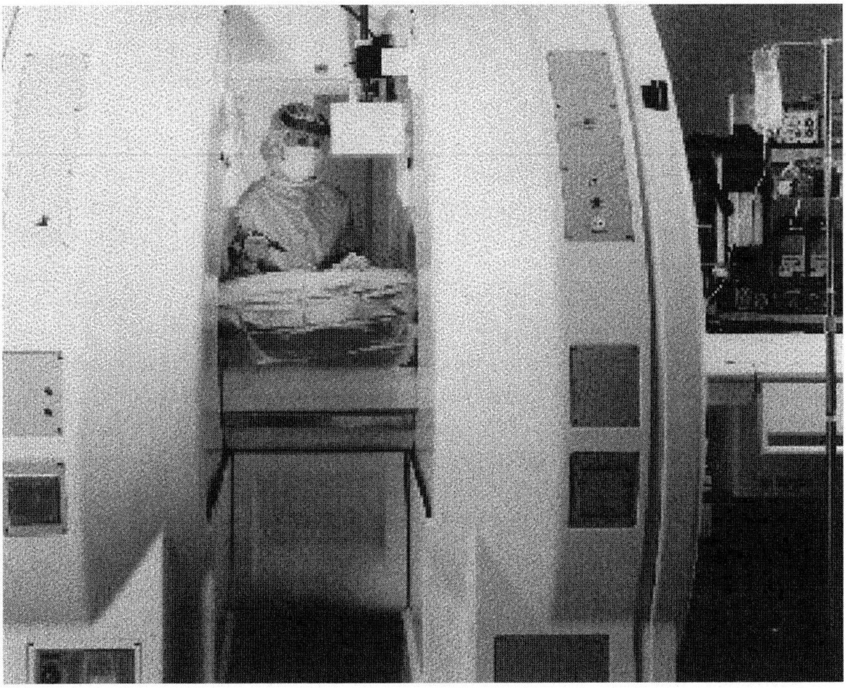

FIG. 2.3 The GE Intraoperative MRI developed at the Brigham and Women's Hospital (107).

cryostats that result in a 56-cm wide vertical gap at the center of the magnet. This allows surgeons to stand on either side of a patient placed within the imager. Flexible radiofrequency coils are contoured around the head and frame the planned craniotomy incision. This design gives a spherical imaging volume of 30 centimeters and no significant reduction in the gradient strength or linearity over the field of view. Multiplanar images can be obtained in any of the sequences performed in standard diagnostic MRI. A set of images in one plane takes between 60–120 seconds to obtain.

The device is housed within a magnetically shielded surgical suite. MRI compatible neurosurgical instruments and equipment for monitoring and the administration of anesthesia have been developed. Video monitors and two-way audiovisual communication devices allow communication between surgeon and MR console. The patient is usually positioned within the bore of the magnet as in standard MRI machines, but can also be positioned perpendicular to the magnet or within an adjustable chair. An MRI-compatible microscope (Studor Medical Engineering Ag, Rhenfall, Switzerland) can be positioned between the magnets and over the shoulder of the surgeon. Images can be obtained with the microscope in position.

Confirmation of the extent of resection, accommodation to intraoperative changes, and monitoring of potential intraoperative complications are routine with craniotomies performed in this device. A light emitting diode (LED) based navigational system is an integrated component of the MRI unit and provides tracking capabilities within the three-dimensional space at the center of the magnet (Integrated Technologies, Boulder, CO). The surgeon can achieve real-time localization when the navigational system is used in conjunction with MRI acquisition. Uniplanar real-time images are acquired in 2–14 seconds.

This system acts as a remarkable stereotactic frame that allows real-time monitoring of probe placement and a novel way of evaluating surgical resection. It has also led to new treatment modalities. Implantation of I-125 seeds can be done after resection of recurrent malignant gliomas, a technique that may be as effective as radiosurgery and applicable to large lesions. Laser technology can be used to ablate a target with direct visualization of energy deposition (58, 59). These extend the surgical power of the neurosurgical oncologist considerably.

In the past five years, our group has performed over 300 craniotomies in this device. Pathologic diagnoses have included glioblastomas, anaplastic gliomas, low-grade gliomas, astrocytomas, oligodendrogliomas, gangliogliomas, pineoblastoma, meningiomas, and metastatic lesions. Patients whose tumors are particularly appropriate for resection in the intraoperative MRI include:

1. Patients with primary gliomas in or adjacent to sensitive cortical areas, such as the sensory or motor strip, where knowledge of the tumor extent and location is critical during resection. This is particularly important for low-grade gliomas whose margins may not be adequately visualized in other way.
2. Patients with deep lesions difficult to biopsy in the white matter or brain stem in which the trajectory of the approach must be optimized and confirmation of target entry is critical. Here it is the visualization of the final site that is so important.
3. Patients with small intraparenchymal lesions that might be difficult to locate accurately with other systems.
4. Patients with recurrent gliomas that blend with surrounding tissue. Schwartz et al. showed that reoperation on malignant gliomas can increase survival time, but this must be done with accurate knowledge of tumor margins (92).
5. Patients with skull base and pituitary tumors, especially if recurrent.

A cardiac pacemaker or other implanted ferromagnetic device is a contraindication to this surgery.

Craniotomies are performed in a standard fashion. Operating within the magnet does not limit the surgeon's ability to perform the procedure. The size of the bone flap and dural opening can be decreased with an assurance that adequate exposure will be achieved. Marking shifting (> 1 cm) of the brain parenchyma is regularly seen on serial images as surgery progresses. Accuracy in the localization, targeting, and guidance of the resection is maintained as these anatomic changes occur by constantly updating images and correlating this with the surgical field of view. In about 50% of cases, tumor imaging reveals residual tumor unsuspected from visual guidance, and five to eight updates are used per case.

Other imaging modalities, including plain films, fluoroscopy, and ultrasound, have been used intraoperatively to supplement surgical judgment. Radiographs and CT are limited to two-dimensional information, may be less sensitive than MR, and have the problem of radiation exposure for the patient and the surgical team. Ultrasound provides real-time information but may have difficulty adequalty delimiting tumor margins; it is, however, an important adjunct to surgery (8, 9).

Several other MRI systems allow updates of imaging during surgery. These include those by Philips, Siemens, and Toshiba. Virtually all of them, however, require transportation in and out of the scanner. Transporting a patient from the operating room to a CT or MRI during surgery is time consuming and cumbersome, and does not provide the surgeon with real time, up-to-date imaging information as the surgery continues.

With the ability to visualize the brain with MRI during surgery, we have seen the future of glioma surgery. In craniotomies or biopsy for gliomas, it has been remarkably accurate.

Based on our experience thus far, we believe that intraoperative imaging provides the following major advances in the management of gliomas:

1. The imaged abnormality in most low-grade gliomas can be successfully resected, with only 11% of tumors being truly unresectable (22).
2. The morbidity after one month in major resection of high- and low-grade gliomas is 4% (37).
3. There appears to be a change in mortality based on these approaches. We reviewed 56 patients with low-grade astrocytomas treated either by biopsy, resection, or complete removal. These patients all had diffuse astrocytomas with no pilocytic or anaplastic features. Nineteen of them had biopsy only, had partial resection and 19 had greater than 90% resection. With a four year follow-up, a significant difference in mortality among the groups, was found with significantly longer survival ($p < 0.05$) in patients with greater resection (81).

These data are not surprising, since our biological understanding tells us that low-grade astrocyomas are unstable lesions that tend to progress irrevocably to higher-grade tumors (22, 63). It has been suggested that the majority of glioblastomas arise from transformation of lower-grade lesions (64). One of the major hypotheses to test in this next generation is whether resecting the imaged tumor in a low-grade glioma might delay the development of its higher-grade successor. If these tumors are not extensively invasive, this would make particularly good sense. In low-grade gliomas, image-guided resection may make a significant difference in survival (10, 81). For malignant gliomas, degree of resection has an important effect on prognosis as well (2, 49, 50). The understanding of biology will need to guide our surgical technology. It is clear that new approaches need to be made in the biology of malignant gliomas using such concepts as antiangiogenic therapy and immune therapy. However, along with these should come the concept of new approaches for the delivery techniques to be discussed.

Biology

The understanding of glioma biology has increased significantly in the last decade (23, 63). Zlokovic and Apuzzo described how the increased understanding of cellular and molecular neurosurgery may revolutionize the care of these and other neurosurgical diseases in the next century (106). Every oncologic front is now witnessing major advances, whether in molecular genetics (68), transcription and growth factors (62), cell cycle control (84), or angiogenesis (67). These understandings have led to new initiatives in therapy, such as using cell cycle control agents for gene therapy (84).

One important implication of present techniques is to reconsider the classification of gliomas. For example, it is possible that developmental markers may be used for these tumors and that they arise from multipotential precursor cells (82). This feature may lead to reconsidering the complex subtypes in low-grade gliomas, the invasiveness of these tumors, and the resistance of tumors to radiation. This developmental analysis may be important since the tumors may retain an appropriate response to developmental stimuli, such as retinoic acid (83).

Preventing angiogenesis may help to overcome heterogeneity and invasion in gliomas. Angiogenesis is a balance between stimulation and inhibition (74). Most malignant brain tumors appear to require new blood vessel formation and inhibitors of such formation may stop tumor growth. Leon et al. showed that microvessel count in gliomas correlates with grade and is an independent prognostic indicator in these tumors (67). Kirsch et al. showed that angiostatin, an inhibitor of angiogensis, can markedly increase survival in a nude mouse model of glioblastoma (61).

Technology and Biology in Glioma Neurosurgery— The Concept of Epicentric Tumor Therapy

Traditionally, intravenous and intra-arterial administration have been the major techniques for delivery of chemotherapeutic agents. However, agents delivered in this way may have important systemic side effects and also require much greater concentrations of the therapeutic compound than might be needed with local application. Burke et al. recently summarized problems of drug delivery to the central nervous system, and reviewed the impediments created by the blood-brain barrier, blood-cerebrospinal fluid barrier, and blood-tumor barrier (31).

There are a number of strategies that have attempted to avoid these impediments—enhancing blood-brain barrier permeability by opening it with osmotic or biochemical agents, increasing lipophilicity of a drug, using large neutral amino acids to enhance carrier-mediated drug delivery, or using liposomes. None of these techniques has been shown to be useful for brain tumor treatment, however.

Application of therapeutic agents in local or "epicentric" therapy—that is, therapy that works from the center of the tumor—is a particularly important alternative to systemic therapy for the neurosurgeon. Below are a number of examples of such "epicentric" techniques:

1. Gene therapy, which requires stereotactic injection into the tumor. One technique used the combination of HSV TK gene and ganciclovir in a retrovirus system. Initial study showed some evidence of efficacy and little toxicity. The major challenge is getting the virus to move beyond the local neighborhood in which it is injected. Non-viral transfection agents are also used to transfer genetic material (104).
2. Intratumoral infusion of agents, which may use slow infusion pumps, such as the Infusaid system (Infusaid Corp. Norwood, MA), MiniMed PIMS system (MiniMed, Sylmo, CA), or the Medtronics Synchromed system (Medtronics, Minneapolis, MN). Hall et al. demonstrated prolonged survival in a rat glioma model using intratumoral topotecan (48). A number of clinical trials have been mounted using these systems, as summarized by Burke et al. (31). Oldfield's laboratory has been particularly important in evaluating the usefulness of these systems.
3. Application of radiolabeled antibodies in the tumor cavity (105). The concept of immune-linked chemotherapy also has been investigated extensively.
4. Xenotransplantation. Thompson et al. created a line of melanoma cells engineered to produce granulocyte-macrophage colony stimulating factor (GM-CSF) or interleukin-2. They then transplanted these into the brains of mice who were then given melanoma. The researchers found a significant therapeutic effect. A variant of this concept is to enclose transplanted tissue in polymeric membrane with a defined pore size, which permits the passage of nutrients and small molecules but is impermeable to cells, complement, antibodies, and viruses (55).
5. Stem cell therapy. There is evidence that, unlike viruses, stem cells will travel through the brain to a tumor and can be infected with a therapeutic agent. Aboody et al. demonstrated this to be an effective way of delivering the thymidine kinase-ganciclovir system to gliomas in a nude mouse model (1).
6. Slow-release polymers embedded with chemotherapeutic agents. This is a particularly attractive option for surgeons because of its extensive development by Henry Brem and the Johns Hopkins group (29, 30, 31). The best example is BCNU-impregnated polyanhidride wafers (Gliadel, Rhone-Poulenc Rhorer). In an early phase I-II study in patients with recurrent malignant gliomas, these

were placed in the lining of the tumor cavity after surgical resection. Median survival was 46 weeks, and 8 of 21 patients survived over one year (29). A prospective multicenter trial treated 222 patients with recurrent malignant glioma using 3.85% BCNU wafers. For patients with glioblastoma, six-month survival for patients with wafers was twice that without. The wafers were approved for use by the FDA in 1996 and now have been used in initial management of glioblastoma as well. A phase III trial by Valtonen et al. in Finland treated 32 patients with gliadel or placebo wafers at initial surgery. Median survival was 53 weeks for BCNU and 40 weeks for placebo. A phase I study in children and a phase II in adults are currently in progress. Other trials currently in progress include combinations of wafer with systemic chemotherapy, with permanent I-125 seeds, and with a number of radiation therapy protocols. Other drugs also being embedded in the wafer and tested in animals include taxol, camptothecin, adriamycin, carboplatin, methotrexate, and minocycine (as an antiangiogenic agent). A variant system using polymer microspheres is also under consideration.

Advantages of epicentric therapy include the avoidance of systemic toxicity, and a concentration gradient of drug, which is the same as the gradient of neoplastic cells around the tumor core. As more systems are developed, this will be an increasingly promising field.

The Neurosurgeon as Local Oncologist

The concept of epicentric therapy is important because it places the neurosurgeon squarely at the center of future brain tumor chemo- and biological therapies. The problem of getting therapeutic agents across the blood-brain barrier and of flooding the body with materials targeted at a small area of brain is a significant one. Epicentric therapy allows a focused and precise "minimally invasive" approach to the pharmacotherapy of brain tumors that may be as effective as the minimally invasive surgical techniques of our present era. It should be possible to use new cell cycle agents, anti-invasive agents, and gene therapies as local treatments. It seems particularly important that the glioma surgeon of tomorrow be interested not only in extirpation of a tumor but also in new delivery methods for destroying it with molecular biological techniques. In this way, invasiveness and heterogeneity may be overcome "from the inside out," and the neurosurgical oncologist will be able to explore new frontiers of effective therapy. This combination of technology and biology may truly then be the "beginning of the end" for the devastation that gliomas create. It will create a bright and significant future for glioma surgery.

REFERENCES

1. Aboody KS, Bower KA, Shivji S, McDonough CB, Brown A, Rainov NG, Black PM, Breakefield XO, Snyder EY: A novel strategy for gene therapy delivery to brain tumors: Foreign gene expressing neural stem cells (NCSc) display tropism for intracranial gliomas. *Abstract,* AANS Annual Meeting 2000, San Francisco.
2. Albert FK, Forsting M, Sartor K, Adams H-P, Kunz S: Early postoperative magnetic resonance imaging after resection of malignant glioma: Objective evaluation of residual tumor and its influence on regrowth and prognosis. **Neurosurgery** 34:45–60, 1994.
3. Alexander E., Black P, Martin C, Kikinis R, Jolesz F: Interventional magnetic resonance imaging: The MRT System in Alexander and Maciunas (ed). *Advanced Neurosurgical Navigation,* New York, Thieme, 1998.
4. Allam A, Taghian A, Gioioso D, Duffy M, Suit HD: Intratumoral heterogeneity of malignant gliomas measured in vitro. **Int J Radiat Oncol Biol Phys** 27:303–8, 1993.
5. Apuzzo ML, Sabshin JK: Computed tomographic guidance stereotaxis in the management of intracranial mass lesions. **Neurosurgery** 12:277–285, 1983.
6. Barnett GH: Frameless stereotactic systems, in, Kay A, Black PM (ed): *Operative Neurosurgery.* London: Churchill Livingstone, 2000.
7. Barnett GH, Kormos DW, Steiner CP, Weisenberger J: Intraoperative localization using an armless, frameless stereotactiic wand. **J Neurosurg** 78:510–514, 1993.
8. Berger MS: Ultrasound guided stereotaxis biopsy using a new apparatus. **Neurosurg** 15:550–554, 1986.
9. Berger MS: The impact of technical adjuncts in the surgical management of cerebral hemispheric low-grade gliomas of childhood. **J Neurooncol** 28:129–155, 1996.
10. Berger MS, Deliganis, AV, Dobbins J, Keles GE: The effect of extent of resection on recurrence in patients with low grade cerebral hemisphere gliomas. Cancer 74:1784–1791, 1994.
11. Berger M, Wilson C: *The Gliomas.* Philadelphia, WB Saunders, 1999.
12. Bigner DD, Bigner SH, Ponten J, Westermark B, Mahaley MS, Rouslahti E, Herschman H, Eng LG, Wikstrand CH: Heterogeneity of genotypic and phenotypic characteristics of fifteen permanent cell lines derived from human gliomas. **J Exp Neuropathol Exp Neurol** 40:201–229, 1991.
13. Black PM: Historical Vignette–Peter Bent Brigham Hospital. **J Neurosurg** 75: 987–988, 1991.
14. Black P, Martin C, Wong T, Moriarty T, Alexander E, Steig P, Woodard E, Schwartz R, Jolesz F: Imaging of the nervous system during surgery: General considerations and limitations in Crockard A. (ed). *Neurosurgery. The Scientific Basis of Clinical Practice. 3rd Edition.* London: Blackwell Science 1999.
15. Black P, Mehta V: Craniopharyngioma (Adult) in Winn HR (ed). *Youmans Neurological Surgery. 5th edition.* Seattle, W. B. Saunders Company (in press).
16. Black PM. Surgery for astrocytomas, in Black PM, Schoene WC, Lampson L (ed): *Astrocytomas: Diagnosis, Treatment, and Biology.* Boston, Blackwell Scientific 1993.
17. Black PM, ed: *The Surgical Art of Harvey Cushing.* Park Ridge, IL: American Association of Neurological Surgeons, 1992.
18. Black PM, Alexander E III, Tarbell N, Shrieve D, Goumnerova LC, Leffler JS: Lienar accelerator based radiosurgery for malignant tumors of the central nervous system. **Crit Rev Neurosurg** 6:225–231, 1996.

19. Black PM, Moore MR, Rossitch E: Harvey Cushing at the Brigham. Park Ridge, Illinois: American Association of Neurological Surgeons, 1993.
20. Black PM, Moriarty T, Alexander E, Stieg P, Woodard EJ, et al. Development and implementation of intraoperative magnetic resonance imaging and its neurosurgical applications. **Neurosurgery** 41:831–845, 1997.
21. Black Peter McL, Alexander Eben III, Claudia Martin, et al: Craniotomy for tumor treatment in an intraoperative magnetic resonance imaging unit. **Neurosurgery** 45:423–433, 1999.
22. Black PM, Nikas D: Neurosurgical considerations in low grade gliomas. *Eleventh International Congress of Neurological Surgery.* Bologna, Monduzzi, 1997.
23. Black PM, Nomura K, Cavanee WK, Kakizoe T, Mukai K: Report of the Ninth International Symposium of the Foundation for Promotion of Cancer Research: Basic and Clinical Research in Brain Tumors. **Jpn J Clin Oncol** 26:277–282, 1996.
24. Black PM, Ronner SF: Cortical mapping for defining the limits of tumor resection. **Neurosrugery** 20:914–919, 1987.
25. Black PM, Schoene WC, Lampson L, (ed): Astrocytomas: *Diagnosis, Management and Biology.* Boston: Blackwell Scientific Publications, 1993.
26. Black PM, Tarbell N, Loeffler J, Scott RM, Fine H, Wen P, Sallen S: Hemisphere astroglial neoplasms in adults and children, in, Black PM, Schoene WC, Lampson L, (ed). *Astrocytomas.* Boston: Blackwell, 1993.
27. Black PM, Wen PY: Clinical, imaging and laboratory diagnosis of brain tumors, in Laws E, Kaye A (ed). *Brain Tumors: An Encyclopedic Approach.* Edinburgh, Churchill Livingstone, 1995, pp. 191–214.
28. Black P McL. Harvey Cushing at the Peter Bent Brigham Hospital. **Neurosurgery** 45:990–1001, 1999.
29. Brem H, Piantadosi S, Burger P, Walker M, Selker R, Vick NA, Black K, Sisti M, Brem S, Mohr G, Muller P, Morawtetz R, Schold SC: Placebo-controlled trial of safety and efficacy of intraoperative controlled delivery by biodegradable polymers of chemotherapy for recurrent gliomas. **Lancet** 345:1008–1011, 1995.
30. Brem H, Walter KA, Tamargo RJ, Olici A, Langer R: Polymeric Site-Specific Phaermacotherapy. John Wiley and Sons, 1994, pp. 1176–1239.
31. Burke M, Brem H, Langer R: Drug delivery to the central nervous system; Encyclopedia of controlled drug delivery 1999, (in press).
32. Chabrerie A, Ozlen F, Nakajima S, Leventon M, Atsumi H, Grimson E, Jolesz F, Kikinis R, Black PM: Three-dimensional image reconstruction for low-grade glioma surgery. **Neurosurg Focus** 4(4): Article 7, 1998.
33. Chicoine MR, Silbergeld DL: Invading C6 glioma cells maintaining tumorigenicity. **J Neurosurg** Oct, 83(4):665–671, 1995.
34. Ciric I, Ammirati M, Vick N et al: Supratentorial gliomas: Surgical considerations and immediate postoperative results. **Neurosurgery** 21:21–26, 1987.
35. Couldwell WT, Apuzzo MLJ: Initial experience related to the use of the Cosman-Roberts-Wells stereotactic instrument. **J Neurosurg** 72:145–148, 1990.
36. Cushing H. *Intracranial Tumors: Notes Upon a Series of 2000 Verified Cases with Surgical-Mortality Percentages Pertaining Thereto.* Philadelphia, CC Thomas and Sons, 1932.
37. Danks RA, Aglio LS, Gugino V, et al: Craniotomy under local anesthesia and monitored conscious sedation for the resection of tumors involving eloquent cortex. **J Neurooncol** (in press).
38. Danks RA, Rogers M, Aglio LS, Gugino LD, Black PM: Patient tolerance of craniotomy performed with the patient under local anesthesia and monitored conscious sedation. **Neurosurgery** 42:1:28–36, 1998.

39. Darling JL, Thomas DGT, Paul EA, Finn AGP: Heterogeneity in response of short-term glioma cell cultures to cytotoxic drugs; correlation of in vitro chemosensitivity and relapse-free interval. Walker MD, Thomas DGT, (ed): *Biology of Brain Tumour.* Boston, Martinus Nijhoff, 1986, pp 457–464.
40. Davey LM, Harvey Cushing: The New Haven Years. **Neurosurgery** 45:1002–1009, 1999.
41. deRidder L, Laerum OD, Mork SJ, Bigner DD: Invasiveness of human glioma cell lines in vitro: Relation to tumorigenicity in athymic mice. **Acta Neuropathol** 72:207–213, 1987.
42. Division of Neuropathology, Brigham and Women's Hospital. Neuropathology of Central Nervous System Tumors, Chapter 2, in Black P, Loeffler J (ed): *Cancer of the Nervous System.* Cambridge, Blackwell 1998, pp 25–53.
43. El-Azouzi M, Chung RY, Farmer GE, Martuza RL, Black PM, Rouleau GA, Hettlich C, Hedley-Whyte ET, Zervas NT: Loss of distinct regions on the short arm of chromosome 17 associated with tumorigenesis of human astrocytomas. **Proc Natl Acad Sci USA** 86:7186–7190, 1989.
44. Fine H, Dear K, Loeffler JS, Black PM, Canellos GP: Meta-analysis of radiotherapy with and without adjuvant chemotherapy for malignant gliomas in adults. **Cancer** 71:2585–2597, 1993.
45. Gugino LD, Aglio LS, Black PM: Cortical stimulation techniques, Chapter 7, in Black PM, Kaye AH (ed): *Operative Neurosurgery.* London, Harcourt Publishers Limited 2000, pp 85–97.
46. Guha A, Dashner K, Black PM, Wagner JA, Stiles CD: Expression of PDGF and PDGF receptors in human astrocytoma operation specimens supports the existence of an autocrine loop. **Int J Cancer** 60:168–173, 1995.
47. Hakim R, Loeffler JS, Anthony DC, Black PM: Gangliogliomas in Adults. **Cancer** 79:1:127–131, 1997.
48. Hall JS, Kaiser M, Chakrabarti IK, Parsa A, Yon F, Bruce JN: Topotecan via intracerebral clysis prolongs survival in a rat glioma model. *AANS.* Philadelphia, 1998.
49. Harbaugh KS, Black PM: Strategies in the Surgical Management of Malignant Gliomas. **Semi Surg Oncol** 14:26–33, 1998.
50. Harsh GR, Levin VA, Gutin PH, et al: Reoperation for recurrent glioblastoma and anaplastic astrocytoma. **Neurosurgery** 21:615–621, 1987.
51. Heilbrun MP, Roberts TS, Apuzzo MLJ, Wells TH, Sabshin JK: Preliminary experience with the Brown-Roberts-Wells computerized tomography stereotaxic guidance system. **J Neurosurg** 59:217–222, 1983.
52. Heppner GH. Tumor heterogeneity. **Cancer Res** 44:2259–2265, 1984.
53. Horsley V, Clarke RH: The structure and function of the cerebellum examined by new method. **Brain** 45–124, 1908.
54. Joki T, Carroll R, Black P: Encapsulation of endostatin-transfected BHK cells as therapy for malignant glioma., submitted.
55. Jolesz FA, Shtern F: The operating room of the future. Imaging guided stereotactic tumor diagnosis and treatment. Report of the National Cancer Institute Workshop. **Invest Radiol** 27:326–328, 1992T.
56. Kassis AI, Van den Abbeele AD, Wen PY, Baranowska-Kortylewicz J, Aaronson RA, DeSisto WC, Lampson LA, Black PM, Adelstein SJ: Specific uptake of the auger electron-emitting thymidine analogue 5[^{123}I/^{125}I]iodo-2'-deoxyuridine in rat brain tumors: Diagnostic and therapeutic implications in humans. **Cancer Res** 50:5199–5203, 1990.
57. Kelly PK, Kall BA, Goerss S, Earnest F IV: Computer-assisted stereotaxic laser resection of intra-axial brain neoplasms. **J Neursurg** 64:427–439, 1986.

58. Kettenbach J, Kuroda K, Hata N, Morrison P, McDannold NJ, Gering D, Saiviroonporn P, Zientara GP, Black PM, Kikinis R, Jolesz FA: Laser-indued thermotherapy of cerebral neoplasia under MR tomographic control. **Min Invas Ther Allied Technol** 7/6:589–598, 1998.
59. Kettenbach J, Silverman SG, Hata N, Kuroda K, Saiviroonporn P, Zientara GP, Morrison PR, Hushek SG, Black PM, Kikinis R, Jolesz FA: Monitoring and visualization techniques for MR-guided laser ablations in an open MR system. **J Magn Reson Imaging** 8:933–943, 1998.
60. Kikinis R, Gleason LP, Moriarty TM, Moore MR, Alexander E III, Steig PE, Matsumae M, Lorensen WE, Cline HE, Black P McL, Jolesz FA: Computer-assisted interactive three-dimensional planning for neurosurgical procedures. **Neurosurgery** 4:640–651, 1996.
61. Kirsch M, Strasser J, Allende R, Bello L, Zhang J, Black PM: Angiostatin suppresses malignant glioma growth in vivo. **Cancer Res** 58:4654–4659, 1998.
62. Kirsch M, Wilson JC, Black PM: Platelet-derived growth factor in human brain tumors. **J Neurooncol** 35:289–301, 1997.
63. Kirsch M, Zhu JJ, Black PM: Theory of Pathogenesis in Human Brain Tumors, in J Loeffler, P Black (ed): *Tumors of the Central Nervous System*. 1997.
64. Kleihues P, Burger PC, Scheithauer BW: Histological typing of tumours of the central nervous systems, 2nd edition. Berlin: Springer-Verlag, World Health Organization, 1993.
65. Laws ER, Jr: *Neurosurgery's* Man of the Century: Harvy Cushing—The man and his legacy. **Neurosurgery** 45:977–982, 1999.
66. Leksell LA: Stereotactic apparatus for intracerebral surgery. **Acta Chir Scan** 99:229–233, 1949.
67. Leon S, Folkerth R, Black P: Microvessel density is a prognostic indicator for patients with astroglial brain tumor. **Cancer** 77:362–72, 1996.
68. Leon S, Zhu J, Black PM: Genetic aberations in human brain tumors. **Neurosurgery** 34:708–722, 1993.
69. Loeffler JS, Alexander E III, Hochberg FH, Wen PY, Morris JH, Schoene WC, Siddon RL, Morse RH, Black PM: Clinical patterns of failure following stereotactic interstitial irradiation for malignant gliomas. **Int J Radiat Oncol Biol Phys** 19:1455–1462, 1990.
70. Loeffler JS, Alexander E III, Wen PY, Shea WM, Coleman CN, Kooy HM, Fine HA, Nedzi LA, Silver B, Riese NE, Black PM: Results of stereotactic brachytherapy used in the initial management of patients with glioblastoma. **J Natl Cancer Inst** 82:1918–1921, 1990.
71. Long DM: Harvey Cushing at Johns Hopkins. **Neurosurgery** 45:983–989, 1999.
72. Martin C, Alexander E III, Wong T, Schwartz R, Jolesz F, Black P: Surgical treatment of low-grade gliomas in the intraoperative magnetic resonance imager. **Neurosurg Focus** 4(4):Article 8, 1998.
73. Martin C, Schwartz R, Jolesz F, Black P: Neurosurgical procedures in the intraoperative MRI, in Black P, Kaye A (ed). *Operative Neurosurgery,* London, Churchill Livingstone (in press).
74. Maruyama T, Black PM: The inibition and stimulation of angiogenesis in gliomas. **Crit Rev Neurosurg** 5:150–156, 1996.
75. Maxwell M, Naber SP, Wolfe HJ, Galanopoulos T, Hedley-Whyte ET, Black PM, Antoniades HN: Coexpression of platelet-derived growth factor (PDGF) and PDGF-receptor genres by primary human astrocytomas may contribute to their development and maintenance. **J Clin Invest** 86:131–140, 1990.
76. McCord D: The Fabrick of Man. Portland, Maine: Atheneum, 1963.

77. Mikkelsen T, Yan PS, Ho KL, Sameni M, Sloane BF, Rosenblum ML: Immunolocalization of cathepsin B in human glioma: Implications for tumor invasion and angiogenesis. **J Neurosurg** 83:285–90, 1995.
78. Moore MR, Black PM, Ellenbogen R, Gall CM, Eldredge E: Stereotactic craniotomy: Methods and results using the Brown-Roberts-Wells stereotactic frame. **Neurosurgery** 25:572–577, 1989.
79. Moriarty TM, Kikinis R, Jolesz FA, Black PM, Alexander E III: Magnetic resonance imaging therapy: Intraoperative MR imaging. **Neurosurg Clin N Am** 7(2): 323–331, 1996.
80. Nakajima S, Atsumi H, Moriarty TM, Kikinis R, Jolesz FA, Black PMcL: The use of cortical surface vessel registration for image-guided neurosurgery. **Neurosurgery** 40(6):1021–1210, 1997.
81. Nikas DC, Bello L, Zamani AA, Black PM: Neurosurgical considerations in supratentorial low-grade gliomas: Experience with 175 patients. **Neurosurg Focus** 4(4):Article 4, 1998.
82. Noll E, Welsh DK, Fan MH, Canales M, Black PM: Towards a lineage-based classification system for gliomas: Innovation or imagination? **Crit Rev Neurosurg** 8:6–18, 1998.
83. Noll EN, Black PM: Retention of an appropriate astrocytic response to retinoids by human brain tumors composed of predominantly glial fibrillary acidic protein-positice cells. **Neurosurg Focus** 4(4):Article 2, 1998.
84. Parr MJ, Manomie Y, Tanaka T, Wen P, Kue DW, Kaelin WG, Fine H: Tumor-selective transgene expression in vivo mediated by an E2F-responsive adenoviral vector. **Nat Med** 3:1145–1149, 1997.
85. Paulus W, Tonn JC: Basement membrane invasion of glioma cells mediated by integrin receptors: **J Neurosurg** 80:515–519, 1994.
86. Pedersen P-H, Edvardsen K, Garcia-Cabrera I, Mahesparan R, Thorsen J, Mathisen B, Rosenblum ML, Bjerkvig T: Migratory patterns of lac-z transfected human glioma cells in the rat brain. **Int J Cancer** 62:767–771, 1995.
87. Pederson PH, Ness GO, Engebraaten O, Bjerkvig R, Lillehaug JR, Laerum OD: Heterogeneous response to the growth factors (EGF, PDGF bb, TGF-alpha, bFGF, IL-2) on glioma spheroid growth, migration, and invasion. **Int J Cancer** 56:255–261, 1994.
88. Rosenblum M, Eisenburg A, Norman D: Brain tumor invasion: Clinical patterns of malignant astrocytoma spread. **Proc Annu Meet Am Soc Clin Oncol** 11:A414, 1992.
89. Rutka JT, Apodaca G, Stern R, Rosenblum M: The extracellular matrix of the central and peripheral nervous system: Structure and function. **J Neurosurg** 69:155–70, 1988.
90. Salcman M: Malignant glioma management. **Neurosurg Clin N Am** 1:49–63, 1990.
91. Schulder M, Loeffler JS, Howes AE, Alexander E, Black PM: Historical vignette: The radium bomb: Harvey Cushing and the interstitial irradiation of gliomas. **J Neurosurg** 84:530–532, 1996.
92. Schwartz MS, Loeffler JS, Black PM, Shrieve DC, Wen PY, Fine HA, Alexander E III: Reoperation following radiosurgery of glioblastoma: Impact on survival and neurologic status. Radiosurgery 1:141–157, 1996.
93. Schwartz RB, Hsu L, Wong TZ, Kacher DF, Zamani AA, Black PM, Alexander EA III, Stieg PE, Moriarty TM, Martin CA, Kikinis R, Jolesz FA: Intraoperative MR imaging guidance for intracranial neurosurgery: Experience with the first 200 cases. **Neuroradiology in Radiology.** 477–488, 1999.
94. Shapiro JR, Yung WKA and Shapiro WR: Isolation, karyotype, and clonal growth of

heterogeneous subpopulations of human malignant gliomas. **Cancer Res** 41: 2349–2359.

95. Shrieve D, Alexander E, Black PM, Wen P, Fine H, Kooy H, Loeffler J: Treatment of patients with primary glioblastoma multiforme with standard postoperative radiotherapy and radiosurgical boost: Prognostic factors and long-term outcome. **J Neurol** 72–77, 1999.
96. Silbergeld DL, Chicoine MR: Isolation and characterization of human malignant glioma cells from histologically normal brain. **J Neurosurg** 86:525–531, 1997.
97. Spiegel EA, Wycis HT: Stereoencephalotomy: Thalamotomy and related procedures. **JAMA** 148:446–451, 1952a.
98. Stavrou D, Bise K, Groeneveld J, Stocker U, Kretzschkmar HA, Keiditsch E, Mehraein P: Antigenic heterogeneity of human brain tumors defined by monoclonal antibodies. **Anticancer Res** 9:1489–1496, 1989.
99. Strommer K, Hamou MF, Diggelmann H, de Tribolet N: Cellular and tumoural heterogeneity of EGR gene amplification in human malignant gliomas. **Acta Neurochir (Wien)** 107:82–87, 1990.
100. Tew JM, JR., M Gazi Yasargil: *Neurosurgery's* Man of the Century. **Neurosurgery** 45:1010–1014, 1999.
101. Wen PY, Fine HA, Black PM, Shrieve CD, Alexander E, Loeffler JS: High-grade astrocytomas in, Wen P, Black PM, (ed). *Neurologic Clinics: Brain Tumors in Adults.* Philadelphia: W. B. Saunders, November, 1995, vol. 13, no. 4, pp 875–900.
102. Wong T, Schwartz R, Nabavi A, Pergolizzi R, Black PM, Alexander E, Jolesz F: *Neurosurgical Procedures Monitored by Intraoperative MRI. Nuclear Magnetic Resonance Imaging and Spectroscopy in Medicine and Biology.* Young IR (ed), 1999.
103. Yasargil MG: A legacy of microneurosurgery. **Neurosurgery** 45:1025–1091, 1999.
104. Zhu J, Zhang L, Hanisch UK, Felgner PL, Reszka R: A continuous intracerebral gene delivery system for in vivo liposome-mediated gene therapy. **Gene Ther** 3:472–476, 1996.
105. Zhu J, Takahashi H, Nakazawa S: Human monoclonal antibody-drug conjugates in the experimental treatment of malignant gliomas. **Neurol Med Cir** 34:279–285, 1994.
106. Zlokovic BV, Apuzzo ML: Cellular and molecular neurosurgery: Pathways from concept to reality—part II: Vector systems and delivery methodologies for gene therapy of the central nervous system. **Neurosurgery** 40:805–812, 1997.
107. http://www.ge.com/medical/mr/iomri/index.htm

CHAPTER

3

Developmental Glial Biology: The Key to Understanding Glial Tumors

MARK E. LINSKEY, M.D.

Over the last 20 years, tremendous advances have been made in the science of developmental glial biology. We have witnessed the identification and characterization of multipotential and restricted-potential glial precursor cells, as well as the elucidation of the basic steps in the progression and growth factor (GF) control of gliogenesis. We are now making early inroads towards an understanding of glial precursor cell migration. During the same 20 year period, we have experienced very little progress in improving the clinical outlook for patients with malignant gliomas despite extensive experimental and clinical efforts. Currently, the median survival for unselected patients with glioblastoma multiforme (GBM) is not significantly greater than in 1978, when the results of the first prospective, randomized, malignant glioma trial was published (106, 107).

There are at least four possible ways that the science and principles of developmental glial biology may substantively and positively impact upon our understanding of glioma biology and potentially improve our ability to care for patients with malignant gliomas (Table 3.1). The first would be the development and validation of a glioma classification system based on the cellular lineage and stage of differentiation of the cells comprising the glial tumor (ontogeny-based tumor classification system). The second would be significant improvement of the fidelity of our in vitro glioma modeling systems in order to optimize the translational validity of experimental results to the clinical setting. Third would be significant improvement of the fidelity of our in vivo glioma modeling systems in order to optimize the translational validity of experimental results to the clinical setting. Fourth would be the identification of potentially fruitful biological levers or targets for new glioma therapies.

This presentation will draw heavily upon several previously published manuscripts (55–58, 71, 72), but will not attempt to review the totality of our current understanding of the progression and control of developmental glial biology. For this purpose, the reader is referred to

TABLE 3.1
Potentially Beneficial Applications of Developmental Glial Biology in the Study of Glioma Biology

- Ontogeny-based glioma classification system
  - Better prediction of prognosis?
  - More successful assignment of patients to alternative treatments?
- Improved in vitro glioma modeling
  - Better prediction of translational success of new treatments
- Improved in vivo glioma modeling
  - Better prediction of translational success of new treatments
- A more sophisticated approach to studying growth factor/cytokine interactions for Biological targeting purposes

several recent and detailed reviews of the topic (16, 35, 55–57, 63, 83, 93–95).

ONTOGENY-BASED TUMOR CLASSIFICATION SYSTEM

In general, cellular malignant transformation is associated with the loss of genetic material (chromosomal deletions), relocation of genetic material (chromosomal translocation), transformation of a normal gene(s) to an abnormal gene(s) (point mutation), or the insertion of foreign genetic material (viral transfection with possible oncogene acquisition). Only the latter option would involve the actual acquisition of new genetic material, and the amount of genetic material in a virus is very small in comparison with the amount contained in the target cell genome. In addition, the genes controlling normal cellular developmental processes are still present in the genome of mature cells. Rapid proliferation, active cellular migration, and loss of contact inhibition are just some of the characteristics essential for malignancy and which are normal processes during glial development. It seems most probable, therefore, that oncogenesis involves the reactivation and the loss of control of normal, or subtly altered developmental genes.

Ideally, we should be able to accurately assign a cell of origin, as well as state of differentiation, to any neoplasm that arises in the central nervous system (CNS). Understanding the biology of mitogenic control, potential differentiation fates (as well as the factors that influence fate determination), and the control of apoptosis for the normal cell of origin would provide important information for specifically tailoring therapy to control and/or eliminate the resultant neoplasm. Choosing the appropriate treatment modality for each tumor based on a thorough understanding of the normal biology of the cell that has undergone transformation would almost certainly improve our ability to predict tumor responsiveness to alternative forms of therapy and optimize patient outcome. More accurate predictions of patient prognosis might also be possible with such an ontogeny-based classification system.

To date, we have only been able to approach this ideal situation for the hematopoietic system. In the hematopoietic system, the use of an ontogeny-based neoplastic classification system has led to significant improvements in our ability to predict clinical prognosis and to assign patients to the most effective treatment protocols (25, 32, 36, 37, 104). Significant progress towards this end has also been achieved in gastrointestinal neoplasia (particularly colon cancer) and in dermatological malignancies. Currently, however, neither of the latter classification systems has supplanted more traditional descriptive histological classification systems for clinical utility.

Ontological neoplastic classification systems are most powerful for organ systems that contain stem cells that provide a source for ongoing replenishment of terminally differentiated cells. This is presumably so because malignant transformation can occur not only in the terminally differentiated cell, but also in the stem cell or one of its progeny which has not yet reached full maturity. In organ systems where terminally-differentiated cells have a very short life span (e.g., the hematopoietic system), or where the terminally-differentiated cells are constantly being sloughed off (e.g., skin and gastrointestinal tract), the stem cell pool must represent a significant proportion of the organ's adult cell population in order for constant cell renewal to keep up with constant cell loss. As a result, the persistence of stem cells into adulthood in these organ systems has been relatively easy to confirm. In contrast, an organ system such as the CNS, where significant cell loss only comes about from pathological conditions or injury, the role of a persistent stem cell population would only be one of occasional organ repair. Since the need for their assistance would not be constant, the population of persistent stem cells would only need to represent a very small percentage (1 to 3%?) of the total organ cellular population, so long as that stem cell population could be rapidly amplified via humoral stimulation in time of need.

An important distinction must also be made between stem cells and precursor, or "progenitor" cells (Table 3.2). Stem cells are a self-sustaining, permanent, and replenishable cell population that persists throughout life. Precursor cells are a transient cell population that only exists during development and early childhood. While both are potential targets for neoplastic transformation, precursor cell tumors would most likely be found in children, whereas stem cell origin tumors might be identified throughout life. However, reality is not that clean and simple. We are discovering more and more that the differentiation path is

TABLE 3.2
Characteristics of Stem Cells versus Progenitor or "Precursor" Cells

Stem Cells	Progenitor ("Precursor") Cells
• Long cell cycle time	• Short cell cycle time
• Asymmetric division - one progeny destined to terminally differentiate - one progeny another stem cell	• Symmetric division - both progeny additional progenitor cells - both progeny destined to terminally differentiate
• A self-sustaining, replenishable cell population throughout life	• A transient cell population during organ development

a "two-way street" and that "terminal differentiation" may not be so "terminal." Under conditions of humoral amplification, adult glial stem cells will revert to a precursor cell phenotype (see Table 3.2), and display all the characteristic of glial precursor cells (114, 115). Even mature astrocytes may revert to a multipotential precursor cell phenotype in vitro under proper humoral amplification conditions (28, 50, 53).

Current glioma classification systems are based more on tumor architectural features, such as endothelial proliferation and necrosis, than individual cellular features. Part of the reason for currently relying more on tumor architectural features than on cellular features to classify gliomas is the morphological heterogeneity of glioma tumor cell population. Another reason is the lack of good antigenic markers for cell type when analyzing formalin-fixed, paraffin-embedded tissue. Glial fibrillary acidic protein (GFAP) expression is often weak and/or incomplete in many astrocytomas and is positive to some extent in at least 50% of tumors classified as "oligodendrogliomas," whereas we have no antigenic marker for oligodendrogliomas for formalin-fixed, paraffin-embedded tissue.

At least four astrocytoma classification systems are currently in use in the United States (Table 3.3). Three of them divide tumors into "grades I–IV." Since all three of these classification systems use differ-

TABLE 3.3
Current Descriptive Glioma Classification Systems

Astrocytoma
• Three-Tiered System (astrocytoma, AA, GBM)
• World Health Organization, Grades I–IV
• St. Anne/Mayo, Grades I–IV
• Kernohan, Grades I–IV

ent criteria for each grade, there is often a great deal of confusion as to the meaning of a "grade II" or "grade III" designation unless the specific classification system utilized is specifically stated. The situation for oligodendrogliomas is even more controversial. A great deal of disagreement exists as to whether "low grade" oligodendrogliomas go on to become GBMs, malignant oligodendrogliomas, or both. Given the recent recognition of the increased chemotherapy sensitivity of anaplastic oligodendrogliomas, there is increasingly greater pressure on neuropathologists to diagnose "malignant oligodendroglioma" over GBM, or at least to recognize an "oligodendroglial component" in a mixed anaplastic glioma. This phenomenon is manifesting itself in the recent development of significant regional variation in the diagnosis of GBM versus malignant oligodendroglioma. One has to wonder what impact this will have on the comparability of clinical research results from one region to another.

Normal Glial Ontogeny

A detailed account of the antigenic progression and biological control of normal glial ontogeny is beyond the scope of this presentation. For a complete account, the reader is referred to several recent comprehensive reviews of the subject [55–57, 93]. What follows here is a brief schematic outline. A summary of the antigenic phenotype of each cell type as well as the role of GFs and cytokines in the progression and control of gliogenesis are presented in Tables 3.4 and 3.5.

The production of mature adult glial cells begins with the formation of multipotential neuronal-glial precursor cells from the neuroepithelial cells of the neural tube. These cells can go on to produce neurons, astrocytes, or oligodendrocytes. Their existence has been proven by in vivo retroviral gene transfer studies using the (β-galactosidase gene [81, 82, 100, 108, 109, 112], by in vitro "neurosphere" three-dimensional culture techniques [90, 91], and by in vitro clonal analysis [46, 98]. Multipotential neuronal-glial precursor cells appear to arise and reside predominantly in the ventricular and subventricular zones of the developing CNS.

Multipotential neuronal-glial precursor cells give rise to glial precursor cells that are more restricted in their potential cellular fate [88]. Two glial lineages have been well worked out. In the Type-1 astrocyte (T1A) lineage, T1A precursor cells go on to form T1As, which are the dominant mature astrocyte in the adult population. In the oligodendrocyte-Type-2 astrocyte (O2A) lineage, perinatal O2A progenitor cells go on to form oligodendrocytes. O2A progenitor cells have the capacity to form Type-2 astrocytes (T2A) in vitro: however, we have no evidence

TABLE 3.4
Glial Cell Lineage and Stage of Maturation by Antigenic Phenotype

Cell Type	GD3	A2B5	RAN-2	O4	GalC	O1	Nestin	Vimentin	GFAP	NF
Multipotential Neuronal-Glial Precursor Cell	?	?	?	−	−	−	+	−	−	−
Type-1 Astrocyte Precursor Cell	?	−	+	−	−	−	+	+	−	−
Mature Type-1 Astrocyte	−	−	+	−	−	−	−	+	+	−
Perinatal O2A Progenitor Cell	+	+	−	−	−	−	+	+	−	−
Adult O2A Progenitor Cell	+	+	−	−	−	−	?	−	−	−
Immature Oligodendrocyte	+	+	−	+	−	−	−	±	−	−
Mature Oligodendrocyte	−	−	−	+	+	+	−	−	−	−
Type-2 Astrocyte	−	+	−	−	−	−	−	−	+	+
Ependymal Cell	−	−	−	−	−	−	−	+	−	−

TABLE 3.5

Growth Factor and Cytokine Effects on the Progression and Control of Gliogenesis

Factor	Cell(s) Stimulated to Proliferate	Cell(s) Stimulated to Differentiate	Cell(s) Dependent on the Factor for Survival
PDGF	Type-1 Astrocyte Perinatal O2A Progenitor Adult O2A Progenitor	—	Perinatal O2A Progenitor Immature Oligodendrocyte
IGF-1	Perinatal O2A Progenitor	Perinatal O2A Progenitor (Oligodendrocyte)	Perinatal O2A Progenitor Oligodendrocyte
IGF-2	—	?	Oligodendrocyte
CNTF	Multipotential Neuronal-Glial Precursor	Perinatal O2A Progenitor	Oligodendrocyte
NT-3	Perinatal O2A Progenitor	?	Oligodendrocyte
BDNF	Perinatal O2A Progenitor	?	?
LIF	Multipotential Neuronal-Glial Precursor	Type-1 Astrocyte Precursor	Oligodendrocyte
IL-6	?	?	Oligodendrocyte
TGF α	Multipotential Neuronal-Glial Precursor	—	—
TGF β	?	Type-1 Astrocyte Precursor	?
BMP	?	Multipotential Neuronal-Glial Precursor (Astrocyte) Type-1 Astrocyte Precursor	?
EGF	Multipotential Neuronal-Glial Precursor Type-1 Astrocyte Precursor	—	—
bFGF	Multipotential Neuronal-Glial Precursor Type-1 Astrocyte Precursor Perinatal O2A Progenitor Adult O2A Progenitor	—	—
aFGF	Type-1 Astrocyte	?	—
Sonic Hedgehog	Multipotential Neuronal-Glial Precursor Perinatal O2A Progenitor	Perinatal O2A Progenitor (Oligodendrocyte)	?
Thyroid Hormone	Perinatal O2A Progenitor	?	?

that they do so in vivo under normal (non-pathological) conditions. The ontogeny of ependymal cells and specialized glia, such as tanycytes, cerebellar Bergmann glia, and retinal Muller cells, has not yet been well worked out.

Multipotential neuronal-glial precursor cells, T1A precursor cells, and perinatal O2A progenitor cells have all been demonstrated to be present in the developing CNS of humans and other mammals (44, 46, 76, 81, 82, 90, 91, 96, 98, 100, 101, 108, 109, 112). Multipotential neuronal-glial stem cells have now been demonstrated to be present in both human and other mammalian adult brain (41, 50, 52). Adult O2A "progenitor" cells (oligodendrocyte "precursor" cells) have likewise been demonstrated to be present in both human and other mammalian adult brain (1, 3, 48, 56, 111, 113, 115). Interestingly, while adult CNS stem cells were first isolated from the subventricular zone of adult brains (27, 28, 34, 38, 49–51), they have now been shown to be present in both white matter tracts (adult O2A "progenitor" cells) (48, 105) and cortical areas (multipotential neuronal-glial stem cells) (50, 53). Even more interesting is the observation that apparently mature astrocytes from adult CNS can revert to a multipotential neuronal-glial stem cell phenotype under proper in vitro humoral amplification conditions (27). Stem cells do indeed represent a very small but important subset of the adult CNS glial cell population (probably ~1%).

Current Status for Gliomas

Malignant transformation of an astrocyte would most likely lead to formation of an astrocytoma, while malignant transformation of an oligodendrocyte would most likely lead to formation of an oligodendroglioma. However, if seemingly mature astrocytes retain the capacity to revert to a multipotential neuronal-glial precursor cell under proper humoral conditions (27), then it remains possible that transformation of an astrocyte could lead to other types of gliomas as well. Presumably, malignant transformation of an adult O2A "progenitor" cell could lead to either an oligodendroglioma or an astrocytoma (or a mixed tumor), since O2A progenitor cells retain the capacity to form astrocytes under abnormal conditions. Type-1 astrocyte precursor cells and perinatal O2A progenitor cells are only realistic as transformation targets in children, but could account for the genesis of certain pediatric gliomas.

While a few of the developmental glial biology antigens listed in Table 3.4 are intracellular proteins, the majority are cell surface gangliosides, sulfatides, cerebrosides, or the carbohydrate moieties attached to them. While this is an advantage for in vitro work since they are resistant to trypsin digestion used to dissociate tissue into individual cells, it is a distinct disadvantage for tissue staining. Cell surface gangliosides, sulfatides, cerebrosides, or the carbohydrate moieties attached to them are best detected on live cells. Freshly frozen tissue yields marginal results for immunohistochemistry. Formalin fixation and/or paraffin embedding are suboptimal and unreliable for immunohistochemistry of these antigens.

An optimal approach to attempting an ontogeny-based classification of gliomas would be to dissociate live cells from a portion of the tumor and screen these cells for a battery of developmental glial biology antigens with a fluorescence activated cell sorter (FACS). The next best option would be to quickly freeze a fresh portion of the tumor, section the tumor by cryotome, and then stain for a battery of developmental glial biology antigens using immunohistochemical methods. To date, neither of these approaches has been pursued and no results have been published.

Currently, four studies of formalin fixed, paraffin embedded glioma tissue have been undertaken to try to classify gliomas according to lineage of origin (11, 22, 24, 77). Each study relied predominantly on the presence or absence of A2B5 staining to assign gliomas to either the T1A or the O2A glial lineage. It was concluded that oligodendrogliomas were uniformly of O2A lineage (24), that medulloblastomas were uniformly of O2A lineage (22), and that astrocytomas could arise either from T1A or O2A lineage (11, 77). These results must be considered preliminary given their limited antigenic screening and the fact that they were obtained from studies of formalin fixed, paraffin embedded glioma tissue. Furthermore, since the researchers predominantly examined A2B5, no further distinction of degree of differentiation within the lineage of origin could be made.

Given that all normal oligodendrocytes are of O2A lineage, the lineage findings for oligodendrogliomas are not very surprising. The possibility that medulloblastomas (which also express the neuronal markers neuron-specific enolase and synaptophysin) could also be of O2A lineage, is controversial. A2B5 was first described as a marker for neurons and not O2A lineage glia (29). It remains possible that medulloblastomas arise from an earlier, less restricted, multipotential neuronal-glial precursor cell rather than from a perinatal O2A progenitor cell. The findings for a possible dual origin of astrocytomas from two separate glial lineages is intriguing, and would be in keeping with findings from primary culture of human GBM specimens under serum-free conditions (56, 72). Bishop and de la Monte estimated that approximately 24% of astrocytomas were of O2A lineage, and that this subset of as-

TABLE 3.6
Status of Attempts to Investigate and Establish an Ontogeny-Based Glioma Classification System

Number of published studies analyzing fresh, live, and glioma cell samples antigenically by fluorescence activated cell sorting	0
Number of published studies analyzing freshly frozen glioma tissue samples antigenically by immunohistochemistry	0
Number of published studies correlating ontological classification of gliomas with patient prognosis	1
Number of published studies correlating ontological classification of gliomas with patient treatment outcome	0

trocytomas may have a more favorable prognosis than astrocytomas of T1A lineage (11) (Table 3.6). Our own findings, however, suggest that even a subset of GBMs is likely to be of O2A lineage (56, 72).

In addition to screening cellular antigenic phenotype, another means of determining glioma lineage origin may be in vivo ^{1}H-NMR metabolite spectroscopy. Neurons and O2A progenitor cells show high N-acetyl-aspartate on ^{1}H-NMR spectroscopy. Oligodendroglia and O2A progenitor cells demonstrate high glycine levels on ^{1}H-NMR spectroscopy. T1As , on the other hand, can be distinguished by their high choline-to-amino acid ratios (102, 103) (Table 3.7). Very few radiologists realize that an N-acetyl-aspartate peak on ^{1}H-NMR spectroscopy of a tumor voxel may represent a true finding of O2A origin tumor cells displaying an O2A progenitor cell phenotype, rather than simply contamination of the voxel by trapped neurons.

TABLE 3.7
Distinguishing Neuroglial Cell Types According to Metabolic Concentrations and Metabolite Ratios as Determined by ^{1}H-NMR Spectroscopy

Metabolite/ Metabolite Ratio	Neurons	O2A Progenitor Cells	Oligodendrocytes	Type-1 Astrocytes
β-Hydroxybutyrate	High	Barely Detectable	Barely Detectable	Barely Detectable
N-acetyl-aspartate	High	High	Absent	Absent
Glycine	Low	High	High	Low
Choline: aspartate ratio	Low	Low	Low	High
Choline: glutamate ratio	Low	Low	Low	High
Choline: glycine ratio	Low	Low	Low	High

HIGH FIDELITY IN VITRO AND IN VIVO GLIOMA MODELING

Molecular biology studies on fresh or snap frozen glioma samples have the advantage of providing truly representative tumor cells, proteins, and nucleic acids for study. The results obtained from these studies have direct applicability to the in situ glioma condition and have the highest validity of all current experimental human glioma studies. Unfortunately, molecular biology techniques have the disadvantages of quickly exhausting the original supply of tumor under study and of not being able to study the living biology of gliomas, glioma progression, or glioma response to new treatments. Ideally, one should be able to screen and identify promising new treatment strategies in the laboratory and confirm their translational effectiveness in high fidelity in vitro models and in vivo animal models before bringing the treatments to expensive and time consuming clinical trial. Low passage in vitro primary culture and in vitro cell lines have the advantage of being a consistent and renewable source of human glioma cells for study either in cell culture or as transplanted xenografts in appropriate animal hosts.

Unfortunately, anyone who has tried to establish human glioma cell lines in cell culture has been struck by the paradox that cells which show progressive and inexorable growth in vivo, grow poorly, if at all, in culture media lacking animal serum or other endogenous mitogens. It would seem from this observation that glioma cells are provided in vivo with factors that they themselves cannot produce, which are necessary for these cells to survive and/or undergo cell division. This difficulty has led to heavy reliance on animal serum (usually fetal calf serum [FCS]) as an undefined media additive for maintaining the few primary glioma cultures that survive to become established glioma cell lines. It is our hypothesis that one of the major reasons for our lack of advancement in glioma translational research is the fatal flaw inherent in most in vitro and in vivo glioma experimental models of exposing the glioma cells to the profound and irreversible effects of FCS and/or other animal serum in culture media.

The Tragedy of Fetal Calf Serum

Glioma cell lines are difficult to establish in cell culture. Most grown in FCS go on to lose GFAP reactivity and become populated by cells with a spindle-shaped morphology that express fibronectin [10, 45]. This mesenchymal phenotype is not seen in the natural in vivo setting. Ironically, almost all of the GFAP positive cultures were derived from the most malignant glioma specimens (9 GFAP+ cultures from 68 Grade IV astrocytomas, and only one GFAP+ culture from 19 Grade I and II astrocytomas). This is the exact opposite of what one would expect from the state of differentiation of the original tumor specimen (45).

By growing and serially passaging cells in media containing FCS, we are introducing a foreign selection pressure on cell growth, which leads to domination by cells with a mesenchymal, rather than a glial, phenotype. This effect becomes permanent and irreversible within one cell division. Not only do these cells assume a spindle-shaped morphology and express fibronectin-like sarcoma cells, they also behave like sarcomas rather than gliomas when confronted with neuropil as a substrate. When multicellular tumor spheroids (39, 116) of these "gliosarcoma" cell lines are confronted with neuropil in the form of fetal rat brain aggregates (12, 13) in three-dimensional culture, they invade the neuropil in a sarcomatous fashion. The tumor spheroid invades the brain aggregate with a homogeneous destructive wave front, creating a sharp tumor-neuropil border (30, 31, 60, 99), rather than as individual infiltrating cells with a transition zone from tumor to neuropil, as one would expect from a GBM. Likewise, while these "gliosarcoma" cells do yield tumors when they are transplanted into the CNS of animal hosts, they produce densely cellular "blue tumors" without the normal nuclear-to-cytoplasmic ratio, cytoplasmic processes, and extracellular space usually seen with GBMs. The typical architectural features of necrosis with pseudopalisading and/or endothelial proliferation are generally absent.

These observations seriously call into question the validity of relying on cells grown in culture with FCS as a valid experimental model for studying glioma biology. Under these circumstances, testing the effectiveness of new treatment modalities for translational implementation are bound to misfire. We seriously question the validity of many observations and findings that have been published using these glioma models.

Treating Glioma Cell like Glial Precursor Cells

Exposing glioma cells to FCS is a very abnormal and unnatural state of affairs. Once the blood-brain barrier forms during development, serum proteins are for the most part excluded from the extracellular space in the CNS. This means that growth media containing animal serum does not accurately reflect the CNS extracellular microenvironment in vivo. Indeed, it was only after the abandonment of FCS and a switch to chemically defined serum-free media that GFs were proven to be mitogenic for human gliomas (80).

We know from developmental glial biology, that FCS has profound and irreversible effects on the biology of precursor cells of O2A lineage (54, 84, 86, 87). Exposing either perinatal O2A progenitor cells or immature oligodendrocytes to FCS in culture will induce early 100% of both cell types to permanently express GFAP within three days of exposure. These so called "Type-2 astrocytes" (T2As) appear to be an in vitro artifact with no in vivo correlate under normal developmental conditions. We know that the astrocyte is the cell predominantly responsible for regulating the extracellular environment in the CNS under normal in vivo conditions. Indeed, the development and use of astrocyte-conditioned serum-free media (ACM) was the major break through that led to the identification and characterization of the first glial precursor cells in vitro. Why not treat glioma cells like glial precursor cells in cell culture, eliminating animal serum from growth media and growing cells in either ACM or chemically-defined serum-free media (56, 57, 69–72)? Rapid proliferation, active cellular migration, and loss of contact inhibition are just some of the characteristics essential for malignancy, which are normal processes for glial precursor cells. ACM remains an undefined media, however, since the cell producing the undefined factor(s) is the appropriate cell for the corresponding in vivo setting.

Abandoning FCS-containing media for ACM and adopting this philosophical approach has drawbacks. It would require a major break with established cell culture tradition. It would require abandoning many well-characterized "gliosarcoma" cell lines and calling into question the results that have been obtained based through studying their biology. It would mean accepting a lower cell survival yield and cell line establishment yield from attempts at primary glioma culture. It would mean an increase in laboratory expense and logistical difficulties since ACM cannot be purchased but must be produced through periodic dissection and primary astrocyte culture with the culling of partially depleted media from T1A monolayer "breeder" cultures. It would require regular quality control for the ACM produced, as well as more frequent experimental media changes since ACM is partially depleted media. No wonder this "purist" approach has been slow to catch on in glioma biology labs.

Adopting this purist approach will improve our in vitro and in vivo glioma models so that they more accurately reflect the in situ glioma setting (Table 3.8). This in turn should improve our ability to study glioma biology and accurately predict the effects and efficacy of new treatment modalities before bringing them to clinical trial.

Hu-O-2A/Gb1

Mark Noble and Karen Bevan were the first to apply this purist approach to glioma biology. Out of the first 20 human GBM samples grown using only ACM, they were able to produce one human GBM cell line (70). This cell line is the first human GBM cell line to be convincingly demonstrated to arise from the O2A glial lineage (Hu-O-2A/Gb1). It has

TABLE 3.8
Fetal Calf Serum versus Astrocyte-Conditioned, Serum-Free Glioma Modeling

Characteristic	Fetal Calf Serum-Containing Model	Astrocyte-Conditioned, Serum-Free Model
In vitro Cellular Morphology	Mesenchymal	Glial
Antigenic Phenotype	Mesenchymal (Fibronectin+)	Glial (Fibronectin−)
Invasion pattern when confronted with neuropil substrate in vitro	Sharply-defined, homogeneous, destructive wave front (Sarcoma)	Individual cellular migration & invasion with a transition zone (Glioma)
Tumor formed upon intracerebral	Densely cellular "blue" tumor	Appropriate Nu/cytoplasmic ratio, neuropil development, & cellular density
Transplantation in animals	Absent secondary glioma architectural features	Secondary glioma architectural features
	Invasion as a sharply-defined, homogeneous, destructive wave front (Sarcoma)	Presence of a tumor transition zone with individual cell invasion at the leading edge (Glioma)

the same ^{1}H-NMR metabolic spectrum as perinatal O2A progenitor cells, responds to GFs in vitro in a similar way to O2A progenitor cells, expresses all the appropriate O2A lineage antigens, and can be manipulated in culture either towards a more oligodendrocytic or a more astrocytic phenotype (56, 57, 71, 72). Like most human GBMs (33, 89, 105, 110), it demonstrates clonal chromosomal aberrations on chromosome 10 (61). Even more importantly, it behaves biologically like a GBM when confronted by neuropil. When a Hu-O-2A/Gb1 multicellular tumor spheroid is confronted with a fetal rat brain aggregate in vitro, the cells first migrate over the surface of the brain aggregate to coat it like an "M & M". Individual cells then invade the neuropil in a radial direction, insinuating themselves among the normal cells until the brain aggregate is gradually taken over and consumed (56). When Hu-O-2A/Gb1 multicellular tumor spheroids are transplanted intracerebrally in nude rats, they produce tumors with many cytological features typical for human GBMs (M. O'Leary, personal communication, 1995).

Fine-Tuning Biological Targeting

Most malignant gliomas are not surgically curable due to their diffusely infiltrative nature and occasional multicentricity, while even the subset of "benign" or "low grade" gliomas that are not diffusely infiltrative may not be amenable to surgical excision due to critical location in the CNS. Unfortunately, the dominant nonsurgical treatment modalities currently available involve various forms of radiation therapy and/or cytotoxic chemotherapy. Both of these modalities solely exploit a difference in proliferation rate between tumor and normal cells for their effectiveness. As a result, their therapeutic index (the ratio of effectiveness to treatment-limiting toxicity) is low, and improvement in survival is often achieved at the expense of distressing and sometimes dehumanizing CNS toxicity.

Glioma researchers are actively searching for more specific "biological targets" in order to improve the outcome as well as the therapeutic index for patients with malignant gliomas. Efforts have focused upon both extracellular and intracellular interactions. Extracellular interactions that may serve as effective biological targets include the processes of malignant cell invasion and/or migration, as well as the process of recruitment of additional blood supply for the growing tumor (angiogenesis). Agents targeting both processes (e.g., metalloproteinase inhibitors and anti-angiogenesis agents) are currently undergoing clinical trial. Intracellular efforts have focused upon cellular proliferation signaling pathways, with a primary focus upon the mitogenic effects of individual GFs and cytokines, as well as their down stream signaling pathways. Agents under investigation and/or started into early clinical trials include individual GF antagonists, protein kinase C inhibitors (pharmacological and antisense oligos), and farnesyl transferase inhibitors (pharmacological and antisense oligos).

Many of the GFs and cytokines that are listed in Table 3.5 have been individually investigated as possible mitogens and/or autocrine factors for malignant gliomas. Developmental glial biology has, however, recently identified two additional factors (bone morphogenic protein and sonic hedgehog) as important factors in glial development that have not yet been explored as potential autocrine/paracrine for gliomas. Bone morphogenic protein has been found to be important in promoting the astroglial commitment of multipotential neuronal-glial precursor cells [117, 118]. Sonic hedgehog has been recently shown to promote both multipotential neuronal-glial precursor cell proliferation, but also induce oligodendrocytic differentiation [42, 92]. The potential role of these two factors for glioma biology is as yet unknown.

Whether one is talking about intracellular steroid receptor signaling pathways, the G protein/cyclic AMP/A kinase pathway, the phospholipase C pathway, the protein kinase C pathway, or the ras/raf-1 pathway, we are discussing final common signaling pathways that are ubiquitously present in all cells. These pathways affect the control of a host of cellular biological processes, in addition to cellular proliferation. Thus, simply targeting one GF or cytokine or these final common signaling pathways may not provide the improved therapeutic index we seek. However, we may be able to take a more sophisticated approach to targeting the actions of GFs and cytokines. Developmental glial biology has clearly demonstrated that GFs and cytokines have pleotrophic effects on glial precursor cells that go well beyond that of being simple individual mitogens (Table 3.9). In addition, the cellular source of these GFs and cytokines may be very different from the cells manifesting their effects.

Growth Factor Combinations and Factor-Factor Interactions

One of the major discoveries to arise from the study of developmental glial biology is that GFs often have their greatest effects when applied *in combinations,* either in series or simultaneously. Examples of simultaneous synergistic effects include: 1) the effects of bFGF and EGF (as well as the combination of bFGF, EGF, and LIF) in promoting the growth and division of multipotential neuronal-glial precursor cells in three-dimensional "neurosphere" culture (18, 21, 23, 97,) 2) the effects of PDGF in combination with bFGF in perpetuating the self-renewal of perinatal and adult O2A progenitor cells [14, 65, 68, 69, 114], 3) the effect of PDGF in combination with NT-3 in perpetuating the self-renewal of perinatal O2A progenitor cells (7) and, 4) the effect of IGF-1 with NT-3 and either LIF, CNTF, or IL-6 in promoting the survival of oligodendrocytes (8). Examples of the sequential action of GFs to serve as possible "priming" or "competency" factors, which allows a subsequently enhanced response from the second GF (even if the first GF is withdrawn), include: 1) the need for neuronal precursor cells to be first exposed to FGF in order to make them competent to respond to NGF at a later time (19, 40) and, 2) the response of multipotential neuronal-glial precursor cells to bFGF and EGF (bFGF then EGF equivalent to

TABLE 3.9
Biological Roles for Growth Factors and Cytokines in Developmental Glial Biology

Individual Mitogens
Synergistic Mitogens (multiple GFs at the same time)
"Priming" or "Competency" Factors (GFs acting sequentially)
Survival Factors
Differentiation Inhibitors
Differentiation Factors

bFGF +EGF, EGF alone less effective) [17, 21]. The role of GF cooperation in combination in glioma biology remains relatively unexplored. However, perturbing these interactions as a biological target may prove to be a more specific target for biological therapies than targeting individual GF pathways.

Survival Factor Role as it may Apply to Glioma Treatment Resistance

During gliogenesis, glial cell numbers can be increased by staving off apoptosis as easily as by increasing glial cell division. In malignant gliomas, apoptosis is the final common pathway for the therapeutic effects of both cytotoxic chemotherapy and radiation therapy. Resistance to apoptosis may be a major mechanism that promotes the resistance of gliomas to standard therapies, favoring tumor persistence and progression. To date, the majority of attention on apoptosis in gliomas has focused upon the p53 genomic surveillance system and the bcl-2 family of apoptosis resistance genes.

Developmental glial biology, however, would suggest that GFs and cytokines may play a major role in preventing apoptosis in glial cells by serving as survival factors. Factors that have been found to prevent apoptosis for normal oligodendrocytes during gliogenesis include IGF-1, IGF-2, insulin (but only at concentrations that secondarily saturate IGF-1 receptors), CNTF, LIF, NT-3, and IL-6 (at very high doses) [6, 8, 59, 62]. If a humoral factor was exerting its major pathological affect as a survival factor rather than as a mitogen, these positive growth effects would not be detectable with standard tritiated thymidine and/or BrDu assays, but would only be detectable using a cell death assay like the MTT assay [67]. The role of individual GFs as survival factors in glioma biology and glioma treatment resistance remains relatively unexplored.

Differentiation Inhibition as a Transformational Phenomenon

Glial precursor cell numbers can be increased by staving off differentiation as easily as by increasing glial cell division. Examples from developmental glial biology include PDGF and bFGF in combination perpetuating the self-renewal of O2A progenitor cells [14], as well as transforming adult O2A "progenitor" cells into self-renewing cells with the characteristics of perinatal O2A progenitor cells [115]. It is interesting to note that transfection of perinatal O2A progenitor cells with either of the nuclear oncogenes c-myc or SV 40 large T antigen will produce identical effects as exposing these cells simultaneously to PDGF and bFGF [4, 5]. It would seem likely that certain types of oncogene-mediated cellular transformation might share certain common mechanisms with GF-mediated progenitor cell differentiation inhibition.

If certain malignant transformations do involve inducing and perpetuating a precursor cell phenotype in normal glia or even glial stem cells, it remains possible that we may yet be able to override this differentiation "block" and induce differentiation in the tumor [55, 56]. So far, attempts at developing and utilizing "differentiation agents" for malignant gliomas have been mostly limited to empiric trials of retinoic acid [26, 43]. A better understanding of the GF and cytokine mechanism for blocking the precursor cell differentiation program would go a long way towards identifying additional targets for improved pharmacological manipulation.

Humoral Interplay with Normal Stromal Cells

It is a fundamental fact in developmental glial biology that the GFs that critically influence a given glial cell type are often supplied and secreted by a different glial cell type, or even from non-glial cells in the CNS, such as endothelial cells [62, 66]. The glial cell supplying and secreting the critical factor may even be from a different glial lineage, as in the case of T1As secreting PDGF as a mitogen for perinatal O2A progenitor cells [73, 74, 85]. To date, most glioma biology investigation into GF humoral feedback loops has focused upon potential self-perpetuating glioma autocrine phenomena. What if a rate-limiting step in glioma survival and progression was a humoral feedback loop with normal cells surrounding the tumor or within the tumor stroma? While glioma cells are heterogeneous in phenotype and difficult to consistently and predictably control, the normal cellular response in the critical humoral feedback loop may be easier to control or eliminate in a consistent and predictable manner.

Gliomas growing in situ contain normal astrocytes, oligodendrocytes, and endothelial cells intermixed within their stroma. The observations that gliomas are almost impossible to grow in primary culture in austere chemically-defined media, and that ACM can serve as a substitute for FCS-containing media in supporting glioma cells in vitro, suggests that a major factor controlling glioma growth in situ may be the humoral interplay and positive feedback loops working between the neoplastic cells and the normal cells of the immediate tumor stromal microenvironment. Certain effects of tumor cells on normal cells, such as glioma cells effecting the blood-brain barrier [9, 15, 20, 75] and/or producing tumor angiogenesis factor(s), are under active investigation [2, 47, 78, 79]. However, the potential positive growth and survival effects of normal astrocytes, oligodendrocytes, and endothelial cells on glioma cells and ways to interrupt or turn off their support from the normal cell side of the feedback loop, remain unexplored for malignant gliomas.

CONCLUSION

Rapid proliferation, active cellular migration, and loss of contact inhibition are just some of the characteristics essential for malignancy, which are normal processes during glial development. The genes controlling normal cellular developmental processes are still present in the genome of mature cells. It is very probable that oncogenesis involves the reactivation and loss of control of normal, or subtly altered developmental genes. It would, therefore, seem likely that the study of gliomas might very well benefit from developmental glial biology findings, as well as the application of developmental glial biology principles in neuropathology and the glioma laboratory.

While it remains an attractive scientific and clinical goal, at the present time we have insufficient evidence to say with certainty that an ontogeny-based glioma classification system would be an improvement over currently available classification systems. On the other hand, it is a logical fallacy to assume that "absence of evidence" equates with "evidence of absence." The key work in this area remains to be completed. We can only hope that a positive result will be achieved to the benefit of our patients.

The in vitro and in vivo biological behavior of Hu-O-2A/Gb1 (the first human O2A origin GBM cell line), suggests that applying developmental glial biology principles, treating glioma cells like glial precursor cells, and using only astrocyte-conditioned, serum-free media may yield in vitro and in vivo glioma models with much higher fidelity to the in situ human glioma condition. It remains to be proven that improving the experimental model will improve the results of translational glioma research for fast-tracking new treatment modalities to the clinical setting. If successful, however, the outcome will justify the additional cost and logistical difficulties inherent in the approach.

Lessons learned and observations obtained from the study of developmental glial biology may direct us to potentially fertile new areas of glioma research for identifying new biological targets for glioma treatment. Examples of potential ways to increase the sophistication of our biological targeting include: 1) exploring perturbations of specific GF interactions rather than just targeting ubiquitous individual GF signaling pathways, 2) exploring the role of GFs and cytokines as survival factors rather than just glioma mitogens, 3) developing more specific ways to overcome differentiation inhibition in cases where transformation may have occurred from a "block" in the differentiation program of a glial stem cell, and 4) exploring means of perturbing positive humoral feedback loops between glioma cells and stromal normal cells from the normal cell side of the equation. These strategies, taken by analogy from the study of developmental glial biology, suggest new avenues for trying to improve the specificity, and therefore the therapeutic index, of future biological therapies.

REFERENCES

1. Aloisi F, Giampaolo A, Russo G, Peschle C, Levi G: Developmental appearance, antigenic profile, and proliferation of glial cells of the human embryonic spinal cord: An immunocytochemical study using dissociated cultured cells. **Glia** 5:171–181, 1992.
2. Alvarez JA, Baird A, Tatum A, Daucher J, Chorsky R, Gonzalez AM, Stopa EG: Localization of basic fibroblast growth factor and vascular endothelial growth factor in human glial neoplasms. **Mod Pathol** 5:303–307, 1992.
3. Armstrong RC, Harvath L, Dubois-Dalcq ME: Type 1 astrocytes and oligodendrocyte-type 2 astrocyte glial progenitors migrate towards distinct molecules. **J Neurosci Res** 27:400–407, 1990.
4. Barnett SC, Crouch DH: The effect of oncogenes on the growth and differentiation of oligodendrocyte type 2 astrocyte progenitor cells. **Cell Growth Differ** 6:69–80, 1995.
5. Barnett SC, Franklin RJ, Blakemore WF: *In vitro* and *in vivo* analysis of rat bipotential O-2A progenitor cell line containing the temperature sensitive mutant gene of the SV40 large T antigen. **Eur J Neurosci** 5:1247–1260, 1993.
6. Barres BA, Hart IK, Coles HSR, Burne JF, Voyvodic JT, Richardson WD, Raff ML: Cell death and control of cell survival in the oligodendrocyte lineage. **Cell** 70:31–46, 1992.
7. Barres BA, Raff MC, Gaese F, Bartke I, Dechant G, Barde YA: A crucial role for neurotrophin-3 in oligodendrocyte development. **Nature** 367:371–375, 1994.
8. Barres BA, Schmid R, Sendnter M, Raff MC: Multiple extracellular signals are required for long-term oligodendrocyte survival. **Development** 118:283–295, 1993.
9. Berkman RA, Merrill MJ, Reinhold WC, Monacci WT, Saxena A, Clark WC, Robertson JT, Ali IU, Oldfield E: Expression of the vascular permeability factor/vascular endothelial growth factor gene in central nervous system neoplasms. **J Clin Invest** 91:153–159, 1993.
10. Bigner DD, Bigner SH, Ponten J, Westermark B, Mahaley MS Jr, Ruoslahti E, Herschman H, Eng LF, Wikstrand CJ: Heterogeneity of genotypic and phenotypic characteristics of fifteen permanent cell lines derived from human gliomas. **J Neuropath Exp Neurol** 40:201–229, 1981.
11. Bishop M, de la Monte SM: Dual lineage of astrocytomas. **Am J Pathol** 135:517–527, 1989.
12. Bjerkvig R, Steinsvag SK, Laerum OD: Reaggregation of fetal rat brain cells in a stationary culture system. I: Methodology and cell identification. **In Vitro** 22: 180–192, 1986.
13. Bjerkvig R: Reaggregation of fetal rat brain cells in a stationary culture system. II: Itrastructural characterization. **In Vitro** 22:193–200, 1986.
14. Bogler O, Wren D, Barnett S, Land H, Noble M: Cooperation between two growth factors promotes extended self-renewal and inhibits differentiation of oligodendro-

cyte-type-2 astrocyte (O-2A) progenitor cells. **Proc Natl Acad Sci USA** 87:6368–6372, 1990.

15. Bruce JN, Crisuolo GR, Merrill MJ, Moquin R, Blacklock JB, Oldfield EH: Vascular permeability induced by protein product of malignant brain tumors: Inhibition by dexamethasone. **J Neurosurg** 67:880–884, 1987.
16. Cameron RS, Rakic P: Glial cell lineage in the cerebral cortex: A review and synthesis. **Glia** 4:124–137, 1991.
17. Cardenas-Aguavo MC, Santa-Olalla J, Fregoso-Lomas M, Salgado L, Covarrubias L: Characterization of bFGF and EGF-responsive neural precursor cells (NPCs) along the anterior-posterior (AP) axis of the developing nervous system. **Soc Neurosci** 25:94.2, 1999. [Abstract]
18. Carpenter MK, Cui X, Hu ZY, Jackson J, Sherman S, Seiger A, Wahlberg LU: In vitro expansion of a multipotent population of human neural progenitor cells. **Exp Neurol** 158(2):265–278, 1999.
19. Catteneo E, McKay R: Proliferation and differentiation of neuronal stem cells regulated by nerve growth factor. **Nature** 347:762–765, 1990.
20. Criscuolo GR, Merrill MJ, Oldfield EH: Further characterization of malignant glioma-derived vascular permeability factor. **J Neurosurg** 69:254–262, 1988.
21. Croft CM, Turnerfand DA, Shetty AK: In vitro proliferation and differentiation of embryonic day 15 cortical stem cells responsive to EGF and FGF. **Soc Neurosci** 25:296.3, 1999. [Abstract]
22. Cudkowicz M, de la Monte SM: Histogenesis and cell lineage analysis of medulloblastomas. **J Neurol Sci** 94:221–229, 1989.
23. Cui X, Seiger A, Almquist P, Wahlberg L: The effects of LIF family cytokines on Human Neural Progenitor cell cultures. **Soc Neurosci** 25:812.14, 1999. [Abstract]
24. de la Monte SM: Uniform lineage of oligodendrogliomas. **Am J Pathol** 135:529–540, 1989.
25. Deegan MJ: Membrane antigen analysis in the diagnosis of lymphoid leukemias and lymphomas: Differential diagnosis, prognosis as related to phenotype, and recommendations for testing. **Arch Pathol Lab Med** 113:606–618, 1989.
26. Defer GL, Adle-Biassette H, Ricolfi F, Martin L, Authier FJ, Chomienne C, Degos L, Degos JD: All-trans retinoic acid in relapsing malignant gliomas: Clinical and radiological stabilization associated with the appearance of intratumoral calcificaitons. **J Neurooncol** 34(2):169–177, 1997.
27. Doetsch F, Caille I, Lim DA, Garcia-Verdugo JM, Alvarez-Buylla A: Subventricular zone astrocytes are neural stem cells in the adult mammalian brain. **Cell** 97(6):703–716, 1999.
28. Doetsch F, Garcia-Verdugo JM, Alvarez-Buylla A: Cellular composition and three-dimensional organization of the subventricular germinal zone in the adult mammalian brain. **J Neurosci** 17(13):5046–5061, 1997.
29. Eisenbarth GS, Walsh FS, Nirenberg M: Monoclonal antibody to a plasma membrane antigen of neurons. **Proc Natl Acad Sci USA** 76:4913–4917, 1979.
30. Engebraaten O, Bjerkvig R, Lund-Johansen M, Wetsre K, Pederson PH, Mork S, Backlund EO, Laerum OD: Interaction between human brain tumor biopsies and fetal rat brain tissue *in vitro*. **Acta Neuropathol** 81:130–140, 1990.
31. Engebraaten O, Bjerkvig R, Pedersen PH, Laerum OD: Effects of EGF, bFGF, NGF, and PDGF (bb) on cell proliferation, migratory and invasive capacities of human brain tumor biopsies *in vitro*. **Int J Cancer** 53:209–214, 1993.
32. Foon KA, Todd RF III: Immunological classification of leukemia and lymphoma. **Blood** 68:1–31, 1986.
33. Fults DD, Brockmeyer D, Tullous MW, Redone CA, Lawthorne RM: p53 Mutation and

loss of heterozygosity on chromosones 17 and 10 during human astrocytoma progression. **Cancer Res** 52:674–679, 1992.

34. Garcia-Verdugo JM, Doetsch F, Wichterle H, Lim DA, Alvarez-Buylla A: Architecture and cell types of the adult subventricular zone: In search of the stem cells. **J Neurobiol** 36(2):234–248, 1998.
35. Goldman JE, Vayesse PJ: Racing glial cell lineages in the mammalian forebrain. **Glia** 4:149–156, 1991.
36. Greaves MF: Analysis of the clinical and biological significance of lymphoid phenotypes in acute leukemia. **Cancer Res** 41:4752–4766, 1981.
37. Griffin JD, Davis R, Nelson DA, Davey FR, Mayer RJ, Schiffer C, McIntyre OR, Bloomfield CD: Use of surface marker analysis to predict outcome of acute lymphoblasticleukemia. **Blood** 68:1232–1241, 1986.
38. Gritti A, Parati EA, Cova L, Frolinchsthal P, Galli R, Wanke E, Faravelli L, Morassutti DJ, Roisen F, Michel DD, Vescovi AL: Multipotential stem cells from the adult mouse brain proliferate and self-renew in response to basic fibroblast growth factor. **J Neurosci** 16(3):1091–1100, 1996.
39. Haji-Karim M, Carlssom J: Proliferation and viability in cellular spheroids of human origin. **Cancer Res** 38:1457–1464, 1978.
40. Heuer JG, van Bartheld CS, Kinoshita Y, Evers PC, Bothwell M: Alternating phases of FGF receptor and NGF receptor expression in developing chick nervous system. **Neuron** 5:283–296, 1990.
41. Honsou D, Kato T, Akiyama Y, Kocsis JD, Uede T, Hash K: Clonal analysis of neural stem cells derived from adult human brain. **Soc Neurosci** 25:914.7, 1999. [Abstract]
42. Ji B, Reilly J, Ranciato R, Allendoerfer K, Dudek H: Regulation of CNS neurological lineage cells by sonic hedgehog signaling. **Soc Neurosci** 25:204.5, 1999. [Abstract]
43. Kaba SE, Kyritsis AP, Conrad C, Gleason MJ, Newman R, Levin VA, Yung WK: The treatment of recurrent cerebral gliomas with all-trans-retinoic acid (tretinoin). **J Neurooncol** 34(2):145–151, 1997.
44. Kennedy PGE, Fok-Seang J: Studies on the development, antigenic phenotype and function of human glial cells in tissue culture. **Brain** 109:1261–1277, 1986.
45. Kennedy PGE, Watkins BA, Thomas DGT, Noble M: Antogenic expression by cells derived from gliomas does not correlate with morphological classification. **Neuropath Appl Neurobiol** 13:327–347, 1987.
46. Kilpatrick TJ, Bartlett PF: Cloning and growth of multipotential neural precursors: Requirements for proliferation and differentiation. **Neuron** 10:255–265, 1993.
47. Kim KJ, Li B, Winer J, Armanini M, Gillet N, Phillips HS, Ferrara H: Inhibition of vascular endothelial growth factor-induced angiogenesis suppresses tumour growth *in vitro*. **Nature** 362:841–844, 1993.
48. Kim SU: Antigenic expression by glial cells grown in culture. **J Neuroimmunol** 8:255–282, 1983.
49. Kirschenbaum B, Doetsch F, Lois C, Alvarez-Buylla A: Adult subventricular zone neuronal precursors continue to proliferate and migrate in the absence of the olfactory bulb. **J Neurosci** 19(6):2171–2180, 1999.
50. Kukekov VG, Laywell ED, Suslov O, Davies K, Scheffler B, Thomas LB, O'Brien TF, Kusakabe M, Steindler DA: Multipotent stem/progenitor cells with similar properties arise from two neurogenic regions of adult human brain. **Exp Neurol** 156(2):333–344, 1999.
51. Kukekov VG, Laywell ED, Thomas LB, Steindler DA. A nestin-negative precursor cell from the adult mouse brain gives rise to neurons and glia. **Glia** 21(4)399–407, 1997.

52. Laywell ED, Kukekov VG, Steindler DA: Multipotent neurospheres can be derived from forebrain subependymal zone and spinal cord of adult mice after protracted postmortem intervals. **Exp Neurol** 156(2):430–433, 1999.
53. Laywell ED, Kukekov VG, Steindler DA: Evidence that cultured astrocytes from diverse CNS areas of the mouse produce neurospheres *in vitro*. **Soc Neurosci** 25:224.13, 1999. [Abstract]
54. Levison SW, McCarthy KD: Characterization and partial purification of AIM: A plasma protein that induces rat cerebral type-2 astroglaia from bipotential glial progenitors. **J Neurochem** 57:782–794, 1991.
55. Linskey ME, Gilbert MR: Glial differentiation: A review with implications for new directions in neuro-oncology. **Neurosurg** 36:1–22, 1995.
56. Linskey ME: The developmental biology of glial cells and its relation to the study of glioma biology, in, Apuzzo MLJ (ed): *Benign Cerebral Glioma, Vol 1.* Park Ridge, IL: American Association of Neurological Surgeons, 1995, pp 13–53.
57. Linskey ME: Advances in the study of glial lineage, in, Kornblith PL, Walker M (ed): *Advances in Neuro-Oncology, Vol II.* New York: Futura Publishing Co., 1997, pp 3–33.
58. Linskey ME: Glial ontogeny and glial neoplasia: The search for closure. **J Neurooncol** 34:5–22, 1997.
59. Louis JC, Magal E, Takayama S, Varon S: CNTF protection of oligodendrocytes against natural and tumor necrosis factor-induced death. **Science** 259:689–692, 1993.
60. Lund-Johansen M, Bjerkvig R, Humphrey PA, Bigner SH, Bigner DD, Laerum OD: Effect of epidermal growth factor on glioma cell growth, migration, and invasion *in vitro*. **Cancer Res** 50:6039–6044, 1990.
61. Mao X, Jones TA, Tomlinson I, Rowan AJ, Fedorova LI, Zelenin AV, Mao JI, Gutowski NJ, Noble M, Sheer D: Genetic aberrations in glioblastoma multiformé: Translocation of chromosome 10 in an O-2A-like cell line. **Br J Cancer** 79(5–6):724–731, 1999.
62. Mayer M, Bhakoo K, Noble M: Ciliary neurotrophic factor and leukemia inhibitory factor promote the generation, maturation, and survival of oligodendrocytes *in vitro*. **Development** 120:143–153, 1994.
63. McKay RD: The origins of cellular diversity in the mammalian central nervous system. **Cell** 58:815–821, 1989.
64. McKay R: Stem cells in the central nervous system (Review). **Science** 276(5309): 66–71, 1997.
65. McKinnon RD, Matsui T, Dubois-Dalcq M, Aaronson SA: FGF modulates the PDGF-driven pathway of oligodendrocyte development. **Neuron** 5:603–614, 1990.
66. Mi H, Barres BA: Induction of astrocyte differentiation by vascular endothelial cells via LIF in the developing rat optic nerve. **Soc Neurosci** 25:308.13, 1999. [Abstract]
67. Mosman T: Rapid calorimetric assay for cellular growth and survival: Application to proliferation and cytotoxicity assay. **J Immunol Meth** 65:55–63, 1983.
68. Noble M: Points of controversy in the O-2A lineage: clocks and type-2 astrocytes. **Glia** 4:157–164, 1991.
69. Noble M, Ataliotis P, Barnett SC, Bevan K, Bogler O, Groves A, Jat P, Wolswijk G, Wren G: Development, regeneration, and neoplasia of glial cells in the central nervous system. **Ann NY Acad Sci** 633:35–47, 1991.
70. Noble M, Bevan K, Venter D: Cellular and molecular approaches to the study of gliomas and glial development, in, Thomas DGT, Graham DI (ed): *Malignant Brain Tumours.* New York: Springer-Verlag, 1995, pp 1–12.

71. Noble, M, Gutowski N, Bevan K, Engle U, Linskey M, Urenjak J, Bhakoo K, Williams S: From rodent glial precursor cell to human glial neoplasia in the oligodendrocyte-type-2 astrocyte lineage. **Glia** 15:222–230, 1995.
72. Noble M, Mayer-Proschel M: Growth factors, glia and gliomas [Review]. **J Neurooncol** 35(3):193–209, 1997.
73. Noble M, Murray K: Purified astrocytes promote the *in vitro* division of a bipotential glial progenitor cell. **EMBO J** 3:10:2243–2247, 1984.
74. Noble M, Murray K, Stroobant P, Waterfield MD, Riddle P: Platelet-derived growth factor promotes division and motility and inhibits premature differentiation of the oligodendrocyte/type-2 astrocyte progenitor cell. **Nature** 333:560–562, 1988.
75. Ohnishi T, Sher PB, Posner JB, Shapiro WR: Capillary permeability factor secreted by malignant brain tumor: role in peritumoral edema and possible mechanism for antiedema effect of glucocorticoids. **J Neurosurg** 72:245–251, 1990.
76. Pagano SF, Galli R, Girelli M, Cova L, Parati EA, Mora M, Vescovi AL: Epigenetic regulation of differentiation in human neural stem cells. **Soc Neurosci** 25:914.5, 1999. [Abstract]
77. Piepmeier J, Fried I, Makuch R: Low grade astrocytomas may arise from different astrocyte lineages. **Neurosurg** 33:627–632, 1993.
78. Plate KJ, Breier G, Farrell CL, Risau W: Platelet-derived growth factor receptor-B is induced during tumor development and upregulated during tumor progression in endothelial cells in human gliomas. **Lab Invest** 67:529–534, 1992.
79. Plate KH, Breier G, Weich HA, Risau W: Vascular endothelial growth factor is a potential tumour angiogenesis factor in human gliomas in vivo. **Nature** 359:845–848, 1992.
80. Pollack IF, Randall MS, Kristofik MP, Kelly RH, Solker RG, Vortosick FT Jr: Response of low passage human malignant gliomas *in vitro* to stimulation and selective inhibition of growth factor—-mediated pathways. **J Neurosurg** 75:284–293, 1991.
81. Price J, Thurlow L: Cell lineage in the rat cerebral cortex: A study using retroviral-mediated gene transfer. **Development** 104:473–482, 1988.
82. Price J, Williams B, Grove E: Cell lineage in the cerebral cortex. **Development** (Suppl 2):23–28, 1991.
83. Raff MC: Glial cell diversification in the rat optic nerve. **Science** 243:1450–1455, 1989.
84. Raff MC, Abney ER, Cohen J, Lindsay R, Noble M: Two types of astrocytes in cultures of developing rat white matter: Differences in morphology, surface gangliosides, and growth characteristics. **J Neurosci** 3:1289–1300, 1983.
85. Raff MC, Lillien LE, Richardson WD, Burne JF, Noble MD: Platelet-derived growth factor from astrocytes drives the clock that times oligodendrocyte development in culture. **Nature** 333:562–565, 1988.
86. Raff MC, Miller RH, Noble M: A glial progenitor cell that develop *in vitro* into an astrocyte or an oligodendrocyte depending on culture medium. **Nature** 303:390–396, 1983.
87. Raff MC, Williams BP, Miller RH: The *in vitro* differentiation of a bipotential glial progenitor cell. **EMBO J** 3:8:1857–1864, 1984.
88. Rao MS, Mayer-Proschel M: Glial-restricted precursors are derived from multipotent neuroepithelial stem cells. **Dev Bio** (Orlando) 188(1):48–63, 1997.
89. Rasheed BK, Fuller GN, Friedman AH, Bigner DD, Bigner SH: Loss of heterozygosity for 10q loci in human gliomas. **Genes Chromosomes Cancer** 5:75–82, 1992.
90. Reynolds BA, Tetzlaff W, Weiss S: A multipotent EGF-responsive striatal embryonic progenitor cell produces neurons and astrocytes. **J Neurosci** 12:4563–4574, 1992.

91. Reynolds BA, Weiss S: Generation of neurons and astrocytes from isolated cells of the adult mammalian central nervous system. **Science** 255:1707–1710, 1992.
92. Roukampt CA, Murray K, Dubois-Dalcq M: Sonic hedgehog regulates the development of telencephalic rat oligodendrocytes. **Soc Neurosci** 25:83.5, 1999. [Abstract]
93. Scheffler B, Horn M, Blumcke I, Laywell ED, Coomes D, Kukekov VG, Steindler DA: Narrow-mindedness: A perspective on neuropoiesis [Review]. **Trends Neurosci** 22(8):348–357, 1999.
94. Skoff RP, Knapp PE: Division of astroblasts and oligodendroblasts in postnatal rat brain: Evidence for separate astrocyte and oligodendrocyte lineages. **Glia** 4:165–174, 1991.
95. Skoff RP, Knapp PE: Lineage and differentiation of oligodendrocytes in the brain. **Ann NY Acad Sci** 633:48–55, 1991.
96. Svendsen CN, Prowse KR, Linskens MHK, Jauniaux E: Precursor cells isolated from the developing human CNS show regional specificity and lack telomerase expression. **Soc Neurosci** 25:102.5, 1999. [Abstract]
97. Svendsen CN, ter Borg MF, Armstrong RJ, Rosser AE, Chandran S, Ostenfeld T, Caldwell MA: A new method for the rapid and long term growth of human neural precursor cells. **J Neurosci Methods** 85(2):141–152, 1998.
98. Temple S: Division and differentiation of isolated CNS blast cells in microculture. **Nature** 340:471–473, 1989.
99. Terzis AJ, Fiskerstrand T, Regsum H, Ueland PM, Arnold H, Bjerkvig R: Proliferation, migration and invasion of human glioma cells exposed to antifolate drugs. **Int J Cancer** 54:112–118, 1993.
100. Turner DL, Cepko CL: A common progenitor for neurons and glia persists in rat retina late in development. **Nature** 328:131–136, 1987.
101. Uchida N, He D, Reitsma MJ, Masek M, Weissman L, Gage F, Buck D: Direct isolation of human neural stem cells from fetal brain by cell sorting. **Soc Neurosci** 25:701.3, 1999. [Abstract]
102. Urenjak J, Williams SR, Gagian DG, Noble M: Proton nuclear magnetic resonance spectroscopy unambiguously identifies different neural cell types. **J Neurosci** 13:981–989, 1993.
103. Urenjak J, Williams SR, Gagian DG, Noble M: Specific expression of N-acetylaspartate in neurons, oligodendrocyte-type-2 astrocyte progenitors, and immature oligodendrocytes *in vitro*. **J Neurochem** 59:55–61, 1992.
104. van Eys J, Pullen J, Head D, Boyett J, Crist W, Falleta J, Humphrey GB, Jackson J, Riccardi V, Brock B: The French-American-British (FAB) classification of leukemia: The Pediatric Oncology Group experience with lymphocytic leukemia. **Cancer** 57:1046–1051, 1986.
105. Venter DJ, Thomas DGT: Multiple sequential abnormalities in the evolution of human gliomas. **Br J Cancer Res** 63:445–448, 1991.
106. Walker MD, Alexander E Jr, Hunt WE: Evaluation of BCNU and/or radiotherapy in the treatment of anaplastic gliomas: A cooperative clinical trial. **J Neurosurg** 49:333=-343, 1978.
107. Walker MD, Green SB, Byar DP: Randomized comparisons of radiotherapy and nitrosoureas for the management of malignant glioma after surgery. **New Eng J Med** 303:1323–1329, 1980.
108. Walsh C, Cepko CL: Clonally related cortical cells show several migration patterns. **Science** 241:1342–1345, 1988.
109. Walsh C, Cepko CL: Widespread dispersion of neuronal clones across functional regions of the cerebral cortex. **Science** 255:434–440, 1992.

110. Watanabe KM, Nagai M, Wakai S, Arai T, Kawashima K: Loss of constitutional heterozygosity in chromosome IO in human glioblastoma. **Acta Neuropathol** 80:251–254, 1990.
111. Whittemore SR, Sanson HR, Wood PM: Concurrent isolation and characterization of oligodendrocytes, mecroglia, and astrocytes from adult human spinal cord. **Int J Dev Neurosci** 11:755–764, 1993.
112. Williams BP, Read J, Price J: The generation of neurons and oligodendrocytes from a common precursor cell. **Neuron** 7:685–693, 1991.
113. Wolswijk G, Noble M: Identification of an adult-specific glial progenitor cell. **Development** 105:387–400, 1989.
114. Wolswijk G, Noble M: Cooperation between PDGF and FGF converts slowly dividing O-2A ^{adult} progenitor cells to rapidly dividing cells with characteristics of O-2A ^{perinatal} progenitor cells. **J Cell Biol** 118:889–900, 1992.
115. Wilswijk G, Noble M: In vitro studies on the development and maintenance of the oligodendrocyte-type-2 astrocyte (O-2A) lineage in the adult central nervous system, in, Kettenmann H, Ransom BR (ed): *Neuro-Glial Cells.* Oxford University Press (in press).
116. Yuhas JM, Li AP, Martinez AO, Ladman AJ: A simplified method for the production and growth of multicellular tumor spheroids. **Cancer Res** 37: 3639–3643, 1977.
117. Yung SY, Zhang D, Kessler JA: Identification of genes involved in progenitor cell lineage commitment and responses to bone morphogenetic proteins. **Soc Neurosci** 25:413.2, 1999. [Abstract]
118. Zhang D, Mehler MF, Kessler JA: Bone morphogenetic protein (BMP) 2 and 4 up regulate the basic helix-loop-helix transcriptional repressors Id4 and Id2 in subventricular zone pregenitor cells. **Soc Neurosci** 25:93.16, 1999. [Abstract]

CHAPTER

4

BEHAB/brevican: An Extracellular Matrix Component Associated with Invasive Glioma

SYDNEY C. GARY, PH.D., SUSAN HOCKFIELD, PH.D.

SUMMARY

The extracellular matrix (ECM) has a prominent role in many physiological processes, including organ development, wound healing, and neoplastic growth and invasion. In each of these processes, changes in the composition of the matrix can lead to increased cell movement. In this review, we discuss the role of ECM components in glioma invasion, with special emphasis on the brain-specific proteoglycan, Brain-Enriched Hyaluronan Binding (BEHAB)/brevican.

INTRODUCTION

Primary brain tumors, including astrocytoma, oligodendroglioma, and glioblastoma, are all derived from glial cells and are collectively referred to as gliomas. These cells are highly motile and move away from the primary tumor locus and invade normal brain tissue to set up new tumor focii. The invasive nature of glioma makes these tumors refractory to conventional therapies.

The composition of the ECM is a critical factor in determining the invasive potential of cancer cells. Tumor cells not only utilize existing ECM molecules as substrates to migrate through normal tissue, but also produce their own matrix elements to facilitate invasion. Invasion of tumor cells into normal tissue is a multistep process that requires adhesion of tumor cells to matrix components, proteolytic degradation of ECM, and migration of tumor cells. These events are carried out by a variety of cell:matrix interactions. Cell surface receptors such as CD44 and the integrins facilitate binding of tumor cells to the ECM; matrix elements that serve as substrates for this interaction include tenascin, hyaluronic acid, and laminin (6). Degradation of ECM is carried out by proteases produced by the invading tumor cells. Included in the growing list of tumor-associated proteases are cysteine and serine proteinases, as well as many matrix metalloproteinases (29). Once the matrix is enzymatically altered, migration of the tumor cells occurs and new cell:matrix connections are established. This multistep process is a general mechanism utilized by most invasive cancer cells, including invasive glioma cells in the brain.

THE ECM OF THE BRAIN IS DISTINCT FROM THAT OF OTHER TISSUES

Brain ECM has very low levels of collagen, fibronectin, and laminin (ECM components common to most tissues) and high levels of chondroitin sulfate proteoglycans (CSPG) and the glycosaminoglycan, hyaluronan (HA) (23). Different structures in the brain have different ECM constituents. At the external surface of the brain, the glial limitans externa is primarily composed of collagen (Types I, III, and IV), laminin, fibronectin, and heparin sulfate proteoglycans (HSPG). The vascular basement membrane contains types IV and V collagen, laminin, entactin, vitronectin, and HSPG. The main components of the brain parenchymal ECM are HA, CSPGs, tenascin, and BEHAB/brevican. Perineuronal nets, ECM structures surrounding neurons, are extremely heterogeneous, with different members of a family of CSPGs expressed on distinct subsets of neurons (3).

The composition of the ECM of the brain changes over the course of development (10, 11, 27). In the developing brain, the ECM is soluble and permissive for cell proliferation and migration. In contrast, the matrix in the normal adult brain is less soluble and limits cell motility and stabilizes cell-cell relationships. For example, soluble HA is abundant in the embryonic brain, which allows for increased cell movement, but is far less abundant in normal adult brain (4). In contrast, Cat-301, a perineuronal CSPG implicated in the stabilization of synaptic relationships, is not expressed embryonically but is upregulated during the postnatal period to reach adult levels around the end of the period for synaptic plasticity (28). Therefore, changes in the levels of ECM molecules can affect a cell's environment and favor increased motility and proliferation, the hallmarks of glioma.

THE BEHAB/BREVICAN PROTEOGLYCAN

BEHAB/brevican is a member of the lectican family of CSPGs, a family that includes aggrecan, versican, and neurocan (Fig. 4.1) (12). Lecticans, also known as hyalectans, are complex macromolecules with a core protein modified by the addition of one or more types of glycosaminoglycan (GAG) chains (7, 30). The core proteins of all the lecticans have several common structural features. At the N-terminus, an immunoglobulin-like loop and two proteoglycan tandem repeats com-

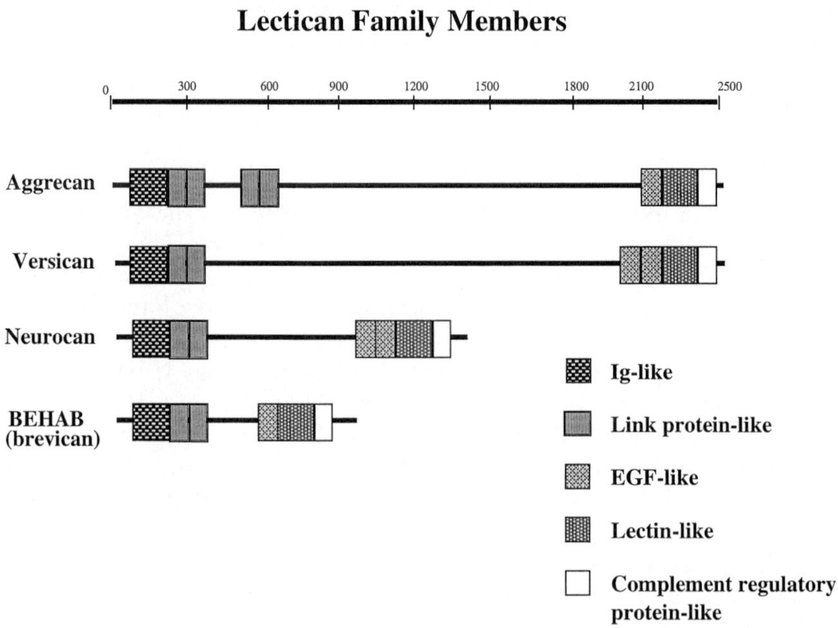

FIG. 4.1 BEHAB/brevican is a member of the lectican family of proteoglycans. The core proteins of the lecticans have several common structural features, with all members of this family sharing several highly conserved domains. Each lectican has both an N-terminal HA-binding domain (comprised of an Ig-like loop and two link proteoglycan-like repeats) and a C-terminal lectin-binding domain (comprised of an EGF-like repeat, a C-type lectin like domain, and a CRP-like domain). A central, non-homologous region that contains attachment sites for chrondroitin sulfate chains, joins the two termini. HA, hyaluronic acid; Ig, immunoglobulin; EGF, epidermal growth factor; CRP, complement regulatory protein.

prise an HA-binding domain. An epidermal growth factor (EGF)-like repeat, a C-type lectin-like domain, and a complement regulatory protein-like domain comprise the C-terminal region. The central region joining the two termini contains attachment sites for chondroitin sulfate chains. Unlike the N- and C-terminal domains, the central region is not conserved among lectican family members. Aggrecan and versican are expressed in brain as well as in other tissues, while both neurocan and BEHAB/brevican are expressed exclusively in brain (2, 9, 15, 20, 21).

BEHAB/brevican expression is markedly upregulated in human glioma. Here, we review the identification and characterization of this CNS-specific ECM element and address the possible role of BEHAB/brevican in mediating glioma invasion.

IDENTIFICATION OF THE BEHAB/BREVICAN GENE, ISOFORMS, AND PROTEIN

BEHAB/brevican was identified simultaneously by two independent laboratories. Yamada et al. used an antibody to a brain proteoglycan fraction to isolate a cDNA from a bovine brain expression library encoding brevican (32). Our laboratory, using polymerase chain reaction (PCR) and hybridization strategies based on the structure of the cartilage proteoglycan, aggrecan, isolated a cDNA encoding BEHAB from a rat brain library (13). Subsequent analysis demonstrated an identity between the 5' end of brevican (nucleotides 1-1381 of rat sequence) and BEHAB, which indicated that BEHAB and brevican are the same (14). Both laboratories identified a 3.6 kb mRNA whose sequence predicts a secreted member of the lectican family. A genomic clone of mouse BEHAB/brevican has been identified and characterized, and reveals a gene approximately 13 kb in length spanning 14 exons and located on murine chromosome 3 (22).

Following the initial identification of the BEHAB/brevican transcript, a second isoform was isolated by expression cloning using antisera to synaptic junction proteins (26). A 3.3 kb mRNA gives rise to this second isoform, with a sequence that predicts a glycophosphatidylinositol (GPI)–anchored protein. The genomic organization indicates that this alternative transcript is generated by a "no splice" event after exon 8, which results in a read-through of the transcript into intron 8. The resulting protein lacks all of the C-terminal domains found in the full length protein and has a unique C-terminus comprised of 21 amino acids, encoded by otherwise intronic sequence, that contains the signal for the GPI anchor. This is the only example of a GPI-anchored isoform among the lectican family.

The full-length rat BEHAB/brevican transcript encodes an 883 amino acid secreted protein that migrates at approximately 145 kDa (26, 27, 32). Structurally, the BEHAB/brevican protein is similar to the other lectican family members, with an N-terminal signal sequence followed by an HA-binding domain, a non-homologous central domain, and a C-terminus with an EGF repeat, a lectin-like domain, and a complement regulatory protein-like domain. The central domain contains 2 potential N-glycosylation sites, 4 potential GAG attachment sites, and a highly acidic, glutamate-rich region. A large proportion (approximately 20 to 50%) of both rat and bovine BEHAB/brevican does not have GAG chains, which results in the classification of BEHAB/brevican as a "part time" proteoglycan (27, 32).

In addition to post-translational processing of the BEHAB/brevican protein, proteolytic processing also occurs (23) (Fig. 4.2). While the central domain of BEHAB/brevican is largely non-homologous between species (68%

rat versus bovine), a stretch of 54 amino acids within the central domain shows 94% identity between rat and bovine. This highly conserved region harbors a 22 amino acid sequence that is 50% identical to a proteolytic cleavage site found in another lectican family member, aggrecan. Yamada et al. showed that BEHAB/brevican can be cleaved at this site and produces a 50 kD N-terminal fragment that contains the HA-binding domain, and a 80 kD C-terminal fragment (33). The protease that cleaves BEHAB/brevican at this site has been identified as a member of the ADAMTS family (Matthews et al., in press). The potential functional significance of this cleavage event will be discussed.

Based on the domain structure and similarities to other lecticans, the major functional roles of BEHAB/brevican are predicted to be binding of HA at the N-terminus and binding of lectins at the C-terminus. At the C-terminus, it has been shown that the lectin domain of BEHAB/brevican can mediate binding to tenascin-R and specific cell surface glycolipids (1, 19).

BEHAB/BREVICAN IN THE ADULT BRAIN

The adult rat, bovine, and cat brain express BEHAB/brevican at moderate levels (13, 32). In the rat brain, mRNA expression is relatively diffuse, with some regions (hippocampus, cerebellum, and some

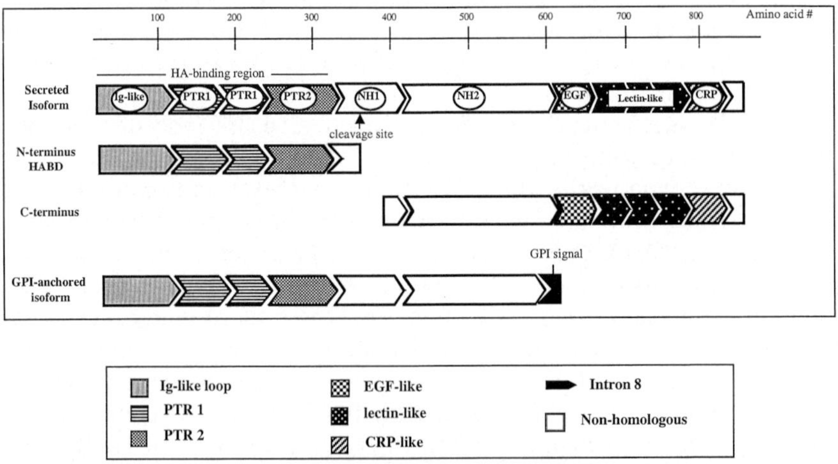

FIG. 4.2 Schematic diagram of BEHAB/brevican isoforms and proteolytic cleavage products. The cleavage site in the NH1 domain of the secreted isoform is indicated; the GPI-anchor signal is labeled on the GPI-anchored isoform. NH, nonhomologous; PTR, proteoglycan tandem repeat; GPI, glycosylphosphatidylinositol.

brainstem nuclei) exhibiting higher levels of expression. In the cerebellar cortex, the BEHAB/brevican protein is detected on the surface of astrocytes that form neuroglia sheaths around glomeruli (31). An in situ hybridization study has indicated that there is cell type-specific processing of the BEHAB/brevican transcript in the adult rat, with the secreted isoform expressed predominantly by neurons, and the GPI-anchored isoform expressed predominantly by glia (25).

BEHAB/BREVICAN SHOWS MARKED UPREGULATION AT TIMES OF INCREASED GLIAL CELL MOTILITY

During development, neurons and glia are highly motile as they migrate through the soluble, immature matrix to reach their mature locations. In the rat, BEHAB/brevican expression increases during the first two weeks after birth, reaching adult levels by postnatal day 21 (13, 15, 26, 31). While the overall level of BEHAB/brevican mRNA is low during the late embryonic and early postnatal period, a very high level of expression is concentrated in the proliferative ventricular zone. The highest level of BEHAB/brevican expression coincides with the peak of gliogenesis in each region of the brain examined (15).

In response to CNS injury, glial cell processes extend into and around the injury site. This increase in glial cell motility is accompanied by an upregulation of proteins expressed by mature glia, such as glial fibrillary acidic protein (GFAP), as well as reexpression of proteins normally found in immature glia, such as nestin (8, 5, 31). In a CNS-injury model, BEHAB/brevican is upregulated in glial cells immediately adjacent to the site of injury, with a time course and distribution that parallel the upregulation of nestin (16). Only the secreted isoform is upregulated in response to injury; the level of expression of the GPI-anchored isoform shows no regulation.

In addition to injury, glial cells also assume a more immature, motile state in primary brain tumors. Primary brain tumors, including astrocytoma, oligodendroglioma, and glioblastoma, are all derived from glial cells and are collectively referred to as gliomas. These cells are highly motile and move away from the primary tumor locus to invade normal brain tissue and establish new tumor focii. The highly invasive nature of glioma makes these tumors refractory to conventional therapies. BEHAB/brevican expression is upregulated in these invasive tumors.

CHARACTERIZATION OF BEHAB/BREVICAN IN HUMAN GLIOMA

In surgical samples of human gliomas, BEHAB/brevican expression is dramatically and consistently upregulated over the level of expression in the normal adult brain (17). Over 65 surgical samples of neuropathologically confirmed gliomas were examined and all showed an upregulation of BEHAB/brevican. Importantly, BEHAB/brevican mRNA is undetectable in tumors that are not of glial origin, including CNS lymphoma, meningioma, and primary cancers of the lung, colon, and breast. Non-glial tumors from peripheral locations growing within the brain, such as brain metastases of breast cancer, do not express detectable levels of BEHAB/brevican. Therefore, BEHAB/brevican is expressed selectively and specifically by brain tumors of glial origin.

The expression of BEHAB/brevican in surgical samples of human glioma has interesting parallels in experimental glioma models. When grown under standard tissue culture conditions, none of over 20 differ-

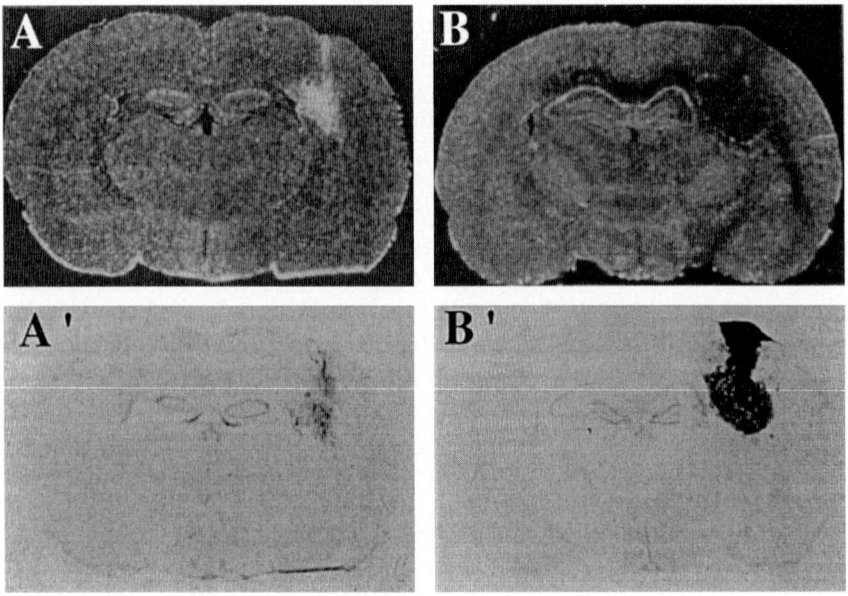

FIG. 4.3 Intracranial tumors of cell lines that show an invasive phenotype express BEHAB/brevican mRNA, whereas tumors of cell lines that show a noninvasive phenotype do not. Top panels show in situ hybridization with a ^{35}S-labeled BEHAB/brevican cRNA probe on sections through the forebrain of animals 2 to 4 weeks following intracranial injections of CNS-1 (A) and 9L (B) cells. Lower panels show corresponding sections stained with cresyl violet to visualize regions of high cell density, demonstrating the location of tumors that developed from the injected cells. The intracranial cell mass in animals injected with CNS-1 cells has indistinct boundaries, with cells invading the surrounding brain tissue (A'); these invasive tumors express BEHAB/brevican (A). In contrast, the cell mass in an animal injected with 9L cells has relatively distinct boundaries, with cells confined to an area corresponding to the injection site (B'); these noninvasive tumors do not express BEHAB/brevican (B).

ent human and rodent glioma cell lines expresses BEHAB/brevican (17). When glioma cell lines are grown as rodent intracranial grafts, two distinct tumor phenotypes are observed—a non-invasive growth pattern, which resembles that of brain metastases of non-glial-derived tumors and an invasive phenotype that resembles the diffuse growth pattern of human gliomas (Fig. 4.3). Those cell lines with an invasive tumor phenotype express BEHAB/brevican in vivo; cell lines that grow as non-invasive tumors do not express it. Moreover, the same cell lines that upregulate BEHAB/brevican expression as invasive intracranial tumors do not express BEHAB/brevican when grown as subcutaneous tumors (17). From these results we have concluded that expression of BEHAB/brevican correlates with an invasive phenotype and that this expression is regulated by a brain-derived factor. The high levels of BEHAB/brevican expression coincident with gliogenesis, in response to injury, and in both human and rodent glioma suggest that the upregulation of this matrix molecule reflects the elaboration of an ECM that is permissive for increased cell movement, an important step in the progression of primary brain tumor.

CLEAVAGE OF BEHAB/BREVICAN AND GLIOMA INVASION

The BEHAB/brevican protein is cleaved in the normal rat brain (as previously described) and in both human glioma and invasive rodent glioma models. To study the role of BEHAB/brevican expression and cleavage in glioma invasion, we used a rat brain tumor model (35). The non-invasive, 9L gliosarcoma cell line does not express BEHAB/brevican in culture or as intracranial grafts. 9L cells were transfected with transgenes encoding either full-length BEHAB/brevican or an amino-terminal fragment containing the HA-binding domain (HABD). The full-length BEHAB/brevican protein produced in 9L cells was not cleaved in culture or in intracranial grafts, thus providing a system to differentiate the effects of full-length BEHAB/brevican from the effects of the cleavage products. When grown as intracranial grafts, 9L cells expressing full-length, uncleaved, BEHAB/brevican produced non-invasive tumors similar to the tumors produced by control 9L cells, with very few cell clusters located beyond the border of the tumor. In contrast, 9L cells expressing the HABD fragment produced invasive tumors with cell clusters extending well beyond the main tumor mass.

These results, together with the observation that cleavage of BEHAB/brevican occurs in invasive rodent and human gliomas, strongly suggest that the products of BEHAB/brevican cleavage are associated with an invasive phenotype. Moreover, they are consistent with a two-component mechanism for BEHAB/brevican's role in brain tumor cell invasion, which requires both an upregulation of BEHAB/brevican expression and proteolytic cleavage of the protein.

CONCLUSIONS

The glioma-specific expression of BEHAB/brevican in humans makes this molecule a potential therapeutic target. In addition to strategies based on the BEHAB/brevican gene or its products, the apparent requirement of cleavage for invasion suggests another therapeutic avenue—targeting the protease responsible for this cleavage. Functional inhibition of BEHAB/brevican might slow the migration of tumor cells from the original tumor site(s), thereby increasing the efficacy of regional therapies, such as surgery or focal irradiation.

REFERENCES

1. Asperg A, Miura R, Bourdoulous S, Shimonaka M, Heinegard D, Schachner M, Ruoslahti E, Yamaguchi Y: The C-type lectin domains of lecticans, a family of aggregating chondroitin sulfate proteoglycans, bind tenascin-R by protein-protein interactions independent of carbohydrate moiety. **Proc Natl Acad Sci** 94: 10116–10121, 1997.
2. Bignami A, Perides G, Rahemtulla F: Versican, a hyaluronate-binding proteoglycan of embryonal precartilaginous mesenchyme is mainly expressed postnatally in rat brain. **J Neurosci** 34:97–106, 1993.
3. Celio MR, Spreafico R, De Biasi S, Vitellaro-Zuccarello L: Perineuronal nets: Past and present. **Trends Neurosci** 21:510–515, 1998.
4. Delpech B, Delpech A, Bruckner G, Girard N, Maingonnat C: Hyaluronan and hyaluronectin in the nervous system, in Evered D, Whelan J, (ed). *The Biology of Hyaluronan, Ciba Foundation Symposium No. 143.* Wiley, Chichester, 1989, pp 208–232.
5. Giordana MT, Attanasio A, Cavalla P, Migheli A, Vigliani MC, Schiffer D: Reactive cell proliferation and microglia following injury to rat brain. **Neuropath Appl Neurobiol** 20:163–174, 1994.
6. Goldbrunner RH, Bernstein JJ, Tonn JC: Cell-extracellular matrix interactions in glioma invasion. **Acta Neurochir** 141:295–305, 1999.
7. Hardingham TE, Fosang AJ: Proteoglycans: Many forms and many functions. **Fed Am Soc Exp Biol** 6:861–870, 1992.
8. Hatten ME, Liem RKH, Shelanski ML, Mason CA: Astroglia in CNS injury. **Glia** 4:233–243, 1991.
9. Hennig AK, Mangoura D, Schwartz NB: Large chondroitin sulfate proteoglycans of developing chick CNS are expressed in cerebral hemisphere neuronal cultures. **Dev Brain Res** 73:261–272, 1993.
10. Herndon ME, Lander AD: A diverse set of developmentally regulated proteoglycans is expressed in the rat central nervous system. **Neuron** 4:949–961, 1990.
11. Hockfield S, Zaremba S, Kalb RG, Fryer H: Expression of neural proteoglycans correlates with the acquisition of mature neuronal properties in the mammalian brain. **Cold Spring Harb Symp Quant Biol** 55:505–514, 1990.
12. Iozzo RV: Matrix proteoglycans: From molecular design to cellular function. **Annu Rev Biochem** 67:609–652, 1998.
13. Jaworski DM, Kelly GM, Hockfield S: BEHAB, a new member of the proteoglycan

tandem repeat family of hyaluronan binding proteins, is restricted to the brain. **J Cell Biol** 125:495–509, 1994.
14. Jaworski DM, Kelly GM, Hockfield S: The CNS-specific hyaluronan binding protein, BEHAB, is expressed during periods of glial cell generation and motility. **Semin Neurosci** 8:391–396, 1996.
15. Jaworski DM, Kelly GM, Hockfield S: The CNS specific hyaluronan-binding protein, BEHAB, is expressed in ventricular zones coincident with gliogenesis. **J Neurosci** 15:1352–1362, 1995.
16. Jaworski DM, Kelly GM, Hockfield S: Intracranial injury acutely induces the expression of the secreted isoform of the CNS-specific hyaluronan-binding protein BEHAB/brevican. **Exp Neurol** 157:327–337, 1999.
17. Jaworski DM, Kelly GM, Piepmeier JM, Hockfield S: BEHAB (brain enriched hyaluronan binding) is expressed in surgical samples of glioma oand intracranial grafts of invasive glioma cell lines. **Cancer Res** 56:2293–2298, 1996.
18. LeBaron RG, Zimmermann DR, Ruoslahti E: Hyaluronate binding properties of versican. **J Biol Chem** 267:10003–10010, 1992.
19. Miura R, Aspberg A, Ethell IM et al: The proteoglycan lectin domain binds sulfated cell surface glycolipids and promotes cell adhesion. J Biol Chem 274:11431–11438, 1999.
20. Rauch U, Gao P, Janetzko A, Flaccus A, Hilgenberg L, Tekotte H, Margolis RK, Margolis RU: Isolation and characterization of developmentally regulated chondroitin sulfate and chondroitin/keratan sulfate proteoglycans of brain identified with monoclonal antibodies. **J Biol Chem** 266:14785–14801, 1991.
21. Rauch U, Karthikeyan L, Maurel P, Margolis RU, Margolis RK: Cloning and primary structure of neurocan, a developmentally regulated, aggregating chondroitin sulfate proteoglycan of brain. **J Biol Chem** 267:19536–19547, 1992.
22. Rauch U, Meyer H, Brakebusch C, Seidenbecher C, Gundelfinger ED, Beier DR, Fässler R: Sequence and chromosomal localization of the mouse brevican gene. **Genomics** 44:15–21, 1997.
23. Rutka JT, Apadaca G, Stern R, Rosenblum M: The extracellular matrix of the central and peripheral nervous systems: Structure and function. **J Neurosurg** 69: 155–170, 1992.
24. Schiffer D, Giordana MT, Cavalla P, Vigliani MC Attanasio A: Immunohistochemistry of glial reaction after injury in the rat: Double stainings and markers of cell proliferation. **Int J Dev Neurosci** 11:269–280, 1993.
25. Seidenbecher CI, Gundelfinger ED, Böckers TM, Trotter J, Kreutz M: Transcripts for secreted and GPI-anchored brevican are differentially distributed in rat brain. **Eur J Neurosci** 10:1621–1630, 1998.
26. Seidenbecher CI, Richter K, Rauch U, Fassler R, Garner CC, Gundelfinger ED: Brevican, a chondroitin sulfate proteoglycan of rat brain, occurs as secreted and cell surface glycosylphosphatidylinositol-anchored isoforms. **J Biol Chem** 270: 27206–27212, 1995.
27. Sheppard AM, Hamilton SK, Perlman AL: Changes in distribution of extracellular matrix components accompany early morphogenetic events of mammalian cortical development. **J Neurosci** 11:3928–3942, 1991.
28. Sur M, Frost D, Hockfield S: Expression of a cell surface antigen in Y-cells in the cat lateral geniculate nucleus is regulated by visual experience. **J Neurosci** 8:874–882, 1988.
29. Uhm JH, Dooley NP, Villemure GJ, Yong VW: Mechanisms of glioma invasion: Role of matrix metalloproteinases. **Can J Neurol** 24:3–15, 1997.
30. Wight TN, Heinegard DK, Hascall VC: Proteoglycans: Structure and function, in Hay

ED (ed). *Cell Biology of Extracellular Matrix, 2nd Edition.* New York, Plenum Press, 1991, pp 45–78.
31. Yamada H, Fredette B, Shitara K, Hagihara K, Miura R, Ranscht B, Stallcup WB, Yamaguchi Y: The brain chondroitin sulfate proteoglycan brevican associates with astrocytes ensheathing cerebellar glomeruli and inhibits neurite outgrowth from granule neurons. **J Neurosci** 17:7784–7795, 1997.
32. Yamada H, Watanabe K, Shimonaka M, Yamaguchi Y: Molecular cloning of brevican, a novel brain proteoglycan of aggrecan/versican family. **J Biol Chem** 269: 10119–10126, 1994.
33. Yamada H, Watanabe K, Shimonaka M, Yamasaki M, Yamaguchi Y: cDNA cloning and the identification of an aggrecanase-like cleavage site in rate brevican. **Biochem Biophys Res Commun** 216:957–963, 1995.
34. Yamaguchi Y: Brevican: A major proteoglycan in adult brain. **Perspect Dev Neurobiol** 93:307–317, 1996.
35. Zhang H, Kelly G, Zerillo C, Jaworski DM, Hockfield S: Expression of a cleaved brain-specific extracellular matrix protein mediates glioma cell invasion in vivo. **J Neurosci** 18:2370–2376, 1998.

CHAPTER

5

The Future of Pituitary Surgery

HAE-DONG JHO, M.D., PH.D., IN-SUNG PARK, M.D., PH.D., ALESSANDRA ALFIERI, M.D.

INTRODUCTION

Various routes of surgical access to the pituitary fossa (transcranial and transsphenoidal) were explored in the early developmental stages of the 1900s, with the modern surgical techniques of transsphenoidal surgery being developed around 1910. Among those surgical techniques, sublabial transseptal transsphenoidal surgery became the most favored. Although transcranial surgery had been the preference in the treatment of sellar disorders between the 1930s to 1960s, transsphenoidal surgery was revived in the 1960s. When the operating microscope was adopted in transsphenoidal surgery in the 1960s, microscopic transsphenoidal surgery became the standard conventional surgical treatment for pituitary tumors (7). Mucosal dissection from the nasal septum, the use of a transsphenoidal retractor, postoperative nasal packing for two to three days, and an average of three to five days of hospitalization have been routine in standard microscopic transsphenoidal surgery. Among the various neurosurgical cranial operations, microscopic transsphenoidal surgery is known to be relatively benign, with good surgical outcomes and minimal morbidities (2).

Although the treatment modality for pituitary adenomas will continue to change from surgical to medical, in the meantime, the well-known benign nature of microscopic transsphenoidal surgery still requires further improvement. Microadenomas that cause Cushing's disease are sometimes difficult to locate intraoperatively, and sometimes are not consistent with localized findings suggested by preoperative petrosal venous sampling. When a pituitary adenoma produces excessive amounts of a hormone, the completeness of tumor removal can not be assured intraoperatively. Balancing complete tumor removal with the preservation of normal pituitary gland function has been the struggle for surgeons when removing those types of adenomas. The surgical outcome with large hormonally hyperactive pituitary adenomas that are extended beyond the pituitary fossa is dismal when compared to that of microadenomas. Removal of large pituitary adenomas, even if they are hormonally nonfunctioning, often results in subtotal resection by microscopic transsphenoidal surgery. Although the surgical treatment of pituitary adenomas invading the cavernous sinus has been reported sporadically, those tumors are generally regarded as surgically incurable. The complication rates related to microscopic transsphenoidal surgery have been known to be low; however, further reduction is also desirable.

The surgical results involving pituitary adenomas may improve further in the future, even if marginal, by the adoption of intraoperative imaging-guidance or real-time imaging, intraoperative immunoradiometric hormonal assay for the assurance of complete tumor removal, and better surgical exposure and visualization of the pathology intraoperatively. The adoption of an endonasal surgical route will eliminate the use of nasal packing and subsequently provide comfort to patients. The low surgical complication rates of microscopic pituitary surgery may be further reduced by adoption of an endonasal route, intraoperative image-guidance or real-time magnetic resonance imaging (MRI), improved surgical instruments, and direct endoscopic visualization of the hidden surgical site. In this paper, the authors present their view on how the use of endoscopy will make further improvements in transsphenoidal pituitary surgery and include a brief review of other current developments.

THE CONCEPT OF BIOECOLOGICAL SURGERY

Over the years, neurosurgeons have been debating radicalism versus minimalism as surgical strategies in the treatment of neurosurgical disorders. Radicalists believe that when serious cranial and spinal disorders are dealt with, extensive radical exposure towards pathology is a correct and justifiable approach, despite increased risks and protracted recovery time. Minimalists argue that minimally invasive strategy provides maximum benefits with quick recovery. The "moderates" have intervened into the debate and state that that surgical exposure should be adequate and precise, neither less nor excessive. Although all share a similar ideology to provide the "best care" to patients via their respective surgical strategies, their ideologies of surgical treatment do not accurately connote the intent of surgeons.

Just as the ecosystem maintains its balance in nature, the human body has a balanced homeostatic equilibrium of organs named the "bioecology of the human body." When this balance is well maintained, it may be called healthy. When the balance is disrupted locally or systemically, it becomes a diseased condition. When this diseased condition requires repair, repair should be performed in an ideal manner with "bioecological surgery." The ideal treatment should render complete restoration of "bioecology," or "cure." The treatment itself should only, or if at all, minimally disturb the remaining bioecology. The treatment itself should not carry significant risk to the patient in the process. Quick, full functional recovery should follow. The treatment must be cost-effective as well. Each treatment modality for certain diseases can be graded or given a score (range 0–100) relative to these criteria: 1) the ability of the treatment to restore "bioecology," 2) factors of the treatment that will disturb the remaining bioecology, 3) treatment risk, 4) estimated recovery, and 5) degree of cost effectiveness.

When different surgical treatments are compared to each other for the treatment of certain disease, the grading of each of these items may vary from treatment to treatment. For example, when microsurgery is compared to gamma-knife surgery for the treatment of acoustic neurilemmomas, each of the criteria would be scored quite differently. Microsurgery may eliminate tumors completely but with increased disturbance to the remaining bioecology, increased surgical risk, and delayed recovery. Gamma-knife surgery rates are proportionately opposite. When microscopic transsphenoidal surgery is judged by the criteria set for "bioecological surgery," it seems to be quite satisfactory when compared to other neurosurgical treatments. Long-term cure rates of microadenomas range from 70% to 90%. Impact on the body by the surgical procedure itself is relatively minimal when compared to that performed by transcranial surgery. The incidences of mortality and major morbidity related to this operation are acceptable. Functional recovery is fairly quick and the hospital stay is relatively short. The treatment cost for microscopic transsphenoidal surgery has been modest. It would seem that the maximal benefit from surgical treatment has already been accomplished by pioneering microneurosurgeons. There seems to be no further room for improvement that could be obtained by any other surgical means. However, the authors believe that this already excellent procedure could be improved.

INTRAOPERATIVE IMAGE-GUIDANCE OR REAL-TIME IMAGING

The surgical trajectory of microscopic transsphenoidal surgery has been traditionally guided by the use of intraoperative fluoroscopic C-arm imaging. Fluoroscopic lateral-view imaging of the head directs the surgeon straight toward the sella when performing the mucosal dissection of the nasal septum. Since this fluoroscopic imaging provides only the lateral view of the head, lateral deviation of the surgical trajectory can occur when the nasal septum is deviated to one side or when the sphenoidal sinus is not well pneumatized. This deviation of the midline surgical trajectory in microscopic transsphenoidal surgery can result in devastating surgical complications. Recently, an intraoperative frameless image guidance system has been used instead of a fluoroscopic C-arm (4). The advantage of an intraoperative image guidance system is its capability to provide three-dimensional anatomical information related to preobtained images that are most often MR images. This information can guide the surgeon to a precise surgical trajectory as well as disclose the dimensions of the tumor. In addition to added cost, mandatory preoperative image acquisition with the placement of fiducial markers is one of the drawbacks of its use. Image-guided systems that do not require fiducial markers exist; however, their accuracy remains to be proven.

Intraoperative real-time MRI has been used to assist surgeons in achieving complete tumor removal. Recently, two centers reported the usefulness of intraoperative MRI to confirm successful tumor removal (15, 18) Although intraoperative MRI can document gross residual pathology, the image quality of the MRI seems to require further improvement in order for one to comprehend the minute details at the operative area. Ghost images related to the operation itself, such as a blood filled tumor-resection-cavity, may mimic residual tumor. However, the concept of real-time intraoperative imaging seems to be promising once a user-friendly, improved version of an MR unit can be installed in the operating room. Recently, a 1.5-tesla mobile MR unit was reported to provide improved quality of images (19). The use of intraoperative ultrasound imaging has been reported to be useful in detection of a minute adenoma that causes Cushing's disease. Further technological advances seem to be required in order to create a doppler probe that can be placed through a narrow surgical corridor. The use of a transcranial doppler has been reported as the means to verify improved blood flow through the anterior cerebral artery system when adequate decompression is accomplished by the removal of a suprasellar tumor (17). However, direct visualization of the suprasellar tumor via an angled endoscope seems to be the better way for such verification.

INTRAOPERATIVE HORMONAL ASSAY

The half-life of adrenocorticotropic hormone (ACTH), growth hormone, and prolactin is relatively short, ranging from 15 to 30 minutes. The use of intraoperative radioimmunoassay of ACTH from the peritumoral blood has been reported as a means of tumor detection (14). Recently, immunoradiometric assay of ACTH has been used as an indicator of complete tumor removal when ACTH-secreting bronchial carcinoid tumors were removed. The rapid intraoperative measurement of hormonal levels enables the surgeon to assure the completeness of tumor removal when intraoperative hormonal levels are measured prior to and after tumor removal (16). When intraoperative ACTH measurements were performed after tumor removal in 18 patients with Cushing's disease, a sensitivity value of 82%, specificity of 71% and, diagnostic accuracy of 78% were observed (5). Although a significant decrease of ACTH value was noted intraoperatively after tumor removal in the cured group, the conclusion of that report was that the decline of intraoperative ACTH after tumor removal did not accurately predict complete tumor removal. In this study, the first intraoperative ACTH value was measured after tumor removal and blood samples were obtained serially thereafter to compare to the first measurement. The predictive power of the ACTH value after tumor removal might have been stronger if the first measurement would have been started earlier than with actual tumor removal. Although there have been no reports regarding intraoperative measurement of prolactin and growth hormone levels, these measurements can be performed in less than half the time required to measure an ACTH level. This report is still encouraging in that the rapid intraoperative measurement of ACTH, prolactin, and growth hormone may assist the surgeon in assuring the completeness of tumor removal intraoperatively. Hormonal assay can be performed either as a plain measurement or as provocative testing.

ENDOSCOPY IN PITUITARY SURGERY

Although pituitary endoscopy is still in a developmental stage, the use of an endoscope in pituitary surgery has proven to be quite promising since adopted by Jho in 1993. (1, 8–13). The adoption of an endoscope in transsphenoidal surgery allows the easy use of an endonasal route as a surgical corridor. Its use eliminates the use of a transsphenoidal retractor, intraoperative fluoroscopic C-arm, and postoperative nasal packing. In addition, it provides a wide panoramic view at the posterior wall of the sphenoidal sinus, has the capability of providing a view inside the sella or tumor cavity, renders a direct angled view at the suprasellar region as well as other anatomical corners, and allows flexibility in approaching the anterior cranial base, cavernous sinus, and clival posterior fossa. The authors strongly believe that endoscopic pituitary surgery will become the future surgical technique for transsphenoidal pituitary surgery. The wide range of surgical accessibility by this endoscopic technique will make rare the occasional indication of craniotomy for treatment of pituitary tumors. The following are the advantages of endoscopic endonasal transsphenoidal pituitary surgery that we have observed.

The Use of an Endonasal Route

An endonasal route has been reported for microscopic transsphenoidal surgery (3, 6). Microscopic surgery requires a straight surgical corridor. From the surgical target to the objective lens of the operating microscope, the cross-sectional diameter of the straight surgical corridor has to be sufficient in size in order to allow the target image to travel through the optical system. The minimal width of a surgical corridor required for microscopic surgery depends proportionally on its length to the surgical target. To serve that purpose, the use of a transsphenoidal retractor is essential for microscopic surgery. An endoscope has the physical advantage in that the light source and target images travel through the endoscope shaft, which is only a few millimeters in diameter. The natural anatomical curves along the nasal cavity accommodate the passage of an endoscope. The tip of the endoscope is the only essential part of the instrument that needs to be placed close to the surgical target. This intrinsic optical advantage eliminates the use of a transsphenoidal retractor when an endonasal route is adopted to reach the pituitary. When the tip of an endoscope is placed in front of the sella through a small anterior sphenoidotomy hole via one nostril, surgical instruments are passed next to the endoscope shaft through the same nostril. The surgical landmark that leads to the sella is the middle turbinate. Direct posterior extension of the inferior margin of the middle turbinate will lead to the clival indentation at 10 mm below the sellar floor. An anterior sphenoidotomy is tailored approximately 10 to 15 mm rostrally from the inferior margin of the middle turbinate. Although the sphenoidal ostium is identifiable during the surgical procedure, it is difficult to use as a useful surgical landmark. This distinct nasal anatomy eliminates the use of a fluoroscopic C-arm or image-guidance stereotaxy in approaching the sella. The adoption of an endonasal route completely eliminates the traditional use of nasal packing, which has been used to approximate the dissected septal mucosa together when a transseptal route is used for microscopic surgery. Adoption of this endonasal route in transsphenoidal pituitary surgery makes postoperative nasal packing unnecessary, provides patient comfort postoperatively, and enhances quick postoperative recovery.

Endoscopic Panoramic View at the Posterior Wall of the Sphenoidal Sinus

Another reason why the use of an intraoperative fluoroscopic C-arm is not necessary in ordinary pituitary adenoma surgery is that an endoscope provides a wide panoramic view at the posterior wall of the sphenoidal sinus, as long as the sphenoidal sinus is well pneumatized. When an endoscope is placed through an anterior sphenoidotomy hole, the first recognizable structure is the clival indentation. Rostral to the clival indentation is the sellar floor, sella, tuberculum sellae, and planum sphenoidale (in that order) as the midline vertical compartment. At the lateral banks of the clival indentation, the carotid artery protuberances are also easily recognizable. Rostral to the carotid protuberances, the paramedian vertical compartment is the broader bony wall that covers the carotid siphon just lateral to the sella, optic nerve protuberance, and lateral planum sphenoidale, in that order. The carotico-optic recess is another consistent landmark that leads to the identification of the optic nerve, carotid artery, and cavernous sinus apex.

When an endoscope is directed laterally, the lateral vertical compartment of the posterior wall of the sphenoidal sinus is under the surgeon's direct view. This includes the optic nerve, cavernous sinus anterior apex, superior orbital fissure, orbital apex, maxillary trigeminal nerve, vidian nerve, foramen lacerum, mandibular trigeminal nerve, and eustachian tube in order from a rostral to caudal direction (Figure 5.1). This obvious anatomy eliminates the use of a fluoroscopic C-arm when the surgeon approaches the sella. It may reduce unexpected damage of the carotid artery, which rarely occurs during a microscopic transseptal approach, which only provides narrow, limited exposure at the sella.

Close-up View Inside Pathology

When tumor in the sella is removed and pituitary tissue in the sella is preserved, an endoscope can be advanced into the sella or tumor resection cavity. This will provide a close-up view at the juncture of tumor and pituitary tissue. Minute crumbs of tumor can be identified and removed. Most often, this tiny tumor tissue can be visualized at the folded region of the diaphragma sella when this diaphragma, or dome of the tumor, descends down into the sella. A cotton patty can be inserted into the sella or tumor cavity and pushed against the descending diaphragma or tumor dome in order to inspect various corners inside the tumor cavity. This thorough direct inspection may improve surgical outcome for macroadenomas.

Direct Angled View of Hidden Anatomical Corners

In microscopic surgery, the visualization of the sellar content is along the surgical trajectory in a slightly cephalad-inclined anteroposterior direction. Although a highly magnified microscopic view may provide more clearly defined images of the anatomy at the directed surgical tar-

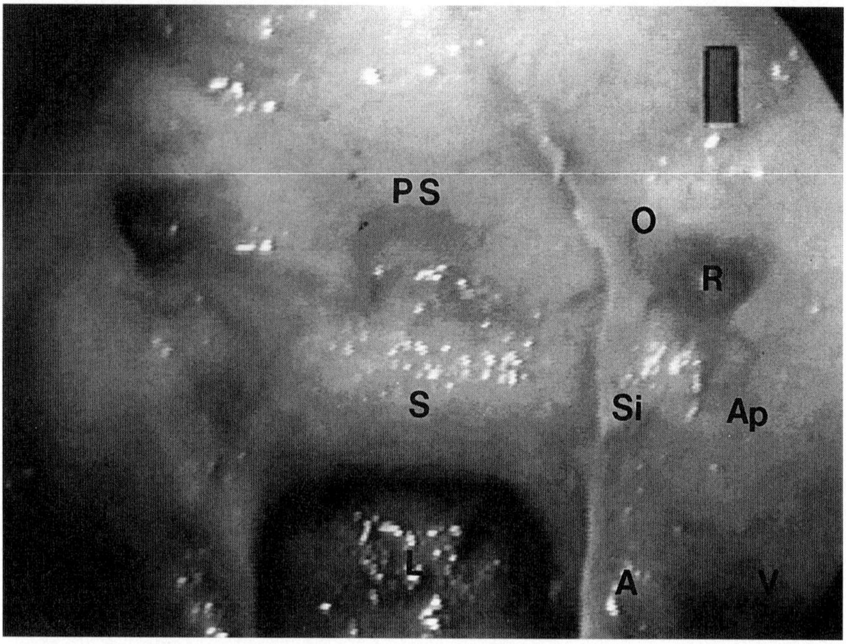

FIG. 5.1 Panoramic view: When an endoscope is inserted into the sphenoidal sinus, a panoramic endoscopic view discloses the clival indentation (L), sella (S), and planum sphenoidale (PS) at the midline vertical compartment; the carotid protuberances (A), cavernous sinuses (Si), and medial optic protuberances (O) at the paramedian vertical compartment; and the carotico-optic recess (R), lateral optic canal, cavernous sinus anterior apex (Ap), maxillary division of the trigeminal nerve (V) at the lateral vertical compartment. These clear anatomical landmarks make intraoperative use of the fluoroscopic C-arm unnecessary.

get than an endoscopic view, the microscopic view can not directly visualize the suprasellar region or lateral wall of the sella. In endoscopic pituitary tumor surgery, a pituitary adenoma located in the sella is removed under a 0-degree endoscope, which still provides a wider angled view than the operating microscope. When a suprasellar tumor does not descend down by brain pulsation even after tumor removal in the sella, an angled endoscope can be directed toward the suprasellar region. This angled endoscope will provide a direct view of the suprasellar portion of the tumor. This suprasellar portion of the tumor is excised under direct endoscopic visualization. When an angled endoscope is rotated to the lateral wall, the medial wall of the cavernous sinus will be under direct view (Figure 5.2). When the endoscope is rotated toward the sellar floor, it also can visualize the floor of the sella. However, this

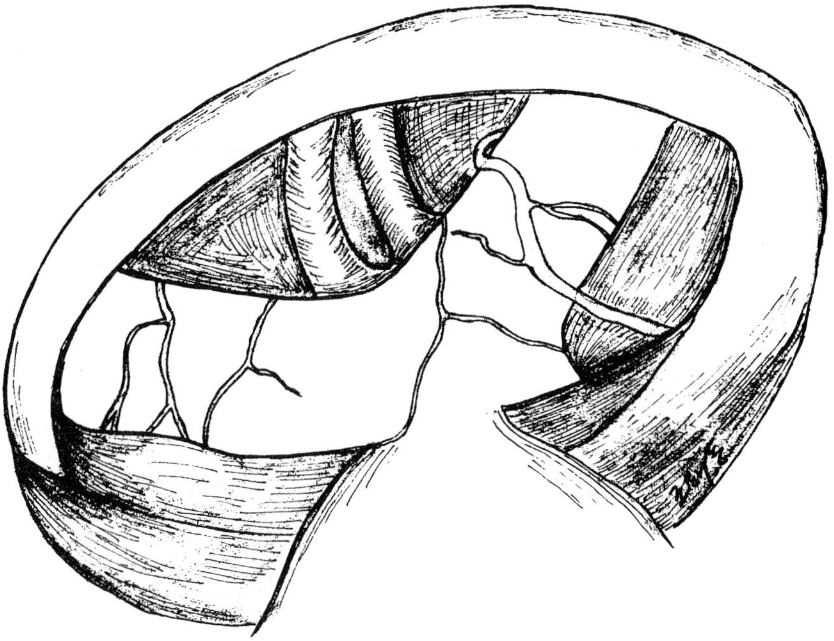

FIG. 5.2 Angled view to hidden anatomical corners: When an angled endoscope (usually a 30 degree lens endoscope) is directed towards the surgical target, it will visualize the object directly. The suprasellar region can be visualized by directing an angled endoscope rostrally and the medial wall of the cavernous sinus can be visualized by directing it laterally. This schematic drawing depicts the optic system and anterior cerebral arteries through the diaphragma sella after tumor removal.

method of visualizing the sellar floor is not necessary since endoscopic pituitary surgery exposes the floor of the sella completely from the onset of tumor removal. The capability for angled endoscopic viewing may make intraoperative MRI unnecessary.

Flexibility of an Endoscopic Surgical Trajectory

When angled endoscopic visualization still does not allow complete tumor removal due to the solid, fibrotic nature of a tumor, direct surgical exposure can be easily made toward the anterior cranial fossa to access the suprasellar portion of the tumor, as well as toward the cavernous sinus or clival region (Figure 5.3).

A surgical approach to the anterior cranial base can be made with an ethmoidectomy in addition to an anterior sphenoidotomy. An endoscopic endonasal surgical approach can access the anterior cranial fossa up to the crista galli rostrally. Among the three different surgical

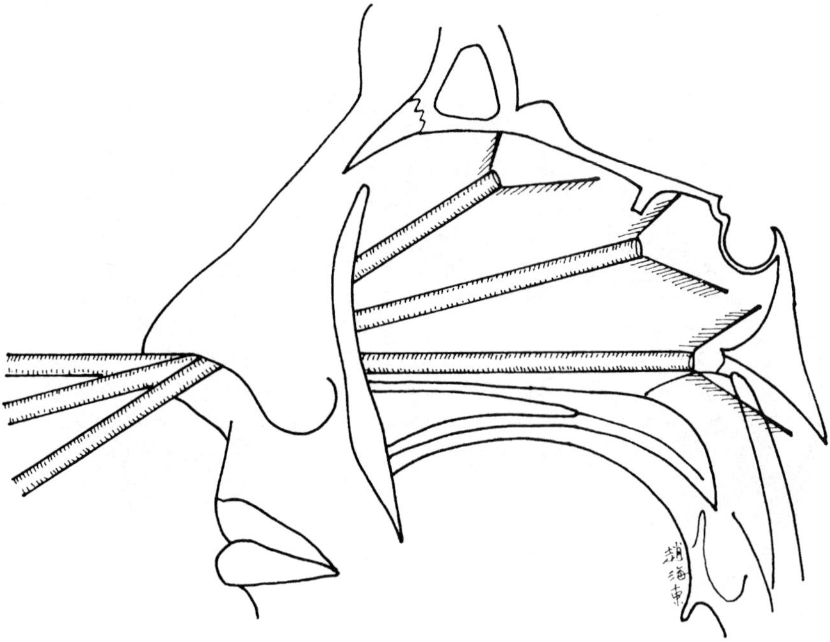

FIG. 5.3 This schematic drawing demonstrates various surgical trajectories that allow a direct endoscopic endonasal approach to the anterior cranial fossa, cavernous sinus, and clivus, respectively, ranging from the crista galli to the foramen magnum

approaches, such as the middle meatal, middle turbinectomy, and paraseptal, we prefer the paraseptal approach that is used most commonly in transsphenoidal surgery. Once an anterior sphenoidotomy is finished through a paraseptal approach, as previously described, further rostral exposure is made by removal of the ethmoidal air cells. The exposure of the planum sphenoidale can be easily made by an additional posterior ethmoidectomy. However, the floor of the olfactory groove at the anterior cranial fossa base presents a relatively steep angled floor toward the surgeon. This direct surgical exposure of the anterior cranial fossa will allow the surgeon to dissect the suprasellar portion of the tumor from the surrounding neurovascular structures with microdissection techniques. This direct surgical exposure carries the burden of reconstruction of the anterior skull base to prevent cerebrospinal fluid (CSF) leak. Dural reconstruction has been performed with direct graft placement with nonpenetrating titanium microclips. However, these dural clips do not serve this function adequately because the shaft of the clip applier is often too short to reach the anterior skull base through an endonasal route. Further instrument development is necessary for dural suturing. Anterior skull base bone is reconstructed with autogenous bone or titanium mesh. The ethmoidectomy site and sphenoidal sinus are filled with abdominal fat graft to enforce the supportive structure.

The cavernous sinus is another common compartment into which pituitary adenomas extend. Pituitary adenomas can invade the cavernous sinus by simple bulging toward the lateral wall of the cavernous sinus inside the C-shaped carotid siphon, extension into the cavernous sinus cavity via a defect of the medial wall of the cavernous sinus, or by direct invasion of the surrounding dura mater. A bulged tumor can be removed without entering the cavernous sinus itself. As described earlier, an angled lens endoscope, when it is directed toward the medial wall of the cavernous sinus, will directly visualize the tumor and will confirm complete removal of tumor. When the medial wall of the cavernous sinus is not deeply laterally bulged, even a 0-degree lens endoscope can visualize the medial wall of the cavernous sinus directly due to the wide angled nature of an endoscopic view. When a tumor extends through a defect of the medial wall of the cavernous sinus, the tumor can be removed under direct visualization, as previously described. Often, the tumor removal is performed inside the C-shaped carotid loop. At the center of this carotid artery, the oculomotor and trochlear nerves pass toward the cavernous sinus anterior apex. Complete tumor removal is possible when the tumor extension occurs into the cavernous sinus through a medial wall defect. When tumor invades the cavernous sinus through direct invasion of the dura mater, complete tumor removal may not be possible; however, tumor mass reduction is still possible through direct exploration into the cavernous sinus, medial and lateral, to the carotid artery. This tumor reduction will allow focused radiation treatment, such as gamma-knife surgery, to be used as postoperative adjunctive therapy instead of fractionated conventional radiation treatment. When the carotid artery is exposed into the sphenoidal sinus after tumor removal at the cavernous sinus, the carotid artery is protected with an abdominal fat graft to prevent possible later erosion of the artery.

When a pituitary tumor invades the clival bone further caudally to the sella, this clival tumor also can be approached through an endonasal endoscopic approach. Caudal exploration can be performed up to the foramen magnum. Surgical exploration can be limited by lateral anatomy of the carotid artery and the hypoglossal nerve when the pathology is extended into the posterior cranial fossa. Tumor that has extended into the pterygoid fossa, infratemporal fossa, and temporal middle cranial fossa also can be approached through this endonasal endoscopic approach. The great flexibility of an endonasal endoscopic approach is quite promising when the surgeon desires to avoid extensive skull base approaches to the pathology.

Facets of Endoscopic Endonasal Transsphenoidal Surgery that Require Further Development

An endoscopic endonasal approach requires different surgical maneuvering techniques when compared to microscopic surgery. Neurosurgeons who are well-trained and familiar with microscopic transsphenoidal surgery will still require practice to overcome the steep learning curve that can be encountered in the use of an endoscope. An endoscope visualizes at deep anatomical corners effectively; however, operating under endoscopic visualization entails more than simple inspection of the site. The endoscopic shaft can be a continual hindrance when the surgeon tries to maneuver surgical instruments at the target area. This learning curve can be overcome only by practice.

Surgical instruments that are designed particularly for endoscopic surgery have to be developed to accommodate the physical characteristics of an endoscope. The tips of the surgical instruments have to be curved accordingly in order to be placed in front of the endoscope tip toward the surgical target. The ideal endoscope for transsphenoidal pituitary surgery has yet to be developed. The endoscopes that we have used are rod-lens sinonasal endoscopes that are 4 mm in diameter and 18 cm in length. The diameter of the rod-lens endoscope affects the clarity of the monitored image. Four or 5 mm diameter rod-lens endoscopes have proven to be adequate for this endonasal procedure. A flexible fibro-optic endoscope does not provide clear images. Since a working channel endoscope has very limited value in pituitary surgery, the rod-lens endoscope is used without adopting a working-channel metallic sheath. A three-chip camera has improved the image quality over that of a one-chip camera; furthermore, when a high definition camera is eventually adopted with a brighter light source, the image quality of the monitored endoscopic images will improve further. Various image monitor systems are in the process of development, such as a head-mounted goggle monitor, a large screen projection monitor, a wide screen picture tube monitor, etc. Three-dimensional endoscopes have been useful. We have noted that wearing the spectacles for viewing three-dimensional endoscopic images for extended periods causes visual fatigue. We have used 5 mm three-dimensional endoscopes; however, at this time they are not commercially available. An ideally shaped endoscope has yet to be developed, particularly for endoscopic endonasal pituitary surgery.

The endoscope holder is an essential tool for endoscopic pituitary surgery. After anterior sphenoidotomy is completed, the endoscope is mounted to a rigid endoscope holder. This endoscope holder allows the neurosurgeon to use two hands to perform delicate dissection of tumor tissue from surrounding normal anatomy. Currently, two different types of endoscope holders are available. One is a manually locking type and the other is a pneumatic powered type. The manually locking holder is inexpensive and does not sag when the joints are tightened; however, multiple joints have to be released and tightened when the endoscope is repositioned. The joints and the endoscope holding terminal are not yet ergonomically designed. The pneumatic powered holder offers the convenience of easy control of the joints by the release of one button. However, when the button is released, the endoscope sags significantly enough to displace the endoscope tip from the point at which it was focused. Further improvement in the balance of the holding arm may solve this problem. In addition, a pneumatic powered holder is relatively expensive. A high-speed drill also has to be designed so it can accomplish efficient bone drilling through this particularly narrow, deep surgical corridor. As mentioned earlier, a dural suturing instrument also has to be developed for dural reconstruction at the skull base when a wide dural opening is made for extensive resection of tumors. When image-guided stereotaxy is used, its attachment has to be designed so it can function like an endoscope holder so as to display the anatomy on the computer screen without obstruction.

Although an endoscope cleansing device may not be essential in sinonasal operations, it is required for pituitary tumor operations when the surgeon desires to perform a relatively uninterrupted operation. The authors have used both first and second generation endoscope cleansing devices. The device consists of an irrigation pump, a disposable fluid-carrying tube, and an endoscope sheath. At one end, a disposable tube is connected into a saline bag that is hung on an pole, and then the proximal portion of this disposable tube is anchored to the irrigation pump. The other end of the tube is connected to the endoscope sheath through which an endoscope is inserted. The irrigation pump is controlled by a foot pedal. When the foot pedal is pressed, the irrigation pump passes saline fluid forward to the endoscope lens. When the foot pedal is released, the irrigation pump automatically draws back the fluid drops from the endoscope lens by reverse flow for a brief moment. Although it is not yet satisfactory, this endoscope cleansing device helps to maintain clarity of the endoscope lens during surgery. When the endoscopic image is blurry despite repeated irrigation with this cleansing device, the endoscope has to be withdrawn and cleaned manually. Overall, the future of endonasal endoscopic transsphenoidal surgery seems to be promising with the advent of high definition video monitors, improved computer technology, and newly refined surgical instruments.

Surgical Outcome in our Patient Series

Among our 160 patients who underwent endoscopic endonasal operations from 1993 through 1999, 128 patients had pituitary adenomas and the remaining patients had other skull base lesions. Among 128 patients with pituitary adenomas, 24 patients had recurrent tumors after previous transsphenoidal surgery. Hormone nonsecreting adenomas numbered 68, prolactinomas numbered 35, ACTH-secreting adenomas numbered 16, and growth-hormone secreting adenomas numbered 9. Thirty patients had microadenomas (23%). There were 24 intrasellar macroadenomas (19%), 41 macroadenomas with suprasellar extension (32%), and 33 invasive adenomas involving the cavernous sinus (26%). Among 68 patients with hormone nonsecreting adenomas, total removal was achieved in 53 (78%) patients and subtotal resection in 15 (22%) patients. Among 35 patients with prolactimonas, 21 (60%) patients had normal postoperative prolactin levels, 6 (17%) patients had mildly elevated prolactin levels, and 8 (23%) patients still required other treatment for elevated prolactin postoperatively. Among 16 patients with Cushing's disease, 11 patients completely resolved their symptoms with normalized 24-hour urinary-free cortisol and 5 patients had incomplete treatment that required other treatment, including gamma-knife surgery and medications. Among nine patients with acromegaly, eight patients had less than 2 ng/ml of postoperative growth hormone levels and one patient required gamma-knife surgery for incomplete treatment. Outpatient surgery was performed on two patients and 67% of 160 patients who underwent endonasal endoscopic surgery only stayed overnight in the hospital.The complications we encountered in our series included deterioration of anterior pituitary function (11%), CSF leak (4.5%), transient diabetes insipidus (4%), sinusitis (1%), synechia of the middle turbinate (1%) and delayed nasal bleeding (1%).

CONCLUSIONS

Although overall surgical outcome in our series of patients with endoscopic endonasal transsphenoidal surgery is comparable to that of microscopic surgery, we are very much encouraged by our patients' quick recovery and minimal postoperative discomfort. Surgical results of endoscopic pituitary surgery may further improve when surgical instrumentation is fully developed and the learning curve is overcome.

The authors believe that endoscopic endonasal surgery will be the future surgical technique for pituitary surgery.

ACKNOWLEDGMENTS

The authors wish to thank Arthur P. Nestler, B.S.N. and Robin Coret, B.A. for their assistance with preparation of the manuscript.

REFERENCES

1. Carrau RL, Jho HD, Ko Y: Transnasal-transsphenoidal endoscopic surgery of the pituitary gland. **Laryngoscope** 106:914–918, 1996.
2. Ciric I, Ragin A, Baumgartner C, Pierce D: Complication of transsphenoidal surgery: Results of a national survey, review of literature, and personal experience. **Neurosurgery** 40:225–237, 1997.
3. Cooke RS, Jones RAC: Experience with the direct transnasal transsphenoidal approach to the pituitary fossa. **Br J Neurosurg** 8:193–196, 1994.
4. Elias WJ, Chadduck JB, Alden TD, Laws ER Jr: Frameless stereotaxy for transsphenoidal surgery. **Neurosurgery** 45:271–277, 1999.
5. Graham KE, Samuels MH, Raff H, Barnwell SL, Cook DM: Intraoperative adrenocorticotropin levels during transsphenoidal surgery for Cushing's disease do not predict cure. **J Clin Endocrinol Metab** 82:1776–1779, 1997.
6. Griffith HB, Veerapen R: A direct transnasal approach to the sphenoid sinus. Technical note. **Neurosurgery** 66:140–142, 1987.
7. Hardy J: Transsphenoidal approach to the pituitary gland, in, Wilkins RH, Rengachary SS (ed): *Neurosurgery. 2nd Edition.* McGraw-Hill, 1996, pp 1375–1384.
8. Jho HD: Endoscopic endonasal pituitary surgery: Technical aspects. **Contemp Neurosurg** 19(6):1–7, 1997.
9. Jho HD, Carrau RL: Endoscopy assisted transsphenoidal surgery for pituitary adenoma. Technical note. **Acta Neurochir (Wien)** 138:1416–1425, 1996.
10. Jho HD, Carrau RL: Endoscopic endonasal transsphenoidal surgery: Experience with 50 patients. **J Neurosurg** 87:44–51, 1997.
11. Jho HD, Carrau RL, Ko Y: Endoscopic pituitary surgery, in, Wilkins RH, Rengachary SS(ed): *Neurosurgical Operative Atlas.* Baltimore: Williams & Wilkins, 1996, vol 5(1) pp 1–12.
12. Jho HD, Carrau RL, Ko Y, Daly M: Endoscopic pituitary surgery: An early experience. **Surg Neurol** 47:213–223, 1997.
13. Jho HD, Carrau RL, Mclaughlin ML, Somaza SC: Endoscopic transsphenoidal resection of a large chordoma in the posterior fossa. **Acta Neurochir (Wien)** 139:343–348, 1997.
14. Ludecke DK: Intraoperative measurement of adrenocorticotropic hormone in peripituitary blood in Cushing's disease. **Neurosurg** 24:201–205, 1989.
15. Martin CH, Schwartz R, Jolesz F, Black PM: Transsphenoidal resection of pituitary adenomas in an intraoperative MRI unit. **Pituitary** 2:155–162, 1999.
16. Raff H, Shaker JL, Seifert PE, Werner PH, Hazelrigg SR, Findling JW: Intraoperative measurement of adrenocorticotropin (ACTH) during removal of ACTH-secreting bronchial carcinoid tumors. **J Clin Endocrinol Meta** 80:1036–1039, 1995.
17. Ram Z, Bruck B, Hadani M: Ultrasound in pituitary tumor surgery. **Pituitary** 2:133–138, 1999.
18. Steinmeier R, Fahlbusch R, Ganslandt O, et al: Intraoperative magnetic resonance

imaging with the magnetom open scanner: Concepts, neurosurgical indications, and procedures: A preliminary report. **Neurosurgery** 43:739–748, 1998.
19. Sutherland GR, Kaibara T, Louw D, Hoult DI, Tomanek B, Saunders J: A mobile high-field magnetic resonance system for neurosurgery. **J Neurosurg** 91:804–813, 1999.

CHAPTER

6

Perspective in Pituitary Adenomas: An end of the Century Review of Tumorigenesis, Diagnosis, and Treatment

IVAN CIRIC, M.D., SAMI ROSENBLATT, M.D. WILLIAM KERR, JR., M.D., FRANK LAMARCA, M.D., DEBI PIERCE, B.S., CRAIG BAUMGARTNER, P.A.-C., M.B.A.

INTRODUCTION

This chapter reviews the current knowledge of the origin and present standards in the diagnosis and management of pituitary adenomas.

MOLECULAR PATHOGENESIS OF PITUITARY ADENOMAS

The decade of the 1990s has witnessed a burgeoning expansion of molecular biological approaches toward the pathogenesis of various diseases, including pituitary adenomas. It has been suggested that pituitary adenomas can arise as a consequence of abnormal regulatory influences exerted by the hypothalamus or from intrinsic abnormalities within the pituitary itself. Recent molecular biological research demonstrates that the majority of pituitary adenomas arise as a result of a somatic mutation in a progenitor cells with subsequent monoclonal expansion of the mutated cell into an adenoma (23, 46) Conversely, normal pituitary and hyperplastic pituitary tissue are polyclonal in nature. (5).

The proliferation of a mutated pituicyte into an adenoma occurs as a consequence of a variety of extrinsic and intrinsic factors within the pituitary itself. Genetic alterations that have been implicated in the origin of a variety of other benign and malignant tumors include loss of tumor suppressor genes or the activation of cellular protooncogenes. Recently published data have shown that a loss of expression of p-53 suppressor gene in pituitary adenomas correlates directly with aggressive growth and invasiveness (50). In addition, the loss of chromosome 11q13 sequence, which contains the MEN-1 gene locus, has been found in a certain subset of growth hormone (GH) secreting adenomas. This suggests that the inactivation of a tumor suppressor gene in this region may play a role in pituitary tumorigenesis (27). On the oncogene side, activating mutations have been found in the α-subunit gene (*gsp*) of the stimulatory guanine nucleotide-binding protein (G-protein), in the H-*ras* gene, and proteinkinase Cα (27, 16). The stimulatory G-protein is involved in the activation of adenylyl cyclase which under physiological circumstances, mediates the regulatory action of growth hormone releasing hormone (GHRH) in the stimulation of GH synthesis and secretion. This stimulatory effect of the G-protein is under physiological circumstances tempered, however, by the α-subunit of this protein that inactivates adenylyl cyclase. Mutation in *gsp* will thus result in a persistent activation of the adenylyl cyclase and, consequently, in the continuous autonomous GH secretion by the adenoma (16). Indeed, this is the most commonly described genetic defect associated with pituitary tumors (16, 27).

A novel pituitary transforming gene (*pttg*) was recently discovered (55). Human *pttg* was demonstrated to be more abundant in pituitary tumors when compared with normal controls, and the *pttg* expression was even more elevated in invasive tumors when compared with enclosed tumors. Thus, it was suggested that human *pttg* expression level may be a marker for invasiveness in hyperfunctioning pituitary tumors (54). Furthermore, extrahypothalamic GHRH gene expression has been demonstrated in GH-producing adenomas, which suggests that GHRH may act to stimulate GH adenoma growth and hypersecretion (53). Overexpression of GHRH gene in these tumors correlated directly with the adenoma invasiveness (49).

The recent molecular biological research of prolactin-secreting tumors (42) has shown that a loss of D_2 receptor gene expression is associated with aggressive growth, invasiveness, and resistance to dopamine agonist therapy (8). Furthermore, tissue specimens from such tumors showed a paucity of nerve growth factor (*ngf*) gene expression. Addition of *ngf* to such tumor tissue in vitro and in vivo resulted in an increase in the D_2 receptor gene expression and in a phenotypic change from an aggressively growing, invasive, and dopamine agonists-resistant tumor to a less aggressively growing, non-invasive, and dompamine agonists-sensitive adenoma (39). It is anticipated that such phenotypic changes toward less agressivity and greater responsiveness to pharmacotherapy, under the influence of genetic manipulation, will become an important arm in the management of various pituitary tumors in the next century.

DIAGNOSIS OF PITUITARY ADENOMAS

Prolactinomas

The clinical syndrome of amenorrhea and galactorrhea in women and impotence and gynecomastia in men, associated with a serum prolactin level of >300–400 ng/ml, is diagnostic of a prolactin-secreting adenoma. Prolactin levels of <200 ng/ml are not diagnostic of but are consistent with a prolactin-secreting pituitary adenoma, especially in patients with a microadenoma. Conversely, they are also consistent with the presence of the so-called stalk effect that is secondary to an interference with the free passage of the prolactin inhibiting factor from the hypothalamus via the stalk circulation to the anterior pituitary, as well as with a variety of physiological and pathophysiological conditions other than an adenoma. However, some patients present with the classical clinical syndrome of a prolactinoma and a magnetic resonance imaging scan (MRI) that demonstrates a pituitary adenoma, frequently an invasive one, but whose serum prolactin level may be in the normal range. Yet, the immunocytochemical examination of the removed tumor tissue will show indisputable evidence for a lactotroph adenoma. This discrepancy can be explained by the so-called "high dose hook effect" of the chemiluminometric assay used (4). As for the imaging of prolactin-secreting pituitary adenomas, the majority of macroprolactinomas tend to be invasive and indeed, giant invasive pituitary adenomas are almost invariably prolactinomas in nature.

Growth Hormone-Secreting Tumors

The endocrine diagnosis of acromegaly rests on the clinical presentation and on the laboratory evidence of an elevated insulin growth factor-1 (IGF-1) and the lack of suppressibility of the GH to below the 1 ng/ml level by the glucose load (OGTT). A preoperatively elevated GH level is not necessarily a *conditio sine qua non* in the diagnosis of acromegaly. Indeed, the diagnosis of acromegaly is possible with GH levels under 5 ng/ml (7, 40). Twenty-four hour hourly GH determinations in these patients will show, however, a lack of pulsatility in GH secretion when compared with normal individuals who do exhibit a pulsatile pattern of secretion, with the GH usually reaching its peak in the mid-afternoon hours (26). On the other hand, preoperatively elevated GH levels are an excellent marker for postoperative followups.

ACTH-Secreting Tumors

The endocrine diagnosis of Cushing's disease rests on a sequential series of laboratory tests, that begin with the determination of hypercortisolism and proceed to the evidence that the pituitary-adrenal feedback loop is set at a higher level. Next, the tests check for evidence of a brisk responsiveness of ACTH secretion to the corticotropin releasing hormone (CRH) stimulation and, if indicated, determine the presence of an ACTH gradient >100% between the petrosal and the peripheral venous blood. Hypercortisolism can be established when the urinary free cortisols are elevated and when during the 24 hour half hourly plasma cortisol determination the plasma cortisol is >5–10 mcg/dl in the early morning hours, usually around 2:00 a.m. Under physiological circumstances, this level is always <5 mcg/dl. A normal or intermediately elevated serum ACTH, concordance of ACTH and plasma cortisol secretion, and a suppression of ACTH and plasma cortisol levels with high dexamethasone dosages over a 48 hour period are all evidence that the pituitary-adrenal feedback loop is intact, though set at a higher level. Perhaps most importantly, a brisk stimulation of ACTH secretion by corticotropin-releasing hormone (CRH) infusion is very much diagnostic of a pituitary-dependent Cushing's disease. Given that there is evidence of a pituitary dependent hypercortisolism, a positive MRI study for a pituitary adenoma (most commonly a microadenoma) is sufficient for diagnosis. In this regard, a difficult to detect microadenoma can be shown with increased resolution if the MRI is performed either immediately or after a 20 minute delay following a double dose contrast infusion. In the absence of a positive MRI, the petrosal sinus sampling test in search of an ACTH gradient of >100% between the petrosal and peripheral venous blood should be carried out. If such gradient is found following CRH infusion, the petrosal sinus sampling test can be considered as 100% specific and 100% sensitive. However, this test is only 75% accurate in predicting the laterality of the adenoma. The reason for this is that venous drainage from the sella is not always ipsilateral.

CURRENT CONCEPTS IN THE TREATMENT OF PITUITARY ADENOMAS

Prolactinomas

Dopamine agonists remain the mainstay in the treatment of prolactin-secreting pituitary adenomas. In addition to bromocriptine (Parlodel ®), the availability of cabergoline (Dostinex) has greatly enhanced our ability to treat these tumors. Cabergoline efficacy is reported to be equal or greater than that of bromocriptine (12, 21) and just as importantly, its side effects may be less that those of bromocriptine (5). Indeed, the number of endocrinologists using cabergoline as a start-up medication is growing daily.

It is generally accepted that microprolactinomas are the prime indication for treatment with dopamine agonists. On the other hand, we feel that patients should be made aware of the possibility that approximately 10% of microprolactinomas can grow and that some will become invasive into the surrounding structures, especially if the treatment is stopped at some time in the future. They should also be made aware that invasiveness means incurability in the majority of such patients.

Finally, patients with microprolactinomas should also be informed of the excellent prognosis for cure following transsphenoidal microadenomectomy and of the minimum morbidity associated with this procedure in the hands of an experienced pituitary surgeon. Indications for surgical treatment of microprolactinomas are as follows: (1 the endocrine syndrome must be supported by an unequivocally positive MRI (2 dopamine agonists are ineffective, be it in terms of containing the tumor size or in terms of achieving euprolactinemia, (3 the patient is intolerant to dopamine agonist therapy due to side effects, (4 infertility persists in spite of dopamine agonist therapy, (5 the patient experiences occasional side effects of hyperprolactinemia (galactorrhea, dyspareunia, etc.) and other symptoms of a pituitary adenoma (headaches) not relieved by dopamine agonist therapy and, finally, (6 patient preference after a thorough discussion as to all the treatment options and their implications.

Evidence of a surgical cure with a small or no chance for a recurrence rests on a postoperative prolactin (PRL) level of 5 ng/ml or less (20). In our experience the incidence of recurrences increases to approximately 10 to 20% when the postoperative PRL level is between 5 and 10 ng/ml, with the frequency of recurrences rising even higher when the postoperative PRL levels are between 10 and 20 ng/ml. As for macroprolactinomas, including invasive prolactinomas, surgical decompression is usually the acceptable form of treatment (usually after a pretreatment with a dopamine agonist), but also under certain circumstances, the necessary initial form of treatment. However, our experience indicates that pharmacotherapy of large and certainly of invasive macroprolactinomas is far superior to the surgical therapy in palliating the mass effect and the endocrine abnormality. Giant invasive prolactinomas are usually rather fibrous and tough tumors that are very difficult to remove because a surgical palliation of the mass effect is not only difficult to achieve but frequently hazardous (9). Similarly, an attempt to achieve endocrine palliation in such tumors with surgical means is nearly impossible. In contrast, dopamine agonists are overwhelmingly and rapidly effective in decompressing large invasive prolactinomas and in palliating the endocrine abnormality, even when the patient presents with an advanced neurological deficit (9).

Acromegaly

Surgery remains the main treatment modality for acromegaly. The incidence of surgical cures following transsphenoidal surgery in patients with microadenomas is in the 90th percentile range (15, 48, 51). A few series, however, base their surgical cure rate data on the strict criterion of a postoperative growth hormone level of ≤2.5 ng/ml, normalization of the OGTT test, and on the IGF-1 level (15, 48, 51). Ample evidence in the literature indicates that a GH level of ≤5 ng/ml is consistent with biologically active acromegaly (24). Even more importantly, a comparison of the survival curves in patients with a postoperative or a last follow-up, GH level of ≤2 ng/ml and those with a GH level of higher than 2 ng/ml, shows a statistically significant longer survival in the former group (43). Consequently, reported cure rates in some series that are based on the postoperative basal GH level of ≤5 ng/ml should not be considered as representative of the true value of transsphenoidal surgery in the cure of acromegaly (11). Surgical results in the treatment of enclosed, non-invasive GH-secreting adenomas are also quite good, although the results do not approximate those in microadenomas. The surgical results are significantly better and the procedure much safer in experienced hands (10, 32, 38). Invasive pituitary adenomas are largely incurable with surgical means alone unless there is a limited invasion of the medial wall of the cavernous sinus when they can be occasionally extracted and removed completely.

Medical management of GH-secreting pituitary adenomas has made considerable progress in the last decade. The advent of somatostatin analogue (octreotide) (19), and very recently in the United States of the long acting somatostatin analogue (Sandostatin LAR ®) (22, 29) (injectable on a once in every 28 day basis) has provided physicians with a new treatment modality for acromegaly. It is the conventional wisdom that somatostatin analogues can lower and eventually normalize GH in approximately 65% of all patients and reduce the size of the tumor to about 50% or less of its baseline size in approximately 40 to 50% of patients (41). The preoperative use of somatostatin analogues does not appear to influence the resectability of the tumor, while it does seem to be associated with improved results in both enclosed and invasive adenomas (13, 34, 47). Dopamine agonists bromocroptine and cabergoline, alone or in combination with somatostatin analogues, were also reported as being effective in the treatment of acromegaly (47). Recently, GH receptor antagonists have been tested for efficacy in the treatment of acromegaly. One study reports normalization of IGF-1 in 92% of 38 patients treated with the investigational drug Trovert™.

Radiation therapy has also become one of the important pillars in the treatment of acromegaly. Conventional radiation therapy, however, while capable of lowering GH to about 20% of its pretreatment baseline values over a period of 10 to 20 years, is rarely if ever associated with normalization of the postoperative GH levels or the IGF-1 levels. Consequently, conventional radiation therapy does not prevent the biological ravages of acromegaly in the long run (26). In contrast, radiosurgery, especially with the "Gamma knife," has proven effective in normalizing the postoperative GH level in about 50 to 60% of patients (25). The main indication for radiosurgery is failed surgical therapy with residual acromegaly secondary to non-removed tumor tissue usually in the region of the cavernous sinus (25, 30, 37).

Various guidelines in the treatment of acromegaly have recently been proposed (36). In our practice, patients with large and invasive GH-secreting adenomas are usually pretreated with somatostatin analogues for a period of about 6 to 8 weeks before undergoing transsphenoidal microsurgery. In addition, older patients and those incapable of undergoing surgery are treated with the long acting somatostatin analogue. Transsphenoidal microsurgery is the first treatment choice for all other patients. If cure is achieved, patients are followed lifelong. If cure is not achieved, imaging studies are obtained and treatment with a somatostatin analogue is instituted. A reoperation can be very effective in patients in whom another surgeon may have missed a portion of the tumor for whatever reason (experience, exposure, etc.). Also, patients with recurrent enclosed adenomas can be amendable to surgical cure (41). On the other hand, if the initial surgery was performed adequately, and the residual or recurrent tumor tissue is not readily accessible because of its location and invasiveness, a reoperation tends to be unsuccessful (33). If reoperation is deemed contraindicated, radiosurgery is recommended for the residual/recurrent tumor.

Cushing's Disease

Surgical removal of an ACTH-secreting pituitary adenoma, usually a microadenoma, is by far the single most effective treatment of this disease. The pivotal factor is achieving a surgical cure is localizing the microadenoma on the preoperative imaging studies and finding it at the time of surgery. Clearly, these efforts require the involvement of a sophisticated endocrinologist and neuroradiologist, and the availability of an experienced pituitary surgeon. In the process of removal of the ACTH-secreting pituitary microadenoma, it is important to remove a thin layer of the surrounding compressed normal anterior pituitary tissue in order to assure cure.

The pharmacotherapy of Cushing's disease tends to be ineffective. Focused radiosurgery in the treatment of ACTH-secreting microadenoma is not being used frequently for the simple reason that a microadenoma can usually be removed successfully in the hands of an experienced pituitary surgeon. Additionally, in contrast to GH-secreting adenomas, ACTH-secreting microadenomas do not tend to be invasive.

The cure is defined when the postoperative basal plasma cortisol levels are ≤2.5 mcg/dl. It is our practice not to start steroid replacement therapy for the first 24 hours after surgery and to obtain 6, 18, and 24 hour postoperative plasma cortisol levels. Normalization is usually achieved at the 18 hour drawing, with symptoms of hypocortisolism beginning to emerge between the 18th and 24th hour postoperatively when replacement therapy is started. Steroid replacement therapy is continued for several months until the pituitary-adrenal axis function is reestablished.

Non-Secreting Tumors

Non-secreting tumors diagnosed incidentally, if perceived non-threatening, can be followed with repeat visual examinations and MRI studies, especially in the elderly. If symptomatic, transsphenoidal surgery is performed always with the goal of attempting a gross total removal. This is more often than not possible, especially in patients with tumors that have symmetrical supraseller extension. Consequently, postoperative radiation therapy is rarely necessary immediately after surgery and is usually reserved for when there is evidence of a recurrence. Even then, if this is deemed appropriate, a reoperation is preferred to radiation therapy.

PROGNOSIS

If diagnosed early and appropriately treated by experienced experts, the prognosis for high quality long-term survival in patients with pituitary tumors is excellent. This is especially true for hypersecreting microadenomas. While the percentage of cures diminishes as the tumor size increases, surgical results in the treatment of enclosed macroadenomas, both nonfunctioning and hypersecreting, are also very good. On the other hand, our ability to eradicate and achieve endocrine cure in patients with invasive tumors is nearly impossible. Decompression of the optic chiasm following removal of a macroadenoma is associated with a visual improvement that usually occurs within the first 24 hours after surgery. The incidence of recurrence ranges from 1 to 2% to approximately 10% in long-term follow up studies. We do not advocate immediate postoperative radiation therapy in patients who had a gross total removal of a macroadenoma, and we are deliberate in our recommendation for such therapy in patients with subtotally removed tumors.

Various studies have been proposed to determine future biological behavior of incompletely removed pituitary adenomas (42). Among these, immunohistochemistry using antibodies to the KI-67 and proliferating cell nuclear antigen (PCNA), which are expressed in cells that have entered mitosis, can be used to assess the proportion of the cells in a tumor that is proliferating. The percentage of such cells, the so-called labeling index (LI), has been shown to be proportionate with invasiveness and a tendency toward recurrences. However, the LI has not proven a reliable predictor of future biological behavior of a pituitary adenoma in that there are aggressively growing pituitary adenomas with a low LI. Conversely, there are slow growing tumors with a relatively high LI. On molecular biological grounds, and thus on a less practical side, it has been variously shown that in addition to a loss of the p53 suppressor gene expression (50), invasive behavior of a pituitary adenoma can also be associated with an increased expression of the human pituitary transforming gene (54) of the epidermal growth factor (31) and of fibroblast growth factors-2 and 4 (17). Finally, measurement of DNA ploidy has not been found useful in patients with pituitary adenomas. For example, aneuploidy, usually associated with tumor aggressiveness, was reported in one study as being associated with biologically indolent pituitary adenomas (52).

SURGICAL TECHNIQUE

Transsphenoidal microsurgery is the surgical technique of choice among pituitary surgeons and the only one proven safe (10). Recent technological advances with the frameless stereotaxis and interactive image-guided transsphenoidal microsurgery have further increased the safety of this procedure (44). On the other hand, the use of an intraoperative MRI, while advocated by some (35), has not been widely accepted as a singular advantage.

Concerning the endoscopic transsphenoidal surgical technique, we should be very careful to encourage those who have shown facility with this procedure to continue their work and demonstrate its safety and usefulness, especially in achieving endocrine cures (28). At the same time, our enthusiasm with this procedure should be tempered with our concern for misuse of the technique in the hands of the less initiated and improperly trained. Neurosurgeons have struggled over the years to operate with two eyes and two hands. Definitely, the operating microscope has been a bliss in allowing the neurosurgeons the luxury, beauty, elegance, and yes, magnificence of a three-dimensional view, enlarged at will, in a sunlit field of otherwise under direct vision barely preceptible deep seated structures, including pituitary adenomas. In contrast, endoscopic surgery is monocular and largely one-handed, and thus so counterintuitive to everything neurosurgeons have strived for throughout the past century. If endoscopic surgery is to challenge microscopic surgery to the extent of replacing it, it will have to do so by achieving binocularity (i.e., three dimensionality) and by allowing the surgeon to use both hands in a field that is free of the still rather bulky and cumbersome endoscopic shafts. Yes, there are centers where various holders are being applied to the endoscope in order to allow the surgeon the freedom of using both hands during the operation, but to the best of our knowledge, this has not been duplicated in other centers to the same extent. In short, endoscopic surgery is still in its infancy and it will hopefully rise to its challenges in this century.

We are concerned that many neurosurgeons still advocate craniotomy for any pituitary adenoma that extends into the suprasellar space, with each neurosurgeon setting his own standard as to where the cutoff point is with the transsphenoidal approach in terms of the degree of the suprasellar extension. The reason for this may be actually quite appropriate. Lack of training and subsequent lack of exposure in a center where this procedure is not being done frequently may result in a trepidation toward engaging in a surgical endeavor in an unfamiliar territory and utilizing unfamiliar techniques—simply doing an operation that can be associated with significant complications (10). A change in this attitude toward transsphenoidal microsurgery can only be achieved if neurosurgeons were to specialize in this field by acquiring additional training and devoting their careers toward becoming accomplished pituitary surgeons. Clearly, this would require support from the neurosurgical community at large in terms of other neurosurgeons avoiding performing transsphenoidal surgery on a sporadic basis.

SUMMARY

Significant advances have been made in the molecular biological understanding of pituitary tumorigenesis. These advances will have an impact on the gene therapy of pituitary tumors in the coming century. Transsphenoidal surgery remains the mainstay of treatment for the majority of pituitary adenomas, with endoscopic surgery being used at some centers in select patients. Pharmacotherapy of pituitary adenomas has made great strides in the management of prolactinomas and GH-secreting pituitary adenomas. Finally, radiosurgery has become a very important adjuvant therapy in the treatment of hypersecreting pituitary adenomas.

REFERENCES

1. Abe R, Ludecke DK, Recent results of secondary transnasal surgery for residual or recurring acromegaly. *Neurosurgery* 42:1013–1021, 1998.

2. Amar AP, Hinton DR, Krieger MD, Weiss MH. Invasive pituitary adenomas: Significance of proliferation parameters. *Pituitary* 2:117–122, 1999.
3. Anniko M, Wersall J. DNA studies for prediction of prognosis of pituitary adenomas. Adv Biosci 69:45–52, 1988.
4. Barkan AL, Chandler WF. Giant pituitary prolactinoma with falsely low serum prolactin: The pitfall of the "high-dose hook effect." Case Report. *Neurosurgery* 42:913–915, 1998.
5. Biller BMK, Alexander JM, Zervas NT, Hedley-Whyte ET, Arnold A, Klibanski A. Clonal origins of adrenocorticotropin-secreting pituitary tissue in Cushing's disease. *J Clin Endocrinol Metab* 75:1303–1309, 1992.
6. Biller BM, Molitch ME, Vance ML, et al. Treatment of prolactin-secreting macroadenomas with the once-weekly dopamine agonist cabergoline. *J Clin Endocrinol Metab* 81:2338–2343, 1996.
7. Brockmeier SJ, Buchfelder M, Adams EF, Schott W, Fahlbusch R. Acromegaly with 'normal' serum growth hormone levels. Clinical features, diagnosis and results of transsphenoidal microsurgery. *Horm Metab Res* 24:392–400, 1992.
8. Caccavelli L, Feron F, Morange I, et al. Decreased expression of the two D_2 dopamine receptor isoforms in bromocriptine resistant prolactinomas. *Neuroendocrinol* 60:314–322, 1994.
9. Ciric I. Giant and invasive prolactin-secreting pituitary adenoma, in, Winchester DP, Brennan MF, Dodd GD Jr, Henson DE, Kennedy BJ, Steele GD Jr, Wilson JF (ed): **Tumor Board Case Management.** Philadelphia: Lippincott-Raven, 1997, pp. 631–634.
10. Ciric I, Ragin A, Baumgartner C, Pierce D. Complications of transsphenoidal surgery: Results of a national survey, review of the literature and personal experience. *Neurosurgery* 40:225–237, 1997.
11. Clayton RN. New developments in the management of acromegaly. Should we achieve absolute biochemical cure? *J Endocrinol* 155 Suppl 1:S23–S29, 1997.
12. Colao A, Di Sarno A, Sarnacchiaro F, et al. Prolactinomas resistant to standard dopamine agonists respond to chronic cabergoline treatment. *J Clin Endocrinol Metab* 82:876–883, 1997.
13. Colao A, Ferone D, Cappabianca P, et al. Effect of octreotide pretreatment on surgical outcome in acromegaly. *J Clin Endocrinol Metab* 82:3308–3314, 1997.
14. Colao A, Ferone D, Marzullo P, et al. Effect of different dopaminergic agents in the treatment of acromegaly. *J Clin Endocrinol Metab* 82:518–523, 1997.
15. Davis DH, Laws ER Jr, Ilstrup DM, et al. Results of surgical treatment for growth hormone-secreting pituitary adenomas. *J Neurosurg* 79:70–75, 1993.
16. Drange MR, Melmed S. Molecular pathogenesis of acromegaly. *Pituitary* 2:43–50, 1999.
17. Ezzat S, Smyth HS, Raymar L, Asa SL. Heterogeneous in vivo and in vitro expression of basic fibroblast growth factor by human pituitary adenomas. *J Clin Endocrinol Metab* 80:878–884, 1995.
18. Fahlbusch R, Honegger J, Buchfelder M. Evidence supporting surgery as treatment of choice for acromegaly. *J Endocrinol* 155 Suppl:S53–S55, 1997.
19. Farooqi S, Bevan JS, Sheppard MC, Wass JAH. The therapeutic value of somatostatin and its analogues. *Pituitary* 2:79–88, 1999.
20. Feigenbaum SL, Downey DE, Wilson CB, Jaffe RB. Transsphenoidal pituitary resection for preoperative diagnosis of prolactin-secreting pituitary adenoma in women: Long-term follow up. 81:1711–1719, 1996.
21. Ferrari CI, Abs R, Bevan JS, et al. Treatment of macroprolactinoma with cabergoline: A study of 85 patients. 46:409–413, 1997.

22. Gisslis JC, Noble S, Goa KL: Octreotide long-acting release (LAR). *Drugs* 53:681–699, 1997.
23. Herman V, Fagin J, Gonsky R, Kovacs K, Melmed S. Clonal origin of pituitary adenomas. *J Clin Endocrinol Metab* 71:1427–1433, 1990.
24. Holdaway IM, Rajasoorya C. Epidemiology of acromegaly. *Pituitary* 2:29–41, 1999.
25. Jackson IMD, Norene G. Role of gamma knife radiosurgery in acromegaly. *Pituitary* 2:71–78, 1999.
26. Jaffe CA. Reevaluation of conventional pituitary irradiation in the therapy of acromegaly. *Pituitary* 2:55–62, 1999.
27. Jameson JL. Molecular pathogenesis of pituitary tumors: An overview, in, Melmed S (ed). Molecular and clinical advances in pituitary disorders. **Third International Pituitary Congress.** Marina del Ray, CA, 1993, 15–19.
28. Jho HD, Carrau RL. Endoscopic endonasal transsphenoidal surgery: Experience with 50 patients. *J Neurosurg* 87:44–51, 1997.
29. Lancranjan I, Atkinson AB. Sandostatin LAR® i acromegalic patients: Results of a European multicare study with Sandostatin LAR® in acromegalic patients. *Pituitary* 1:105–114, 1999.
30. Landolt AM, Haller D, Lomax N, et al. Stereotactic radiosurgery for recurrent surgically treated acromegaly: Comparison with fractionate radiotherapy. *J Neurosurg* 88:1002–1008, 1998.
31. LeRiche VK, Asa SL, Ezzat S. Epidermal growth factor and its receptor (EGFR) in human pituitary adenomas: EFG-R correlates with tumor aggressiveness. *J Clin Endocrinol Metab* 81:656–662, 1995.
32. Lisset CA, Peacey SR, Laing I, Tetlow L, Davis JR, Shalet SM. The outcome of surgery for acromegaly: The need for a specialist pituitary surgeon for all types of growth hormone (GH) secreting adenoma [Review]. *Clin Endocrinol* 49:653–657, 1998.
33. Long H, Beauregard H, Somma M, Comtois R, Serri O, Hardy J. Surgical outcome after repeated transsphenoidal surgery in acromegaly. *J Neurosurg* 85:239–247, 1996.
34. Lucas-Morante T, Garcia-Uria J, Estrada J, et al. Treatment of invasive growth hormone pituitary adenomas with long-acting somatostatin analog SMS 201-995 before transsphenoidal surgery. *J Neursurg* 81:10–14, 1994.
35. Martin CH, Schwartz R, Jolesz F, Black PM. Transsphenoidal resection of pituitary adenomas in an intraoperative MRI unit. *Pituitary* 2:155–162, 1999.
36. Melmed S, Jacons I, Kleinberg D, Kilbanski A. Current treatment guidelines for acromegaly. *J Clin Endocrinol Metab* 83:2646–2652, 1998.
37. Morange-Ramos I, Regis J, Defour H, et al. Gamma-knife surgery for secreting pituitary adenomas. Acta Neurochir 140:437–443, 1998.
38. Ross DA, Wilson CB. Results of transsphenoidal microsurgery for growth hormone-secreting pituitary adenoma in a series of 214 patients. *J Neurosurg* 68:854–867, 1988.
39. Missale C, Sigala S, Fiorentini C, et al. Nerve growth factor suppresses the tumoral phenotype of human prolactinomas [Review]. *Horm Res* 47:240–244, 1997.
40. Mohr G, Chen ZP, Schweitzer M. Acromegaly with normal basal growth hormone levels. *Can J Neurol Sci* 24:250–253, 1997.
41. Newman CB. Medical therapy for acromegaly [Review]. *Endocrinol Metab Clin North Am* 28:171–190, 1999.
42. Pellegrini-Boullier I, Morange-Ramos I, Barlier A, et al. Pituitary-1 gene expression in human lactotroph and somatotroph piutitary adenomas is correlated to D_2 receptor gene expression. *J Clin Endocrinol Metab* 81:3390–3396, 1996.

43. Rajasoorya C, Holdaway IM, Wrightson P, Scott DJ, Ibbertson HK. Determinants of clinical outcome and survival in acromegaly. *Clin Endocrinol* 41:95–102, 1994.
44. Sandeman D, Moufid A. Interactive image-guided pituitary surgery: An experience of 101 procedures. Neurochirurgie 44:331–338, 1998.
45. Sheaves R, Jenkins P, Blackburn P, et al. Outcome of transsphenoidal surgery for acromegaly using strict criteria for surgical cure. *Clin Endocrinol* 45:407–413, 1996.
46. Shimon I, Melmed S. Genetic basis of endocrine disease: Piutitary tumor pathogensis. *J Clin Endocrinol Metab* 82:1675–1681, 1997.
47. Stevenaert A, Beckers A. Presurgical octreotide treatment in acromegaly. *Acta Endocrinol* 129Suppl 1:18–20, 1993.
48. Swearingen B, Barker FG II, Katnelson L, et al. Long-term mortality after transsphenoidal surgery and adjunctive therapy for acromegaly [Comment]. *J Clin Endocrinol Metab* 83:3419–3426, 1988.
49. Thapar K, Kovacs K, Stefaneanu L, et al. Overexpression of the growth hormone-releasing hormone gene in acromegaly-associated pituitary tumors. An event associated with neoplastic progression and aggressive behaviour. *Am J Pathol* 151:769–784, 1997.
50. Thapar K, Scheithauer BW, Kovacs K, Pernicone PJ, Laws ER Jr. p53 expression in pituitary adenomas and carcinomas: Correlations with invasiveness and tumor growth fractions. *Neurosurgery* 38:763–770, 1996.
51. Tindall GT, Oyesiku NM, Watts NB, Clark RV, Christy JH, Adams DA. Transsphenoidal adenomectomy for growth hormone-secreting pituitary adenomas in acromegaly: Outcome analysis and determinants of failure. *J Neurosurg* 78:205–215, 1993.
52. Van der Lely AJ, de Herder WW, Lamberts SW. New medical treatment for acromegaly. *Pituitary* 2:89–92, 1999.
53. Wakahayayashi I, Inokuchi K, Hasegawa O, Sugihara H, Minami S. Expression of growth hormone (GH)-releasing factor gene in GH-producing pituitary adenoma. *J Clin Endocrinol Metab* 74:357–361, 1992.
54. Zhang X, Horwitz GA, Heaney A, Prezant TR, Melmed S. Pituitary adenomas: Marker for functional tumor invasiveness. *J Clin Endocrinol Metab* 84:761–767, 1999.
55. Zhang Z, Horwitz GA, Prezant TR, et al. Structure, expression, and function of human pituitary tumors transforming gene (PTTG). *Mol Endrocrinol* 13:156–166, 1999.

CHAPTER

7

The Future of Neuropathology

CATHERINE DAUMAS-DUPORT, M.D.

I am honored to have been asked my impressions on the future of neuropathlogy. However, rather than discuss generalities, I will instead focus on what I know best: cerebral tumors, especially gliomas. Although I certainly cannot predict the future, I will attempt to explain why the traditional classification and method of histological diagnosis of gliomas does not work, and what can be done to improve this situation.

The histological diagnosis of gliomas is unsatisfactory, and the situation is actually worse than one might think. Recent studies' concordant disastrous results involving the reliability of neuropathologists in typing and grading gliomas demonstrate this clearly. For example, in a study by Mittler et al. (11), interobserver disagreement between four experienced neuropathologists from major centers was 21% for gliosis, 60% for pilocytic astrocytomas, and 43%, 64%, and 38% for low-grade astrocytomas, anaplastic astrocytomas, and glioblastomas, respectively. The results were similar when the same slide was evaluated by the same observer several weeks later. Furthermore, as Rorke (13) wrote about a test comparing the interpretation of two experts of the Childhood Brain Tumor Consortium: "the results were shocking; the reliability of those experts was not too much better than the discrepancy observed between the opinions of the referring pathologists." We will not find our way out of this morass unless we question the traditional histological classifications and diagnostic method of neurosurgical surgical pathology.

What is wrong with the traditional histological classification and method of interpretation of gliomas? The answer is long and complicated:

1. Most of the histological criteria used in the World Health Organization (WHO) classification to determine the histological type and degree of malignancy of gliomas are highly subjective.
2. Ordinary gliomas are heterogeneous tumors, but histological diagnosis is determined exclusively according to the features observed on the histological preparations; therefore, the histological diagnosis is highly dependent on the representatitivity of the samples.

3. Ordinary gliomas are infiltrative tumors, but no distinction is made between the cells that belong to the tumor itself from those that belong to the involved parenchyma.
4. Although pediatric neuropathologists, particularly Rorke et al. (14), have long and repeatedly drawn attention to inaccuracies in the present classification of glial tumors in children, the basis of the WHO classification remains the observation of gliomas in adult patients.
5. Because oncologists cannot proceed with treatment plans without a definite histological diagnosis and malignancy grade, tumors that show unusual features are literally forced into one of the existing histological categories.
6. The main role of the pathologist is assessing the prognosis of a tumor, but collecting followup data is not usually considered part of their job. This is like expecting racetrack bettors to put money on a horse although they will never know the results of the race.
7. In surgical pathology, clinicians and pathologists consider their gold standard what is in fact blind histological interpretation without the benefits of clinical or imaging data, forgetting that diagnosis is essentially a synthesis and ignoring that tumors can look very similar on a slide but behave very differently.
8. Most important to understanding the messy present situation, the commonly used classification does not clearly distinguish an oligodendroglioma from an astrocytoma. Still worse, it contributes to misinterpretation of a substantial proportion of tumors in children and young adults that are wrongly thought low- or even high-grade gliomas, and are treated accordingly although they are stable lesions.

These last assertions may sound inflammatory and even provocative. I will attempt to explain why I came to such conclusions and how, in my experience, most of the problems in the histological interpretation of gliomas can be overcome easily.

In my institution, imaging-based serial stereotactic biopsies were initially performed to determine a target volume for the treatment of "ordinary" gliomas by curietherapy. As I was systematically present in operating room for their interpretation, it became a routine practice for me to integrate neurosurgical, imaging, and histological data. The combined diagnostic approach of imaging-based serial stereotactic biopsies provides simple but pivotal data necessary for the understanding and histological interpretation of "ordinary" gliomas.

Gliomas may show two distinct patterns of tumor growth: solid tumor tissue possessing new formed microblood vessels, or isolated tumor cells that permeate intact brain parenchyma and are not associated with microblood vessels (3). These two components are easy to identify with modern imaging; contrast enhancement reflecting the microvascularity of a lesion occurs within the solid tumor tissue but not in the components of the isolated tumor cells. On the other hand, isolated tumor cells usually induce edema, which means that they correspond to a hypodense area on computed tomographic scans, and to an area of hypo-T1 or hyper-T2 signal on magnetic resonance images (3, 10). Glioblastomas are highly angiogenic tumors: they always show both solid tumor tissue and isolated tumor cells. Conversely, oligodendrogliomas are poor angiogenic tumors. They may grow slowly for years, consisting only of isolated tumor cells. Microangiogenesis, and formation of foci of solid tumor tissue, is a delayed but crucial event in the malignant progression of these oligodendrogliomas (6).

The lack of distinction between isolated tumor cells and solid tumor largely explains the inaccuracy of conventional histological classifications of gliomas. The isolated tumor cells induce a reactive gliosis of the parenchyma (fibrillary or gemistocytic), but the reactive astrocytes are interpreted as differentiated tumoral astrocytes.

In my experience, low-grade astrocytomas do not exist. Tumors diagnosed as such are most often purely infiltrative oligodendrogliomas. Anaplastic astrocytomas also do not exist: most often they are oligodendrogliomas with a solid component that does not exhibit a classical "honeycomb" pattern, or they are purely infiltrative oligodendrogliomas that show mitosis.

On nonrepresentative samples, the infiltrative portion of high-grade oligodendrogliomas or glioblastomas also may be interpreted as anaplastic or low-grade astrocytomas according to the presence or absence of mitosis. As a consequence, we may consider that the St. Anne/Mayo grading system of astrocytoma, which was introduced in 1982 and proved to be useful, now has become obsolete.

Since the imaging appearance of gliomas is closely related to their pattern of growth, computed tomography or magnetic resonance imaging can now be used easily by the pathologist as an equivalent to macroscopic examination when assessing the validity of the samples referred for histological examination.

Furthermore, a combined histological-radiological grading system, such as the one we have recently proposed for oligodendrogliomas, now can be used to overcome the problem of representativeness of biopsy sampling (4). This grading system which is based on the observation that endothelial hyperplasia and contrast enhancement both reflect microangiogenesis, discriminates two grades of malignancy as follows: Grade A, endothelial hyperplasia and contrast enhancement are both absent (median survival, 11 years); and Grade B, endothelial hyperplasia and/or contrast enhancement are present (median survival, 3.5 years). This grading system can also be used for tumors that are presently considered mixed oligoastrocytomas (personal communication).

Morphologically, ordinary gliomas are much less complex tumors than their present histological classifications suggest. According to our recent classification, an ordinary glioma may be either a glioblastoma or an oligo (or oligoastrocytoma) Grade A or B. The imaging appearance in each of these tumor categories is much more uniform than currently thought. Therefore, in most instances integration of radiological data (macroscopic data) permits the pathologist to diagnose the most common types of gliomas easily and correctly.

Regarding the problems with the histological diagnosis of gliomas in children, it is well known that the prognosis for patients with low- or high-grade gliomas is markedly better in children than in adults. This phenomenon has been attributed to the "age effect." This is a statistical observation, however, not an explanation. Survival curves in the literature clearly show that tumors diagnosed as ordinary gliomas in this population are actually a mixture of two different categories of tumors, each with a distinct prognosis. The survival curves of high-grade astrocytomas in children regularly show a plateau effect. An example of this is illustrated in a report by Duffner et al. (7), in which a marked decrease in the survival rate during the first 2 postoperative years, similar to that seen in adults, was followed by an abrupt plateau effect. About 40% of the patients were long-term survivors. In a study by Westergaard et al. (15), the survival curves of patients with nonpilocytic, low-grade gliomas (WHO Grade II) show that most patients younger than 20 years of age are long-term survivors, whereas survival in patients older than 20 years is markedly shorter in all age categories. The unexpected long-term survival observed in these young patients is likely attributable, in part, to the fact that the neuronal element of gangliogliomas may not be present in the samples, and in larger part to the misdiagnosis of dysembryoplastic neuroepithelial tumors (DNTs) as ordinary gliomas.

DNTs provide an excellent demonstration of why we must cease to consider diagnosis exclusively a matter of histopathology. Histologically, DNTs closely resemble low- or even high-grade gliomas, but they are stable lesions. These tumors, which arise during embryogenesis, are now more systematically detected by imaging in children or young adults soon after the onset of symptoms. The actual frequency of DNTs still is largely underestimated because our earlier description of these tumors 15 years ago, and accordingly the histological criteria used in the WHO classification, allows for the diagnosis of a minority of supratentorial cortical DNTs (1).

Fortunately, the clinical presentation and radiological appearance of supratentorial cortical DNTs are clearly distinct from those of ordinary gliomas, and are so characteristic that clinicians and radiologists may recognize them easily. On condition that pathologists not consider only what they see on the histological preparation, the misdiagnosis of DNTs as ordinary gliomas can readily be avoided (5).

DNTs are located in many other sites, including the caudate nuclei and the brain stem (2). It is likely that most pilocytic astrocytomas of the cerebellum are in fact DNTs, and that these tumors may arise also in the medulla. The diagnosis of "nonspecific histological forms" of DNTs in extracortical locations remains a challenging problem. However, the hypothesis of a DNT must be considered in a young patient when there is a discordance between the neurological status and the location of the tumor, and when the imaging appearance of the lesion is not typical of an ordinary glioma, particularly when there is no mass effect and no peritumoral edema.

We must understand that 1) not all brain tumors in general, and especially in children, can be accurately classified histologically; 2) the prognosis of a tumor cannot be systematically predicted on the basis of histological examination, because histology gives only a static view of a lesion, and 3) radiation and/or chemotherapy are not curative, so we must agree that there are no objective reasons to justify administering aggressive treatment immediately after a biopsy or surgical removal in children who harbor a tumor not obviously clinically or radiologically malignant. The actual behavior of a tumor can now be accurately assessed on serial magnetic resonance imaging. Such controls should become a more common practice. In the presence of nontypical tumors, pathologists would recommend imaging surveillance before adjunctive treatment may be prescribed. As a consequence, unduly aggressive radiotherapy or chemotherapy in young patients would probably be delayed or cancelled.

This interpretation of brain tumors, based on the integration of clinical and imaging data, is both simple and logical. In most instances it allows even the inexperienced pathologist to make the correct diagnosis. In contrast to the commonly used classifications, which have wrapped the pathologists in esoteric language, the proposed classification is easily understandable by the non-specialist. It defines a limited number of histological categories, which are closely related to what is seen by the neurosurgeon and the radiologist on imaging studies. To speak about the same things is certainly the best way for neurosurgeons, neuropathologists, and neuroradiologists to communicate.

There are, however, several reasons to be pessimistic about meaningful progress in the histological assessment of gliomas occurring in the near future. The main reason is that in the next WHO classification that will be issued, no significant changes have been accepted in the histological typing of gliomas. Certain pathologists see this questioning of the traditional classifications as questioning their own expertise, and most of these experts are not ready to admit that the ultimate truth is not in what is seen only in the histological preparations. Illustrating this state of mind in the neuropathological community is the comment I received after rejection of a paper about nonspecific DNTs: "The point should also be made that these authors work in a highly sophisticated practice setting, one characterized by close integration of neurosurgical, radiological, and pathological arms. This is not real world. Worldwide, most working pathologists do not find themselves in such a practice setting. The histological definitions thus—function admirably as safeguards against inexperience on the part of radiologists and general neurosurgeons."

The tendency among neuropathologists is to consider that the solution to the problems of histological typing of gliomas will come, not from clinical or radiological data, but from molecular biology and genetics. This approach will certainly deepen our understanding of brain tumors. However, I personally do not believe that, **in the present situation**, this approach can resolve the diagnostic problems of gliomas, for the simple reason that the results of molecular biology and genetics are analyzed into categories that first are determined according to the present histological classifications. This is a vicious circle. Therefore, it is not surprising that the results of present molecular biology and genetic analysis are heterogeneous and contradictory. For example, p53 mutations are variably reported present in 0 to 80% of glioblastomas, in 15 to 45% of low-grade astrocytomas, and in 14 to 42% of oligodendrogliomas (8, 9, 12).

Beyond the specific problems of interpreting gliomas, a broader and more fundamental question needs to be addressed: will future pathologists remember that they are basically physicians, or will they consider themselves biologists? The main force that would lead pathologists to achieve this mutation is, of course, the explosion of new information coming from molecular biology and genetics. Pharmaceutical firms are providing laboratories with an increasing panel of tools that would permit such analysis to be performed in daily practice. Molecular biology is considered an exact science; therefore, clinicians and therapists might expect that molecular biology finally will allow neuropathologists to diagnose brain tumors in general and gliomas in particular accurately and reproducibly. Treating physicians share the hope, if not the conviction, that manipulating the biological factors that contribute to the growth and invasiveness of these tumors holds out more possibility for promising treatments than conventional methods. If this promise becomes a reality, in the future the demand will increase for neuropathologists to assess these biological factors in individual patients.

In the recent literature, authors seeking innovation or positions of leadership have focused their research on molecular biology and used the most advanced techniques. Studies and papers emerging from this type of research are much more likely to be published than those using the "horse and buggy" approach based on simple morphological observation and conventional histological techniques. Publish or perish has never sounded so prophetic. For neuropathologists of the future, as well as for those who must publish to obtain positions in hospitals, it would indeed be a risky business to adopt a diagnostic approach involving hunting down clinical data and imaging, or worse yet spending hours in the operating room.

These last considerations lead to a point concerning the selection, training, and cooperation of various specialists concerned with brain tumors. The huge amount of information that we must now have at our fingertips has resulted in our splitting into independent specialties, which causes an increasingly fragmented approach to the pathology as well as to the care of the patient. The result is that our primary mission—the treatment of the patient—may be lost. This is particularly true for the pathologist who does not come into direct contact with the patient, seeing only the microscopic appearance of their lesion.

Neuropathologists have a tendency to forget that we are here to provide service to the clinician and ultimately to the patient. Unfortunately, for many of us, neuropathology seems to have become an end in itself. The WHO classification of tumors gives this impression as well. Neuropathologists must be aware that a given tumor may have variable histological appearances, but does that justify the distinction of multiple histological types if each of the morphological variants has no implications in terms of clinical presentation, imaging features, or prognosis? Neuropathologists have always shown a particular interest in the histogenesis of brain tumors; this has been the basis of the classification of gliomas. We are now attempting to determine the genetic pathways of their evolution. The results of such recent investigations already have been incorporated in the next WHO classification, but neurosurgeons may wonder whether, from a practical standpoint, the putative histogenesis of a tumor is of any value in actually treating the patient.

An intelligent if not ideal classification should taken into account its use by clinicians, not just neuropathologists. Instead of working independently, we must cooperate and communicate systematically; otherwise there is no hope that we understand each other. For example, with regard to the histological classification of tumors, part of the answer lies in the hands of neurosurgeons. They should be active participants in the WHO workshops that determine these classifications. This would be an ideal way for neuropathologists to find out what neurosurgeons find useful as well as useless or unacceptable. For example, a long debate about whether an oligoastrocytoma is a tumor that contains a majority or a substantial part of tumoral oligodendrocytes may be aborted when we all realize that, except to the pathologist, it doesn't make any difference!

With regard to long-term plans, we must fundamentally review the concept of specialty. With respect to neuropathology and neuroradiology, at a time when imaging is becoming so accurate that we can expect results comparable to those obtained with a low-power microscope, we may wonder why the macroscopic and microscopic lesions continue to be interpreted separately. It does not seem logical to have a radiologist, untrained in pathology, propose an initial diagnosis while a pathologist, unaware of the radiological appearance of the lesion, makes the "final" diagnosis. While imaging tools are technologically sophisticated, the images they provide are not very difficult to interpret. Obviously, we can not ask radiologists to become pathologists or ask pathologists to become radiologists. But some sort of dual training can and should be made available to the next generation of doctors.

A top-notch diagnostic team in the future should include physicians who would interpret imaging and histological data, a biomedical engineer, and radiology and pathology technicians. This would be far more efficient than the present system. The practical consequences of such a new organization look extremely promising. Our common patients deserve the benefit of active and permanent cooperation between "radiopathologists" and neurosurgeons in the coming years.

REFERENCES

1. Daumas-Duport C. Dysembryoplastic neuroepithelial tumours. **Brain Pathol** 3:283–295, 1993.
2. Daumas-Duport C, Lantos PL. Dysembryoplastic neuroepithelial tumours, in, Kleihues P (ed): *Tumors of the Nervous System*. Lyon: International Agency for Research on Cancer, 1997, pp 73–76.
3. Daumas-Duport C, Monsaingeon V, Blond S, Munari C, Musolino A, Chodkiewicz JP, Missir O. Serial stereotactic biopsies and CT scan in gliomas: Correlative study in 100 astrocytomas, oligo-astrocytomas and oligodendrocytomas. **J Neurooncol** 4:317–328, 1986.
4. Daumas-Duport C, Tucker ML, Harry K, Cervera P, Beuvon F, Varlet P, Udo N, Koziak M, Chodkiewicz JP. Oligodendrogliomas. Part II. A new grading system based on morphological and imaging criteria. **Journal Neurooncol** 34:61–78, 1997.

5. Daumas-Duport C, Varlet P, Bacha S, Beuvon F, Cervera-Pierot P, Chodkiewicz JP. Dysembryoplastic neuroepithelial tumors: Nonspecific histological forms—A study of 40 cases. **J Neurooncol** 41:267–280, 1999.
6. Daumas-Duport C, Varlet P, Tucker ML, Beuvon F, Cervera P, Chodkiewicz JP. Oligodendrogliomas. Part I—Patterns of growth, histological diagnosis, clinical and imaging correlations: A study of 153 cases. **J Neurooncol** 34:37–59, 1997.
7. Duffner PK, Cohen ME, Myers MH, Heise HW. Survival of children with brain tumors: SEER program, 1973–1980. **Neurology** 36:597–601, 1986.
8. Haapasalo H, Isola J, Sallinen P, Kalimo H, Helin H, Rantala I. Aberrant p53 expression in astrocytic neoplasms of the brain—Association with proliferation. Am **J Pathol** 142:1347–1351, 1993.
9. Hagel C, Laking G, Laas R, Scheil S, Jung R, Milde-Langosch K, Stravrou DK. Demonstration of p53 protein and TP53 gene mutations in oligodendrogliomas. **Eur J Cancer** 32A:2242–2248, 1996.
10. Kelly PJ, Daumas-Duport C, Scheithauer BW, Kall BA, Kispert DB. Stereotactic histologic correlations of computed tomography- and magnetic resonance imaging-defined abnormalities in patients with glial neoplasms. **Mayo Clin Proc** 62:450–459, 1987.
11. Mittler MA, Walters BC, Stopa EG. Observer reliability in histological grading of astrocytoma stereotactic biopsies. **J Neurosurg** 85:1091–1094, 1996.
12. Reifenberger J, Ring GU, Gies U, Cobbers L, Oberstrass J, An HX, Niederacher D, Wechsler W, Reifenberger G. Analysis of p53 mutation and epidermal growth factor receptor amplification in recurrent gliomas with malignant progression. **J Neuropathol Exp Neurol** 55:822–831, 1996.
13. Rorke LB. Pathologic diagnosis as the gold standard. **Cancer** 79:665–667, 1997.
14. Rorke LB, Gilles FH, Davis RL, Becker LE. Revision of the World Health Organization classification of brain tumors for childhood brain tumors. **Cancer** 56 [Suppl 7]:1869–1886, 1985.
15. Westergaard L, Gjerris F, Klinken L. Prognostic parameters in benign astrocytomas. **Acta Neurochir** (Wein) 123:1–7, 1993.

CHAPTER

8

Honored Guest Presentation-Developments in Surgery of Posterior Circulation Aneurysms

DUKE S. SAMSON, M.D.

> *". . . I have been persuaded by many neurosurgeons that because our experience with posterior circulation aneurysms is so large and unique and unlikely to be repeated, that it deserves summation in a book, if for no other than historical reasons." (11)*

Any discussion of the evolution of vertebro-basilar aneurysms must begin with recognition of the accomplishments of Dr. Charles Drake. The successful surgical management of vertebro-basilar aneurysms is the personal neurosurgical legacy of this outstanding surgeon; the magnificent summary of his life's work (11), published in 1996, details the surgical management of over 1760 patients with posterior circulation aneurysms between 1961 and 1995. To place this in humbling prospective, my experience with all aneurysms of the vertebral and basilar arteries barely equals the number of posterior circulation giant aneurysms reported in the landmark publication by Drake et al. (11). A cursory look at this remarkable volume demonstrates that even in 1999 it is almost impossible to operate on any aneurysm of the vertebro-basilar system, from either side of the arterial wall, without direct reliance on Drake's anatomic and technical insights. This body of experience will never be replicated, and despite our most earnest efforts, the clinical results reported from Western Ontario have yet to be equaled. These aneurysms remain our most difficult lesions to treat, carrying the highest therapeutic mortality, and the adequacy of all the treatment options deserves continual scrutiny.

For 25 years, the unique circumstances of Dr. Drake's practice have proven difficult if not impossible to simulate at other centers. No doubt that is attributable in great measure to the quality of those of us making the attempt, but the nature and acuity of the general aneurysm population also have played some role in the disparity.

Table 1
Posterior Circulation Aneurysms

	Drake et al., 1996 (11)	Southwestern/Samson et al., 1999 (28)
Basilar apex	895 (65%)	342 (80%)
Superior cerebellar	266	53
Bas trunk	144	17
Vertebrobasilar junction	116	14
Vertebral	221	48
Postcerebral	125	25
Outcomes (excellent–good)	85%	74%

During the past two decades, we have observed a somewhat different mix of posterior circulation aneurysms at Southwestern (Table 8.1) than that reported by Drake et al.. As a result, and probably predictably, the mistakes we have made and the lessons we have learned provide a more limited and narrowly focused overview than the extensive London experience. The overwhelming majority of our patients have had ruptured lesions of the basilar apex and have been either admitted or referred to our hospitals within 48 hours of ictus. The average admitting Hunt and Hess score has been almost III, and over time, we have taken a progressive proactive approach to early surgical intervention in all but the most critically ill patients, believing it offers the surest protection against recurrent hemorrhage and the optimal physiological background for the aggressive treatment of cerebral vasospasm. Thus, the bulk of our surgical experience has been in the interpeduncular fossa in patients with "hot brains" shortly after acute hemorrhage; in these patients we wanted to simplify operative intervention, diminish brain tissue retraction, and maximize our familiarity with a single operative exposure, ideally one used more routinely for the management of other conditions in and around the basilar subarachnoid cisterns. The classical subtemporal approach (7–9), a technique developed in cadavers and refined in slack brains using hand-held retractors, head lights, and low-power loupes initially, seemed to answer poorly to all of these needs. Furthermore, the steep learning curve associated with operating on vertebrobasilar aneurysms that Dr. Drake (7, 9, 11) mentioned frequently did not lend itself to the rapid development of posterior circulation expertise with a routine aneurysm population. To bring lesions of the basilar artery into the realm of the merely human aneurysm surgeon, a technical revolution was necessary.

MICROVASCULAR SURGERY

Few individuals can be identified in any field of endeavor who have ushered their profession through a true quantum leap, but beginning in the late 1960s Professor Yasargil (41, 42) almost single-handedly launched our surgical subspecialty into its current orbit around the technology of the operating microscope. His almost innumerable contributions to neurological surgery range from imaging to epilepsy, but his most expansive work has formed the literal foundation of the subspecialty of microvascular surgery (42). Yasargil's conceptual visualization of the base of the human brain as a stereotyped labyrinth of interlocking arachnoid chambers, each with precisely defined contents, boundaries, and connections, provided the young surgeon a degree of anatomic certainty previously available only through years of operative experience. The technical advances (42) he pioneered enabled the dedicated student to routinely expose, dissect, and obliterate lesions previously limited to the few acknowledged surgical masters. Subsequently, the microscope and microtechnique brought illumination and definition to the "dark corners of the brain," and for those of us interested in aneurysm surgery, no corner has been deeper or darker than the interpeduncular cistern (11). From a modicum of experience with posterior circulation aneurysms, Yasargil (42) recognized the limitations and restrictions of the subtemporal exposure and rapidly developed an alternative approach, whose popularization has been a critical factor in making the successful treatment of most basilar aneurysms possible for the well-trained microvascular surgeon.

The pterional or transsylvian approach subsequently has become the popular route of exposure of the region of the basilar apex, and almost every aneurysm surgeon has a special modification of this essential microsurgical exposure (30, 34, 37). At Southwestern, we have become comfortable with a relatively routine scalp, muscle, and bony opening involving a limited subtemporal craniectomy and resection of the sphenoid ridge only to the outer limits of the superior orbital fissure. After opening the dura, we routinely tap the frontal horn in the fashion described by Payne et al. (24), and then widely split the sylvian fissure from the middle cerebral bifurcation to the termination of the internal carotid, where one retractor blade is placed just above the carotid bifurcation. The cistern of the anterior cerebral artery is opened sharply into the prechiasmatic cistern, and for large aneurysms, or those that lie well below or far above the posterior clinoid process, we mobilize the temporal pole and uncus posteriorly with a second retractor to expose the IIIrd cranial nerve. Whenever possible, the lateral wing of Liliequist's membrane is opened lateral to the oculomotor nerve, and the superior cerebellar artery is followed retrograde to the basilar trunk. With proximal control of the basilar artery, the inferior margin of the posterior communicating vessel is followed to the P1–P2 junction, the membrane is opened, and the P1 segment of the posterior cerebral artery is tracked back to the basilar summit. At the surgeon's discretion, additional exposure can be obtained by sectioning the posterior communicating artery to mobilize the carotid anteriorly, opening the carotid-optic triangle to improve visualization of the contralateral posterior cerebral origin, or by a performing a small subpial resection of the most medial portion of the uncus to enhance exposure of the rostral limits of the cistern.

Using any surgical approach, final exposure of aneurysm at or near the basilar apex occurs in a tight confined space, which compels the operator to work in close proximity to the fragile lesion, and often necessitates cleavage of clot and arachnoidal scar to permit mobilization of the aneurysm's fundus. Historically, the most dreaded complication of such dissection has been intraoperative aneurysmal rupture. Drake et al. (11) reported a frequency of up to 20% of cases, which has been associated with a two- to threefold increase in operative morbidity and mortality (2). To reduce the incidence of premature hemorrhage, early in his experience Drake (7–9) resorted to the routine use of profound systemic hypotension during aneurysm dissection and ligation. Nonetheless, in the London series the incidence of premature rupture remained at almost 15%, until the reintroduction of routine proximal temporary arterial occlusion (38).

LOCAL AND SYSTEMIC ARTERIAL ARREST

Temporary arterial occlusion represents one of the most important technical innovations in aneurysm surgery during the past 20 years. Initially championed by Suzuki et al. (38) to reduce the complication of intraoperative aneurysmal rupture, it was rapidly adopted by most experienced aneurysm surgeons, including Dr. Drake who had abandoned its use in 1972. Surgeons quickly discovered that not only does this maneuver significantly diminish both the incidence and the significance of premature hemorrhage (27), but equally important it facilitates definitive isolation of the aneurysm neck from normal afferent and efferent vasculature. An excellent example of this last effect occurs in the final dissection of basilar apex aneurysms via the transsylvian approach.

The view of the distal basilar artery provided by all versions of the transsylvian exposure is oblique, displaying the basilar trunk, both superior cerebellar arteries, and the origins of both P1 segments without manipulation of any contents of the interpeduncular cistern. This approach does not offer an unimpeded view of the critical thalamoperforating arteries that are invariably intimately attached to the posterior wall of basilar summit aneurysms, and whose injury is the major source of operative morbidity with this procedure. However, the use of a temporary clip on the distal basilar trunk permits the surgeon to safely reflect even a posteriorly projecting aneurysm out of the depths of the cistern and away from the underlying perforating arteries. Although with diligence the surgeon can routinely identify the origin of the contralateral P1 segment during dissection of non-giant aneurysms, unfortunately proximal occlusion alone is rarely sufficient for the complete definition of very expansive aneurysmal necks or those containing either thrombosis or calcification. This problem is complicated further by the propensity of giant and very large aneurysms to involve a considerable length of each P1 segment in the aneurysm neck.

In the majority of such situations, adequate visualization and definition of the aneurysm neck can only be achieved by complete evacuation and collapse of the aneurysm fundus. Obviously, this necessitates complete isolation of the basilar apex, causing potential flow reductions in the distal posterior cerebral and superior cerebellar territories, and the much more certain and dangerous ischemia of the thalamoperforating arteries. The presence of reasonable posterior communicating collateral flow mitigates the threat to the cortical distributions of the posterior cerebral arteries, and the superior cerebellar territories seem to tolerate protracted proximal occlusion well, but the mesencephalic and diencephalic distributions of the perforating vessels have no collateral input. In general, the temporal threshold for conversion of ischemia to infarction in this situation appears to be approximately 20 minutes (27), with shorter durations routinely well tolerated and more protracted periods associated with both radiographic and clinical evidence of infarction. Data are inconclusive to determine whether intermittent occlusion and reperfusion is somewhat better tolerated, but generally the issue is moot because aneurysm opening and evacuation rarely allow for temporary restoration of antegrade flow.

The abilities of putative "brain protection" agents to enhance clinical toleration of ischemia have been debated since Suzuki et al. (38, 39) reported the "Sendai cocktail," but currently no unanimity of surgical opinion exists on the benefits of such therapies. Laboratory evidence is plentiful to suggest that certain anesthetic agents such as sodium thiopental (33, 40, 43) and etomidate (40), as well as both moderate (36) and profound hypothermia (10, 19) increase the ischemic threshold. Because the clinical use of such regimens is simple and noninjurious, we have routinely employed both burst-suppression barbiturate coma and moderate hypothermia in almost all patients undergoing posterior circulation aneurysm surgery.

The theoretical ultimate in neuronal protection against ischemia is the profound hypothermia offered by cardiac standstill and extracorporeal circulation. Drake et al. (10) experimented with this approach in the late 1960s, but they abandoned it because of problems associated with the obligatory systemic anticoagulation. We operated on two giant apex aneurysms using cardiac standstill in 1978 and 1979; both patients died in the immediate postoperative period from hemorrhagic complications. However, a decade later after the promising reports of Silverberg et al. (32) at Stanford, and bolstered by the large experience of Spetzler et al. (35) and Solomon and Stein (34), we elected to revisit the issue. In light of our explorations of the temporal threshold for the conversion of ischemia to infarction (27), the best indication to use the pump seemed to be our preoperative prediction of the duration of local circulatory arrest necessary to fix the aneurysm. If experience suggested that the time period would equal or exceed 30 minutes, temporary proximal arterial occlusion could not be considered a safe therapeutic alternative. In such situations we have opted for hypothermic cardiac standstill, which theoretically provides an additional 20 minutes of protected ischemia.

We have operated on 26 giant posterior circulation aneurysms under cardiac standstill. Our results in that group of patients include eight deaths and three patients with severe neurological morbidity; only slightly over 50% of patients have had good clinical outcomes. By virtue of our selection criteria, total arrest times have been lengthy (average, 44 min) and the incidence of complications, both systemic and neurological, has been very high. Nonetheless, in very unusual situations profound hypothermic arrest is a helpful surgical adjuvant, but it must be recognized as a costly, high-risk endeavor that often can be avoided by a judicious use of temporary proximal occlusion.

CRANIAL BASE EXPOSURES

Although cranial base surgical techniques (6, 15, 18, 31) emerged during the last third of Dr. Drake's practice lifetime, they seem not to have made a significant alteration in his basic surgical approaches to posterior circulation aneurysms (11). He declined to incorporate either zygomatic resection or orbital roof removal in his routine subtemporal approach to the distal basilar artery, and despite early experience with presigmoid transtentorial exposure, he ultimately recommended a more traditional lateral, suboccipital exposure for almost all lesions from the dural tunnel of the vertebral artery to the vertebral confluens. For those of us less gifted, the evolution of cranial base concepts has made a major contribution to our own surgical experience in the management of posterior circulation aneurysms, especially for lesions of the basilar summit and trunk situated behind the clivus.

More than 85% of all basilar apex and superior cerebellar artery aneurysms lie at or slightly above the height of the posterior clinoid process (29), and as such they can be optimally exposed, along with the immediately proximal basilar trunk, via a standard transsylvian approach. The anatomic structures that limit the ultimate extent of exposure form a narrow operative corridor 10 to 15 millimeters superficial to the basilar artery; these are the carotid artery, the optic tract, the mesial temporal lobe, the IIIrd cranial nerve, the incisura, and the posterior cavernous sinus. The posterior clinoid process and clivus most commonly project anteriorly (to the left) of the critical structures when the right-sided operative approach is performed with the patient's head turned 45 degrees to the left. Occasionally, removal of the clinoid is helpful in exposing the contralateral origin of a low-lying P1 segment or the superior cerebellar artery, but this does not add to the demonstration of either the proximal basilar artery or its bifurcation.

One effective mechanism to increase this exposure is opening the posterior corner of the cavernous sinus (5). With reflection of the body of the sinus anteriorly, the proximal basilar artery frequently can be followed well into the prepontine cistern. When dealing with large or giant low-lying aneurysms, this exposure involves transection of the IVth cranial nerve in its dural leaflet, but no neuro-ophthalmological consequences of such sacrifice have been observed in almost 20 such patients so treated since 1994. The extent of proximal basilar exposure obtained by the maneuver obviously is variable, but often the origin of one or both anteroinferior cerebellar arteries can be observed. When the basilar apex is displaced superiorly over 1 cm above the posterior clinoid process, removal of the zygomatic process as initially described by Neil-Dweyer et al. (22) has proven very helpful in providing a more anterotemporal perspective, which brings the axis of the basilar trunk and the usually posteriorly located aneurysm into excellent view without the necessity for other manipulations. In the Southwestern experience, extension of the craniotomy to include the orbital roof has not enhanced the existing exposure, simply because the carotid artery and the optic tract preclude effective use of the increased superficial exposure.

The cranial base approaches that have proven most beneficial in our exposure of the vertebral and proximal basilar arteries have been the newer modifications of the classic lateral suboccipital exposure. Although without question, aneurysms of the vertebral arteries from the dural tunnel to the confluens can be operated via a median or paramedian exposure in almost any position other than the supine, the degree of surgical access to the entire intracranial vertebral artery is enhanced by any one of the several variations of the "far" lateral approach (16, 17,

37). All of these involve the lateral position, early exposure of the extracranial vertebral segment in the C1–C2 triangle, bony removal of the lateral suboccipital to expose the sigmoid sinus to the jugular bulb, and resection of the lateral aspect of the bony foramen magnum up to and often including the most posterior portion of the occipital condyle. This approach is tailor made for the aneurysm surgeon: it provides early proximal control, access to the cisterna magna, gravitational retraction of the cerebellum, and the ability to work below, through, and above the curtain of the lower cranial nerves. In addition, this exposure offers the best surgical view of the vertebral artery distal to the posteroinferior cerebellar artery (PICA) takeoff, where invariably the vessel turns medially to run toward the midline. Not only is distal vertebral visualization critical to ensure that clip placement does not stenose or occlude the vertebral artery, but in the event of intraoperative hemorrhage, inability to instantly trap the vertebral artery above and below the aneurysm may be disastrous. Even with an extensive exposure of the aneurysm-bearing vertebral segment, the surgical manipulation required to effectively manage even routine ruptured vertebral PICA aneurysms often results in transient but potentially dangerous lower cranial nerve dysfunction, a complication that Dr. Drake emphasized, and which occurred in almost 20% of the London series (11). Horowitz et al. (17) published a recent series from Southwestern documenting the high short-term incidence of such palsy, but they also demonstrated that if managed carefully, the sequelae are minimal and the incidence of protracted palsy is very small, and limited only to craniotomy for giant aneurysms.

The other aneurysm variant observed with striking frequency in the proximal vertebral artery is the vertebral dissection, whose appropriate treatment continues to be a matter of some controversy. Patients with such lesions may present with neck pain only, with distal embolic-based ischemia, or with hemorrhage into the cerebellopontine cistern or foramen of Luschka. Proximal occlusion alone is generally safe, but unfortunately it is frequently ineffective, especially for hemorrhagic dissections; we have observed four recurrent hemorrhages after either clip or coil vertebral occlusion proximal to the PICA. Exclusion of the entire diseased segment of artery from the arterial circulation with preservation of PICA flow is the optimal and definitive goal of treatment, and if the distal vertebral cannot be surgically remodeled adequately to ensure retrograde flow into the PICA, an occipital PICA bypass should be performed.

In our limited experience, this expanded, far lateral exposure has been adequate for lesions up to and including those of the vertebral confluens/basilar origin, where routine saccular aneurysms are infrequent but generally pose no specific surgical difficulty. However, this relatively benign prognosis is markedly different than that of the giant dolichoectatic aneurysms, which increasingly come to surgical attention primarily because of cranial nerve dysfunction, pontine compression, and incipient hydrocephalus. Unfortunately, at least at our institution these aneurysms, only four of which Dr. Drake subjected to surgery (11), form an increasingly large segment of patients referred for treatment.

DOLICHOECTATIC AND SERPENTINE BASILAR ANEURYSMS

Anatomically and pathophysiologically, these aneurysms are variations on a consistent theme. Both distal vertebral arteries and the basilar trunk are involved in an extensive expansion and remodeling in all three axes, a central feature of which is progressive intraluminal thrombosis and recanalization. The resultant S-shaped mass frequently extends from one cerebellopontine angle transversely across the belly of the pons to the contralateral incisura, and the basilar apex generally is located well rostral to its normal position, often indenting the third ventricle. As a rule, collateral circulation to the basilar trunk is limited to very small PICAs, and one vertebral artery may be extremely small. Atherosclerotic changes are common in the carotid arteries in these patients, but not infrequently these monster lesions are found in distressingly young individuals, which raises the unproven possibility that they may represent some chronic form of arterial dissection, or alternatively a forme fruste of a collagen vascular disease such as Ehlers-Danlos syndrome.

Treatment options in this patient population are limited by the extensive segment of arterial involvement, the necessity to maintain perfusion of the pontine penetrating arteries, the calcific/thrombotic nature of the arterial wall, and the limited availability of collateral to the posterior circulation territories. Cerebrospinal fluid diversion generally is the initial intervention, but in our experience as well as that of others, it frequently precipitates a step-wise decline in neurological status, and never is more than transiently effective in the arrest reversal of neurological deficits. Simple although extensive bony decompression of the posterior fossa, and in some cases of the symptomatic cranial nerves, provides transient remission if any, at least in the long tract deficits. Systemic anticoagulation alone has not been shown to be beneficial in altering the disease's natural history.

The most promising therapeutic approach reported to date has been the Anson et al. (1) adaptation of Dr. Drake's extensive experience with the use of Hunterian ligation for giant saccular aneurysms of the basilar trunk and vertebro-basilar junction (11). Dr. Drake selected patients for treatment on the basis of angiographically demonstrated PICAs, and clinical outcome was good in 75% of almost 50 cases. The goal of this treatment process is reversal of flow in the basilar artery, relying on either natural or surgically created collateral for retrograde perfusion of the basilar trunk.

Unfortunately, as mentioned, most patients with dolichoectatic aneurysms have small PICAs. Of the four patients Drake treated, only one survived. The challenges of treatment are twofold: to provide adequate surgical collateral to induce retrograde flow in the basilar artery, and to prevent subsequent thrombosis of the dolichoectatic segment. This generally necessitates performing a high-volume extracranial to intracranial bypass procedure, sacrificing sequential vertebral artery, and using systemic long-term anticoagulation to preclude progressive thrombosis following flow reversal. Although in theory these challenges can be met routinely, the risks of large volume bypasses into the posterior cerebral artery are not insignificant, and even with documented flow reversal, such aneurysms can and do continue to enlarge, occasionally rupturing. Despite the availability of the gamut of microsurgical and endovascular treatment possibilities at Southwestern, we have yet to evolve a consistently successful therapeutic strategy in perhaps our most challenging aneurysm patient population. Part of this inadequacy certainly relates to the end-stage clinical status of many such patients who are treated, or referred for treatment, only at or near the point of incapacitating neurological deficits, especially long tract and bulbar losses. Whether these deficits relate to actual deformation of the brainstem by the progressive enlargement of the dolichoectatic mass or, as postulated by Drake et al. (11) and Anson et al. (1), to the sequential occlusion of the critical penetrating arteries remains an unresolved issue, but reversal of these neurological losses is extremely unlikely regardless of the imaging success of treatment; therefore documented progression of functional loss is a strong indication for therapy.

SURGICAL SUMMARY

Despite the incremental advances, the surgical management of most posterior circulation aneurysms remains a high-risk undertaking. Even in patients who present in good clinical condition, acceptable long-term outcomes are far from assured, the incidence of intraoperative complications remains high, and the learning curve for new aneurysm surgeons is both steep and costly. It is imperative that we continue to ask whether what we do and the way we do it is the best for patients; critical reevaluation is even more important now that there is a viable therapeutic alternative to microsurgical aneurysm clip ligation.

ENDOVASCULAR TREATMENT

During the past decade, endovascular technology and the skill of its proponents have brought this subspecialty into the therapeutic spotlight of aneurysm management, and nowhere so brightly as in lesions of the posterior circulation. Generally straightforward catheter access to the vertebral and basilar arteries, coupled with a high incidence of small-necked, side-wall aneurysms, have made an inviting interventional target of posterior circulation lesions that have been surgically difficult to expose. The diminished anesthetic demands and low morbidity rates associated with the endovascular procedures, in addition to the rapid learning curve and explosion in technology, have resulted in broad enthusiasm for coiling as a primary treatment option in many locations. The relative paucity of centers offering both microvascular and endovascular options has tended to polarize an increasingly acrimonious debate, which is unfortunately fueled, at least in part, by our national frenzy to slash health care compensation. Regrettably, another guest at this feast has been the neurosurgical ego, on one hand reluctant to recognize the virtues of a competitive technique, on the other unwilling to acknowledge our own limitations, but paradoxically anxious to proclaim "if I can't do it, it can't be done surgically—send it to be coiled." When the similar psychological perturbation of the endovascular community is added to the mix, the debate is even more rancorous.

What do we know, if anything, about the current comparative status of the two treatment modalities in managing aneurysms of the vertebrobasilar system? To date, the only comparative study, from the Gruber et al. (13) at the University of Cincinnati, examined some 50 basilar apex aneurysms treatable with either clips or coils. They found a distinct improved short-term clinical outcome in the 50% of patients undergoing endovascular management. Stimulated by the findings of this study, we reviewed the published endovascular results with this most common posterior circulation aneurysm and compared them with our own operative outcomes (28). As of September 1, 2000, we could identity a total of 434 patients reported in 9 studies in the English literature (3, 4, 12, 14, 20, 21, 23, 25, 26) each having a basilar apex aneurysm treated with Guglielmi detachable coiling, with some clinical follow-up after hospitalization. The specifics of those patients' clinical parameters and those of their aneurysms were tabulated and compared with our own patient population. Somewhat surprisingly, the groups are relatively homogeneous in terms of incidence of subarachnoid hemorrhage (67%), acuity of illness (Hunt and Hess Grades I–III, 79% versus 84%), aneurysm size (small, 60% versus 56%), and so on. Even many of the treatment parameters were similar, including the incidence of complications (18% versus 15%), although the negative contribution of such complications to patient outcome was demonstrably less in the endovascular series.

The efficacy of treatment, as judged by a similar percentage of postoperative angiograms (72% versus 74%) was, as expected, much higher in the surgical group; residual aneurysm was identifiable in 9% of postoperative studies, compared with an average of 46% in the endovascular group. However, if neurosurgeons demanded the same intense radiographic scrutiny of our postoperative patients as our endovascular colleagues, almost certainly the actual incidence of residual aneurysm would be between 15 and 20% (11), instead of half that figure. In these two series, retreatment was undertaken for a variety of reasons in over one-third of endovascular patients, and in slightly more than 2% of our series. Clinical outcome was almost identical in the two patient populations (excellent–good, 78% versus 80%), both at the time of discharge and at latest available follow-up. The incidence of posttreatment subarachnoid hemorrhage was significantly different, occurring in approximately 3% of endovascular patients versus none in the smaller surgical group. The potential importance of that isolated difference becomes more evident when the average length of clinical follow-up in the two populations is examined: 18 months in the endovascular group and more than 5 years in the postsurgical patients.

This admittedly inexact comparative study offers no startling insights, but suggests that each technique has distinct strengths and identifiable weaknesses, characteristics that have been recognized and passionately extolled by their individual proponents. In experienced hands, the risks of endovascular treatment seem to be lower than those of microsurgery, although the radiographic efficacy of clip obliteration is greater than coil embolization. Clinically, the short-term efficiency of the two treatment modalities in preventing recurrent bleeding is high, although early postcoiling hemorrhage has been reported occasionally. Currently, the durability of microsurgery remains the therapeutic gold standard, and in the relatively brief follow-up period presently available, the risk of delayed recurrent bleeding from coiled aneurysms seems to be small but significant.

It is unfortunate that in the main, these two treatment options are competitive rather than complimentary. Microvascular surgeons and their endovascular colleagues both prefer to operate on medium-sized aneurysms with small necks that are separate and distinct from the afferent and efferent vasculature. Both perform better on lesions filled with flowing blood rather than atheroma and clot, and a side-wall aneurysm is simpler and easier to eliminate than a lesion at a true bifurcation or quadrification. Currently, both therapeutic schools have poor answers for the riddles of giant saccular aneurysms that incorporate the efferent vessels, as well as for the serpentine monsters of the distal vertebral and proximal basilar arteries. Furthermore, although there are isolated examples of the beneficial effects of the two techniques applied to the same aneurysm sequentially, these successful cooperative ventures are the exception rather than the rule. Usually, inadequate preliminary treatment with one modality compromises the technical effectiveness and clinical outcome of the sequential therapy.

In theory, the two viable treatment options currently available are applicable to most patients with posterior circulation aneurysms. The practical reality of that availability naturally differs from institution to institution, as do the technical skills and acumen of the cerebrovascular clinicians. In some situations, that variability has been ignored, resulting in narrow and strident advocacy of a single therapeutic approach to every aneurysm. At other centers, interventionalists and microvascular surgeons have together elaborated specific therapeutic algorithms focused primarily on factors such as aneurysm location, size, shape, and geometry to guide their treatment selection. Both of these conceptual approaches are valid vehicles for the conveyance of personal opinion, but has the specialty really learned?

We have milked the present partisan debate dry regarding the relative merits of these two treatment techniques. The future of aneurysm treatment, especially that of posterior circulation lesions, begs to be defined by a prospective objective comparison of the applicability, safety, efficacy, and durability of clip versus coil therapy. The information systems, technology, and a sufficient number of recognized experts in both treatment modalities all are at hand. What remains is simply to identify the participating centers and agree on the patient admission criteria; for all the reasons discussed above, lesions of the vertebrobasilar system would form an ideal study population.

How should these most dangerous of all aneurysms he treated in the 21st century? We have the capacity now to answer that critical question. Dr. Charles Drake, the consummate physician, would expect no less of us.

REFERENCES

1. Anson JA, Lawton MT, Spetzler RF. Characteristics and surgical treatment of dolichoectatic and fusiform aneurysms. **J Neurosurg** 84:185–193, 1996.

2. Batjer HH, Samson DS. Causes of morbidity and mortality from surgery of aneurysms of the distal basilar artery. **Neurosurgery** 25:904–916, 1989.
3. Bavinzski G, Killer M, Gruber A, Reinpreclit A, Gross CE, Richling B. Treatment of basilar artery bifurcation aneurysms by using Guglielmi detachable coils: A 6-year experience. **J Neurosurg** 90:843–852, 1999.
4. Byrne JV, Sohn MJ, Molyneux AJ. Five-year experience in using coil embolization for ruptured intracranial aneurysms: Outcomes and incidence of late rebleeding. **J Neurosurg** 90:656–663, 1999.
5. Coimbra C, Landreneau F, Mickey B, Kopitnik T, Samson D. The paramedial transcavernous approach to the basilar artery: A microanatomical study. **Skull Base Surgery** 7:12,1997.
6. Dolenc VV, Skrap M, Sustersic J, Skrbec M, Morina A. A transcavernous-transsellar approach to the basilar tip aneurysms. **Br J Neurosurg** 1:251–259, 1987.
7. Drake CC. Surgical treatment of ruptured aneurysms of the basilar artery: Experience with 14 cases. **J Neurosurg** 23:457–473, 1965.
8. Drake CG. The surgical treatment of the vertebral basilar aneurysms. **Clin Neurosurg** 16:114–169, 1969.
9. Drake CG. The treatment of aneurysms of the posterior circulation. **Clin Neurosurg** 26:96–144, 1979.
10. Drake CG, Barr HWK, Coles JC, Gergely NF. The use of extracorporeal circulation and profound hypothermia in the treatment of ruptured intracranial aneurysms. **J Neurosurg** 21:575–581, 1964.
11. Drake CG, Peerless SJ, Hernesniemi J. Surgery of vertebrobasilar aneurysms. New York: Springer Verlag, 1996.
12. Eskridge JM, Song JK. Endovascular embolization of 150 basilar tip aneurysms with Guglielmi detachable coils: Results of the Food and Drug Administration multicenter clinical trial. **J Neurosurg** 89:81–86, 1998.
13. Gruber DP, Zimmerman TA, Tomsick A, van Loveren HR, Link MJ, Tew JM Jr. A comparison between endovascular and surgical management of basilar artery apex aneurysms. **J Neurosurg** 90:868–874, 1999.
14. Guglielmi G, Vinuela F, Duckwiler G, Dion J, Lylyk P, Berenstein A, Strother C, Graves V, Halbach V, Nichols D, et al. Endovascular treatment of posterior circulation aneurysms by electrothrombosis using electrically detachable coils. **J Neurosurg** 77:515–524, 1992.
15. Hakuba A, Liu S, Nishimura S. The orbitozygomatic infratemporal approach: A new surgical technique. **Surg Neurol** 26:271–276, 1986.
16. Heros RC. Lateral suboccipital approach for vertebral and vertebro basilar aneurysms. **J Neurosurg** 64:559–562, 1986.
17. Horowitz MB, Kopitnik TA, Landreneau F, Krummerman J, Batjer HH, Thomas G, Samson D. Posteroinferior cerebellar artery aneurysms: Surgical results for 38 patients. **Neurosurgery** 43:1026–1032, 1998.
18. Ikeda K, Yamashita J, Hashimoto M, Futami K. Orbitozygomatic temporopolar approach for a high basilar tip aneurysm associated with a short intracranial internal carotid artery: A new surgical approach. **Neurosurgery** 28:105–110, 1991.
19. Lim RA, Rehder K, Harp RA, et al. Circulatory arrest during profound hypothermia induced by direct blood-stream cooling. **Surgery** 49:367–374, 1961.
20. McDougall CF, Halbach VV, Dowd CF, Higashida RT, Larsen DW, Hlieshima GB. Endovascular treatment of basilar tip aneurysms using electrolytically detachable coils. **J Neurosurg** 84:393–399, 1996.
21. Moret J, Cognard C, Weill A, Castaings L, Rey A. The "remodeling technique" in the treatment of wide neck intracranial aneurysms: Angiographic results and clinical follow-up in 56 cases. **Int Neuroradiol** 3:21–35, 1997.

22. Neil-Dwyer G, Sharr M, Haskell R, Currie D, Hosseini M. Zygomaticotemporal approach to the basis cranii and basilar artery. **Neurosurgery** 23:20–22, 1988.
23. Nichols DA, Brown RD Jr., Thielen KR, Meyer FB, Atkinson JL, Piepgras DG. Endovascular treatment of ruptured posterior circulation aneurysms using electolytically detachable coils. **J Neurosurg** 87:374–380, 1997.
24. Paine JT, Batjer HH, Samson DS. Intraoperative ventricular puncture. **Neurosurgery** 22:1107–1109, 1988.
25. Pierot L, Boulin A, Castaings L, Rey A, Moret J. Selective occlusion of basilar artery aneurysms using controlled detachable coils: report of 35 cases. **Neurosurgery** 38:948–954, 1997.
26. Raymond J, Roy D, Bojanowski M, Moumdjian R, L'Esperance G. Endovascular treatment of acutely ruptured and unruptured aneurysms of the basilar bifurcation. **J Neurosurg** 86:211–219, 1997.
27. Samson DS, Batjer HH, Bowman G, Mootz L, Krippner WJ Jr, Meyer YJ, Allen BC. A clinical study of the parameters and effects of temporary arterial occlusion in the management of intracranial aneurysms. **Neurosurgery** 34:22–29, 1994.
28. Samson D, Batjer HH, Kopitnik TA Jr. Current results of the surgical management of aneurysms of the basilar apex. **Neurosurgery** 44:697–704, 1999.
29. Samson DS, Hodosh RM, Clark WK. Microsurgical evaluation of the pterional approach to aneurysms of the distal basilar circulation. **Neurosurgery** 3:135–141, 1978.
30. Sano K. Temporopolar approach to aneurysms of the basilar artery at and around the distal bifurcation: Technical note. **Neurol Res** 2:361–367, 1980.
31. Shiokawa Y, Saito I, Aoki N, Mizutani H. Zygomatic temporopolar approach for basilar artery aneurysms. **Neurosurgery** 24:385–391, 1989.
32. Silverberg E, Reitz BA, Ream AK. Hypothermia and cardiac arrest in the treatment of giant aneurysms of the cerebral circulation and hemangioblastoma of the medulla. **J Neurosurg** 55:337–346, 1981.
33. Smith DS, Rehincrona S, Siesjo BK. Barbiturates as protective agents in brain ischemia and as free radical scavengers in vitro. **Acta Physiol Scand Suppl** 492:129–134, 1980.
34. Solomon RA, Stein BM. Surgical approaches to aneurysms of the vertebral and basilar arteries. **Neurosurgery** 23:203–208, 1988.
35. Spetzler RF, Hadley MN, Rigamonti D, Carter LP, Raudzens PA, Shedd SA, Wilkinson E. Aneurysms of the basilar artery treated with circulatory arrest, hypothermia, and barbiturate cerebral protection. **J Neurosurg** 68:868–879, 1988.
36. Steen PA, Michenfelder JD. Barbiturate protection in tolerant and nontolerant hypoxic mice: Comparison with hypothermic protection. **Anesthesiology** 50:404–408, 1979.
37. Sugita K, Kobayashi S, Shintani A, Mutsuga N. Microneurosurgery for aneurysms of the basilar artery. **J Neurosurg** 51:615–620, 1979.
38. Suzuki J, Kwak R, Okudaira Y. The safe time limit of temporary clamping of cerebral arteries in the direct surgical treatment of intracranial aneurysm under moderate hypothermia, in, Suzuki J (ed). *Cerebral Aneurysms: Experiences with 1000 Directly Operated Cases.* Tokyo: Tokyo Press, 1979, pp 325–329.
39. Suzuki J, Yoshimoto T. The effect of mannitol in prolongation of permissible occlusion time of cerebral artery: Clinical data of aneurysm surgery. **Neurosurg Rev** 1:13–19, 1979.
40. Wauquier A, Aston D, Clincke G, Niemegeers CJ. Anti-hypoxic effects of etomidate, thiopental, and methohexital. **Arch Int Pharmacodyn Ther** 249:330–334, 1981.
41. Yasargil MG, Antic J, Lagica R, Jain KK, Hodosh RM, Smith RD. Microneurosurgical

pterional approach to aneurysms of the basilar bifurcation. **Surg Neurol** 6:83–91, 1976.
42. Yasargil MG. Vertebrobasilar aneurysms, in, *Microneurosurgery.* Stuttgart: George Thieme, 1986, vol 2, p. 232–255.
43. Yatsu FM. Pharmacologic protection against ischemic brain damage. **Neurol Clin** 1:37–53, 1983.

II

General Scientific Session II Neurovascular Decision Making

CHAPTER

9

Aneurysms Requiring Extended Cranial Base Approaches

DANIEL L. BARROW, M.D., C. MICHAEL CAWLEY, M.D.

The goals of surgery for intracranial aneurysms usually include elimination of the aneurysm from the circulation, maintenance of blood flow to the normal circulation, and avoidance of damage to neural tissue. As with most operations, adequate exposure is essential to success. Cranial base surgical exposures are one of a variety of adjuncts available to the neurovascular surgeon that assist in accomplishing these goals.

Cranial base exposures are accomplished by removing nonvital bone at the cranial base to maximize exposure yet minimize the extent of brain retraction. Using cranial base techniques, a deep, narrow exposure can be converted into a wider, shallower exposure through more caudally located windows. This will facilitate proximal vascular control and clip application.

The standard approaches to most intracranial aneurysms include frontotemporal (pterional), subtemporal, and retrosigmoid suboccipital craniotomies. Performed properly, each of these exposures involves removal of bone from the cranial base to improve exposure, create a wider and shallower window, and minimize retraction; therefore, these are cranial base approaches. In a variety of circumstances, each standard approach can be converted into a more expanded or extended cranial base approach for selected aneurysms as outlined in *Table 9.1*. The selection of a particular approach or combination of approaches is based on careful consideration of the location, size, and configuration of the aneurysm, the presence of calcification or intraluminal thrombus within the aneurysm, and the neurological status of the patient. The aneurysm locations for which extended cranial base approaches are commonly used are outlined in *Table 9.2*.

ANTERIOR CIRCULATION

Internal Carotid Artery Aneurysms

The overwhelming majority of internal carotid artery (ICA) aneurysms are approached through a frontotemporal (pterional) craniotomy. Even for

Table 9.1
Skull Base Extensions of Standard Approaches to Intracranial Aneurysms

Pterional
Anterior clinoidectomy
Orbitozygomatic approach
Posterior cliniodectomy
Transapical
Transcavernous approach
Posterior clinoidectomy
Transapical
Subtemporal
Medial petrosectomy
Combined middle and posterior fossa approaches
Presigmoid petrosal
Retrolabyrinthine
Translabyrinthine
Transcochlear
Suboccipital
Retrolabyrinthine-transsigmoid
Transcondylar (far lateral)
Extreme Lateral Inferior Transcondylar Exposure (ELITE)

a standard pterional craniotomy, extensive extradural removal of the lesser wing of the sphenoid improves exposure and minimizes brain retraction. Those aneurysms arising on the proximal portion of the ICA, including the cavernous, clinoidal, and ophthalmic segments, usually require extended cranial base techniques for adequate exposure and management.

Table 9.2
Aneurysms Requiring Extended Skull Base Approaches

Anterior circulation
Internal carotid artery
Cavernous segment
Clinoidal segment
Ophthalmic artery
Superior hypophyseal artery
Anterior communicating artery
Posterior circulation
Basilar artery
Basilar bifurcation[a]
P1 segment of posterior cerebral artery[a]
Superior cerebellar artery[a]
Basilar trunk
Vertebral artery
Posterior inferior cerebellar artery

[a]Cranial base approaches required for high or low basilar bifurcations.

Aneurysms confined to the cavernous segment of the ICA are associated with a significantly more benign natural history than their subarachnoid counterparts. When progressively symptomatic, these lesions are most commonly treated using ICA sacrifice with or without an extracranial-to-intracranial bypass to augment collateral blood flow (1). Determining the safety of therapeutic carotid sacrifice and the need for extracranial-to-intracranial bypass can be assisted by a balloon test occlusion. On rare occasions, a direct surgical approach to an aneurysm of the cavernous sinus is indicated. In this unusual circumstance, the standard pterional craniotomy is expanded by more aggressive removal of the lesser wing of the sphenoid, as well as aggressive resection of the temporal bone to the floor of the middle fossa to expose the superior orbital fissure and the foramina ovale, rotundum, and spinosum. The petrous segment of the ICA is exposed in the cranial base for proximal control before the cavernous sinus is opened.

Adequate exposure of aneurysms on the clinoidal and ophthalmic segments requires a thorough knowledge of the anatomy of the anterior clinoid process and dural rings, so that the clinoid may be removed in its entirety, the optic canal may be unroofed, and the dural rings opened. On rare occasions, a posterior communicating artery aneurysm will lie below the internal dural ring, and removal of the anterior clinoid process and opening of the dural ring will be necessary for adequate exposure of the proximal portion of the neck, proximal control of the ICA, and satisfactory clip application. Anterior clinoidectomy, extradural optic nerve exposure, and dural ring sectioning are necessary for clip ligation of all clinoidal segment aneurysms and the vast majority of ophthalmic and superior hypophyseal aneurysms. For these aneurysms, proximal control can be obtained by exposing the clinoidal segment of the ICA or exposing the ICA in the cervical region.

Anterior communicating artery aneurysms

Most anterior communicating artery aneurysms are adequately exposed through a standard pterional craniotomy with additional extension of the frontal cut more medially just above the orbital ridge. Some surgeons use an orbitozygomatic extension of the pterional craniotomy for selected anterior communicating artery aneurysms, which provides a more shallow approach to the lesion.

POSTERIOR CIRCULATION

Rostral Basilar Artery Aneurysms

Aneurysms of the rostral basilar artery are most often adequately exposed by either frontotemporal (transsylvian) (28) or subtemporal approaches. This includes aneurysms arising at the basilar bifurcation, proximal posterior cerebral artery aneurysms, and those sacs arising on the basilar trunk at the origin of the superior cerebellar artery. There are advantages and disadvantages with each of these approaches, and different surgeons have personal preferences for similar aneurysms. Transsylvian exposures offer the advantages of familiar anatomy, a better view of the contralateral P1 segment of the posterior cerebral artery, and multiple avenues of exposure through the same approach. Compared with subtemporal approaches, transsylvian exposures allow the basilar bifurcation to be seen from a more anterior angle, they provide early visualization of the basilar trunk for initial proximal control, clot can be removed from a wider area of the basilar cisterns, and multiple aneurysms in the anterior circulation can be treated. Disadvantages of the transsylvian approach to the rostral basilar artery include the more oblique clip application, a requirement for some retraction of the optic nerve, ICA, and middle cerebral artery, some difficulty seeing the perforators on the back wall of the sac, and obscuration of the basilar trunk by the posterior clinoid process in patients with low-lying basilar bifurcations.

The subtemporal exposure offers a better view of the posterior wall of the basilar artery and important perforators that may be attached to the posterior aspect of the sac. The exposure of the basilar artery is at least 1 cm more shallow using this approach than the transsylvian route (17, 27). The requirement of a degree of temporal lobe retraction and poor visualization of the contralateral P1 and its perforators are detractors of the subtemporal approach.

Extended cranial base exposures are required when the basilar artery has a high or low bifurcation (*Figure 9.1*). Anatomic studies demonstrate that the top of the basilar artery is located within 1 cm of the level of the dorsum sellae in 87% of individuals. The apex of the basilar bifurcation is below the tip of the dorsum sellae in 19% of specimens, at about the same height in 51%, and superior to the dorsum sellae in 30% (14, 30). The bifurcation of the basilar artery is quite variable and may be located as low as 10 cm below the pontomesencephalic junction and as far rostrally as the mamillary bodies (19).

A high basilar bifurcation requires excessive retraction of the temporal lobe for exposure by a subtemporal approach, and the anterior cranial base limits the view up into the interpeduncular cistern through a transsylvian approach. In situations where the basilar bifurcation is above the sella turcica, exposure can be improved significantly by performing a transsylvian approach combined with an orbitozygomatic extension. This markedly improves the angle of the operating microscope pointing from below the orbital ridge high up into the interpeduncular fossa.

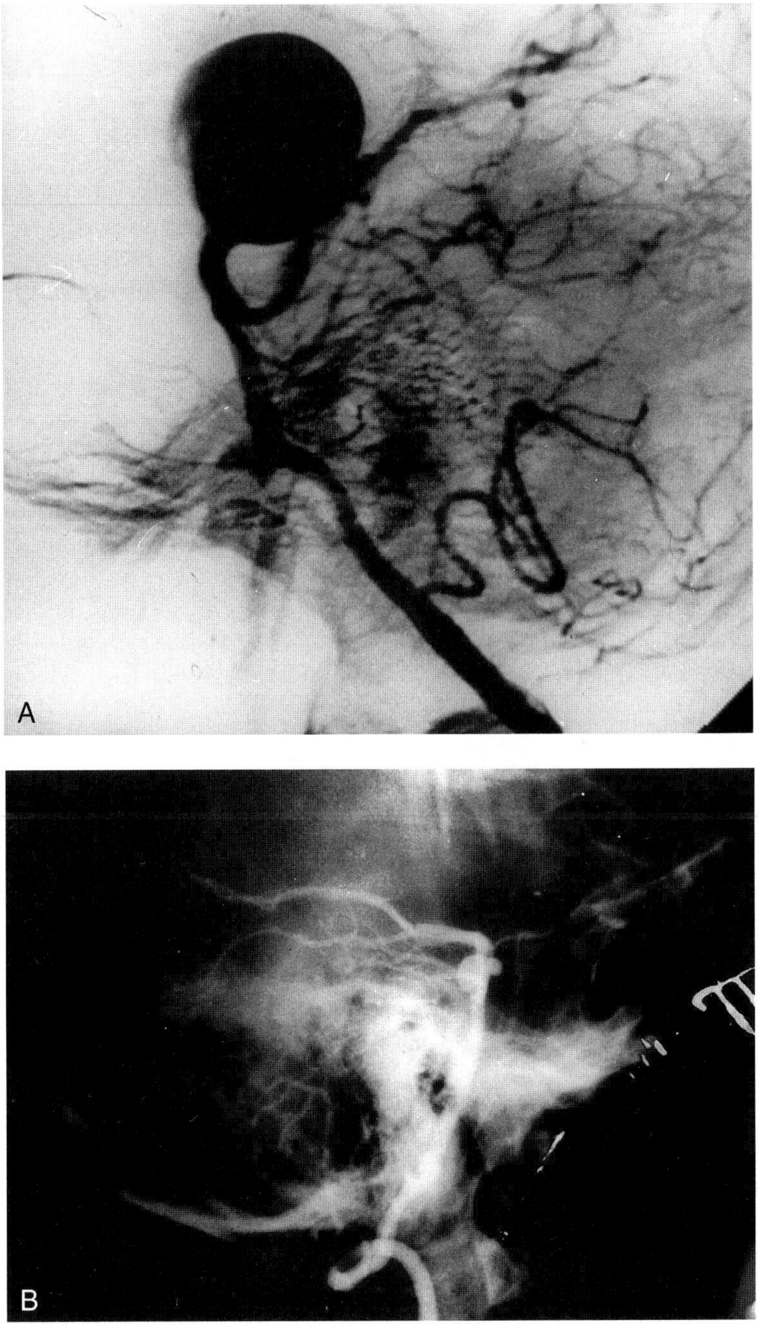

FIG. 9.1 Lateral vertebral angiograms of basilar tip aneurysms. *A*, high basilar bifurcation. *B*, low basilar bifurcation. Adequate visualization of each of these aneurysms is enhanced by extended cranial base approaches.

If the basilar bifurcation is low, i.e., below the sella turcica, the posterior clinoid process obscures the view of aneurysms arising in this region that are exposed through a transsylvian approach. In this situation, the surgeon can combine a frontotemporal approach with a posterior clinoidectomy to improve caudal exposure of the basilar artery. Another option in this situation is to divide the posterior portion of the cavernous sinus to improve caudal exposure through a frontotemporal approach. Although this improves exposure, it often requires sacrifice of the trochlear nerve. An orbitozygomatic extension, in combination with an extended pterional craniotomy and posterior clinoidectomy, will significantly improve exposure of a low-lying basilar bifurcation. When using a subtemporal approach to a rostral basilar aneurysm associated with a low-lying bifurcation, a medial petrosectomy will provide significantly more proximal exposure of the basilar artery.

For many aneurysms arising on the rostral basilar artery, the "half-and-half" procedure combines the advantages of the transsylvian and anterior subtemporal exposures. In this procedure, the basilar apex is approached under an elevated temporal lobe rather than an opened sylvian fissure (20, 22, 26). Dolenc et al. (3, 4) have advocated the transcavernous transsellar approach to enhance exposure of the upper basilar artery complex.

Basilar Trunk Aneurysms

Virtually all aneurysms occurring on the trunk of the basilar artery require some type of extended cranial base approach for adequate exposure. Some neurosurgeons advocate a frontotemporal, transsylvian approach with orbitozygomatic extension combined with posterior clinoidectomy to expose the upper basilar trunk (24). Subtemporal transtentorial and various combined supra- and infratentorial approaches have been used with good results. These combined approaches may be used with varying degrees of mastoid resection as popularized by Spetzler et al. (25). Retrolabyrinthine, translabyrinthine, and transcochlear extensions progressively enhance exposure and create an anterior-to-posterior approach to the basilar artery. A variety of modifications of Kawase's medial petrosectomy have been described to expose the basilar trunk. MacDonald et al. (15) have described the subtemporal, medial transpetrosal approach to the basilar artery that combines the wide view of the subtemporal approach with the more proximal exposure afforded by a medial petrosectomy.

Vertebral Artery Aneurysms

The origin of the posteroinferior cerebellar artery is the most common location for vertebral artery aneurysms. Aneurysms arising at this level up to the vertebral confluence may be exposed through a suboccipital, transcondylar (far lateral) approach. This approach provides early proximal control of the extradural and intradural vertebral artery and a flat view across the anterior aspect of the brainstem by removing the medial one-third of the occipital condyle and suboccipital bone to the sinus. The extreme lateral inferior transcondylar exposure (known as the ELITE approach) has been developed to enhance the retrosigmoid approach and alter the trajectory to lower brainstem pathologies from a posterior orientation to a more lateral and inferior orientation (2, 11, 21).

SURGICAL APPROACHES

The standard exposures for anterior and posterior circulation aneurysms include frontotemporal (pterional), subtemporal, and retrosigmoid suboccipital approaches. Each of these standard exposures will be described and the various cranial base extensions and modifications that we have found useful will be detailed.

Anterior Fossa Cranial Base Approaches

FRONTOTEMPORAL (PTERIONAL)

The head is turned from 10 to 60 degrees away from the side of the approach, depending on the location of the aneurysm, with the head held in place with a radiolucent headholder. The standard frontotemporal (pterional) craniotomy is performed by making an incision from the midline to the ipsilateral zygomatic arch within the patient's hairline. The temporalis muscle is divided beneath the skin incision and reflected anteriorly, held in place with rubberbanded fishhooks attached to a Leyla bar (V. Mueller, Deerfield, IL), and placed on stretch. A single burr hole is placed just above the zygomatic arch. A second burr hole placed over the orbitofrontal angle is used for elderly patients with potentially thinned dura. The Midas Rex drill (Midas Rex Institute, Fort Worth, TX) with a B1 attachment and footplate is used to create a frontotemporal craniotomy. For anterior communicating artery aneurysms, the frontal portion of the craniotomy is carried more medially to the midpupillary line and inferiorly to the supraorbital ridge. The lesser wing of the sphenoid is removed with rongeurs and a high-speed drill until the frontal and middle fossae are flat with each other across the sphenoid ridge. For middle cerebral artery aneurysms, the bone overlying the temporal lobe is removed more aggressively to expose the floor of the middle fossa. The dura is then opened in a curvilinear fashion over the sylvian fissure, and is opened posteriorly to expose the remainder of the fissure.

Anterior Clinoidectomy

When the surgeon anticipates the need to remove the anterior clinoid process, the lesser wing of the sphenoid is removed more aggressively and the posterior one-third of the orbit is unroofed extradurally. The entire anterior clinoid process may be removed from an extradural approach by following the lesser wing of the sphenoid medially and separating the clinoid from the dura. The clinoid may then be removed with small rongeurs or drilled away with a small diamond burr. In the presence of an aneurysm on the proximal carotid artery, it is much safer to unroof the posterior one-third of the orbit extradurally and remove the anterior clinoid process under direct visualization after the dura has been opened.

Once the dura has been opened, the sylvian fissure is opened sharply to allow the egress of cerebrospinal fluid (CSF) and to minimize retraction of the frontal and temporal lobes. Self-retaining retractors are used to maintain exposure and protect the brain once the fissure has been opened to expose the carotid bifurcation, optic nerve, and proximal ICA. The dura over the anterior clinoid process and optic nerve is opened with a No. 11 knife blade in a curvilinear fashion based posteriorly, or in a cruciate fashion (*Figure 9.2A*). A high-speed drill with a diamond burr is used to thin the anterior clinoid process, optic strut, and optic canal under constant irrigation to minimize the risk of thermal damage to the optic nerve. The entire anterior clinoid process is removed and the optic nerve is unroofed to its medial edge (*Figure 9.2B*). This exposes the clinoidal segment of the ICA, that 5- to 6-mm segment of the ICA that is neither intradural nor intracavernous, but lies between the two dural rings. The dural ring is sharply divided and its continuation with the falciform ligament over the optic nerve is sharply cut to free and mobilize the optic nerve. The surgeon now has a view of the clinoidal segment of the ICA, the origin of the ophthalmic artery, the intra- and extradural optic nerve, and any aneurysm of the clinoidal or ophthalmic segments of the ICA. Clinoidal segment aneurysms may extend either medially into the "carotid cave" or laterally toward the cavernous sinus. Adequate exposure for clipping may require more extensive opening of the dural ring in a circumferential manner to mobilize the ICA. Ophthalmic segment aneurysms include the ophthalmic artery aneurysms that arise on the superior wall of the ICA immediately distal to the origin of the ophthalmic artery (*Figure 9.2C*). The superior hypophyseal aneurysm arises on the medial and ventral wall of the ICA slightly more distal to the ophthalmic artery (*Figure 9.2D*). In this situation, the ICA lies between the surgeon and the aneurysm, requiring the use of a fenestrated clip for reconstruction of the ICA and obliteration of the aneurysm (*Figure 9.3.*)

Orbitozygomatic Approach

The orbitozygomatic approach is an extension of the frontotemporal craniotomy that has proven extremely versatile in expanding the exposure for a variety of intracranial aneurysms (*Figure 9.4*). Many different methods for performing this procedure have been reported since the first description by Pellerin et al. (18) and Hakuba et al. (8). The patient is placed in a position similar to that for a standard frontotemporal craniotomy. The head is rotated from 30 to 60 degrees depending on the location of the target. Less rotation is used for exposure of the clivus and posterior fossa, and more rotation is used for anterior circulation aneurysms. The neck is slightly extended so that the malar eminence is the most superior point, which allows gravity to assist in the frontal lobe falling away from the roof of the orbit. As described by Zabramski et al. (29), we prefer to extend the scalp incision from the inferior margin of the ipsilateral zygomatic arch to the contralateral midpupillary line, within the patient's hairline (*Figure 9.4A*). As the scalp incision is elevated, care is taken to avoid dissection of the subgaleal fat pad, within which runs the frontal branch of the facial nerve. The temporal fascia along the frontotemporal insertion of the temporalis muscle is exposed and incised sharply along this insertion, leaving a small cuff for later reattachment. The temporal fascia is elevated in the plane between the muscle and deep fascia to expose the zygoma and superior orbital rim. Where the temporal fascia fuses with the periosteum of the zygomatic arch, the fascia is sharply divided to expose the zygomatic arch. The underlying temporalis muscle is sharply divided along the fascial edges and elevated. The skin flap is retracted inferiorly and held in place with rubberbanded fishhooks attached to a Leyla bar (V. Mueller). A small periosteal elevator is used to elevate the periorbita from the lateral and superior walls of the orbit. The inferior wall of the supraorbital canal may be fractured gently with a small chisel to free the supraorbital nerve and protect it.

A burr hole is placed in the temporal bone just above the zygomatic arch, and the Midas Rex drill with B1 attachment and footplate is used to create a generous frontotemporal craniotomy that includes the temporalis myofascial cuff (*Figure 9.4B*). The exact size of the craniotomy depends on the location of the aneurysm. A variety of methods for performing orbital and zygomatic osteotomies have been used and described. We prefer the method described by Zabramski et al. (29). The periorbita is carefully elevated from the lateral and superior walls of the orbit. While the freed periorbita is protected, a reciprocating saw is used to complete six bone cuts that free the orbitozygomatic bone flap in one piece. The first cut is made obliquely across the most posterior

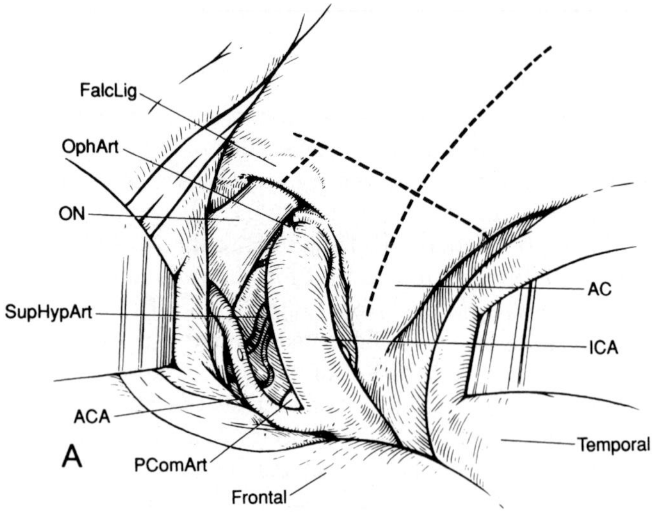

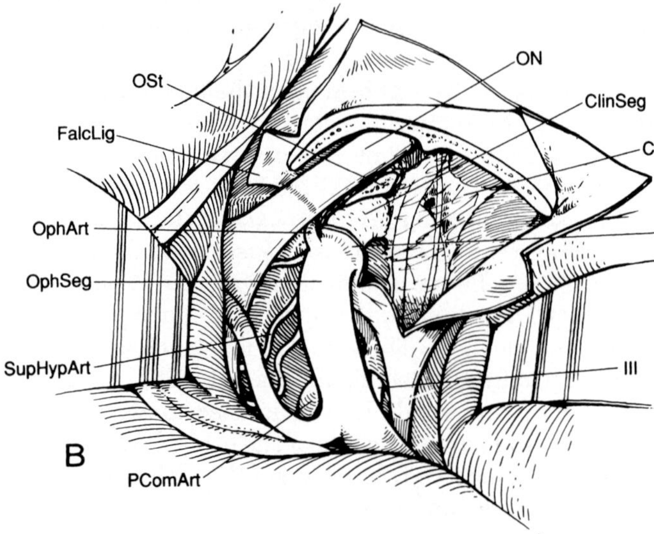

FIG. 9.2 Anterior clinoidectomy. *A,* illustration of exposure of the internal carotid artery (*ICA*) and anterior clinoid (*AC*) process through a frontotemporal craniotomy. *Dotted line* indicates the dural opening over the anterior clinoid process and sectioning of the falciform ligament (*FalcLig*) over the optic nerve (*ON*). *B,* exposure of the origin of the ophthalmic artery (*OphArt*) and clinoidal segment (*ClinSeg*) of the ICA after removal of the anterior clinoid, roof, and lateral wall of the optic canal. The dural ring (*DR*) surrounds the ICA and marks its entrance into the subarachnoid space. The carotid-oculomotor membrane (*COM*) covers the cavernous sinus (*CavSin*). *C,* exposure provided for an ophthalmic artery aneurysm clipped with a side-angled clip. *D,* exposure of a superior hypophyseal artery (*SupHypophArt*) aneurysm clipped with a fenestrated clip using the fenestration to encircle the ICA. *ACA,* anterior cerebral artery; *PcomArt,* posterior communicating artery; *III,* oculomotor nerve; *Ost,* optic strut. (*See* Day AD: Ophthalmic segment aneurysms. *Neurosurgical Operative Atlas.* Park Ridge: AANS, vol 2, no 1.)

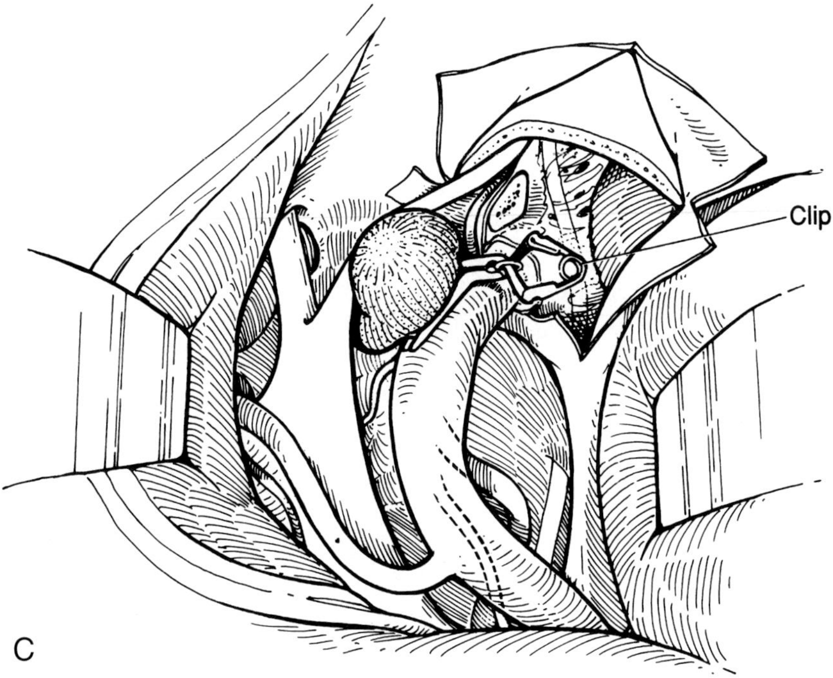

C

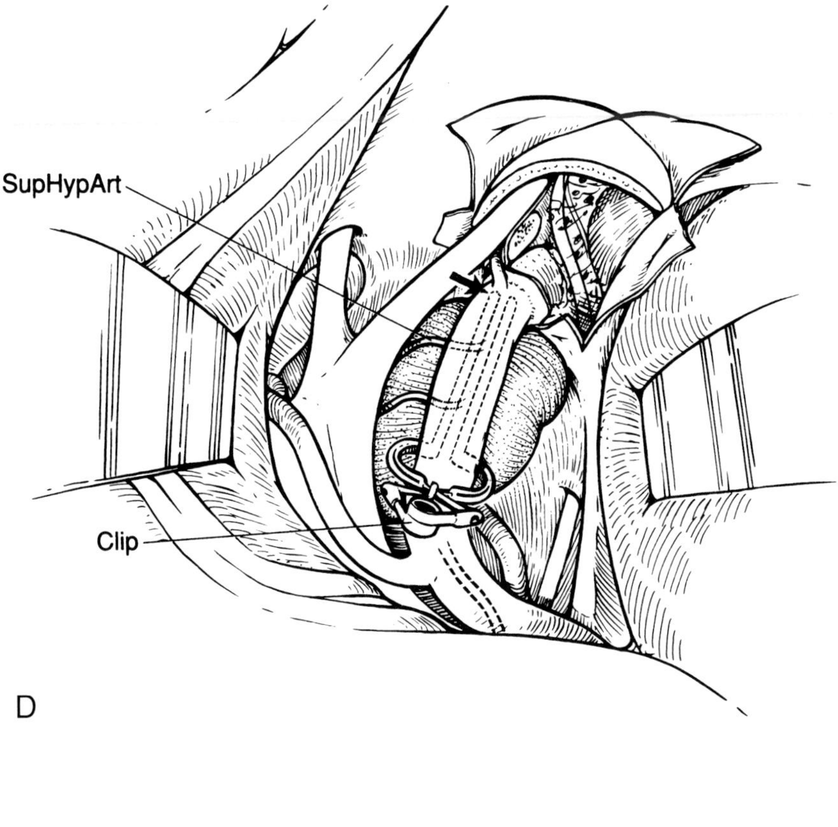

D

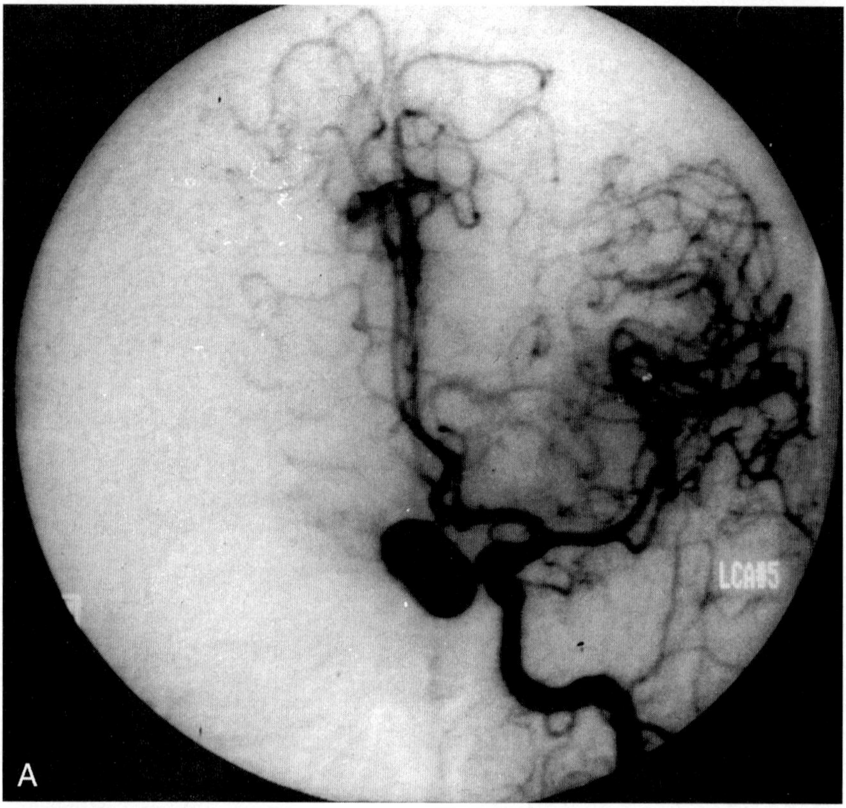

FIG. 9.3 Proximal ICA aneurysms frequently require removal of the anterior clinoid process and opening of the dural ring for adequate exposure. Examples of such aneurysms are demonstrated. *A,* anteroposterior left carotid angiogram of aneurysm arising on the medial aspect of the clinoidal segment of the carotid. *B,* left lateral carotid angiogram of an ophthalmic aneurysm arising just distal to the origin of the ophthalmic artery. *C,* right lateral carotid angiogram of superior hypophyseal aneurysm arising on the ventral and medial aspect of the proximal carotid.

part of the zygomatic process. The second and third cuts separate the zygomatic bone just above the malar eminence. The second cut divides the zygomatic bone from its inferolateral margin toward the lateral orbital rim. The third cut begins intraorbitally with the tip of the saw in the inferior orbital fissure, and it extends laterally and posteriorly to join the second cut, thus dividing the zygomatic bone from the cranium. The dura is elevated from the roof of the orbit and temporal fossa to expose the superior and lateral walls of the orbit. The fourth cut divides the superior orbital rim and roof of the orbit. The cut is initiated by

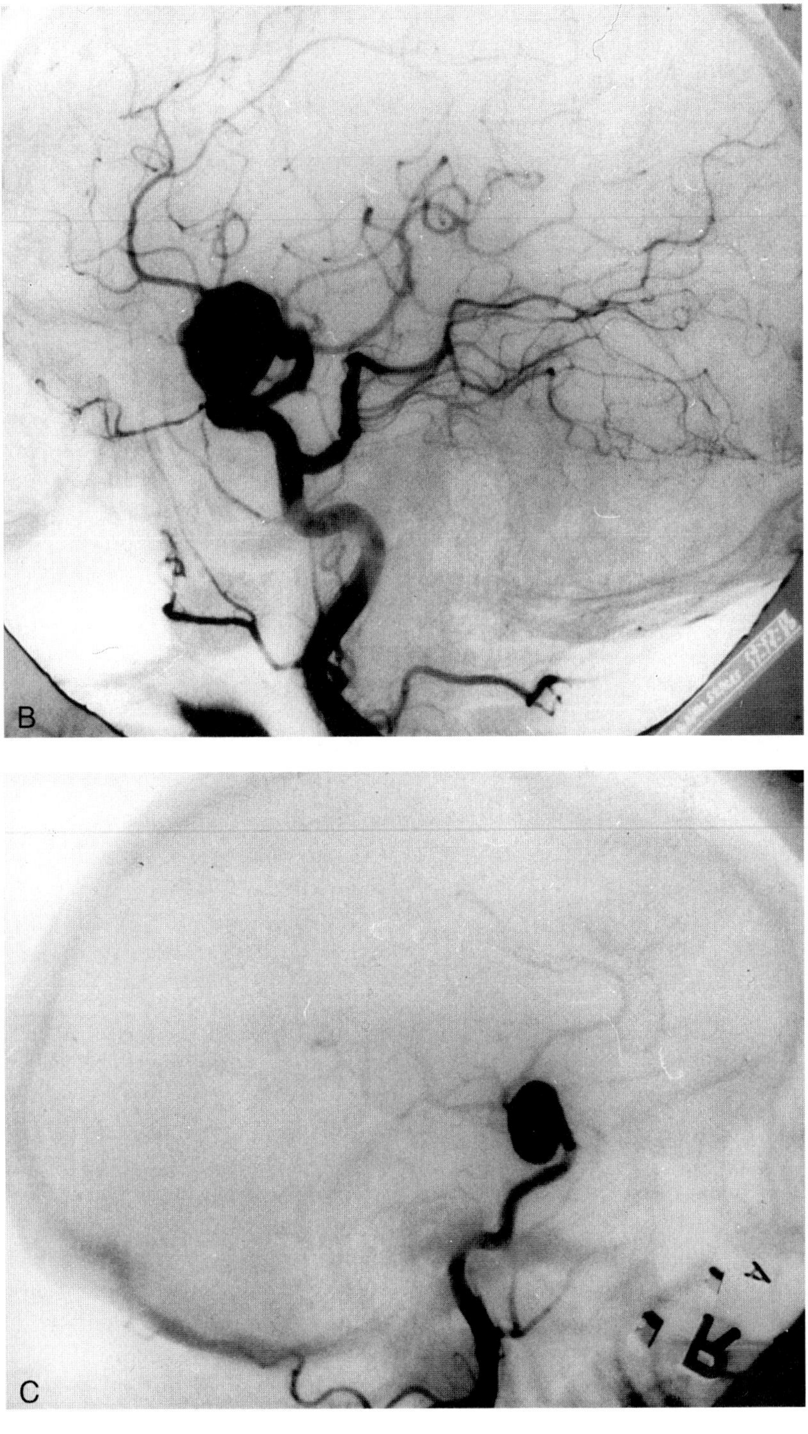
B
C

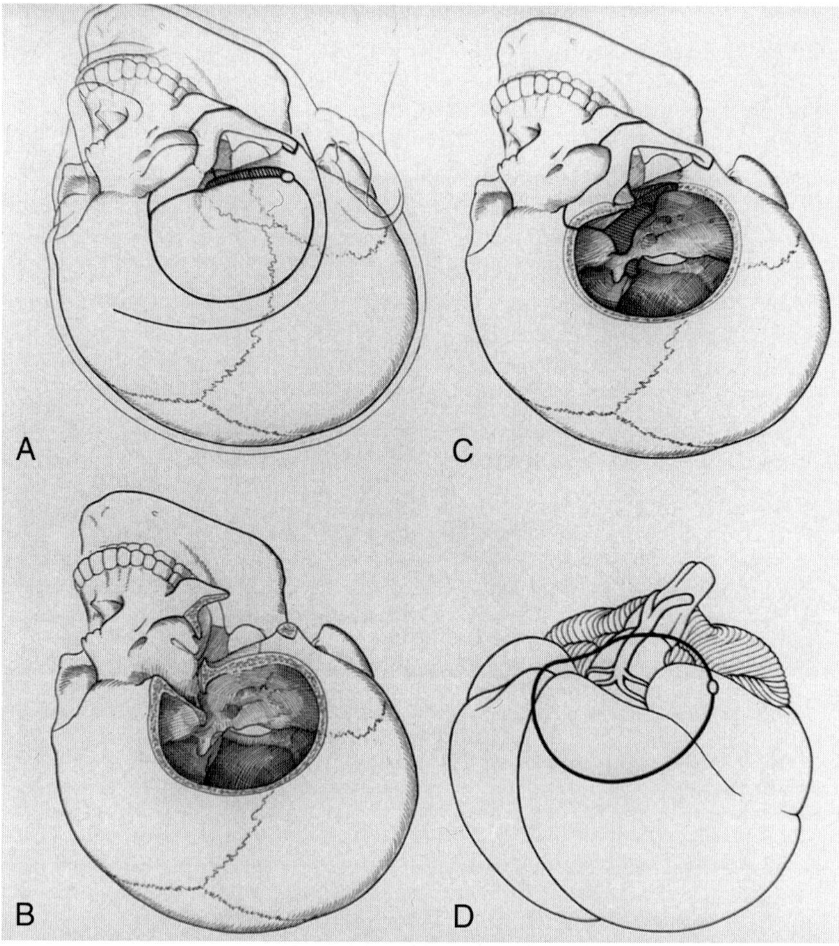

FIG. 9.4 *A*, drawing of scalp incision and bone removal for orbitozygomatic approach. *B*, completion of frontotemporal (pterional) craniotomy. *C*, completed orbitozygomatic osteotomy. *D*, exposure provided by this approach. (*See* Spetzler RF, Koos WT: Color Atlas of Microneurosurgery, Stuttgart: Georg Theime Verlag, 1997, ed 2).

placing the blade perpendicular to the superior orbital rim and dividing the rim. The blade is then placed perpendicular to the orbital roof to cut through to the superior periorbita while protecting the latter with a small, thin retractor. The fifth and sixth cuts free the lateral orbital wall by connecting the inferior and superior orbital fissures. The fifth cut is made by placing the tip of the saw in the inferior orbital fissure and cutting toward the temporal fossa. The final cut extends from the lateral margin of the superior margin of the superior orbital fissure to join the fifth cut from the inferior orbital fissure while the intraorbital contents are protected with a thin retractor (*Figure 9.4C*).

The entire orbitozygomatic bone flap is now free. Occasionally, a small island of bone between the medial edge of the superior orbital fissure and the orbital roof osteotomy prevents complete removal of the flap and must be carefully drilled away. As the orbitozygomatic flap is elevated, care is taken to protect the periorbita. For access to high-lying, rostral basilar aneurysms, the lateral temporal bone is drilled flush to the floor of the middle fossa. The dura is tacked to the surrounding bone flap and opened widely. By tacking the dural opening anteriorly, the orbital contents are retracted inferiorly to improve exposure.

After the aneurysm is appropriately clipped, the dura is closed in a watertight fashion. The frontotemporal and orbitozygomatic bone flaps are replaced and fixed with miniplates and miniscrews. The temporalis muscle and fascia are reapproximated to the myofascial cuff. *Figure 9.5* shows a high basilar aneurysm clipped through an orbitozygomatic approach.

Posterior Clinoidectomy

Removal of the posterior clinoid process is advantageous in the treatment of rostral basilar aneurysms associated with a low basilar bifurcation and proximal basilar trunk lesions. Removal of the posterior clinoid provides more proximal exposure of the basilar trunk from a transsylvian approach. The frontotemporal or orbitozygomatic craniotomy is performed as described above, and the sylvian fissure is opened widely to expose the middle cerebral artery, ICA bifurcation, oculomotor nerve, and free edge of the tentorium. Using a No. 11 knife on a long, thin handle, the dura over the ipsilateral posterior clinoid process is opened, and a small curette is used to peel the dura away from the underlying bone. A high-speed drill with angled handpiece and diamond burr is used to drill away the top of the posterior clinoid process down to the clivus. It is not uncommon for bleeding to occur from the bone or dura. This can be controlled using a small piece of wax on a microdissector or hemostatic agents such as Avitene (Davol, Inc., Cranston, RI). Once the posterior clinoid is removed, the surgeon has an improved angle through the microscope down the clivus.

Transapical (Medial Petrosectomy)

Once the frontotemporal or orbitozygomatic craniotomy and osteotomies have been performed, the medial apex of the petrous bone can be drilled down extradurally or intradurally to enhance exposure

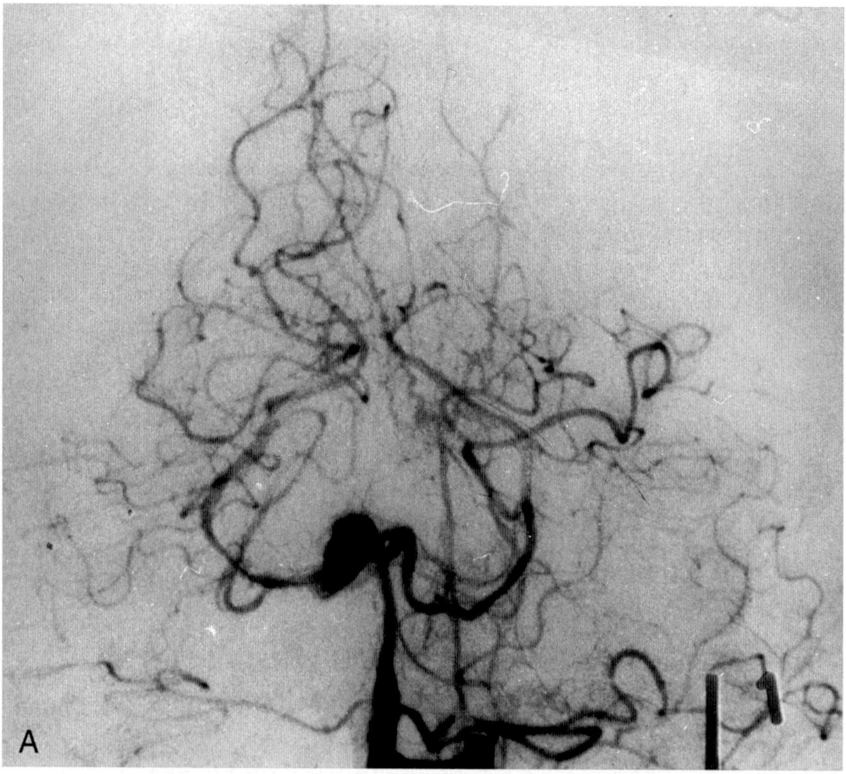

FIG. 9.5 *A*, anteroposterior vertebral angiogram showing a basilar tip aneurysm with a relatively high basilar bifurcation. This aneurysm was exposed by an orbitozygomatic frontotemporal approach to improve visualization up into the interpeduncular fossa.

of the midclivus. We prefer to perform the drilling of the petrous apex extradurally. If performed in combination with a posterior clinoidectomy, a wide exposure of the basilar apex and the upper and midclivus is achieved. Anatomic landmarks for resection of the petrous apex are the trigeminal nerve anteriorly, the greater superficial nerve laterally, the ICA inferiorly, and the inferior petrosal sinus medially. Posteriorly, the cochlea should be avoided.

Transcavernous-Transsellar

Dolenc et al. (3, 4) popularized an expansion of the pterional approach that further expands the exposure and circumvents the obstruction created by the posterior clinoid process and the dorsum sellae. After a standard pterional craniotomy, the sphenoid wing is drilled away and the posterior roof of the orbit is removed extradurally.

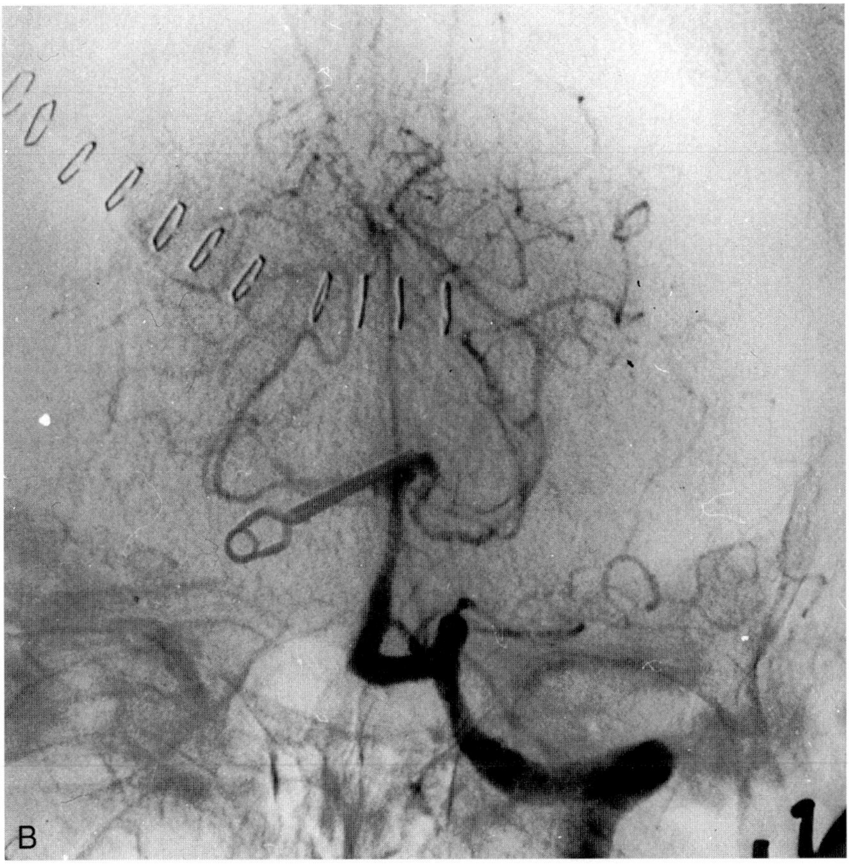

FIG. 9.5 *B*, postoperative anteroposterior angiogram documenting complete clip ligation and demonstrating the upward angle of the clip to the basilar bifurcation.

Although Dolenc advocated an extradural removal of the anterior clinoid process and opening of the superior orbital fissure, we prefer to do this intradurally as described for anterior clinoidectomy (*Figure 6*). A dural incision is then made lateral and parallel to the optic nerve through the distal dural ring and falciform ligament. This mobilizes the optic nerve and ICA and exposes the origin of the ophthalmic artery. An incision is made in the outer layer of the dura that forms the lateral wall of the cavernous sinus, mobilizing the IIIrd and IVth cranial nerves. Bleeding from the cavernous sinus is controlled by gently packing with Surgicel (Johnson and Johnson Products, Chicago, IL). The carotid and chiasmatic cisterns are opened and Liliequest's membrane is divided to expose the posterior communi-

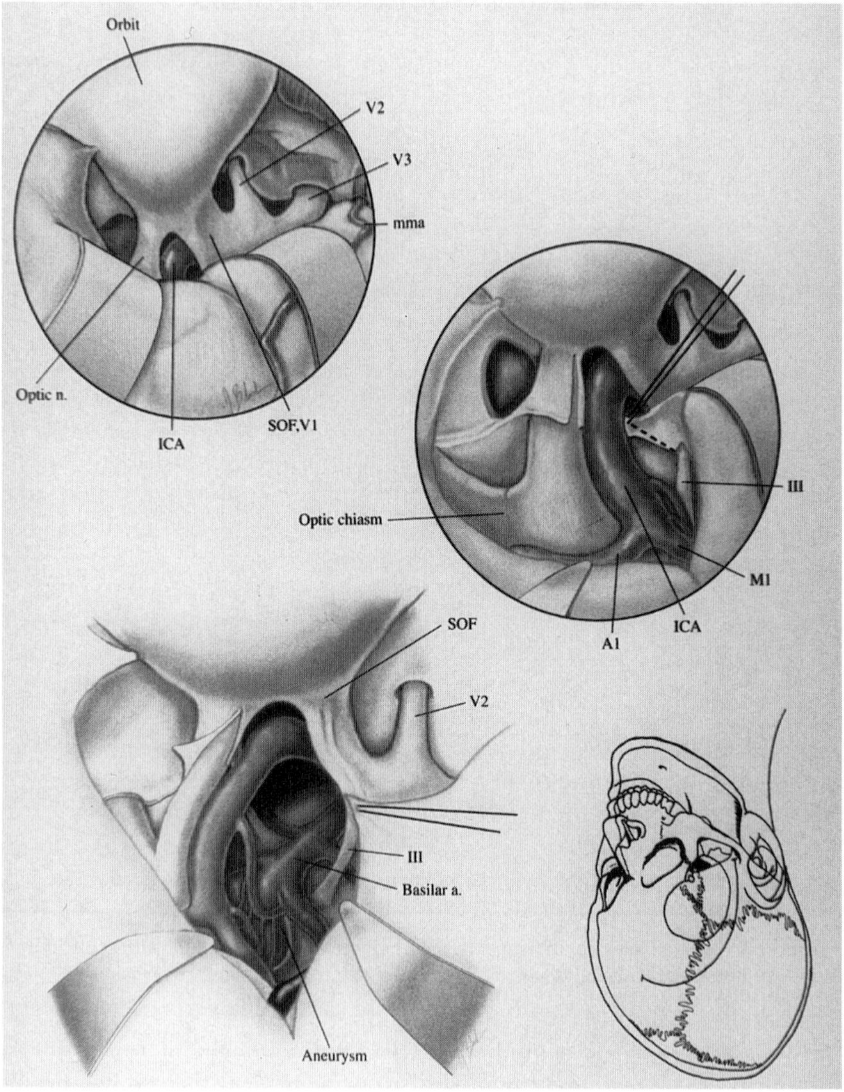

FIG. 9.6 Drawings illustrating the defining maneuvers of the transcavernous-transsellar or temporopolar approach. *A,* extensive extradural bone removal and extradural dissection of the cavernous sinus result in posterior displacement of the temporal lobe under protection of the dura. *B,* after dural incision, the fibrous carotid ring is dissected in addition to the opening of the anterior petroclinoidal ligament (*dotted line*) and liberation of the proximal segment of the oculomotor nerve to widen exposure of the basilar caput and the aneurysm (*C*). *D,* line drawing illustrating the scalp incision and typical pterional type bone flap made for the approach. *a,* artery; *ICA,* internal carotid artery; *mma,* middle meningeal artery; *n,* nerve; *SOF,* superior orbital fissure; *V1, V2, V3,* first, second, and third division of the trigeminal nerve; *III,* Cranial Nerve III. (*See* Day JD, Fukushima T, Giannotta SL: Cranial base approaches to posterior circulation aneurysms. **J Neurosurg** 87:544–554, 1997.)

cating artery from its origin to the posterior cerebral artery. The space between the carotid artery and the oculomotor nerve is enlarged. The diaphragm sellae is divided transversely in front of the posterior clinoid process to expose its tip and base. The posterior clinoid process is drilled away extensively, and if necessary the removal of bone can continue down the clivus, if care is taken not to injure the VIth nerve. This provides excellent exposure of the basilar apex and upper- to midclivus with minimal retraction.

Middle Fossa Cranial Base Approaches

SUBTEMPORAL APPROACHES

Subtemporal approaches are useful for selected rostral basilar aneurysms, particularly those arising at a low-lying basilar bifurcation. A subtemporal approach is chosen for a basilar tip aneurysm pointing posteriorly into the midbrain, allowing a better view of the perforators on the back side of the sac.

When performing a subtemporal exposure for aneurysms, we place a lumbar subarachnoid drain if the patient does not already have an external ventricular drain in place. This allows for the drainage of CSF to minimize the amount of temporal lobe retraction. The patient is then placed in the supine position, with the ipsilateral shoulder slightly elevated with a roll and the head turned sharply to the side opposite the approach, parallel to the floor with the vertex slightly angled downward to allow gravity to assist the temporal lobe falling away from the floor of the middle fossa. A curvilinear incision is made from the zygomatic arch, sweeping around the auricle of the ear within the patient's hairline, and extending to a point near the mastoid process. The temporalis muscle is opened beneath the flap and turned inferiorly to expose the temporal region. Alternatively, a question-mark incision is made from just below the zygoma to the midline, and the temporalis muscle is reflected anteriorly with the scalp to expose the frontotemporal region and superior edge of the zygomatic arch. A single burr hole is created immediately above the zygomatic arch, and the Midas Rex drill with a B1 attachment and footplate is used to create a craniotomy based on the floor of the middle fossa. The inferior extent of the craniotomy is drilled so that the opening is flush with the floor of the middle fossa. The superior surface of the zygomatic arch is drilled flat to further facilitate the subtemporal view with minimal temporal lobe retraction. After CSF is drained, multiple self-retaining retractors are used to gently and evenly retract the temporal lobe and expose the free edge of the tentorium. To further enhance exposure, the tentorium may be divided and tacked back with a few 4–0 silk sutures.

Subtemporal Transtentorial

Peerless and Drake (5, 6, 16, 17) popularized the subtemporal transtentorial approach to aneurysms arising on the middle one-third of the basilar artery. This exposure involves dividing the tentorium 1 to 2 cm behind the petrous ridge and tacking the anterior leaflet to the floor of the middle fossa dura. The petrosal vein is coagulated and divided. Retractors are placed along the anterior cerebellum and the pons is gently retracted from the petrous bone and clivus to expose the VIIth and VIIIth cranial nerves. The working space provided by this approach is quite limited.

Medial Petrosectomy

Exposure of the midbasilar artery and upper clival area may be greatly enhanced by resecting the petrous pyramid, as described originally by Kawase et al. (13). We prefer the anterior subtemporal approach combined with a medial petrosectomy as detailed by MacDonald et al. (15), which yields a broader and more generous exposure of the upper basilar artery and clivus (*Figure 9.7*). After performing a standard anterior subtemporal exposure as outlined in *Figure 9.7A,* the dura is elevated from the middle fossa to expose the middle meningeal artery at the foramen spinosum (*Figure 9.7B*). The vessel is divided, and the edge of the mandibular division of the trigeminal nerve and the greater superficial petrosal nerve (GSPN) are identified. The medial petrous bone is resected with a high-speed drill using cutting and polishing burrs under constant irrigation. The landmarks for the petrous resection are the GSPN laterally, the superior semicircular canal inferiorly, the geniculate ganglion of the facial nerve posteriorly, and the medial surface of the petrous internal carotid artery anteriorly (*Figure 9.7c*). Drilling of the porous bone between the GSPN and the medial petrous cortex is accomplished by working anterior and medial to the internal auditory meatus and cochlea. Medial to the ICA, bone is resected to the petroclival suture until the overlying inferior petrosal sinus can be visualized within the dura. Resection is continued anteriorly and medially beneath the trigeminal ganglion and mandibular division to the cavernous sinus. The dura is opened and the temporal lobe is retracted superiorly with multiple retractors to expose the free edge of the tentorium. The trochlear nerve is dissected free of the arachnoid, and the tentorium is divided just posterior to the entry point of the trochlear nerve. The tentorial incision is continued laterally and obliquely posterior so that it is parallel to the superior petrosal sinus. A second tentorial incision is made perpendicular to the first and just lateral to the trigeminal nerve. This tentorial cut divides the superior

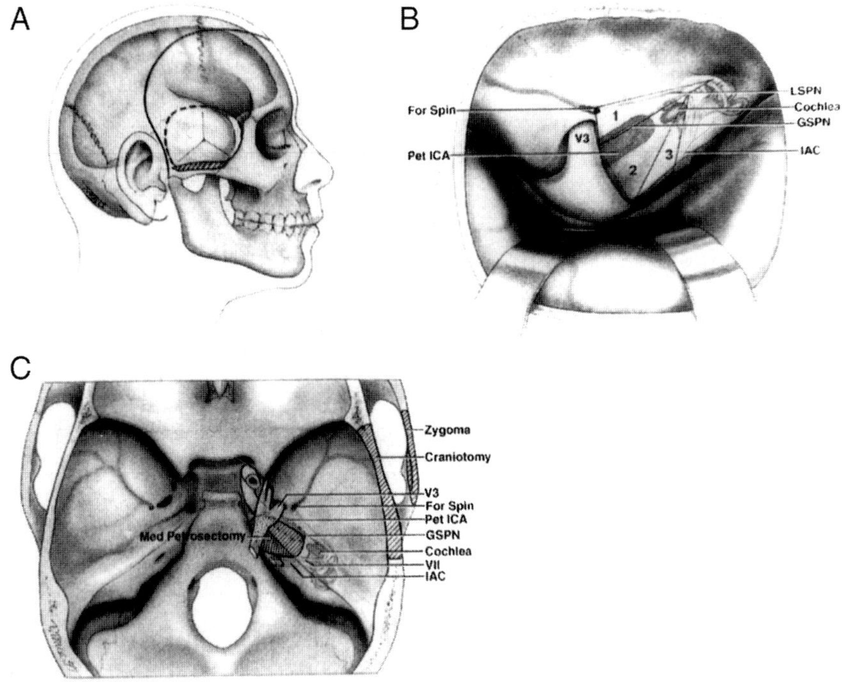

FIG. 9.7 Illustration of subtemporal approach with medial petrosectomy. *A,* scalp incision (solid line) and initial craniotomy (dashed line). The superior portion of the zygoma is drilled away and the dura is opened in an inverted Y-shape to provide a flat approach to the floor of the middle fossa. *B,* the dura has been elevated to the edge of the mandibular division (*V3*) of the trigeminal nerve to expose the extradural middle fossa anatomy. The middle meningeal artery has been divided at the foramen spinosum (*For Spin*). *C,* schematic showing the medial (*Med*) petrosectomy bony defect. The *shaded areas* represent zygoma, craniotomy, and petrous bone removal. The GSPN has been preserved and represents the lateral limit of bone removal. The bone overlying and medial to the petrous segment of the petrous ICA and beneath the mandibular division of the trigeminal nerve has been drilled away, allowing the trigeminal nerve to sag into the petrosectomy defect to further enhance visualization. *GSPN,* greater superficial petrosal nerve; *LSPN,* lesser superficial petrosal nerve; *IAC,* internal auditory canal; *Pet ICA,* petrous internal carotid artery; *1,* Glasscock's triangle; *2,* Kawase's triangle; *3,* posterolateral portion of the medial petrous apex, often added to Kawase's triangle to form a rhomboid-shaped resection area. (*See* Reference 15).

petrosal sinus. The anterior tentorial leaf is tacked anteriorly to expose the middle one-third of the clivus and basilar trunk between the oculomotor and trigeminal nerves. *Figure 9.8* demonstrates the additional exposure provided by a medial petrosectomy. *Figure 9.9* shows a giant rostral basilar artery aneurysm that was exposed through a temporal craniotomy with medial petrosectomy.

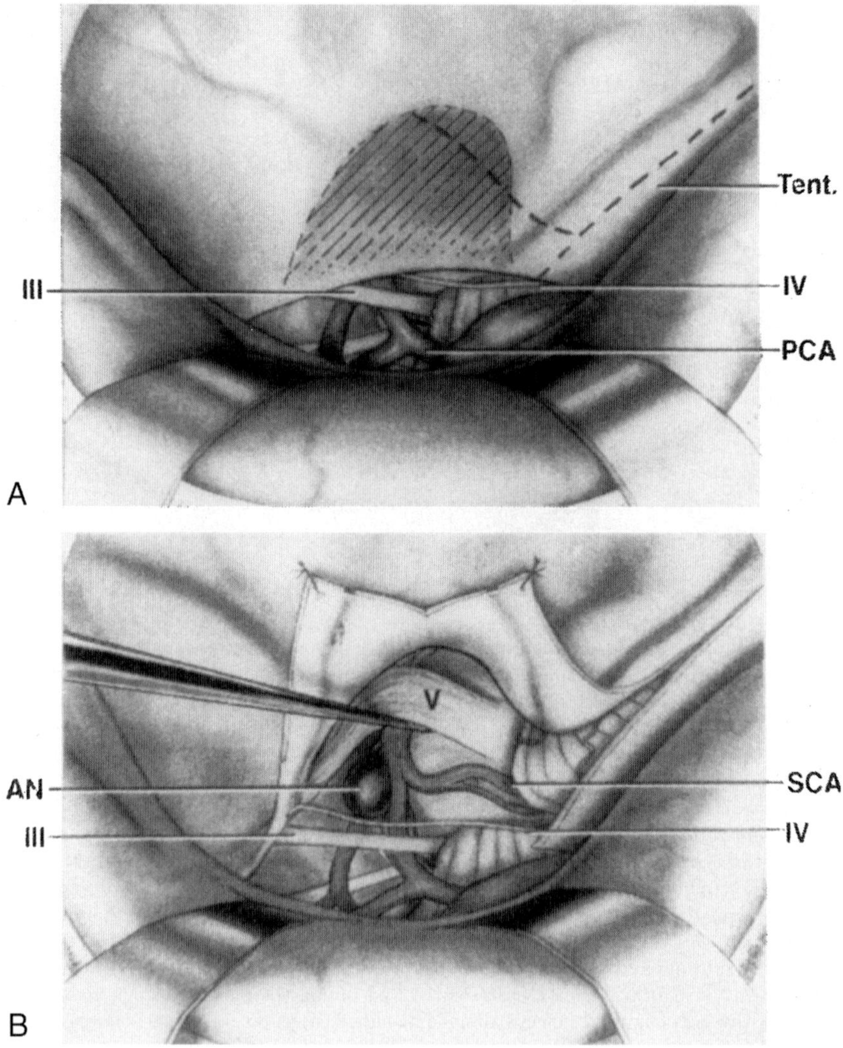

FIG. 9.8 Schematic showing the anterior subtemporal exposure alone (*A*) compared with a similar opening combined with medial petrosectomy (*B*). The *shaded ar*ea represents bony removal. *Dotted lines* represent tentorial and dural incisions. *Tent,* tentorium; *III,* oculomotor nerve; *IV,* trochlear nerve; *PCA,* posterior cerebral artery; *V,* trigeminal nerve; *AN,* aneurysm; *SCA,* superior cerebellar artery. (*See* Reference 15).

Combined Middle and Posterior Fossa Cranial Base Approaches

COMBINED TEMPORAL AND SUBOCCIPITAL CRANIOTOMIES

Kasdon and Stein (12) described a combined supratentorial and infratentorial exposure for low-lying basilar aneurysms, particularly sacs located between the vertebral confluence and the anterior inferior cerebellar artery. Because the transverse sinus is sacrificed with this exposure, it is important to ensure that adequate collateral venous drainage exists.

The patient is placed in the lateral position, with the ipsilateral shoulder elevated so that the head is parallel to the floor with the vertex of the head angled slightly downward. Alternatively, the patient may be placed in the park-bench position. An incision is made beginning anterior to the ear at the level of the zygomatic arch. The incision is carried around the auricle of the ear and extended as a paramedian suboccipital incision to just below the mastoid tip. A temporal and suboccipital craniotomy is created, skeletonizing the transverse sinus. The dura is opened over the temporal lobe and cerebellum. The transverse sinus is ligated and divided posterior to the entrance of Labbé's vein. Retractors are placed to elevate the temporal lobe and displace the cerebellum and pons posteriorly, which provides a wide view of the brainstem and basilar artery. Depending on the level of the aneurysm, the surgeon works between various cranial nerves.

Presigmoid (Petrosal) Exposure

Hashi et al. (10) modified the combined approach to avoid the need to ligate the transverse sinus. This is accomplished by drilling the mastoid more aggressively to expose the dura anterior to the sigmoid sinus and to expose the junction of the superior petrosal and the sigmoid sinuses (*Figure 9.10*). Following the bony drilling, the dura is opened anterior and parallel to the sigmoid sinus, the superior petrosal sinus is divided, and the tentorium is cut to the incisura posterior to the entrance of the trochlear nerve into the free edge of the tentorium. The temporal lobe is retracted superiorly and the cerebellar hemisphere and sigmoid sinus are retracted posteriorly to allow access to the basilar artery from the vertebral confluence to the basilar trunk. The primary problem with this approach for aneurysms is that the trajectory to the basilar artery is posterior to anterior, thus requiring significant cerebellar and brainstem retraction to visualize the vascular anatomy. Spetzler et al. (25) and Hamilton et al. (9) have modified the presigmoid combined approach by adding more radical resection of the mastoid. These include the retrolabyrinthine, translabyrinthine, and

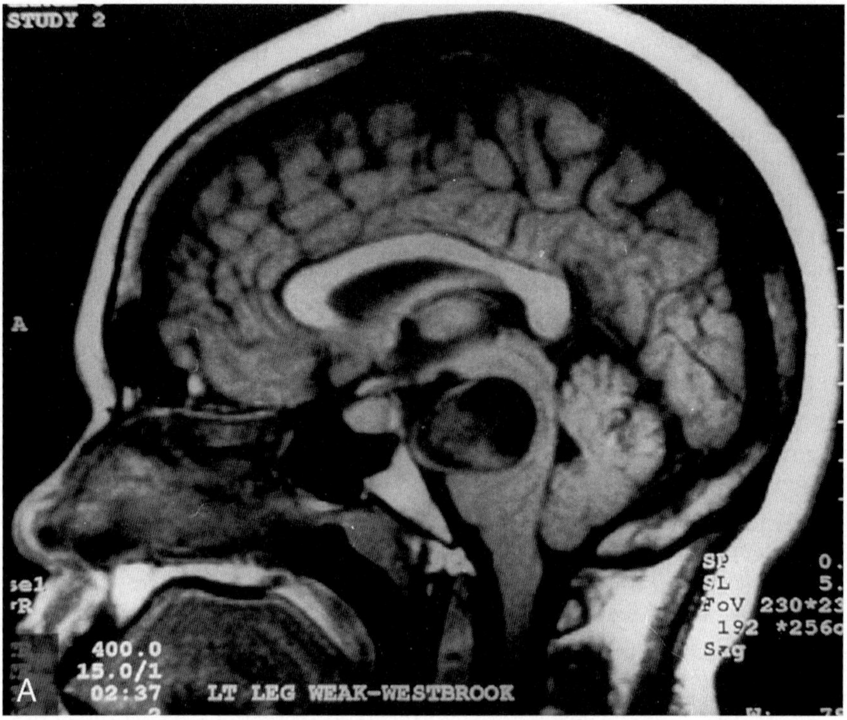

FIG. 9.9 *A,* sagittal magnetic resonance image showing a giant rostral basilar artery aneurysm extending below the petrous bone and markedly compressing the brainstem. *B,* lateral vertebral angiogram illustrating the sac extending inferiorly well below the posterior clinoid processes. The aneurysm was exposed through a temporal craniotomy with medial petrosectomy using deep hypothermic circulatory arrest. *C,* intraoperative angiogram demonstrating complete obliteration of the aneurysm and normal filling of the surrounding vasculature.

transcochlear approaches, each involving progressively greater mastoid removal and accomplishing greater lateral and anterior trajectories (*Figure 9.11*).

Retrolabyrinthine Approach

The retrolabyrinthine approach maintains the integrity of the labyrinth to preserve hearing. The lateral, posterior, and superior canals are skeletonized, with drilling extended as far anterior as possible to expose as much dura as possible in front of the sigmoid sinus. This approach provides good exposure of the cerebellopontine angle but a limited view of the anterior brainstem.

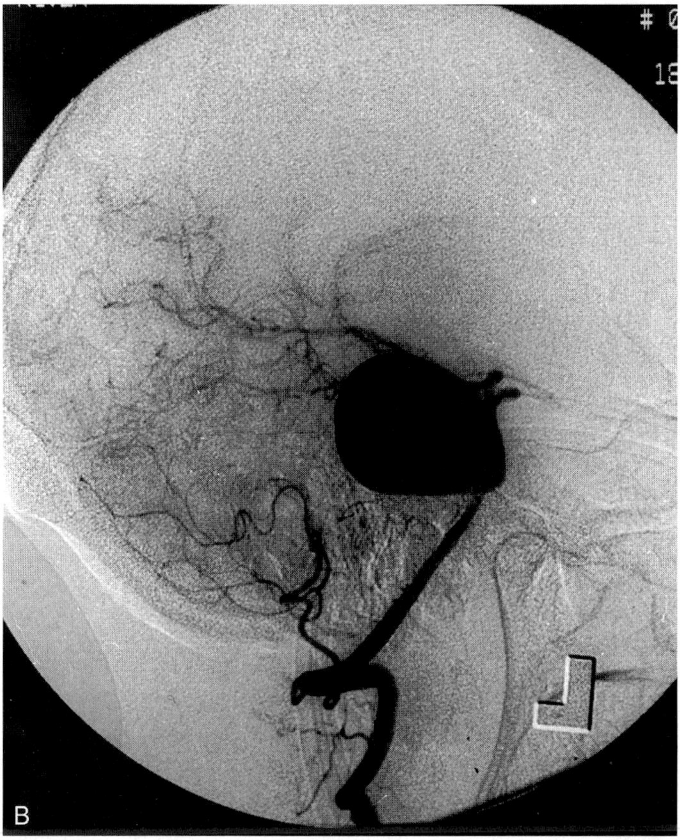
B

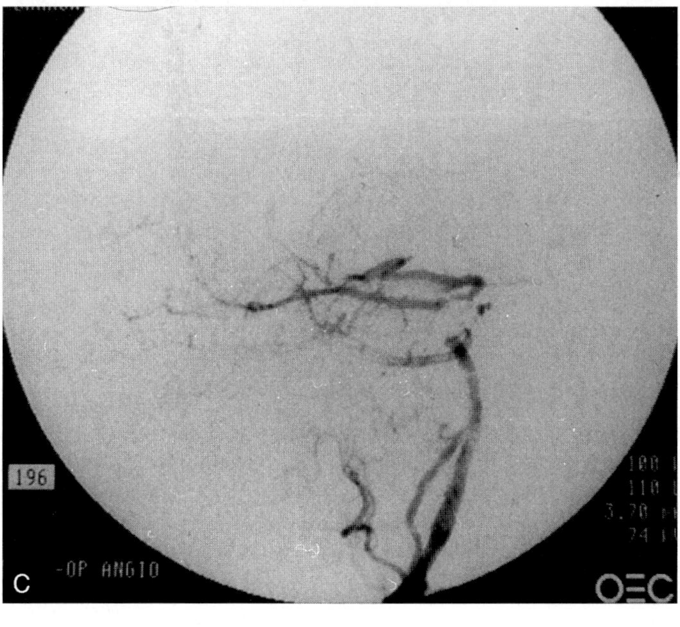
196
-OP ANGIO
C
OEC

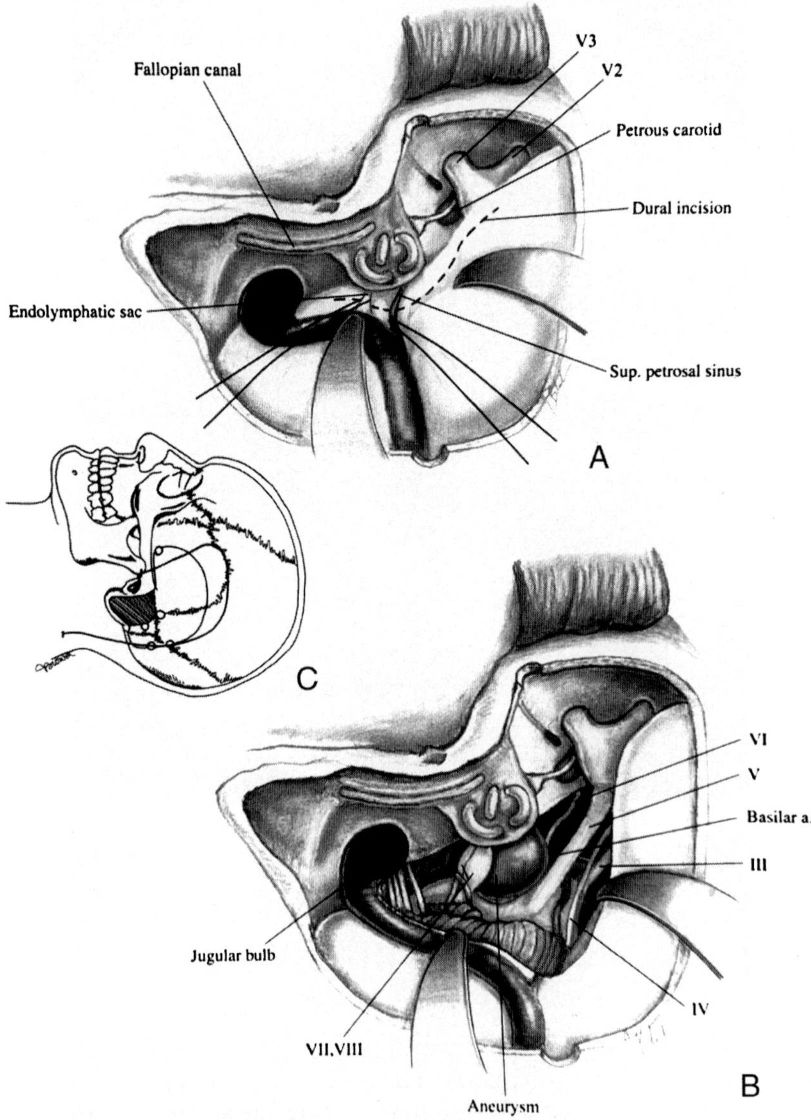

FIG. 9.10 Drawings illustrating procedures used in the combined petrosal approach. *A,* after the extradural bone resection is completed, the dura is incised as shown by the dashed line. *B,* this incision is placed deep, such that the temporal lobe is mostly covered by dura under the retractor blades. The approach provides multiple viewing trajectories for optimum clip placement at the aneurysm neck. *C,* drawing showing the scalp incision and bone opening for a left-sided approach. *a,* artery; *Sup,* superior; *V2, V3,* second and third divisions of the trigeminal nerve; *III, IV, V, VI, VII, VIII,* cranial nerves. (*See* Day JD, Fukushima T, Giannotta SL: Cranial base approaches to posterior circulation aneurysms. **J Neurosurg** 87:544–554, 1997.)

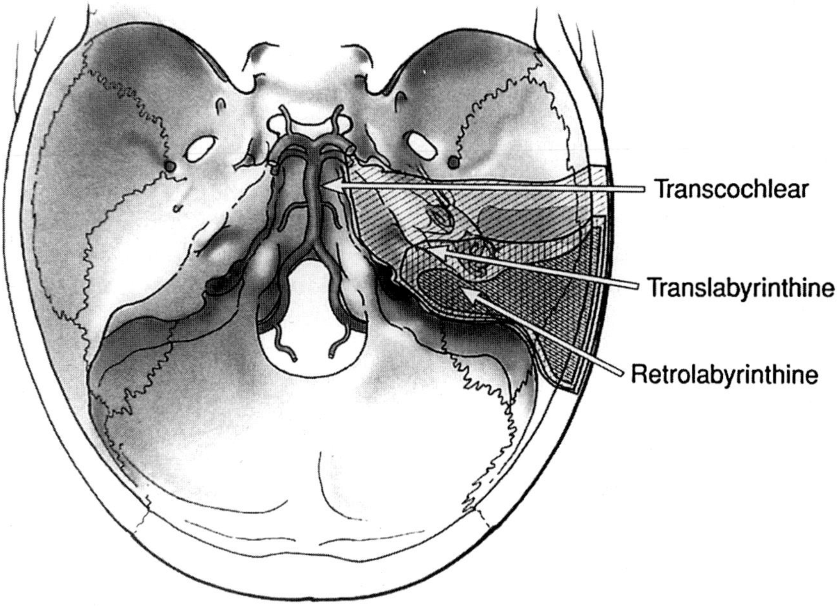

FIG. 9.11 Various options for extending the petrosectomy approach. (From the Barrow Neurological Institute.)

Translabyrinthine Approach

The translabyrinthine approach uses the same basic mastoidectomy as described previously, but it involves removal of the semicircular canals. Drilling is performed anteriorly to skeletonize the posterior aspect of the internal auditory canal and the facial nerve. This approach provides more extensive exposure of the anterior brainstem but sacrifices hearing.

Transcochlear Approach

This approach optimizes exposure of the anterior brainstem by removing the entire petrous bone. The external auditory canal is transected and oversewn. In addition to removing the same bone as for the translabyrinthine approach, the facial nerve canal is skeletonized and opened to mobilize the facial nerve. The GSPN is divided to allow for posterior transposition of the facial nerve. The internal auditory canal and cochlear apparatus are removed completely. The drilling continues anteriorly to skeletonize the internal carotid artery up to the siphon. This approach provides maximal exposure of the petroclival region but sacrifices hearing, and it is associated with at least temporary paresis, if not permanent weakness, of the face.

Posterior Fossa Cranial Base Approaches

RETROSIGMOID SUBOCCIPITAL CRANIOTOMY

The standard retrosigmoid craniotomy is performed with the patient in the supine position with the head turned away from the operative side and flexed, allowing the vertex to tilt downward. For aneurysms of the vertebral artery, we prefer a modified park-bench position, with the operative side facing upward and the axilla protected with a foam roll. The dependant arm is extended over the end of the table and hangs off the end of the table, cradled with foam padding above the radiolucent three-pin head holder (*Figure 9.12*). The head is positioned with the fol-

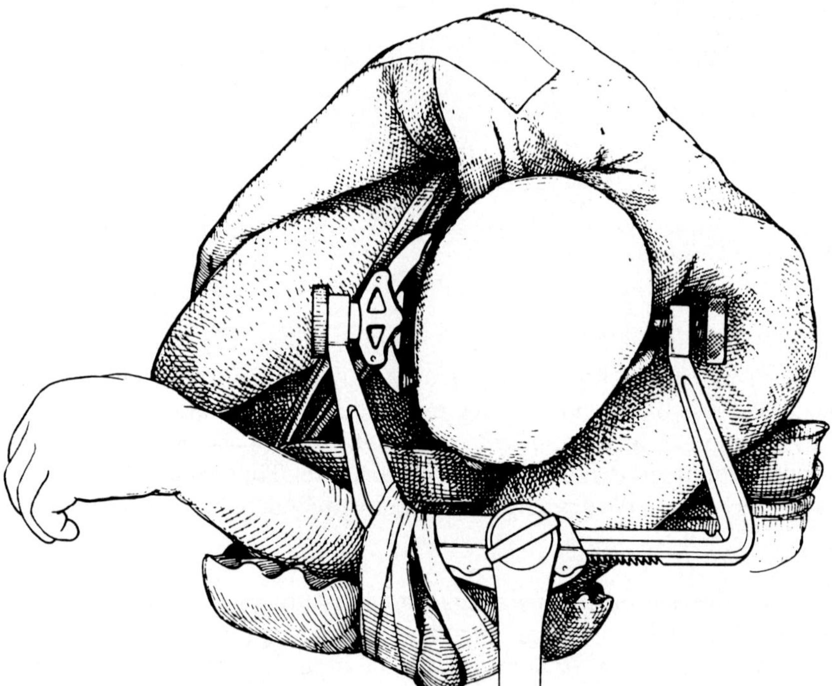

A

FIG. 9.12 *A,* schematic drawing, viewed from the cranial vertex, of a modified park-bench position for a right far lateral approach. The head has been taken through the three maneuvers outlined in the text. Note that the dependent arm has been padded and cradled beneath the head holder. A foam roll is placed under the axilla for extra protection (*not shown*).

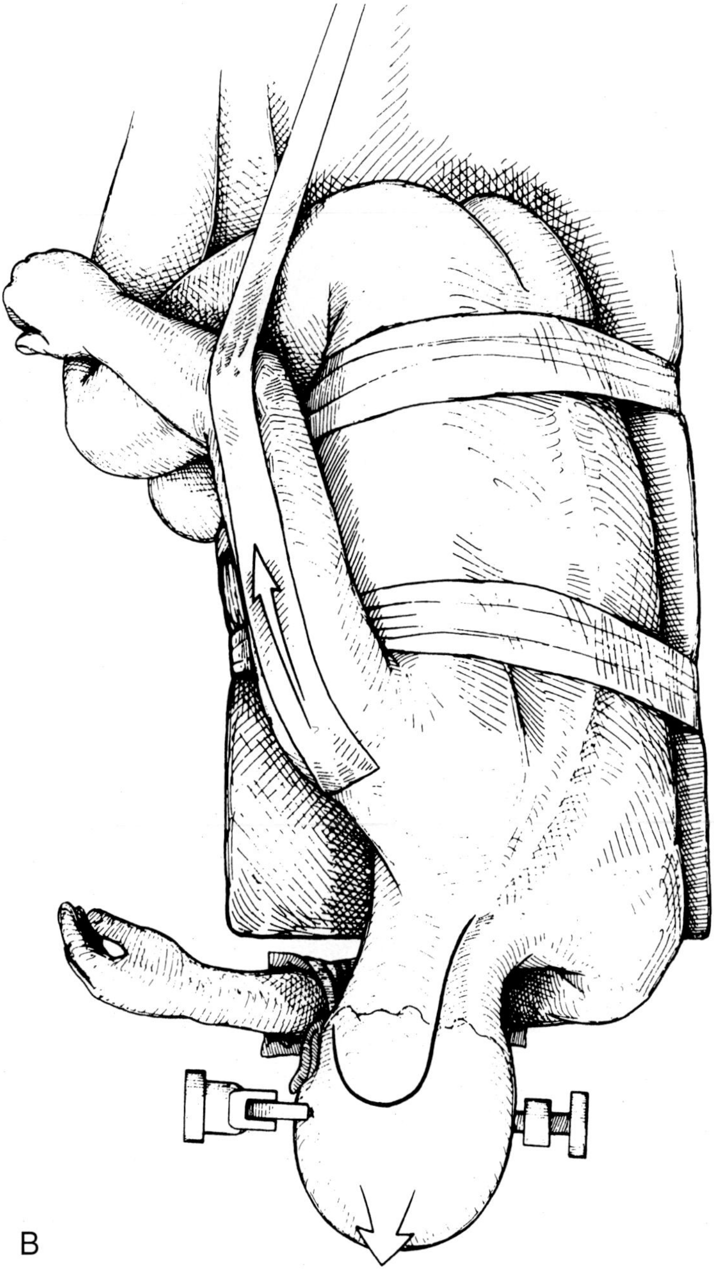
B

FIG. 9.12 *B,* schematic drawing, viewed from above, of patient positioning for the far lateral approach. The right arm is pulled downward with tape to open the craniocervical angle, and the patient is taped securely to the operating table to allow the patient angle to be changed during the operation.

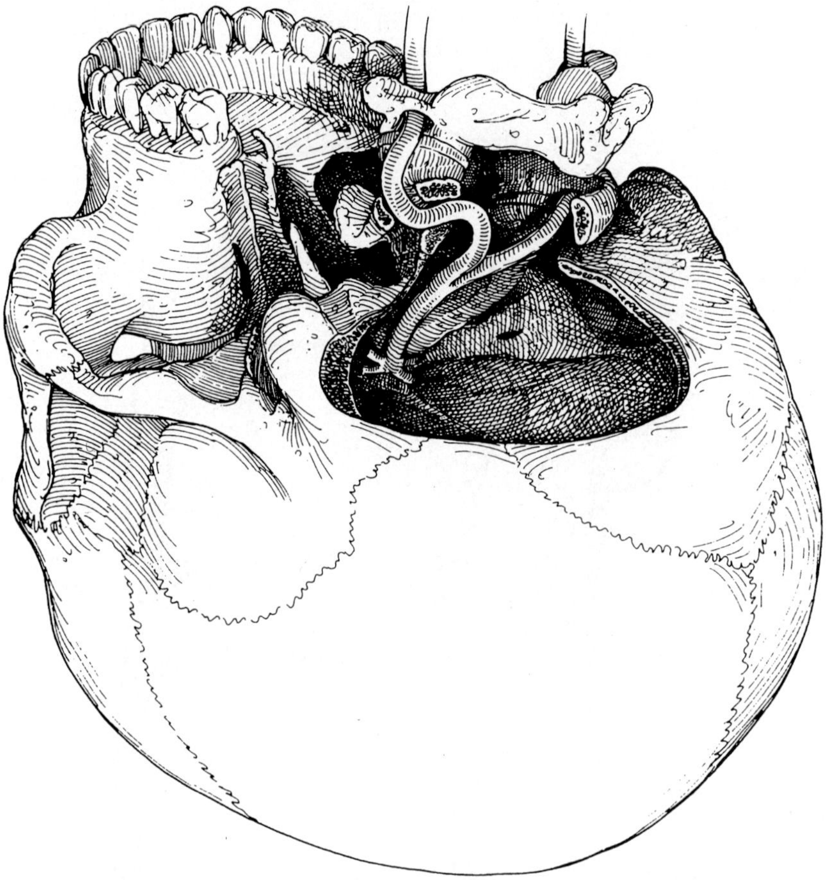

FIG. 9.12 *C,* schematic illustration demonstrating the perspective of the cranium and vessels in relation to the amount of bone resection in the far lateral approach. It is important to resect the occipital and C1 condylar interface so that a gap of 1 cm is present between the extradural vertebral artery and the bone. (*See* Reference 9.)

lowing maneuvers: 1) flexion in the anteroposterior plane until the chin is one finger's breadth from the sternum; 2) rotation 45 degrees away from the side of the lesion; 3) lateral flexion down toward the opposite shoulder; and 4) slight distraction to increase the interval between the foramen magnum and C1. The ipsilateral shoulder is retracted inferiorly with cloth tape to enhance visualization superiorly. As described by Spetzler and Graham (23), this series of maneuvers places the ipsilateral mastoid process at the highest point of the operative field and significantly opens the occipitocervical space.

The skin incision begins in the midline at the level of C2 or C3. It extends superiorly in the midline avascular plane to a point just below the inion and curves laterally to the ipsilateral mastoid process. The suboccipital muscles are divided below the superior nuchal line, and a cuff of muscle and fascia are left for later reapproximation during closure. The subperiosteal dissection exposes the suboccipital region and the arches of C1 and C2. The entire myocutaneous flap is retracted laterally using rubberbanded fishhooks attached to a Leyla bar (V. Mueller).

A suboccipital craniotomy is performed by placing a burr hole and using the B1 attachment and foot plate of the Midas Rex drill to create a craniotomy extending toward the transverse and sigmoid sinuses, and extending inferiorly as far laterally as possible to the foramen magnum just medial to the dural entry of the vertebral artery. The dimensions of the craniotomy are tailored to the patient's individual pathology.

Retrolabyrinthine-Transsigmoid Approach

This approach was originally described by Giannotta and Maceri (7) in 1988 and is useful for exposing aneurysms at the vertebrobasilar junction. The patient is positioned supine with the head turned sharply away from the side of the approach. A curvilinear scalp incision is made in the retroauricular region, and the soft tissues are reflected anteriorly to expose the posterior aspect of the external auditory canal. A retrolabyrinthine mastoidectomy is performed, skeletonizing the sigmoid sinus from the superior petrosal sinus to the jugular bulb. The sigmoid sinus is ligated at those two points, and the resulting dural flap is reflected over the intact labyrinth. By fully skeletonizing the posterior semicircular canals, the exposure can be expanded (*Figure 9.13*). This approach is useful for aneurysms of the upper vertebral artery, vertebrobasilar junction, and lower basilar trunk (*Figure 9.14*).

Transcondylar (Far Lateral) Approach

First described by Heros (11) for aneurysm surgery and later modified by others, the transcondylar approach involves extradural exposure of the vertebral artery and removal of the medial one-third to one-half of the occipital condyle to enhance lateral exposure of the brainstem and vertebral artery up to the vertebral confluence. The initial exposure is as described for the retrosigmoid suboccipital approach. The vertebral artery and its surrounding venous plexus are exposed by subperiosteal dissection along the sulcus arteriosus of C1. Lateral to medial dissection exposes the vertebral artery from the transverse foramen to the atlanto-occipital membrane where it enters the dura. This provides early proximal control of the vertebral artery.

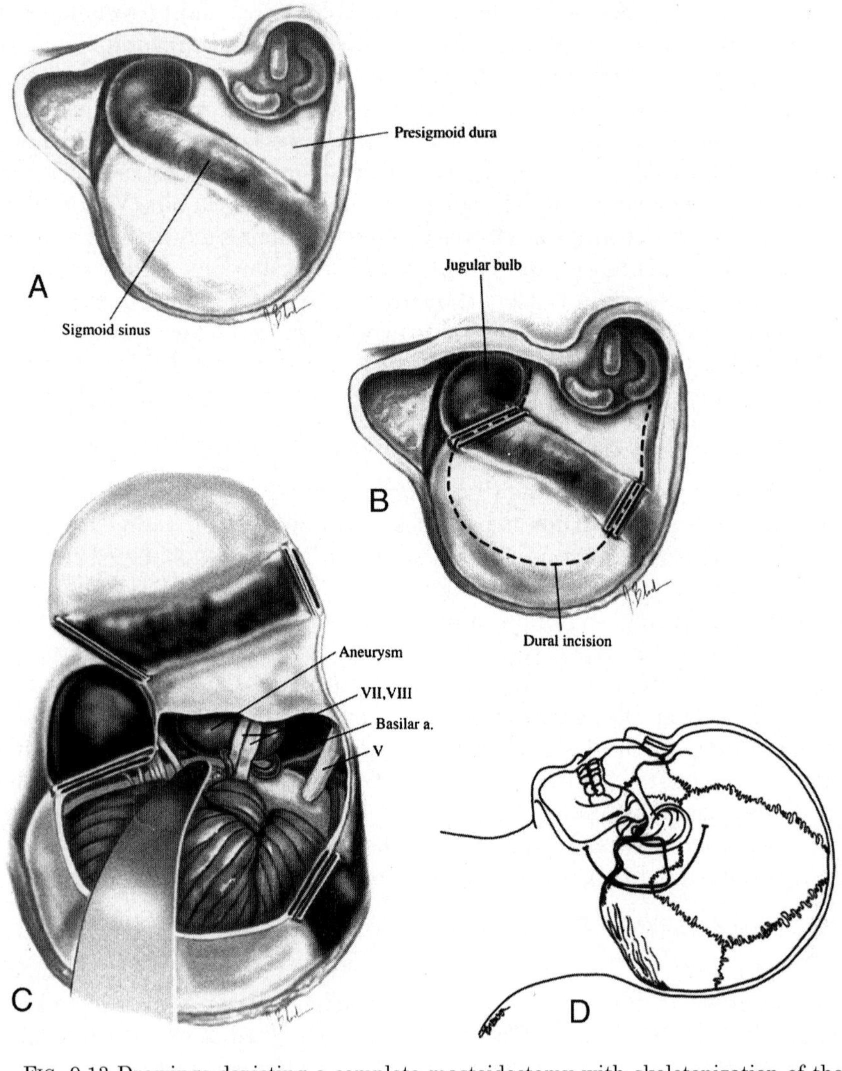

FIG. 9.13 Drawings depicting a complete mastoidectomy with skeletonization of the presigmoid and retrosigmoid dura that is initially performed for the retrolabyrinthine-transsigmoid approach (*A*). The posterior semicircular canal is completely skeletonized. The sigmoid sinus is then ligated superior and inferior as part of dural opening (*B*). A wide retrolabyrinthine exposure of the vertebrobasilar junction area is afforded (*C*). *D,* drawing showing the retroauricular scalp incision and bone opening for a left-sided retrolabyrinthine-transsigmoid approach. *a,* artery; *V, VII, VIII,* cranial nerves. (*See* Day JD, Fukushima T, Giannotta SL: Cranial base approaches to posterior circulation aneurysms. **J Neurosurg** 87:544–554, 1997).

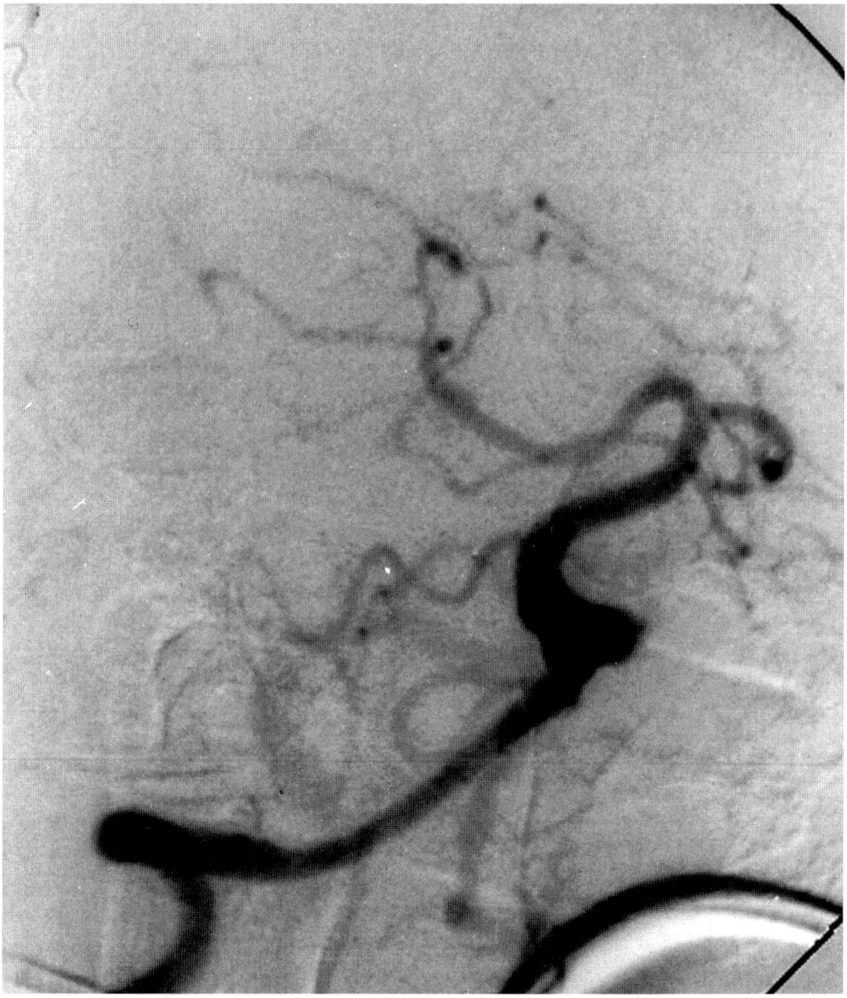

FIG. 9.14 Vertebral angiogram of aneurysm of lower basilar trunk approached by retrolabyrinthine-transsigmoid approach.

A hemilaminectomy of the ipsilateral arch of C1 is performed and a suboccipital craniotomy is created as described above. When the craniotomy is completed, the entire ipsilateral rim of the foramen magnum is removed with small rongeurs (*Figure 9.12C*). While the vertebral artery is protected with a small dissector, the occipital condyle and superior lateral mass and facet of C1 are drilled until a thin cortical shell of bone remains. This shell is then removed with curettes and small

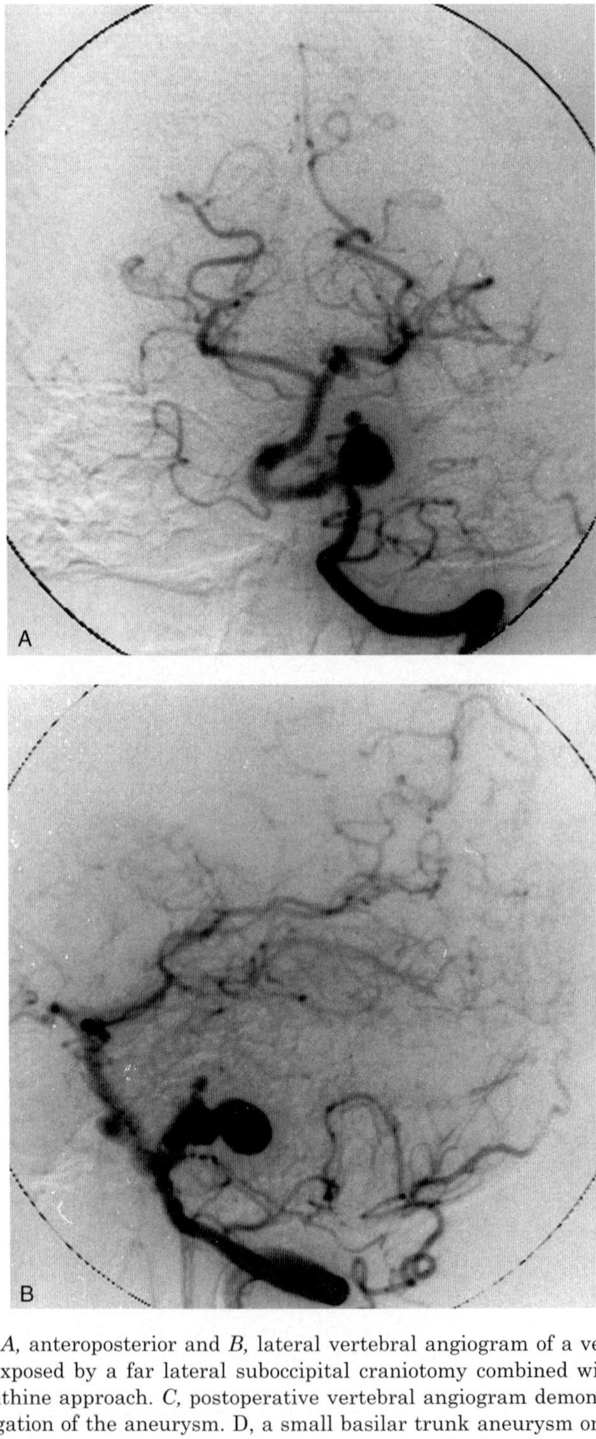

FIG. 9.15 *A,* anteroposterior and *B,* lateral vertebral angiogram of a vertebrobasilar aneurysm exposed by a far lateral suboccipital craniotomy combined with a petrosal retrolabyrinthine approach. *C,* postoperative vertebral angiogram demonstrating complete clip ligation of the aneurysm. D, a small basilar trunk aneurysm on the opposite side of the basilar artery could not be adequately visualized and was treated by endovascular coiling (*arrowhead*).

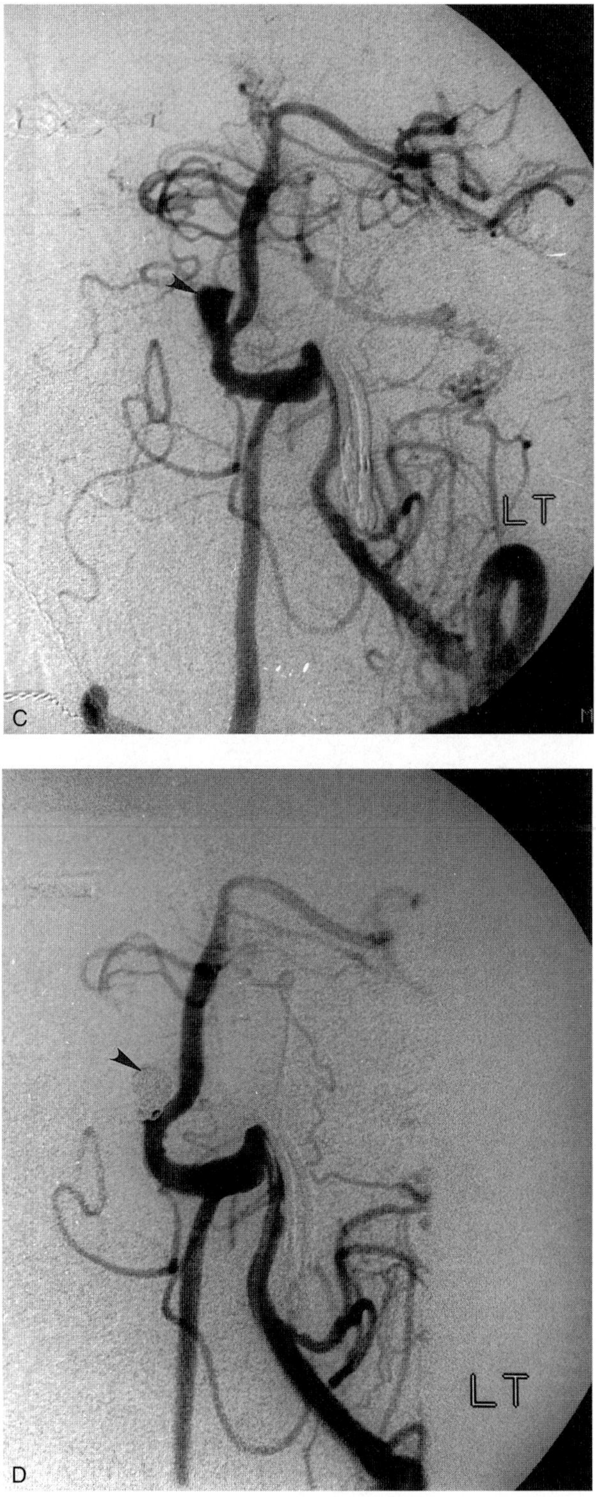
LT
C
LT
D

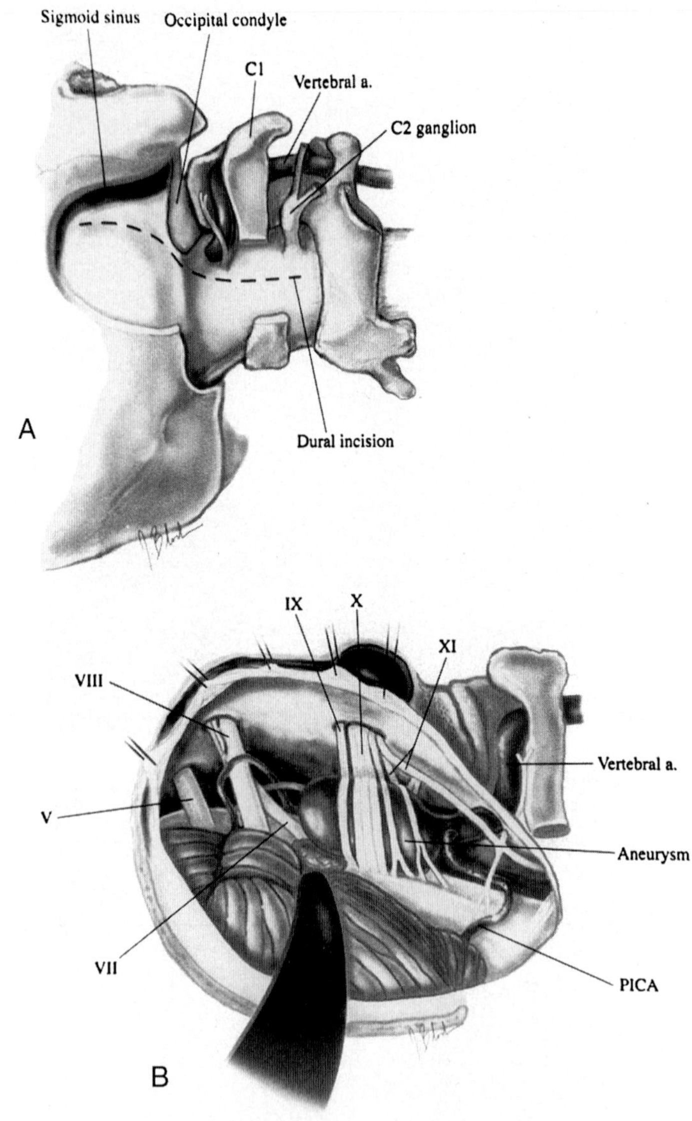

FIG. 9.16 Drawings showing the extreme lateral inferior transcondylar exposure approach beginning with a lateral suboccipital craniectomy through the lateral foramen magnum and removal of the C1 lateral posterior hemiarch in selected cases (*A*). The occipital condyle is subsequently further reduced and the hypoglossal canal is exposed. The jugular tubercle is then reduced by drilling between the hypoglossal canal and the jugular bulb. This approach provides wide exposure anterior to the brainstem with only a minimum of retraction to hold the cerebellar hemisphere away from the field (*B*). *a,* artery; *V, VII, VIII, IX, X, XI,* cranial nerves. (*See* Day JD, Fukushima T, Giannotta SL: Cranial base approaches to posterior circulation aneurysms. **J Neurosurg** 87: 544–554, 1997.)

rongeurs. Removal of the condyle is limited to the medial one-third to one-half to ensure craniocervical stability.

The dura is opened in a curvilinear fashion based laterally. The cisterna magna is opened to allow egress of CSF and brain relaxation. Self-retaining retractors are used to protect the cerebellar hemisphere and tonsil with virtually no retraction required. This approach provides excellent exposure of the anterior foramen magnum and lower clivus. It is an excellent approach for aneurysms of the vertebral artery at the origin of the posterior inferior cerebellar artery up to the vertebral confluence. The far lateral approach may be further extended to include various petrosectomy approaches. *Figure 9.15* shows a vertebrobasilar aneurysm that was exposed through a combined petrosal retrolabyrinthine and far lateral approach.

Extreme Lateral Inferior Transcondylar Exposure

Bertalanffy and Seeger (2) provided a detailed description of this exposure as applied to both neoplastic and vascular lesions. This approach provides more lateral-inferior exposure of the craniovertebral junction and lower brainstem. Following the steps outlined for the transcondylar approach above, the surgeon removes bone laterally to the sigmoid sinus and its junction with the jugular bulb using a high-speed drill. The occipital condyle is drilled until the hypoglossal canal and jugular tubercle are exposed. If necessary, further drilling of the cranial base, including the jugular tubercle, can be performed (*Figure 9.16*).

CONCLUSION

The majority of intracranial aneurysms may be approached and exposed through standard pterional or subtemporal craniotomies. Cranial base extensions are an important adjunct in the management of selected intracranial aneurysms, and may provide opportunities to cure certain rare lesions that were once regarded as untreatable. The neurovascular surgeon should be familiar with the various extensions of standard approaches that provide more optimal avenues to selected complex lesions.

REFERENCES

1. Barrow DL, Alleyne CH Jr: Aneurysms of the intracavernous carotid artery, in, Tindall GT, Cooper PR, Barrow DL (eds). *The Practice of Neurosurgery.* Baltimore: Williams and Wilkins, 1996, vol 2, pp 2013–2032.
2. Bertalanffy H, Seeger W: The dorsolateral, suboccipital, transcondylar approach to the lower clivus and anterior portion of the craniovertebral junction. **Neurosurgery** 29:815–821, 1991.

3. Dolenc VV: Anatomy and surgery of the cavernous sinus. New York: Springer-Verlag, 1989.
4. Dolenc VV, Skrap M, Sustersic J, Skrbec M, Morina A: A transcavernous-transsellar approach to the basilar tip aneurysms. **Br J Neurosurg** 1:251–259, 1987.
5. Drake CG: The surgical treatment of vertebral basilar aneurysms. **Clin Neurosurg** 16:114–169, 1969.
6. Drake CG: The treatment of aneurysms of the posterior circulation. **Clin Neurosurg** 26:96–144, 1979.
7. Giannotta SL, Maceri DR: Retrolabyrinthine transsigmoid approach to basilar trunk and vertebrobasilar artery junction aneurysms: Technical note. **J Neurosurg** 69:461–466, 1988.
8. Hakuba A, Liu SS, Nishimura S: The orbitozygomatic infratemporal approach: A new surgical technique. **Surg Neurol** 26:271–276, 1986.
9. Hamilton MG, Kraus GE, Daspit CP, Spetzler RF: Giant aneurysms of the vertebrobasilar trunk, in Awad IA, Barrow (eds): *Giant Intracranial Aneurysms.* Park Ridge: AANS, 1995, pp 197–221.
10. Hashi K, Nin K, Shimotake K: Transpetrosal combined supratentorial and infratentorial approach for midline vertebro-basilar aneurysms, in, Brock M (ed): *Modern Neurosurgery.* Heidelberg: Springer-Verlag, 1982, vol 1, pp 442–448.
11. Heros RC: Lateral approach for vertebral and vertebrobasilar artery lesions. **J Neurosurg** 64:559–562,1986.
12. Kasdon DL, Stein BM: Combined supratentorial and infratentorial exposure for low-lying basilar aneurysms. **Neurosurgery** 4:422–426, 1979.
13. Kawase T, Toya S, Shiobara R, Mine T: Transpetrosal approach for aneurysms of the lower basilar artery. **J Neurosurg** 68:857–861, 1985.
14. Krayenbuhl HA, Yasargil MG: Cerebral angiography. Philadelphia: J.B. Lippincott, 1963, ed 2.
15. MacDonald JD, Antonelli P, Day AL: The anterior subtemporal, medial transpetrosal approach to the upper basilar artery and ponto-mesencephalic junction. **Neurosurgery** 43:84–89, 1998.
16. Peerless SJ, Drake CG: Management of aneurysms of the posterior circulation, in Youmans JR (ed): *Neurological Surgery.* Philadelphia: W.B. Saunders, 1982, ed 2, vol 3, pp 1715–1733.
17. Peerless SJ, Drake CG: Posterior Circulation Aneurysms, in, Wilkins RH, Rengachary SS (eds): *Neurosurgery.* New York: McGraw-Hill, 1985, pp 1422–1437.
18. Pellerin P, Lesoin F, Dhellemmes P, Donazzan M, Jomin M: Usefulness of the orbitofrontomalar approach associated with bone reconstruction for temporosphenoid meningiomas. **Neurosurgery** 15:715–718, 1984.
19. Saeki N, Rhoton AL Jr: Microsurgical anatomy of the upper basilar artery and the posterior circle of Willis. **J Neurosurg** 46:563–578, 1977.
20. Sano K: Temporo-polar approach to aneurysms of the basilar artery at and around the distal bifurcation: Technical note. **Neurol Res** 2:361–367, 1980.
21. Sen CN, Sekhar LN: An extreme lateral approach to intradural lesions of the cervical spine and foramen magnum. **Neurosurgery** 27:197–204, 1990.
22. Solomon RA, Stein BM: Surgical approaches to aneurysms of the vertebral and basilar arteries. **Neurosurgery** 23:203–208, 1988.
23. Spetzler RF, Graham TW: The far-lateral approach to the inferior clivus and the upper cervical regionL Technical note. **BNI Q** 6:35–38, 1990.
24. Spetzler RF, Schievink W: The anterior subtemporal, medial transpetrosal approach to the upper basilar artery and ponto-mesencephalic junction. **Neurosurgery** 43:89, 1998 (comment).

25. Spetzler RF, Daspit CP, Pappas CTE: The combined supra- and infratentorial approach for lesions of the petrous and clival regions: Experience with 46 cases. **J Neurosurg** 76:588–599, 1992.
26. Sundt TM Jr: Surgical techniques for saccular and giant intracranial aneurysms. Baltimore: Williams & Wilkins, 1990.
27. Weir B: Aneurysms affecting the nervous system. Baltimore: Williams & Wilkins, 1988.
28. Yasargil MG, Antic J, Laciga R, Jain KK, Hodosh RM, Smith RD: Microsurgical pterional approach to aneurysms of the basilar bifurcation. **Surg Neurol** 6:83–91, 1976.
29. Zabramski JM, Kris T, Sankhla SK, Cabiol J, Spetzler RF: Orbitozygomatic craniotomy: Technical note. **J Neurosurg** 89:336–341, 1998.
30. Zeal AA, Rhoton AL Jr: Microsurgical anatomy of the posterior cerebral artery. **J Neurosurg** 48:534–559, 1978.

CHAPTER

10

Selecting Aneurysms for Adequate Exposure without Extended Cranial Base Approaches: Neurovascular Decision-making Counterpoint

T.C. ORIGITANO, M.D., PH.D., FACS

My initial enthusiasm for this task was quenched as its subtleties became more apparent. First and foremost, I consider myself a student of the art and science of aneurysm surgery and management. I am fortunate to have trained and lived during the time of the masters of aneurysm surgery. I Owe special thanks to Professor M. Gazi Yasargil for his enormous contribution to my personal perspective and to this field of neurological surgery. I also consider myself a cranial base surgeon, having mastered the many extended skull base approaches for tumors, and applied and advocated them in aneurysm surgery. I began to wonder what devious conspiracy is this task; to be successful would be to reject the very faith I preach—very much like criticizing your mother, or worse, defending your mother in an argument with your wife . . . a no-win situation.

My position has given me a unique perspective living in both worlds. Often, new techniques arrive on the scene with great fanfair and appeal. They carry the perception of ubiquity and progress evoking the Mount Everest phenomena: we do it because it is there. It is the tradition of neurological surgery to critically analyze and call to task each new pretender to progress, assessing each for its best application as it relates to optimal patient outcome.

GENERAL PHILOSOPHY: COMMON GROUND

Regardless of the approach used, four principles remain constant: 1) early proximal and distal control; 2) see the perforators before, during, and after clip application; 3) it is not the size of the exposure, but the exposure of the critical structure (aneurysm neck, parent artery, and perforator) that counts; and 4) the goal is complete obliteration of the aneurysm with complete patency of the parent artery and perforators.

Furthermore, the operative management of intracranial aneurysms is analogous to bow hunting for grizzly bear. Clearly the bear is an irritable beast, master of its domain, easily aroused to anger and once angered, difficult to bring under control; the bear's lair is a small hostile environment, unforgiving and set with traps for the uninitiated invader. Its seeming tranquility can become a storm in the flash of a second. Finally, if you only wound the bear . . . it will make you pay.

Therefore, a successful hunt is contingent on: A thorough knowledge of the beasts and its habits; an understanding of the intricacies of its variable environment and how it can become hostile; the ability to maneuver for the kill shot; and expertise with the weapon.

UNDERSTANDING THE ENVIRONMENT

Ultimately, the aneurysm and its parent artery reside within the arachnoid space of the intracranial cisterns. No amount of bone removed or soft tissue transposition will change the size or geometry of the aneurysm's lair. You must enter the cistern to attack the aneurysm. The actual working space of individual cisterns can only be modified by its opening and the linkage to its adjacent neighbor. In doing so, the aneurysm becomes vulnerable for attack. This process also leads to the untethering of individual neuronal structures from each other and from the cranial base. With untethering, independent mobilization of one lobe from another can occur without linked traction on the dome of the aneurysm buried within.

The cisterns are also the home of the parent vessels, whose control is vital for safe passage and whose subtle differences in configuration, caliber, and perforator anatomy are critical for a successful hunt. Keeping the cisterns expanded and the brain relaxed improves navigation through them. Critical to this end are two highly underrated adjuvants: patient positioning and spinal drainage.

Optimal patient positioning takes advantage of site lines, which will highlight particular aneurysms by location and orientation. Furthermore, positioning can play an important role in brain relaxation by optimizing venous outflow and gravity retraction.

Spinal drainage can be both a blessing and a bane. When the brain is tense, judicial spinal drainage will permit adequate relaxation for entrance into the cisternal system. Although it yields a relaxed brain, overuse of spinal drainage also collapses the arachnoid space. Flattened cisterns are harder to work through. Cerebrospinal drainage should occur sequentially as each cistern is opened and linked. Premature drainage collapses the arachnoid onto the brain and onto the aneurysm, increasing the chance of pial violation and worse complications.

THE MOST COMMON THINGS ARE COMMON

The vast majority of aneurysms are smaller than 1.0 cm, and are located on the carotid circulation (85–95%) in three locations: anterior communicating (30%); posterior communicating (25%), and middle cerebral (20%). The remaining 5 to 15% of aneurysms are located in posterior fossa are dominated by basilar apex lesions. Therefore, the vast majority of intracranial aneurysms are approachable through a standard pterional, craniotomy with minor modifications. Aneurysms best approached through extend cranial base procedures are shown in *Table 10.1.*

MINIMAL MODIFICATIONS OF THE CLASSICAL PTERIONAL APPROACH

A number of minor and subtle modifications of the classical pterional approach can be safely and easily applied to facilitate entry into the basal cisterns. The inferior translocation of the temporalis muscle permits a robust exposure of the sphenoid wing. This soft tissue transfer requires a transfascial or intrafascial dissection of the temporalis fascia for safe convenience of the frontal branch of the facial nerve out of harm's way. This single manuever provides centimeters of exposure to permit extension of drilling of the sphenoid wing.

Classically, the sphenoid wing is drilled to the level of the orbitomeningeal artery prior to opening the dura. Further gentle drilling of the medial sphenoid wing to expose the superior orbital fissure projects the opening to the carotid cistern. Additional precious millimeters of space can be obtained for anterior midline aneursyms by gentle ex-

TABLE 10.1
Aneurysms Best Approached through Extended Cranial Base Procedures

Location	Approach
Midbasilar	Petrosal
Vertebrobasilar Junction	Petrosal/far lateral transcondylar
Large giant basilar apex	Orbitocranial zygomatic
Low-lying basilar apex	Petrosal
High-lying basilar apex	Orbitocranial zygomatic
Large to giant anterior communicating aneurysms	Orbitocranial zygomatic
Posterior projecting anterior communicating aneurysms	Orbitocranial

tradural elevation of the frontal lobe and flat drilling of the orbital roof, which flattens the anterior fossa. The dura is opened low across the frontal lobe around the anterior surface of the temporal lobe. A second relaxing incision is made along the sylvian fissure. The dura is then pulled taut flush to the surface of the drilled bone, enhancing access to the deep sylvian fissure and carotid cistern.

It should be realized that a pterional craniotomy is a modified subfrontal approach. Dissection of the sylvian fissure and basal cistern is meant to release the frontal lobe from its attachment to the temporal lobe and skull base. Sylvian fissure microdissection can occur proximal to distal or distal to proximal, depending on the anatomy of the individual fissure (balanced, frontal dominant, or temporal dominant). Retractors should be used to tailor the mobilized brain, which avoids the transmission of traction across a fixed structure and possible aneurysm rupture. Placement of refractors changes a dynamic, flexible space into static fixed space, and retractors are best deployed once dissection is completed. Certainly, the retractor-pull technique (placing a frontal and temporal retraction, then pulling) to open the fissure may work, but it is fraught with danger and should be avoided.

HUNTING FOR ANEURYSMS BY SITE

Reconnaissance

Detailed preoperative angiographic evaluation is critical for a successful aneurysm hunt. It is never enough just to find an aneurysm.

Cerebral angiograms should always comprise high-resolution four vessel subtraction angiography, to account for a 20% possibility of multiple aneurysm. Each aneurysm found should have multiple views to detail the size, location, geometry, and orientation of the neck, dome, parent artery, and perforator anatomy.

Collateral circulation, both right to left and back to front, should be performed. This knowledge can be comforting and life saving if intraoperative rupture occurs or temporary clip application is needed. With large, giant, or geometrically complex aneurysms, endovascular microcatheter analysis may prove indispensible in assessing clippability. Three-dimensional computed tomographic angiography or angiographic reconstruction can enhance the spatial relationship of bone to aneurysm dome or neck in microsurgical detail.

The Case for Proximal Control

Cranial base approaches are intended to provide proximal control for aneurysms of the cavernous and ophthalmic segment through exposure of the petrous carotid artery, with the traditional approach including isolation of cervical carotid in the neck. Advocates of petrous carotid exposure and control with a balloon or clip espouse the benefits of single-site exposure and proximity to the operative field, i.e., "it is right there!" Exposure to the petrous carotid requires a detailed knowledge of the middle cranial fossa floor anatomy and its varients.

POTENTIAL RISKS

Potential risks of exposing the petrous carotid include 1) facial nerve injury by traction on the greater superficial petrosal nerve; 2) hearing loss by damage to the cochlea; 3) injury to the carotid if bony canal is dehiscent; and 4) injury to the eustachian tube with a potential cerebrospinal fluid fistula. The carotid artery in petrous bone is thinner because its adventia has blended with the periostium of the bone. The space exposed is small, and the angle for clip placement is acute. In the presence of rupture, the proximal control site is involved in the same microfield. Cervical carotid control is robust and remote, permitting an assistant easy and independent access. Adjuvant retrograde suction and intraoperative angiography also can be performed from this site. As for endovascular or any balloon control, I have observed failure of balloons at the most inopportune times.

The Case for Anterior Clinoid Removal

Aneursyms of the ophthalmic segment (ophthalmic artery, superior hypophyseal, and proximal posterior communicating artery) can require anterior clinoid process removal for optimal visualization and clip application. Extradural cranial base resection has been advocated. Before such an endeavor, a detailed analysis of the bony relationship to the aneurysm must be performed. Aneurysm rupture during extra dural resection can lead to a disappointing day. Direct intradural visualization with resection after proximal and distal control may not be fashionable, but it is sound, safe, and recommended.

Operating on Common Aneurysms that do not require extended Cranial Base Approaches

Aneursyms of the posterior communicating artery, anterior communicating artery complex, and middle cerebral artery constitute nearly 75% of all aneurysms.

THE "SIMPLE" POSTERIOR COMMUNICATING ARTERY AND ANTERIOR CHOROIDAL ARTERY ANEURYSMS

Although they are considered easy to expose, a series of subtle nuances shared by posterior communicating artery and anterior choroidal artery aneurysms must be appreciated for successful surgical outcome. First, their orientation to the carotid artery is found projecting lateral superior into the temporal lobe, lateral inferior under the petroclinoid ligament, or directly posterior under the course of the carotid. With a shortened supraclinoid carotid, the anterior clinoid artery can obstruct the visualization of a posterior communicating artery aneurysm or the vessel its itself, which then requires its intradural resection.

Traction on the temporal lobe can be catastrophic in the treatment of laterally oriented aneurysms and essential for those located posteriorly. If possible, the posterior communicating artery should be isolated before clipping. Sacrifice at its origin is usually well tolerated, except in situations of fetal origin. The anterior choroidal artery (or arteries with multiple vessels) should be identified before clipping is attempted. Inadvertent sacrifice can lead to a severe neurological deficit.

The art of the kill is in the management of the distal end of the clip, which must be free of the underlying perforators from both arteries. Clips that are too long can find the midportion of the posterior communicating artery, the deep running choroidal(s), or perforators of the respected parent arteries.

Posteriorly oriented aneurysms can be difficult to visualize on standard approach vectors. Rolling the carotid can enhance visualization of the neck and rupture of the aneurysm. Attacking through a more lateral subtemporal approach increases visualization of the neck and permits a near perpendicular view of the aneurysm and posterior communicating artery origin and course. This, however, requires mobilization of the temporal lobe laterally and back out of the middle cranial fossa. A solution is the use of a right-angled fenestrated encircling clip maneuvered in front of or under the choroidal complex and closed parallel to the parent artery. This is especially applicable to wide-neck posteriorly oriented aneurysms.

Intraoperative angiography can be especially helpful for interdictive clip adjustment in cases of fetal origin and posterior oriented aneurysms requiring vessel reconstitution. There is no substitution for direct inspection to guarantee perforator patency.

ALL ANTERIOR COMMUNICATING ARTERIES ARE NOT CREATED EQUAL

Surgically, the anterior communicating artery complex is a collection of seven important vascular structures: 1) the ipsilateral A1; 2) the contralateral A1; 3) The ipsilateral A2; 4) the contralateral A_2; 5) the anterior communicating artery (which can be duplicated or fenestrated); 6) the ipsilateral artery of Heubner; and 7) the hypothalamic perforators.

A successful operation is contingent on identification and preservation of all these structures. Aneurysms of the anterior communicating artery complex can project in four different orientations: 1) anterosuperior up and into the interhemispheric fissure above the optic chiasm; 2) anteroinferior, projecting forward and down, often into the optic chiasm; 3) superoposterior, projecting back between both A2 arteries; and 4) posteroinferior toward the hypothalamus.

The pterional craniotomy is used and modified by flattening the orbital roof, which improves the subfrontal view. This is especially advantageous for variants projecting posteriorly. The attack is made along the dominate A1 for more definitive proximal control. a dominate A1 occurs in **70 to 80%** of cases where anterior communicating artery aneursyms occur. Preoperative angiographic collateral assessment is recommended.

Operative attack is facilitated by sylvian fissure dissection. The internal carotid artery bifurcation is visualized and the A1 segment followed to the aneurysm. Dissection along the back wall of the A1 is safe, but care must be taken not to injure the perforators or the recurrent artery of Heubner.

This technique also provides significant, but not total, proximal control. Dissection of the gyrus rectus aids in early A1, A2 junction identification and decreases the amount of tractional force transmitted to the vascular bundle. Once at the aneurysm, a stepwise identification of the seven critical vessels is undertaken. The major difficulty is identifying contralateral structures hidden by the aneurysm. Clip length again becomes crucial; the general a tendency is to select clips that are too long rather than too short.

Management of a posteriorly projecting aneurysm may be enhanced by a more subfrontal look after a standard lateral dissection. Fenestrated encircling clips can be helpful in these cases. After clip application, careful inspection of the clip blades and the seven critical vessels should be revisited. Intraoperative angiography can be helpful to determine major branch occlusion, but only the surgeon can confirm hypothalamic perforator patency, the lack of which can cause profound neurocognitive dysfunction.

MIDDLE CEREBRAL ARTERY ANEURYSMS: THE EXCLUSIVELY SURGICAL ANEURYSMS

Aneurysms of the middle cerebral artery are highly variable in projection, geometry, parent artery configuration, and variability of the sylvian fissure. Sylvian fissure dissection is mandated. The direction of dissection, **distal to proximal versus proximal to distal,** depends on the above mentioned variables. Occasionally, an aneurysm can occur proximally before the main bifurcation at the site of a substantial anterior temporal artery.

In these situations, the dome can rest on the sphenoid wing. Aggressive dissection of the sphenoid wing can led to a disappointing day befor the dura is opened. The neck of these aneurysms will often partially incorporate a major branch. Microvascular tailoring of the neck with low current, bipolar with proximal vessel temporary clip application, may be necessary to construct a clippable neck.

Temporary clip application allows global inspection of the aneursym and dissection of adherent shadow branches. Great care must be exercised with clip application to avoid torsional forces capable of translational occlusion of both major branches and upstream perforators. Intraoperative angiography definitely rules out major branch occlusion. Because of the complex nature of the neck in relation to parent artery anatomy, current endovascular techniques are not advisable.

FINAL CONSIDERATIONS

Intraoperative rupture has a way of accelerating the conclusion of a case. One should do everything in one's power to avoid it and everything in one's power to prepare for it.

Two basic tenets should be followed. First, Be prepared: 1) know the collateral circulation; 2) obtain proximal/distal control early and always; 3) have temporary clips ready; and 4) keep the anesthesia service and the circulator in the room aware of where you are and, second, you have time if you do not hurry. Control **yourself and then the bleeding.** Suction directed on a cottonoid with gentle tamponade followed by proximal artery control will permit recovery and allow definitive clip application.

Obliteration of an intracranial aneursym by clip ligation carries the greatest potential and expectation of a surgical cure. A suboptimal clip application compromises that outcome, with the potential for aneurysm regrowth and subsequent hemorrhage. Intraoperative angiography provides a means to assess a suboptimal clip placement, and intervene and/or confirm optimal clip placement. This opportunity for direct assessment can be lifesaving for the patient and gratifying for the surgeon.

REFERENCES

1. Awad, IA: *Current management of cerebral aneurysms* in: *Neurosurgical Topics.* Park Ridge: AANS, 1993.
2. DeOliveira E, Sequeira M, Tedeschi H, Peace D, *Cerebral aneurysms and skull base lesions,* in *Surgical Anatomy for Microneurosurgery*, 1993, vol 6.
3. Fox JL: *The pterional perspective,* in: *Atlas of Neurosurgical Anatomy.* New York: 1989.
4. LeRoux P, Winn HR: *Current management of cerebral aneurysms: Part II—Techniques of aneurysm occlusion.* **Neurosurg Clin N Am,** 1998.

5. Origitano TC: *The Orbitocranial Zygomatic Approach To Aneurysms Of The Upper Basilar Trunk.* Park Ridge: AANS, 1999.
6. Origitano, TC, Al-Mefty, O. *Treatment of giant aneurysms of the cavernous portion of the internal carotid artery.* **Techniques in Neurosurgery,** 1998.
7. Yasargil, MG: Clinical Considerations, Surgery of the Intracranial Aneurysms and Results, in: *Microneurosurgery.* New York: Georg Theime Verlag, 1984.
8. Yasargil MG: Microsurgical anatomy of the basal cisterns and vessels of the brain: diagnostic studies, general operative techniques and pathological considerations of the intracranial aneurysm in: *Microneurosurgery.* New York: Georg Theime Verlag, 1984.

CHAPTER

11

Which Aneurysms Should Be Referred for Endovascular Therapy?

SUNGHOON LEE, M.D., DANIEL HUDDLE, D.O., ISSAM A. AWAD, M.D.

INTRODUCTION

The first diagnostic visualization of intracranial aneurysms was realized with the contribution of Egaz Moniz and the advent of cerebral angiography in 1933. Contemporary neurosurgeons of that era led the way in the treatment of cerebral aneurysms; Dott was the first to attempt a securing of cerebral aneurysm with a muscle fragment, and later, Dandy became the first to place a clip across the neck of an aneurysm in 1938. Surgical clipping with parent artery preservation has since remained the principal therapy for aneurysms, with the realization that cervical carotid ligation was neither safe nor effective in the treatment of the majority of cases. Neurovascular surgeons have strived to improve outcomes from open surgery over the past 25 years, with the introduction of and expanding expertise with microsurgical techniques, advances in neuroanesthesia, brain protection, and skull base exposure strategies.

At the same time, there was the development of endovascular therapeutic approach, pioneered by Serbinenko and followed by contributions of Debrun, Djindjian, Lasjaunias, Berenstein, Hieshima, and others, achieving secure endovascular navigation and occlusion of parent arteries and attempting aneurysm obliteration with balloons. In the past decade, electrically detachable thrombogenic coils introduced by Guglielmi, Vinuela, and others have allowed the successful occlusion of intracranial aneurysms with parent artery preservation.

Although the feasibility, safety, and long-term efficacy of endovascular therapy for cerebral aneurysms remain yet undefined and subject to ongoing debate, the popularity of this treatment modality has seen rapid growth. The United States Food and Drug Administration (FDA) approval of treatment of cerebral aneurysms with Guglielmi detachable coils (GDC) was specified for those patients with high medical and surgical risk of conventional therapy. Yet, there is no consensus as to the selection of specific patient and aneurysm subgroups for endovascular treatment. Some centers have advocated initial consideration of endovascular treatment whenever possible, while others continue to use this modality primarily for cases not amenable to surgical treatment. The preferences of patients and referring physicians, often without evidence-based guidelines, are heavily weighed in therapeutic decisions. Yet, there is sufficient experience and published literature that should guide rational selection of optimal therapy of the individual case from an armamentorium of open and endovascular treatment options. In this report, we review the current spectrum of endovascular therapies and discuss specific aneurysms and clinical scenarios where this treatment is advantageous and warrants primary consideration.

SPECTRUM OF ENDOVASCULAR THERAPIES FOR ANEURYSMS

The current spectrum of endovascular therapies directed at cerebral aneurysms includes extradural and intradural parent vessel occlusion, endosaccular embolization, and endovascular adjuncts to open surgical therapy.

Parent vessel occlusion of large caliber arteries is usually accomplished with detachable latex or silicone balloons with self-sealing valves. Balloon embolization may be the therapy of choice in cases where extradural carotid occlusion is contemplated for treatment of cavernous segment aneurysms, pseudoaneurysms related to carotid dissection and neoplastic disease, and in certain complex intradural aneurysms. Coils are used for smaller caliber arteries, and intradural parent vessel occlusion may be a reasonable therapeutic option for aneurysms involving distal leptomeningeal arteries that preclude simple clip occlusion. The GDC coils are used with the aim of endosaccular occlusion of aneurysms with parent artery preservation, including clinical scenarios where open surgical intervention might be associated with increased risk. Endovascular adjuncts for preoperative test occlusion and intraoperative proximal control, suction decompression, and angiography have enhanced the safety of surgical management of anatomically complex cerebral aneurysms.

EXTRADURAL PARENT VESSEL OCCLUSION

Extradural parent vessel occlusion has emerged as the principal therapeutic modality for extradural aneurysms and remains a useful option for certain complex intradural aneurysms. Most extradural aneurysms are difficult to treat by direct surgical exposure and clip ligation or by endovascular approach without parent vessel sacrifice. The spectrum of extradural aneurysms includes dissecting aneurysms that may be spontaneous or traumatic in origin, neoplastic pseudoaneurysms, and cavernous segment aneurysms. Arterial occlusion with or without bypass grafting remains the traditional treatment for these aneurysms. Intradural aneurysms that preclude simple clip occlusion, clip reconstruction, or endosaccular coiling may be treated by extradural parent artery occlusion, possibly in conjunction with incomplete endosaccular coiling and/or adjunctive bypass revascularization.

Endovascular detachable balloon technique has been noted to offer several advantages over abrupt or gradual surgical arterial ligation. A transfemoral arterial catheter approach allows the procedure to be performed in the awake patient under local anesthesia. Balloon test occlusion permits close and continuous monitoring of the patient's neurologic status while defining angiographic patterns of collateral supply of the territory of the occluded artery, and documenting cerebral blood flow during occlusion using single photon-emitting computed tomographic (SPECT) isotope techniques or stable xenon-computed tomography. This allows real time definition of the patient's hemodynamic reserve prior to committing permanent arterial occlusion (24, 32, 34). Adjunctive management including peri-procedure anti-coagulation, hemodynamic support, and long-term antiplatelet therapy further enhances the safety of this therapeutic endeavor.

Cavernous Segment Aneurysms

Aneurysms of the cavernous segment of the carotid artery are not rare, representing 3 to 5% of all intracranial aneurysms (30). Until recently, aneurysms involving the cavernous segment of the carotid artery have posed a difficult clinical dilemma. Small aneurysms of this location are usually asymptomatic, whereas large or giant aneurysms of the cavernous segment can cause symptoms related to mass effect, including opthalmoplegia, facial pain, and transient ischemic attacks or strokes from embolic phenomena. Recently, management strategies for cavernous segment aneurysms have been better defined. One significant advance in our understanding of carotid segment aneurysms may be that lesions which are entirely confined to the extradural space have little if any propensity to cause subarachnoid hemorrhage. The natural history and the indications for treatment of cavernous segment aneurysms have been examined in a retrospective fashion by Linskey et al. (30). The authors demonstrated no incidence of subarachnoid hemorrhage in this review, and furthermore, they noted that symptomatic aneurysms may manifest spontaneous symptomatic resolution.

The relatively benign natural history of cavernous segment aneurysms, with a low risk of mortality related to the lesion and its propensity to affect somewhat older patients, demands that any therapeutic strategy carries a low risk of morbidity and mortality. Symptomatic intracavernous carotid aneurysms have been treated to halt their clinical progression. Accepted indications include progressive opthalmoplegia or visual loss, intractable ipsilateral facial or orbital pain, radiographic enlargement of the aneurysm, and subarachnoid hemorrhage or epistaxis (31). Traumatic cavernous segment aneurysms, often associated with basilar skull fracture or previous transphenoidal or paranasal sinus surgery, and aneurysms arising from the anterior genu of the carotid siphon and extending intradurally into the subarachnoid space have been shown to have the potential for causing fatal epistaxis or subarachnoid hemorrhage, respectively (30).

Currently, a number of treatment options are available including direct surgical clipping of the intracavernous aneurysm, therapeutic carotid occlusion with or without prophylactic bypass surgery, or endovascular balloon embolization procedures with parent vessel preservation. Neurosurgical approaches to the cavernous sinus for the therapy of cavernous carotid aneurysm is a relatively recent development, described initially by Dolenc (10). Dolenc's innovative combined extradural-intradural technique to the surgery of the cavernous sinus improved the safety of such an endeavor (10, 26). However, the enthusiasm for intracavernous surgery has been tempered by issues regarding appropriate patient selection criteria and the increasingly safer option of endovascular intervention. Cases where cavernous segment aneurysm presents a definable neck have been successfully treated with detachable coiling technique. Halbach et al. (23) have reported a series of 35 patients that have been treated with endovascular coiling technique with parent vessel preservation for symptomatic cavernous segment aneurysm. These authors reported particularly outstanding outcome in which 96% of the patients presenting with cranial neuropathies had either complete resolution of symptoms or dramatic improvement. All patients that had suffered hemorrhage related to their aneurysms (epistaxis or SAH) had no further episodes of hemorrhage.

Although the low rate morbidity and mortality and the significant success rate of endovascular coiling technique justifies enthusiasm, the mean size of the aneurysms reported in the Halbach series was 11 mm, much smaller than the usually symptomatic cavernous segment lesions. There remains some reservation about generalizability of these results to larger lesions and about potential exacerbation of symptomatic mass effect with coil packing of giant lesions. Even with these alternate therapeutic avenues, therapeutic carotid occlusion remains a principal modality of therapy of the majority of cavernous segment carotid aneurysms (31). The current management regimen including peri-procedural anticoagulation, adjunctive provocative testing, and cerebral blood flow analysis has dramatically improved the safety of therapeutic carotid occlusion (*Fig. 11.1*). Therapeutic endovascular carotid occlusion without prophylactic bypass surgery remains a good option for the subset of patients with adequate hemodynamic reserves to tolerate ipsilateral carotid occlusion. While the debate regarding the usefulness of prophylactic bypass surgery continues, it is clear that if parent vessel occlusion is contemplated in a patient with inadequate hemodynamic reserve, bypass surgery may be prudent, if not necessary. Future advances of stent technology will likely further enhance the role of endovascular treatment of cavernous segment aneurysm and allow parent artery preservation in a larger fraction of cases.

Extradural Dissecting Aneurysms, Traumatic and Neoplastic Pseudoaneurysms, and Carotid Blowout Syndrome

Dissections of the internal carotid artery can occur spontaneously or may be associated with blunt or penetrating trauma. It is rare for cervical carotid dissection to extend cephalad to the skull base and into the

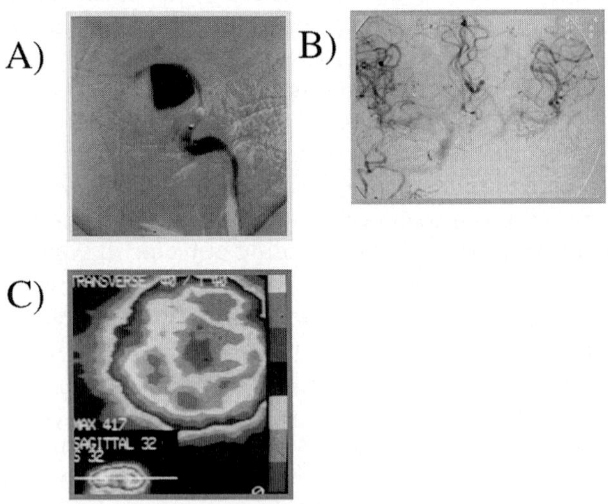

FIG. 11.1 (*A*) Angiogram reveals a giant cavernous segment internal carotid aneurysm. (*B*) Angiogram performed during temporary balloon test occlusion revealed excellent collateral flow, and patient tolerated the occlusion clinically without neurologic sequelae. (*C*) SPECT scan reveals no asymmetry of cerebral blood flow. Patient tolerated permanent carotid occlusion without complications.

subarachnoid space. Typically, conservative therapy with anticoagulation is sufficient in a majority of patients in avoiding ischemic sequelae. Follow-up imaging usually demonstrates recanalization of the involved carotid with or without lumen compromise or residual cervical pseudoaneurysm. These sequelae are typically managed expectantly, with prophylactic antiplatelet therapy and with excellent clinical outcome. Pseudoaneurysms from spontaneous dissection or non-penetrating blunt trauma have never been reported to rupture and do not warrant treatment unless associated with thromboembolism to the brain or retina.

More aggressive approach is indicated if the patient displays ischemic symptoms despite anticoagulation or if the dissection extends into the subarachnoid space, thus precluding the option of anticoagulation. Arterial injury from penetrating trauma may also evolve a dissecting aneurysm with a threatened impending rupture. Analogous situations may be encountered in patients with head and neck neoplastic disease with integral involvement of the carotid artery with impending rupture. Some of these patients present with catastrophic hemorrhage from a carotid blowout syndrome.

In such instances, the optimum treatment is urgent or emergent endovascular carotid occlusion. Nevertheless, the same principles of extradural parent artery occlusion should apply in the management of these patients. Endovascular ligation, rather than open Hunterian ligation, is recommended to allow for the dynamic estimation of the hemodynamic reserve with balloon test occlusion. Peri-procedural anticoagulation, adjunctive cerebral blood flow studies, and appropriate fluid and critical care management will determine the success of stroke prevention. Subsequent open surgical interventions for neoplasm are delayed by several weeks to allow for thrombus organization and hemodynamic adjustment.

COMPLEX INTRADURAL ANEURYSMS

Parent vessel occlusion remains an important adjunct for the management of complex intradural aneurysms. Complex intracranial aneurysms, such as giant or fusiform aneurysms, or aneurysms with difficult surgical exposure can require a multidisciplinary approach requiring combined parent vessel occlusion with surgical clip applications or endosaccular coil embolization. Giant aneurysms are known to progress and grow, despite seemingly adequate endosaccular coiling, as continued arterial flow turbulence prevents its complete thrombotic obliteration. The strategy of parent vessel occlusion can be applied to halt the flow-related failure of endosaccular occlusion in giant aneurysms.

As with the therapy of extradural aneurysms, treatment of complex intradural aneurysms with parent vessel occlusion requires the judicious assessment and supplementation of hemodynamic reserve and the application of anticoagulation to avoid thromboembolic complications. Such strategies in tackling complex intracranial aneurysms may require staging to allow the maturation of hemodynamic reserve following the treatment. For instance, the treatment of a giant vertebrobasilar junction aneurysm may require the first-stage endosaccular coil embolization, which rarely results in permanent cure. This is followed by staged, sequential extradural parent vessel occlusion of both vertebral arteries. If the patient fails balloon test occlusion of the second vertebral artery, there should be a consideration for prophylactic surgical revascularization prior to the completion of extradural arterial occlusion.

INTRADURAL PARENT VESSEL OCCLUSION

Intradural parent vessel occlusion is an important modality of therapy for intradural aneurysms occurring beyond major collateral pathways. Its utility is critical for the management of more distal lesions, such as mycotic aneurysms, and aneurysms associated with arterial feeders of arteriovenous malformations (AVMs). Furthermore, giant aneurysms occurring distal to the Circle of Willis that preclude simple surgical clip obliteration may be managed in part with intradural parent vessel occlusion. The success of intradural parent vessel occlusion depends on the adequate assessment of the eloquence of the cerebrovascular territory of the involved artery. This assessment can be made by the application of temporary balloon test occlusion or provocative testing with superselective sodium amytal injection. Careful neurologic monitoring during these endovascular challenges will help determine if the patient can tolerate distal parent vessel occlusion.

The presence of eloquent branches adjacent to the aneurysmal arterial segment is another critical consideration in the therapeutic paradigm of intradural parent vessel occlusion. Association of eloquent branches from the involved artery may increase the risk of ischemia with endovascular parent artery occlusion. Coil migration or propagating thrombosis of adjacent perforators remains a major source of morbidity from endovascular parent vessel occlusion. In such instances, open microsurgical approach, rather than endovascular occlusion, may be advantageous. Microsurgical occlusion or trapping by precise clip placement may allow preservation of the associated perforators or other eloquent branches. In the absence of adjacent eloquent branches, treatment may proceed with endovascular coil trapping and packing. If the patient is unable to tolerate endovascular test occlusion or mini-Wada test, alternative strategies should be considered including surgical occlusion, trapping, or reconstruction.

Distal Aneurysms of Leptomeningeal Arteries

Intracranial mycotic aneurysms can arise from systemic infections with bacterial or fungal etiologies. Although mycotic aneurysms are rare entities, they pose a signi cant threat of hemorrhage or septic thromboembolism. Because of their propensity to involve multiple distal leptomeningeal arteries, often in eloquent cerebral locations and in view of potential lesion involution with appropriate antibiotic or antifungal therapy, some of these aneurysms are treated conservatively. Aggressive surgical or interventional therapy for mycotic aneurysms may be reserved for clinical aneurysm rupture or the failure of lesion resolution despite appropriate antibiotic therapy. The caveat to a conservative, medical course of therapy is the assumption of the risk of hemorrhage during the treatment interval. Primary therapy with either microsurgical or endovascular approach may be justi ed in solitary lesions where the angioarchitecture of the lesion and the associated anatomy are favorable. Therapeutic intervention is aimed at aneurysm trapping with exclusion of the diseased arterial segment from the circulation. As mycotic aneurysms involve circumferential microbial infestation of the vessel wall, it is not advisable to attempt aneurysm treatment with parent artery preservation (neck clipping or endosaccular occlusion).

The experience with endovascular therapy of mycotic aneurysms is limited (20, 28, 41). The propensity of mycotic aneurysms to occur distal to the major collateral pathways allows the possibility of its successful obliteration with intradural parent vessel occlusion (*Fig. 11.2*). There may be relative dif culty in the surgical management of these lesions, secondary to issues of exposure and localization, making the endovascular alternative reasonable and attractive. Reports of parent vessel occlusions for the treatment of mycotic aneurysms have emphasized the importance of careful patient selection with the use of provocative testing (28, 41). Khayata et al. (28) reported satisfactory occlusion of mycotic aneurysms in three patients applying superselective sodium amytal injections for provocative testing. Scotti et al. (41) also reported three cases of endovascular parent vessel occlusions with successful exclusion of mycotic aneurysms.

Enthusiasm for endovascular management of mycotic aneurysms with intradural parent vessel occlusion must be tempered by a rational consideration of potential complicating sequelae. The possibility of

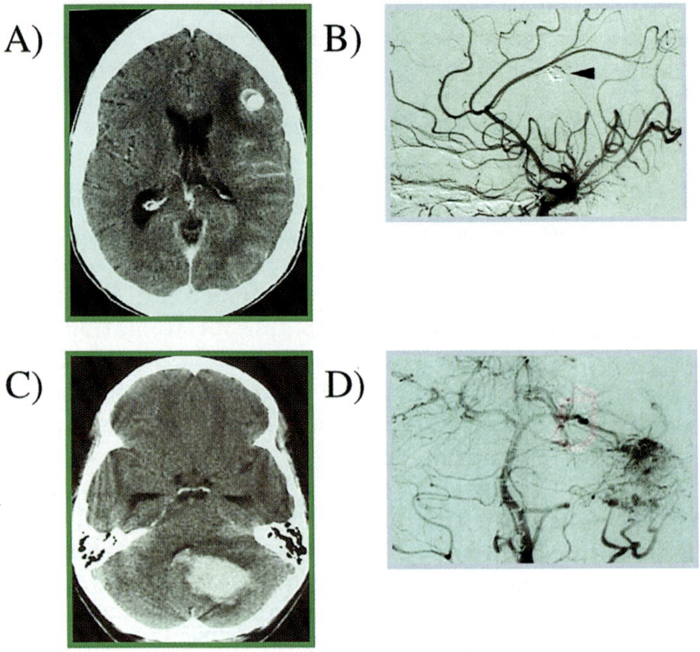

FIG. 11.2 (*A*) Distal mycotic aneurysm is visualized with associated hemorrhage. (*B*) Distal parent artery coiling accomplished aneurysm trapping (*arrowhead*). (*C*) Large posterior fossa hemorrhage from an AVM. (*D*) Associated feeding artery aneurysm (*circle*) was obliterated by endovascular glue at the same setting as embolization of the AVM.

propagation of thrombosis from parent artery occlusion proximal and distal to a coiled segment may preclude its application in situations where the parent artery gives rise to adjacent eloquent branches or perforators. Perforator and eloquent branch preservation are better achieved with microsurgical dissection and clip occlusion or trapping. Cases of mycotic aneurysm at eloquent branches of major leptomeningeal arteries may require microvascular reconstructions (arterial bypass) in conjunction with aneurysm trapping and excision. Careful preoperative assessment of the eloquence of the parent vessel supply with superselective catheterization and provocative testing will assist in determining the appropriate surgical strategy.

Cerebral arterial aneurysm associated with AVM has been described with a variable incidence, averaging 10% of AVM cases (8). Hemorrhagic sequelae in these patients are frequently related to the aneurysms of the feeding arteries rather than from the AVM itself. The treatment of these lesions places the added emphasis on preemptive obliteration of the aneurysm prior to the therapy of the AVM, as the aneurysms are prone to hemorrhage before, during, and following the treatment of the arteriovenous malformations (43). Staged surgical or endovascular therapy of arterial aneurysms associated with AVMs aiming for parent artery preservation may be possible when the aneurysms are proximal to the AVM nidus. Endovascular therapy can be the safer alternative when the aneurysm is closer to the nidus of the AVM. These aneurysms may be amenable to GDC coil packing or obliteration with embolic glue (intradural parent artery occlusion) at the same session as preparatory presurgical endovascular embolization of the AVM nidus (*Fig. 11.2*). This provides immediate protection from hemorrhage and facilitates subsequent staged therapy of the AVM itself.

Surgical obliteration of the aneurysm is preferable when there are associated eloquent branches that may be vulnerable to endovascular treatment. Surgical strategies may be directed toward occlusion of the parent artery distal to the eloquent branches or trapping of the involved aneurysm (*Fig. 11.3*).

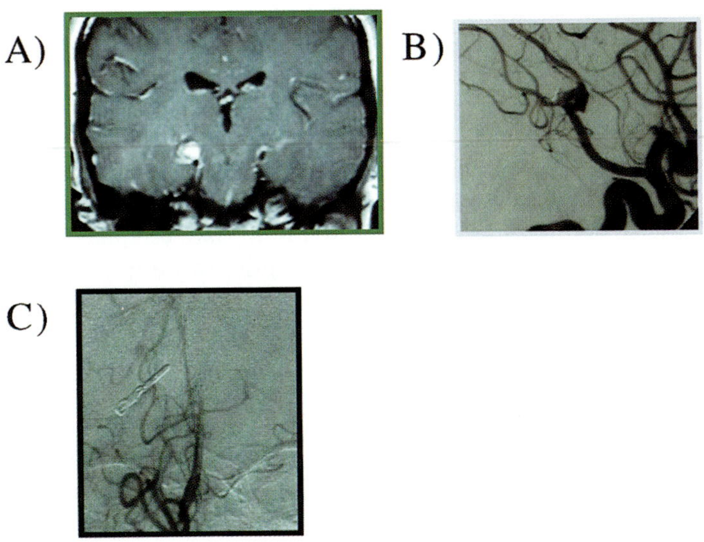

FIG. 11.3 (*A*) Patient presented with hemorrhage from a partially thrombosed right P3—P4 segment aneurysm. (*B*) The aneurysm had a broad neck, intimately associated with temporal branches and brainstem and collicular perforators. Surgical parent vessel occlusion was performed sparing adjacent eloquent branches. (*C*) Postoperative angiogram shows aneurysm obliteration and lling of adjacent branches. The patient has done well without neurologic sequelae at 1 year follow-up.

Adjunct to Management of Giant Aneurysms

Intradural parent vessel occlusion may be an important adjunct to the management of giant aneurysms occurring distal to major collateral pathways. Giant aneurysms of the MCA that preclude direct surgical clip reconstruction and preservation of the parent vessel may be managed with prophylactic extracranial-intracranial bypass and endovascular parent vessel occlusion. Prophylactic revascularizations are justi ed in these instances as patients rarely tolerate MCA branch occlusion without ischemic sequelae and loss of function. Aneurysm occlusion may be accomplished by the ow inversion created by EC—IC revascularization distal to the aneurysm along with proximal endovascular occlusion of the parent artery. Giant MCA aneurysms have been treated with combined revascularization and parent vessel occlusion (46). Hacein-Bey et al. (22) successfully combined surgical and endovascular approaches including EC—IC bypass and parent vessel occlusion, endovascular proximal artery occlusion followed by surgical clipping, and proximal artery occlusion followed by aneurysm decompression for mass effect.

Other contraindications to endovascular parent artery occlusion in the management of intracranial aneurysms are related to the eloquence of the involved arterial territory of the parent artery and associated perforators.

Aneurysms of the distal posterior cerebral artery can often be treated effectively with parent vessel occlusion, as the calcarine cortex is frequently well supplied by leptomeningeal collaterals. However, endovascular coil occlusion of the P3 or P4 segments often results in thromboembolic propagation to anterior temporal and parieto-occipital branches of these segments or vital perforators to the optic tract and brainstem. Clip obliteration of the artery at the aneurysm neck may better preserve these branches and minimize ischemic sequelae (*Fig.11.3*).

Mass effect exerted by the giant aneurysms may not be relieved by endovascular parent vessel occlusion. Cases with compelling symptoms related to mass effect should be considered for microsurgical trapping and decompression of the aneurysm. Giant aneurysms of the proximal anterior cerebral artery are best treated by such microsurgical clip trapping. This is tailored to preserve the anterior communicating complex and adjacent perforators while allowing prompt decompression of mass effect on adjacent optic chiasm (14).

ENDOSACCULAR OCCLUSION (GDC)

Endosaccular occlusion with GDC has become an increasingly accepted therapeutic modality for intracranial aneurysms. Multiple host or aneurysm factors may influence the decision whether the particular case is best managed surgically or by GDC embolization. These factors may include the patient's medical and neurologic condition, angioarchitecture and location of the aneurysm, the capabilities and experience of the surgical and endovascular teams, and patient preference.

Approved Indications

Despite advances in the surgical and critical care of patients with aneurysmal subarachnoid hemorrhage, high rates of morbidity and mortality persist in patients presenting with unstable neurologic condition, serious medical comorbidity, or aneurysms with surgically unfavorable location and morphology. Investigational device exemption approved by the United States FDA has been granted to evaluate the safety and efficacy of GDC embolization in the treatment of ruptured and unruptured intracranial aneurysms in patients deemed to be at *excessive risk for surgery*. The GDC Clinical Trial Summary states that the goal of the trial was to "provide treatment for certain intracranial aneurysms that because of morphology, location, or the patient's general medical condition are considered by the treating neurosurgical team to be either at very high risk for management by traditional operative techniques or are inoperable" (1). The rationale of subsequent FDA device approval was that patients deemed to be at excessive surgical risk may still benefit from the GDC embolization technology because preliminary evidence suggested that the modality may at least offer protection from early rebleeding in the acute period (17).

The practical application of these broadly stated FDA-approved indications calls for the definition of *excessive surgical risk* in relation to a particular case. Subjective interpretations of these guidelines for GDC embolization have varied widely among clinicians. A degree of subjectivity and flexibility in the interpretation of the approved guidelines is desirable in view of variable experience and expertise of the microsurgical and endovascular teams at different centers. Certain aneurysms, notably those with broad sessile neck or partially incorporating parent vessels, are not easily or safely amenable to GDC treatment. Larger and giant lesions have shown serious propensity to aneurysm refilling and growth from coil compaction and hemodynamic stress at the aneurysm inflow zone. Other cases present difficult endovascular access. Hence, better therapeutic boundaries may be defined within the FDA guidelines as to what clinical conditions should and should not define medical and neurologic instability and which aneurysms should be defined as carrying *excessive risk for surgery,* while being suitable for endovascular treatment with GDC.

MEDICAL INSTABILITY

Potential clinical conditions that may meet the criterion of *excessive surgical risk* due to "medical instability" may broadly include hemodynamic instability and shock, respiratory distress syndrome and refractory hypoxemia, intractable coagulopathy, fulminant sepsis, massive cardiac ischemia, and hepatic, renal, or other multisystem failure. Advanced age may further compound the impact of such comorbidity. Pregnancy may also be considered a state of increased medical risk. In these patients, it may be beneficial to consider the option of GDC embolization, weighing the risks involved with an endovascular procedure with those of craniotomy and microsurgery for the particular aneurysm. In the consideration of therapeutic options for this difficult group of patients, it is important to consider the urgency of the planned intervention or whether the aneurysm requires any intervention at all. In this regard, there should be a clear conceptual separation of the "medical instability" guidelines of the FDA approval based on whether the therapy is considered for a ruptured or unruptured aneurysm. In cases with ruptured aneurysm, there is reason to warrant a consideration of urgent intervention despite medical comorbidity.

Unfortunately, the medical conditions that absolutely preclude surgical intervention such as severe hypotension and refractory pulmonary failure may also preclude endovascular therapy. General anesthesia is thought to be required for all cases of GDC embolization, and such treatment is not necessarily associated with shorter anesthetic time, especially in elderly patients with difficult vascular access. A fraction of cases in whom GDC treatment is attempted are found to be untreatable by this modality due to prohibitive access or unfavorable aneurysm morphology, hence necessitating a second anesthetic for definitive treatment.

In considering the therapeutic options for unruptured aneurysm, the treatment may be pursued on an elective basis. If intervention is warranted based on actuarial analysis and the particular size, location, and angioarchitecture of the aneurysm in question, aggressive medical optimization should be pursued in preparation for the planned therapy regardless of whether surgical or endovascular therapy is entertained. For instance, significant comorbid cardiac risk factors may be alleviated by optimization of medication regimen, cessation of smoking, coronary revascularization procedures, and possibly the placement of pacemakers or defibrillators. Peri-operative or peri-procedural risk management can be planned in advance if necessary, such as Swan-Ganz catheter monitoring. In many instances, aggressive comorbid risk modification will allow the selection of the most optimal open or endovascular therapeutic procedure for the particular aneurysm. Surgery should be strongly considered in patients in whom repeated follow-up angiography is contraindicated, such as those patients with renal insufficiency or severe allergies to intravenous contrast.

NEUROLOGIC INSTABILITY

Potential neurologic conditions that would meet the criterion of *excessive surgical risk* are primarily limited to presentations with high clinical grade after subarachnoid hemorrhage (Hunt-Hess grade 4 to 5) and associated raised intracranial pressure. The classical neurosurgical strategy when confronted with ruptured aneurysm of high clinical grades has been to perform delayed surgery, allowing for the decrease in brain swelling and stabilization of neurologic status. The rational foundation of this strategy has been that there is significant potential for neurologic morbidity in the attempt to secure the ruptured aneurysm microsurgically in the setting of swollen brain with lower threshold for permanent injury. The obvious drawback of this strategy has been that the ruptured aneurysm is left unsecured during the period of time with the highest risk of rehemorrhage and during the course of vasospasm.

Endosaccular embolization may offer a favorable therapeutic option in cases of high-grade subarachnoid hemorrhage with elevated intracranial pressure. Whereas brain swelling represents a major barrier in the microsurgical exposure of aneurysms, the endovascular approach is not significantly hindered by the same limitation. With endosaccular occlusion in high-grade patients, early treatment strategy can be pursued for aneurysm protection without incurring the morbidity associated with an open craniotomy in the same clinical setting. If the ruptured aneurysm in question is easily treatable with definitive surgical therapy with the exception of the concurrent elevated intracranial pressure, there should be consideration of planned staged therapy. The aneurysm may be partially secured with GDC embolization, offering some protection from a re-rupture, while the neck of the aneurysm is left clear of coils. When the patient is optimized neurologically, a surgical clip can be placed across the neck of the aneurysm for permanent, definitive therapy.

Endovascular treatment of aneurysm may also be considered in patients who are deteriorating neurologically from symptomatic vasospasm in the setting of unsecured ruptured aneurysm. Endovascular therapy of vasospasm with angioplasty or intraarterial papaverine may be undertaken at the same setting as GDC embolization of aneurysm.

Surgery remains the preferable choice of therapy in cases of significant mass effect from intraparenchymal hematoma associated with the ruptured aneurysm. Surgery may also be indicated in high-grade patients with improving neurologic status, low intracranial pressure, favorable CSF drainage, and facile microsurgical access.

EXCESSIVE SURGICAL DIFFICULTY

In the past four decades, we have witnessed exponential improvements in the technical aspects of neurovascular surgery for intracranial aneurysms. In recent years, innovative skull base approaches, improved neuroanesthetic techniques and brain protection, and better understanding of the neurovascular microanatomy have facilitated surgical therapy for virtually all cerebral aneurysms. Nevertheless, the direct surgical management of aneurysms with unfavorable location, size, and morphology remain a formidable challenge, even in the hands of the most experienced neurovascular surgeons. Aneurysms presenting a greater degree of surgical difficulty and risk in the posterior circulation include those at the basilar summit, trunk, anterior inferior cerebellar aneurysms (AICA), and the vertebral basilar junction. In the anterior circulation, aneurysms involving the paraclinoid segment of the internal carotid artery, especially those involving a ventral and medial projection, and those with partially extradural neck have presented a greater surgical challenge.

Aneurysms with Difficult Surgical Access

The aneurysms of the basilar trunk, the AICA, and the vertebrobasilar junction remain significant challenges to the neurovascular surgeon. The access and exposure are difficult, and the lower cranial nerves and the brain stem complications can produce devastating clinical sequelae. The incidence of these aneurysms is low, and thus, few surgeons other than neurovascular subspecialists have acquired the experience to tackle them. Large or giant aneurysms in these locations are best approached by surgeons in specialized neurovascular centers with availability of various approaches. Adequate support from interventional neuroradiology, skull base surgery, neuroanesthesiology, and cardiac surgery are also critical.

In light of the excessive surgical difficulties involved in the treatments of complex and uncommon posterior circulation aneurysms, endovascular therapy, when feasible, is potentially favorable. Although the lesions are difficult to expose surgically and require complex base of skull approaches that may be unfamiliar to many neurosurgeons, endovascular catheterization of these locations may be possible without extraordinary difficulty. Surgical morbidities encountered in relation to cranial neuropathies and CSF leakage may be avoided with the endovascular approach. Potential therapeutic options with endovascular therapy include endosaccular coiling with GDC embolization, parent vessel embolization, or possibly endosaccular occlusion in conjunction with parent artery occlusion.

These considerations for basilar trunk, AICA, and vertebrobasilar junction aneurysms are not necessarily applicable to lesions involving PICA. Any segment of PICA can be exposed surgically with relative ease, and clip application allows precise and effective occlusion of smaller lesions and reconstruction and decompression of mass effect in larger lesions, while sparing adjacent brainstem perforators and other eloquent branches.

Basilar Summit Aneurysms

Appropriate management of basilar summit aneurysms remains an issue of particular controversy and concern. Despite formidable advances in microsurgical exposure and clipping, the complex features of basilar summit aneurysms continue to present formidable technical challenges for the neurovascular surgeon and frequent complications related to inadequate proximal control, frequent oculomotor palsies, perforator compromise, or brainstem injury. Recent experience with GDC embolization has provided an attractive alternative to microsurgical approach, with possibly lower morbidity. This has initiated a reappraisal as to the optimal therapy for these lesions.

The most extensive series of surgical experience with basilar summit aneurysms belongs to Drake et al. (11). The experience of Dr. Drake and his colleagues represents the current gold standard in the treatment of basilar summit aneurysms. Of the 688 patients treated surgically for ruptured basilar apex lesions, 85% returned to the level of activity enjoyed prior to the hemorrhage. Postoperative angiography noted that only 14% of the treated cases had any residual aneurysmal remnant. The results are particularly outstanding when taking into consideration that the study population included only ruptured aneurysms and a disproportionate representation of large and giant lesions. In the modern era, other accomplished and experienced neurovascular surgery centers have reported comparable outcomes. Samson et al. studied 303 cases of ruptured and unruptured aneurysms; 75% of their patients achieved acceptable outcome (GOS of 4 and 5), 18% were neurologically disabled (GOS of 2 and 3), and 7% had died during the hospitalization (40). Morcos and Heros reported good outcomes in greater than 82% of the cases in a series of 124 patients. Good outcomes were reported in 82% of the cases from the Yarsagil series and from Ojemann and Crowell.

Despite these extensive experiences from leading neurovascular surgeons, reported outcomes still predict that approximately 15 to 20% of the patients will die or suffer some neurologic disability. These morbidities and mortalities are related primarily to the risk of perforator injury, and to a lesser degree poor proximal control and cranial nerve or brainstem injury. In the face of these technical difficulties, endovascular strategies have continued to evolve as a viable alternative to conventional microsurgery. Recently published experience with GDC embolization of basilar summit aneurysms has documented favorable rates of morbidity and mortality while significantly reducing the risk of rebleeding. After the first introduction of detachable platinum coils by Guglielmi and colleagues, the safety and efficacy of the procedure have improved significantly. Guglielmi et al. published their first experience with posterior circulation aneurysms, which yielded a morbidity rate of 8% (19). Other reports have since been published that have confirmed such favorable outcome. Raymond et al. reported a series of 31 patients treated with basilar apex aneurysms. The authors of this experience reported a procedure-related morbidity rate of 3% and mortality rate of 3%. Seven of the aneurysms recanalized during the follow-up period and required additional coil placement. No rebleeding episodes were noted during the follow-up period. Recent series from Nichols et al. and Klein et al. reported comparable excellent rates of morbidity and mortality.

Nevertheless, decreased rates of morbidity and mortality associated with endovascular GDC embolization are tempered by the associated rate of failed complete occlusion of the aneurysm. In various endovascular series, the rates of complete aneurysm occlusion have varied from 21 to 84% (4), depending on the particular morphology of the involved aneurysm. Smaller aneurysms with narrow neck are most easily coiled completely (4), which are also best suited for a curative surgical clip application. The enthusiasm for endovascular therapy for aneurysms must also be tempered by its yet unproven durability to provide long-term protection from hemorrhage. Mid-term follow-up reports of GDC-treated basilar summit aneurysms have reported significant rates of recanalization or coil compaction, especially in large and giant aneurysms with wide aneurysm necks. It is unfortunate that the cases of surgically difficult basilar summit aneurysms (larger lesions with broad neck) are also less amenable to therapy by GDC embolization related to failed occlusion or recanalization.

The current standard of the optimal application of endovascular therapy for basilar summit aneurysms may still be best outlined in cases with neurologic and medical instability or those with excessive surgical risk. In our own institution, we have favored primary GDC treatment in elderly patients and those with increased surgical risk related to a low-lying basilar summit aneurysm neck (*Fig. 11.4*), inferior to the posterior clinoid process, or a posteriorly directed aneurysm dome into the substance of the brainstem. Smaller (<1 cm) basilar summit aneurysms with supraclinoid neck location and superior or anterior-pointing sac are primarily approached through a trans-sylvian corridor, with minimal risk of third nerve or perforator injury–and morbidity rates similar to anterior circulation lesions (*Fig. 11.4*). Larger basilar summit lesions present a challenge to either surgical and endovascular approaches, with the former resulting in higher morbidity but also high obliteration rates, and the latter lower morbidity and also lower effectiveness. Treatment options for these cases are individualized while factoring these considerations.

Ventral Medial Paraclinoid (Superior Hypophyseal) Aneurysms

Paraclinoid aneurysms may arise at the internal carotid artery from its most proximal intradural portion to the origin of the posterior communicating artery. These aneurysms may also arise between the prox-

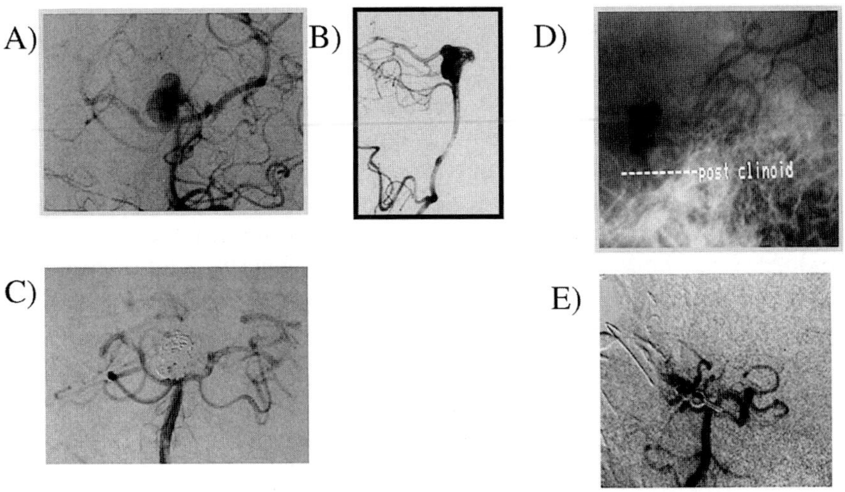

FIG. 11.4 (*A and B*) Dysmorphic basilar summit aneurysm in an elderly patient with unfavorable surgical anatomy, posteriorly pointing sac and inferior to the posterior clinoid. (*C*) The aneurysm was embolized with GDC coils with excellent recovery after transient perforator syndrome. (*D*) Aneurysm of the basilar summit in a young patient. The aneurysm and the basilar summit complex presented superior to the posterior clinoid process. Aneurysm was clipped via trans-sylvian approach without neurologic sequelae. (*E*) Intraoperative angiogram reveals complete aneurysm obliteration.

imal and distal dural rings of the internal carotid artery. Because of the complex anatomy of paraclinoid aneurysms and the associated difficulty of obtaining proximal control intracranially, the difficulty of microsurgical repair of these aneurysms has been well recognized by leading neurovascular surgeons. In the recent years, however, the improved understanding of the involved surgical anatomy and novel adjunctive uses of retrograde suction decompression have enhanced the safety and outcome of surgical treatment of paraclinoid aneurysms (2, 9, 12, 13). Arnautovic et al. (2) have employed aggressive skull-based approaches in conjunction with endovascular balloon occlusion to improve exposure, assure vascular control, and reduce brain retraction. Recently, De Jesus et al. (9) reported satisfactory surgical clipping in 32 of 35 cases of paraclinoid aneurysms.

Despite these advances, the treatment of ventral, medial variant of paraclinoid aneurysms (also known as superior hypophyseal aneurysms) remains a significant technical challenge in microsurgery. These aneurysms project away from the surgeon, pointing ventrally and medially. The sac may be intimately associated or otherwise obscured by the visual apparatus, and the aneurysm neck may be partially extradural. These difficulties can be largely obviated by the endovascular approach.

Endovascular experience with superior hypophyseal aneurysms has been encouraging. Gurian et al. (21) reported the application of GDC embolization to treat superior hypophyseal aneurysms in 11 patients. Seven of the patients in the study population had failed prior surgical intervention, whereas three were considered to be at too high risk for surgery, and the remaining patient refused surgery. The authors reported no technical or clinical complications related to embolization and satisfactory aneurysm occlusion in 10 of 11 cases. Complete aneurysms occlusion was obtained in five cases. Nine of the 10 patients with successful embolizations were noted to have good to excellent outcome. Roy et al. (39) reported comparable results in the endovascular treatment of paraclinoid aneurysms. These authors noted that the superior hypophyseal variant may be most attractive for GDC embolization given its likelihood to present with a small neck. The authors noted a complete occlusion rate of 85% in superior hypophyseal aneurysms. In view of this experience, we currently consider GDC as a primary choice of treatment for small aneurysms with narrow neck at that location (*Fig. 11.5*).

We and others have encountered disastrous complications when GDC technique is applied for larger aneurysms with broad neck. Undertreated lesions will invariably recanalize, whereas overcompacting of aneurysm often results in thromboembolic complications or parent vessel compromise (*Fig. 11.6*). We continue to favor open microsurgical

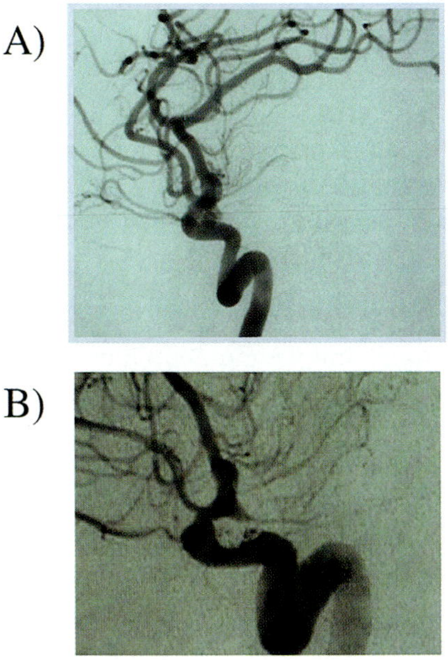

FIG. 11.5 (*A*) Superior hypophyseal aneurysm is noted on a lateral carotid angiogram in a pregnant patient with acute subarachnoid hemorrhage. (*B*) With a narrow aneurysm neck, the case was favorable for endosaccular coiling. Superior to the coil mass is notably a posterior communicating artery infundibulum.

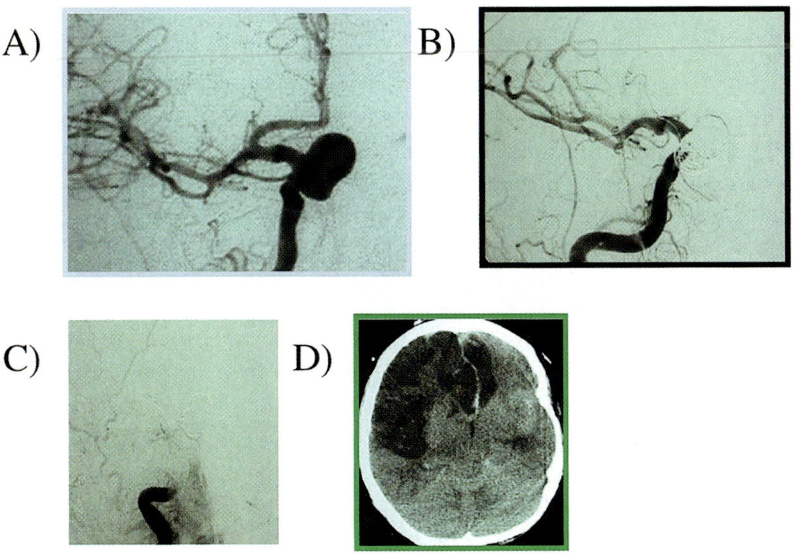

FIG. 11.6 (*A*) Giant paraclinoid aneurysm in an elderly patient with recent hemorrhage. (*B*) Endosaccular embolization was carried out with apparent parent vessel preservation during the initial angiogram. (*C*) Subsequently, the patient became comatose, and repeat angiogram revealed coil mass migration and parent artery occlusion. (*D*) Patient suffered bihemispheric ischemic sequelae and expired.

treatment of larger paraclinoid aneurysms with broad neck those most frequently failing GDC coiling, and the majority of dorsal (ophthalmic segment) aneurysms (except those with neck calci cation). Their treatment is enhanced by microsurgical clinoidectomy and optic canal decompression, opening of the dural ring and endovascular intraoperative adjunct (see below) for proximal control, suction decompression, and intraoperative angiography. Other more distal giant anterior circulation aneurysms are treated effectively with aneurysm thromboendarterectomy and primary clip reconstruction (with or without adjunctive bypass) under focal circulatory arrest (15). Extradural parent vessel occlusion remains an attractive option for giant lesions with neck calci cation or lesions extending into the cavernous sinus.

Expanded Indications

INCOMPLETE PALLIATIVE COILING

The primary causes of morbidity and mortality related to aneurysmal subarachnoid hemorrhage are the effects of initial hemorrhage and subsequent rebleeding and vasospasm. Prior to the advent of endovascular techniques, high-grade subarachnoid hemorrhage patients were managed frequently with delayed surgery. The rationale for this management strategy has been to neurologically and medically stabilize the patient and allow brain swelling to subside prior to surgical intervention. The preoperative morbidity and mortality in high grade patients awaiting delayed surgical therapy have been reported as high as 65% (35), where recurrent hemorrhage was felt to be the principal cause. The rate of rehemorrhage has been estimated at 15 to 30% in the rst 14 days following the initial hemorrhage, with the greatest incidence occurring in the rst 72 hours (5, 27). These data strongly argue for some form of securing of the aneurysm to prevent early rebleeding.

Strong evidence points to the effective early protection that GDC embolization can provide following subarachnoid hemorrhage. Grave et al. reported that no recurrent hemorrhages occurred in 13 patients with early treatment of ruptured aneurysms with GDC embolization (17). The authors noted the only peri-procedural complication from the study was related to incidental parent vessel thrombosis, requiring the institution of urokinase therapy. The report also suggested that the early treatment with GDC allowed the institution of aggressive hemodynamic therapy for ensuing vasospasm. Other authors have reported a similar degree of early protection from rehemorrhage with GDC embolization (6, 37, 44).

As the rupture site is typically from the aneurysm dome or daughter sacs, a strategy of palliative, partial embolization with GDC has recently been pursued in selected cases. This may be particularly useful when the patient is too unstable medically or neurologically to tolerate a completion of embolization, or when geometry of the aneurysm precludes the necessary coil packing to completely exclude the aneurysm from the circulation without compromising parent vessel branches. Such a strategy must be tempered by the clearly documented observation that partially thrombosed aneurysms continue to be at some risk of early rehemorrhage (33). No de nitive study has addressed the degree of protection from rehemorrhage that can be expected from a partially coiled aneurysm. De nitive surgical or endovascular therapy must be pursued at the earliest opportunity when conditions become favorable.

Results from studies of completion treatment of partially coiled or recanalized aneurysms have been generally favorable. Horowitz et al. (25) reported a series of nine patients that underwent aneurysm retreatment following incomplete or failed embolization therapy. Five of the patients were treated surgically, and four of the patients underwent reembolization. It is important to note that during the follow-up period, none of the patients experienced rehemorrhage, suggesting that even partially thrombosed aneurysms confer a signi cant degree of protection from rebleeding. The authors reported excellent anatomic obliteration of the aneurysms and further elucidate speci c management strategies involved in completion treatment of partially coiled aneurysms. The authors suggest that repeat coiling may be the favored treatment modality as the surgical management of partially coil-packed lesions can be dif cult, often encountering the risk of parent vessel injury or occlusion. The authors opted for the surgical approach when the residual angioarchitecture of the aneurysm precluded further endovascular coil packing. The authors noted that the key to successful surgical occlusion was proximal and distal control; temporary clips were applied when coil extraction was necessary for aneurysm obliteration.

Simple clip application without the necessity of coil extraction may be possible, and preferable, when the neck of the aneurysm is available and free from coils. If a staged partial GDC occlusion and subsequent surgery is planned, the neck of the aneurysm may be left with room for clip application without occluding the parent vessel. Gurian et al. (20) reported eight lesions that were treated surgically for residual aneurysmal remnants. Five of the lesions were clipped, two were bypassed and trapped, and one was managed with Hunterian ligation. Gurian et al. also noted that the aneurysms without a coil mass at the base are easier to treat with primary clipping. The authors also noted that secondary to the potentially signi cant surgical dif culty, repeat endovascular therapy should be considered the rst line therapeutic measure. Gurian et al.

suggested the importance of careful considerations of the factors that may contribute to the success of retreatment with surgery such as the degree of neck occlusion, the elapsed time since prior embolization, the patient s age and neurologic condition, and the aneurysm location.

BALLOON-ASSISTED EMBOLIZATION

Utilization of GDC coils has favorably expanded treatment options for certain types of aneurysms that previously may have been considered untreatable. Since inception of GDC system in 1990 (7, 18), evolving experience has shown that predictably the best technical success was achieved in those aneurysms meeting certain anatomic criteria (i.e., small neck size (less than 4 mm), favorable sac to neck ratio). Series reporting suboptimal or incomplete aneurysmal obliteration and/or high rate of recurrence typically attribute this to inability to completely pack the aneurysm sac (42). Continued improvements in the technical application of the GDC system have expanded the spectrum of aneurysm morphology that may be amenable to treatment with this device. A relatively new technique in which non-detachable microballoon catheters are employed to assist placement of the platinum coils is now available. This has been variably referred to as balloon-assisted technique (29), neck-plastic technique (42), and balloon-remodeling technique (36) (*Fig. 11.7*). This requires placement of a second catheter system, introduced through the contralateral femoral artery, within the vessel harboring the aneurysm. A non-detachable balloon is then navigated across the neck of the aneurysm. Various microballoon catheters (e.g., Endeavor, Boston Scienti c/Target Therapeutics, Fremont, CA) can be used for this technique, and selection is based on operator experience and familiarity. The microballoon is temporarily in ated across the neck of the aneurysm during delivery of the coil and immediately d e ated upon successful delivery of the coil. The intent is to prevent inadvertent migration of the coils into the parent artery and to allow for denser packing of the aneurysm sac. Reports of aneurysms treated with this technique have been favorable from both a clinical and technical standpoint (29, 36, 42). As a result of the development and clinical application of the balloon-assisted procedure, more liberal application of GDC embolization in the management of broad-necked aneurysms has been possible.

COILING IN PREPARATION FOR PARENT VESSEL OCCLUSION

Giant aneurysms with broad neck may recanalize even after apparently successful endosaccular obliteration with GDC (with or without balloon bracing as described above). Other giant aneurysms may have

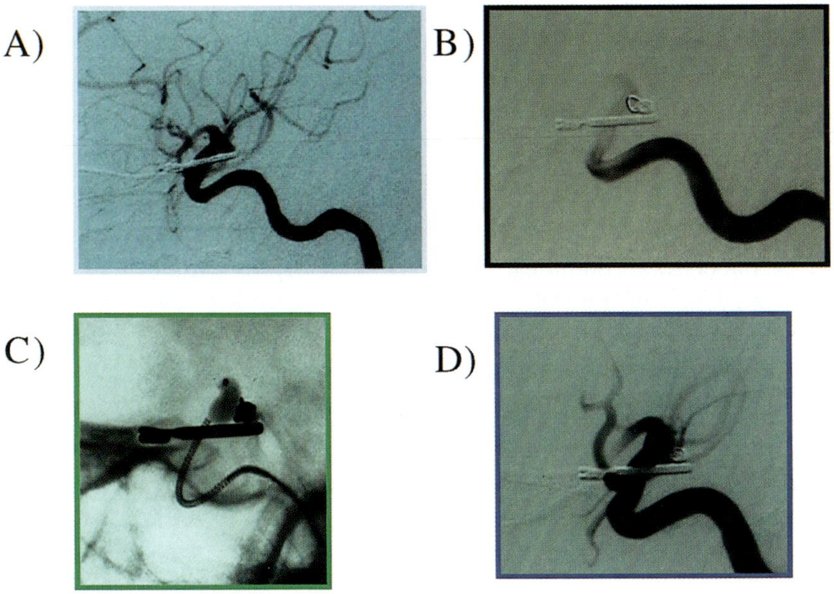

FIG. 11.7 (*A*) Open clipping of posterior communicating artery aneurysm left a small aneurysmal remnant at the base of the aneurysm. The patient elected attempt at endovascular obliteration of aneurysm remnant. (*B*) Secondary to the wide neck of this aneurysmal remnant, endosaccular coils migrated into the parent artery during attempted embolization. (*C*) Balloon-assisted coil compaction achieved recompaction of the coil mass into the aneurysm sac. (*D*) Aneurysm is effectively eliminated from the circulation via the surgical clip and the endosaccular coils, with preservation of adjacent posterior communicating and anterior choroidal arteries.

an eccentric sac but involve the parent vessel more diffusely with fusiform morphology. Treatment of these lesions with GDC may be particularly useful in obliterating eccentric pouches of dilatation from the aneurysm proper. In such cases, thrombosis induced by the aneurysm coil packing can be more de nitively secured with parent artery occlusion. Gobin et al. (16) reported their series of nine patients with large or giant fusiform aneurysms treated endovascularly. Three cases were managed with selective coil occlusion with parent artery preservation, and the remaining six patients were managed with preparatory occlusion of the aneurysm followed by parent artery occlusion. The tolerance to parent artery occlusion was assessed by angiography, balloon test occlusion, and amytal injection. Five of the six patients treated with complete coil occlusion of the aneurysm and the parent artery remained permanently occluded at 6 months to 2 years at angiographic follow-up. Importantly, none of the three cases where aneurysm coil packing was attempted with the preservation of the parent artery showed technically good outcome.

Combined application of endosaccular coil packing and parent artery occlusion may be useful in the management of partially thrombosed giant saccular aneurysms. Completion endosaccular coiling of partially thrombosed giant aneurysms often yields initial satisfactory angiographic occlusion, only to fail in follow-up examinations with a reexpansion of the aneurysm base. Intradural or extradural parent vessel occlusion may complement endosaccular coil packing by enhancing the thrombosis of the coil-packed aneurysm with low afferent ow. We currently consider this technique of combined GDC and staged parent artery occlusion in giant posterior circulation aneurysms where open surgical interventions present formidable risks, where GDC alone routinely fails, and where parent artery occlusion alone might not result in aneurysm involution. We also consider this option in elderly patients with paraclinoid or proximal internal carotid artery aneurysms harboring signi cant neck calci cation.

GDC Embolization in Aneurysms That Are Easily Clippable

The lowest rates of morbidity and the highest rates of aneurysm obliteration with GDC embolization have been reported in smaller lesions with narrow neck and in good grade patients. Not surprisingly, these are also the cases where open surgical intervention provides the best outcome. Practice guidelines in determining the best therapeutic strategy are emerging from recent outcome studies of lesions in speci c locations. The results are favorable for primary endovascular treatment of select cases in the posterior circulation and at the superior hypophyseal artery. A primary strategy of GDC coiling does not yield as favorable an outcome in other clippable anterior circulation aneurysms.

Regli et al. recently examined the ef cacy of coil embolization versus surgical clipping in unruptured MCA aneurysms (38). The authors assigned GDC as the primary modality of therapy in the 34 patients studied. Only two patients could be effectively embolized, and the remaining patients were referred for surgical clipping. Of the 32 patients that had surgical clipping of their MCA aneurysms, 11 patients had failed attempts at GDC embolization, and in 21 patients, primary clipping was performed because of unfavorable angioarchitecture. The authors cited an unfavorable dome to neck ratio and the incorporation of perforating vessels or parent artery branches at the base of the aneurysms as the most signi cant factors for the failure of endovascular embolization. Secondary to the relative dif culty of approaching MCA aneurysms from endovascular standpoint and the generally favorable surgical approach, microsurgery remains the primary modality of therapy for these aneurysms.

The complex anatomy of the region of the anterior communicating artery can make aneurysms in this location dif cult to treat. Re nements of microsurgical technique have dramatically improved the outcomes from direct surgical clipping. Currently, the overall morbidity and mortality of surgery for anterior communicating aneurysms are generally comparable to the outcomes reported from other aneurysms of the anterior circulation. The most comprehensive analysis of outcome based on microsurgery is reported from Yasargil, who reviewed 371 patients that presented with a rupture (47). Yasargil noted good results in 87.8%. There were 22 postoperative deaths, but only ve of the deaths were directly related to the operation. Good outcomes correlated highly with good presenting clinical grade. Inferiorly projecting aneurysms and aneurysms with complex morphology were associated with greater postoperative morbidity and mortality. Cognitive and psychological disturbances were associated with 18.9% of the patients but were permanent in only 1.3%. These excellent results have been well replicated by other neurovascular surgeons, and better results are documented in unruptured cases.

There has been increasing interest in considering endovascular therapy for anterior communicating artery lesions. Moret et al. (37) reported a series of 36 patients who were treated with GDC embolization as the primary modality of therapy. Thirty of the 36 patients had presented with subarachnoid hemorrhage. The authors were able to completely occlude the aneurysm in 23 cases, while partial thrombosis was noted in six cases. Seven cases could not be embolized secondary to either unfavorable anatomy of the aneurysm or the severe atheromatous changes that precluded selective catheterization. Thrombotic complications occurred in three cases while aneurysmal rupture occurred in one case. Although this and other endovascular series represent encouraging preliminary experience with GDC embolization, they do not compare favorably with published results achieved by microsurgery. With the exception of cases involving refractory medical or neurologic instability, the current gold standard for the treatment of anterior communicating aneurysms remains microsurgery.

When considering GDC therapy for clippable aneurysms in the absence of prohibitive medical or neurologic risks, patients must be informed that such treatment is beyond currently approved GDC indications. Also, patients must be aware that the procedure would not avoid general anesthesia, might not be feasible upon nal microcatheterization of the aneurysm, and is not necessarily faster nor safer than conventional microsurgical clipping. They must consent to continued follow-up with serial angiography up to two years or more after treatment and should accept the signi cantly greater risk of incomplete aneurysm obliteration, which might require retreatment. Regardless of initial patient or referring physician inclination, no patient should be denied full information about the option of microsurgical intervention and its demonstrated results of feasibility, treatment morbidity, and obliteration rates and durability in their particular aneurysm.

ENDOVASCULAR ADJUNCTS TO MICROSURGERY

Endovascular adjuncts have improved the safety and ef cacy of microsurgical treatment of complex aneurysms. Routinely, diagnostic angiograms can be performed intraoperatively, post-clipping, to assess completeness of aneurysm obliteration and patency of the parent vessel and its major branches. In larger and giant lesions, intraoperative angiography has been shown to motivate clip reapplication in a significant fraction of cases, including instances of unsuspected parent vessel compromise (45) (*Fig. 11.8*). The technique can also document patency of bypass reconstructions prior to parent artery sacri ce.

Advantages of intraoperative angiography are enhanced in cases of large and giant opthalmic and other paraclinoid aneurysms in which proximal control had in the past necessitated dissection of the cervical carotid artery. Currently, endovascular adjuncts allow the navigation of a temporary balloon proximal to the lesion; its precise in ation can be timed with the intraoperative need for temporary proximal occlusion. A more recent development has been the integration of aneurysm suction decompression with the endovascular technique. Prior to the clip manipulation of the aneurysm, the balloon is in ated proximal to the aneurysm, and a temporary clip is applied immediately distal to the neck of the aneurysm. The catheter is then gently aspirated to achieve suction decompression and facilitate clip application and adjustment (3).

Endovascular adjuncts are not without potential complications, and their application should be preceded by a careful consideration of associated risks and bene ts. There have been reports of thromboembolic sequelae with endovascular and open suction decompression techniques (12). Carotid dissection is also a potential complication (2). Prophylaxis against embolic complications may be possible with a temporary infusion of intravenous heparin intraoperatively during the period of balloon in ation and suction decompression.

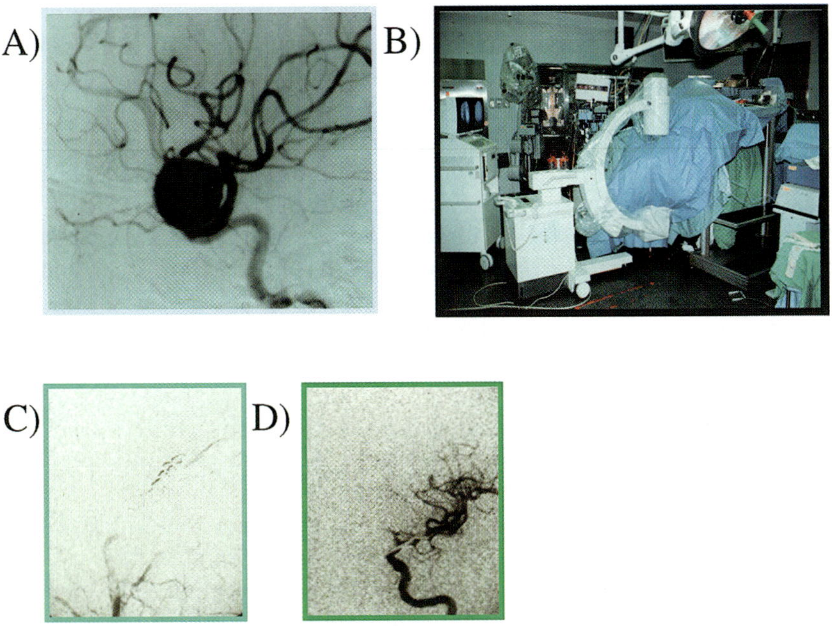

FIG. 11.8 (*A*) Giant opthalmic artery aneurysm is visualized on lateral angiogram. (*B*) For proximal control and veri cation of parent artery preservation, the operating suite is set up for intraoperative angiogram. (*C*) Initial clip placement showed the occlusion of parent vessel by angiogram. (*D*) Replacement of the surgical clip revealed the reconstitution of ow in the parent artery.

SYNTHESIS AND CONCLUSIONS

Endovascular techniques offer innovative and promising strategies for the treatment of intracranial aneurysms. The range of endovascular options and ongoing experience has already resulted in up to half of intracranial aneurysms at large referral centers being treated with this modality. This has allowed the successful treatment of previously inoperable cases and less invasive approaches in lesions that are dif cult to treat surgically and in unstable patients.

Extradural or intradural parent vessel occlusions may be applied in the treatment of selected cases with great effectiveness. The safety of these interventions is further enhanced by appropriate adjunctive measures such as provocative testing, cerebral blow ow studies, and judicious periprocedure management. This has become the undisputed treatment of choice for a wide range of extradural aneurysms including giant, traumatic, and neoplastic lesions. Endovascular parent vessel occlusion allows awake patient monitoring in real time, a range of adjunctive testing of hemodynamic reserve, and continuous periprocedure anticoagulation. In other instances, appropriate patient selection criteria must be applied, and this treatment is reserved for cases where more direct strategies aimed at parent vessel preservation cannot be performed with similar safety. Intradural parent vessel occlusion may best be performed by surgical clipping after preparatory endovascular exploration and provocative testing if there are associated eloquent branches or perforators at the site of proposed occlusion. Direct surgical clip occlusion allows more precise sparing of these vessels and permits decompression of mass effect or adjunctive reconstruction or bypass if indicated.

Endosaccular occlusion of cerebral aneurysms with GDC is enjoying wide application and acceptance. The technique is conceptually appealing, and experience with it is clearly increasing. Newer coils and adjunctive strategies herald even greater promise in the future. Yet, the results of GDC treatment have not been uniformly favorable. Giant aneurysms and those with broad neck are associated with high rates of treatment failure and with unacceptable rates of aneurysm recanalization. GDC treatment of such lesions should not be undertaken primarily without full consideration of microsurgical options by an experienced surgical team with facile application of modern adjunctive surgical options (skull base exposure, brain protection, intraoperative angiography).

Treatment of other aneurysms with GDC has not been demonstrated to be more feasible, ef cacious, safer, or more durable than with open techniques. There is much broader experience and literature involving the microsurgical treatment of cerebral aneurysms, including feasibility and durability of aneurysm obliteration and prospective documentation of morbidity rates in large scienti c trials. There are little data on aneurysm GDC treatment outcomes other than those reported by the endovascular therapy team, often without third-party adjudication or prospective follow-up methodology. In contrast to numerous studies of surgical outcome in widely varying settings, there is serious concern about the generalization of reported best practice performance in endovascular therapy.

Some aneurysms pose a clear challenge to surgical intervention, and it is clear that endovascular option may provide safer treatment alternatives with acceptable effectiveness. These include patients with unstable medical and neurologic condition and aneurysms in less surgically accessible locales such as the basilar trunk, vertebrobasilar junction, and some basilar summit and paraclinoid lesions. Primary selection of endovascular treatment of these aneurysms should consider likely lower obliteration rates and the need for continued patient follow-up to ensure durability of obliteration. Treatment is not always feasible, morbidity is not necessarily lower, and patients are not spared general anesthesia. For these reasons, wider application of GDC treatment to more clippable aneurysms cannot be endorsed at this time outside the scope of investigational clinical trials.

The near future will uncover more rigorous outcome data and hopefully randomized trials and adjudicated registries clarifying which patients should, and should not, be referred for endovascular therapy. Novel management paradigms may dictate that some cases be selected for de nitive microsurgical treatment without diagnostic catheter angiography (based on MR or CT angiography) if this is the most optimal treatment for their aneurysms. Other cases will be considered for the more invasive route of catheter angiography and endovascular treatment, accepting the need for continued post-treatment surveillance with serial angiography.

Endovascular treatment represents a wide range of therapeutic strategies and will likely involve further innovations in the future. Adjunctive multimodality interventions, stent technology, and endovascular delivery of biologic vectors will likely change the face of aneurysm management in upcoming years.

REFERENCES

1. Anonymous: *Gugliemi Detachbale Coil (GDC) U.S. Clinical Study Summary.* Target Therapeutics, Fremont, CA, 1995.
2. Arnautovic KI, Al-Mefty O, Angtuaco E: A combined microsurgical skull-base and endovascular approach to giant and large paraclinoid aneurysms. **Surg Neurol** 50:504—518, 1998; Discussion 518—520.
3. Batjer HH, Samson DS: Retrograde suction decompression of giant paraclinoidal aneurysms: Technical note. **J Neurosurg** 73:305—306, 1990.
4. Bavinzski G, Killer M, Gruber A, Reinprecht A, Gross CE, Richling B: Treatment of basilar artery bifurcation aneurysms by using Guglielmi detachable coils: A 6-year experience. **J Neurosurg** 90:843—852, 1999.
5. Broderick JP, Brott TG, Duldner JE, Tomsick T, Leach A: Initial and recurrent bleeding are the major causes of death following subarachnoid hemorrhage. **Stroke** 25:1342—1347, 1994.
6. Byrne JV, Molyneux AJ, Brennan RP, Renowden SA: Embolisation of recently ruptured intracranial aneurysms. **J Neurol Neurosurg Psychiatry** 59:616—620, 1995.
7. Casasco AE, Aymard A, Gobin YP, Houdart E, Rogopoulos A, George B, Hodes JE, Cophignon J, Merland JJ: Selective endovascular treatment of 71 intracranial aneurysms with platinum coils. **J Neurosurg** 79:3—10, 1993.
8. Cunha e Sa MJ, Stein BM, Solomon RA, McCormick PC: The treatment of associated intracranial aneurysms and arteriovenous malformations. **J Neurosurg** 77: 853—859, 1992.

9. De Jesus O, Sekhar LN, Riedel CJ: Clinoid and paraclinoid aneurysms: Surgical anatomy, operative techniques, and outcome. **Surg Neurol** 51:477—487, 1999; Discussion 487—488.
10. Dolenc VV: Surgery of vascular lesions of the cavernous sinus. **Clin Neurosurg** 36:240—255, 1990.
11. Drake C, Peerless SJ, Hernesniemi J: *Surgery of Vertebrobasilar Aneurysms.* New York, Spring Verlag, 1996.
12. Fahlbusch R, Nimsky C, Huk W: Open surgery of giant paraclinoid aneurysms improved by intraoperative angiography and endovascular retrograde suction decompression. **Acta Neurochir (Wien)** 139:1026—1032, 1997.
13. Fan YW, Chan KH, Lui WM, Hung KN: Retrograde suction decompression of paraclinoid aneurysm: A revised technique. **Surg Neurol** 51:129—131, 1999.
14. Gewirtz RJ, Awad IA: Giant aneurysms of the proximal anterior cerebral artery: Report of three cases. **Neurosurgery** 33:120—124, 1993; Discussion 124—125.
15. Gewirtz RJ, Awad IA: Giant aneurysms of the anterior circle of Willis: Management outcome with open microsurgical treatment. **Surg Neurol** 45:409—420, 1996.
16. Gobin YP, Vinuela F, Gurian JH, Guglielmi G, Duckwiler GR, Massoud TF, Martin NA: Treatment of large and giant fusiform intracranial aneurysms with Guglielmi detachable coils. **J Neurosurg** 84:55—62, 1996.
17. Graves VB, Strother CM, Duff TA, Perl J II: Early treatment of ruptured aneurysms with Guglielmi detachable coils: Effect on subsequent bleeding. **Neurosurgery** 37:640—647, 1995; Discussion 647—648.
18. Gugliemli G: Endovascular treatment of intracranial aneurysms. **Neuroimag Clin North Am** 2:269—278, 1992.
19. Guglielmi G, Vinuela F, Duckwiler G, Dion J, Lylyk P, Berenstein A, Strother C, Graves V, Halbach V, Nichols D, Hopkins N, Ferguson R, Sepetka I: Endovascular treatment of posterior circulation aneurysms by electrothrombosis using electrically detachable coils. **J Neurosurg** 77:515—524, 1992.
20. Gurian JH, Martin NA, King WA, Duckwiler GR, Guglielmi G, Vinuela F: Neurosurgical management of cerebral aneurysms following unsuccessful or incomplete endovascular embolization. **J Neurosurg** 83:843—853, 1995.
21. Gurian JH, Vinuela F, Guglielmi G, Gobin YP, Duckwiler GR: Endovascular embolization of superior hypophyseal artery aneurysms. **Neurosurgery** 39:1150—1154, 1996; Discussion 1154—1156.
22. Hacein-Bey L, Connolly ES Jr, Mayer SA, Young WL, Pile-Spellman J, Solomon RA: Complex intracranial aneurysms: Combined operative and endovascular approaches. **Neurosurgery** 43:1304—1312, 1998; Discussion 1312—1313.
23. Halbach VV, Higashida RT, Dowd CF, Urwin RW, Balousek PA, Lempert TE, Hieshima GB: Cavernous internal carotid artery aneurysms treated with electrolytically detachable coils. **J Neuroophthalmol** 17:231—239, 1997.
24. Higashida RT, Halbach VV, Dowd C, Barnwell SL, Dormandy B, Bell J, Hieshima GB: Endovascular detachable balloon embolization therapy of cavernous carotid artery aneurysms: Results in 87 cases. **J Neurosurg** 72:857—863, 1990.
25. Horowitz M, Purdy P, Kopitnik T, Dutton K, Samson D: Aneurysm retreatment after Guglielmi detachable coil and nondetachable coil embolization: Report of nine cases and review of the literature. **Neurosurgery** 44:712—719, 1999; Discussion 719—720.
26. Jafar JJ, Huang PP: Surgical treatment of carotid cavernous aneurysms. **Neurosurg Clin North Am** 9:755—763, 1998.
27. Kassell NF, Torner JC: Aneurysmal rebleeding: A preliminary report from the Cooperative Aneurysm Study. **Neurosurgery** 13:479—481, 1983.

28. Khayata MH, Aymard A, Casasco A, Herbreteau D, Woimant F, Merland JJ: Selective endovascular techniques in the treatment of cerebral mycotic aneurysms: Report of three cases. **J Neurosurg** 78:661–665, 1993.
29. Levy DI, Ku A: Balloon-assisted coil placement in wide-necked aneurysms: Technical note. **J Neurosurg** 86:724–727, 1997.
30. Linskey ME, Sekhar LN, Hirsch WL Jr, Yonas H, Horton JA: Aneurysms of the intracavernous carotid artery: Natural history and indications for treatment. **Neurosurgery** 26:933–937, 1990; Discussion 937–938.
31. Linskey ME, Sekhar LN, Horton JA, Hirsch WL Jr, Yonas H: Aneurysms of the intracavernous carotid artery: A multidisciplinary approach to treatment. **J Neurosurg** 75:525–534, 1991.
32. Little JR, Rosenfeld JV, Awad IA: Internal carotid artery occlusion for cavernous segment aneurysm. **Neurosurgery** 25:398–404, 1989.
33. Manabe H, Fujita S, Hatayama T, Suzuki S, Yagihashi S: Rerupture of coil-embolized aneurysm during long-term observation: Case report. **J Neurosurg** 88:1096–1098, 1998.
34. Mathis JM, Barr JD, Jungreis CA, Yonas H, Sekhar LN, Vincent D, Pentheny SL, Horton JA: Temporary balloon test occlusion of the internal carotid artery: Experience in 500 cases. **Am J Neuroradiol** 16:749–754, 1995.
35. Milhorat TH, Krautheim M: Results of early and delayed operations for ruptured intracranial aneurysms in two series of 100 consecutive patients. **Surg Neurol** 26:123–128, 1986.
36. Moret J, Cognard C: Angiographic results and clinical follow up in 56 cases. **Intervent Neuroradiol** 3:21–35, 1997.
37. Moret J, Pierot L, Boulin A, Castaings L, Rey A: Endovascular treatment of anterior communicating artery aneurysms using Guglielmi detachable coils. **Neuroradiology** 38:800–805, 1996.
38. Regli L, Uske A, de Tribolet N: Endovascular coil placement compared with surgical clipping for the treatment of unruptured middle cerebral artery aneurysms: A consecutive series. **J Neurosurg** 90:1025–1030, 1999.
39. Roy D, Raymond J, Bouthillier A, Bojanowski MW, Moumdjian R, L'Esperance G: Endovascular treatment of ophthalmic segment aneurysms with Guglielmi detachable coils. **Am J Neuroradiol** 18:1207–1215, 1997.
40. Samson D, Batjer HH, Kopitnik TA Jr: Current results of the surgical management of aneurysms of the basilar apex. **Neurosurgery** 44:697–702, 1999; Discussion 702–704.
41. Scotti G, Li MH, Righi C, Simionato F, Rocca A: Endovascular treatment of bacterial intracranial aneurysms. **Neuroradiology** 38:186–189, 1996.
42. Takahashi A, Ezura M, Yoshimoto T: Broad neck basilar tip aneurysm treated by neck plastic intra-aneurysmal GDC embolization with protective balloon. **Intervent Neuroradiol** 3:167–170, 1997.
43. Thompson RC, Steinberg GK, Levy RP, Marks MP: The management of patients with arteriovenous malformations and associated intracranial aneurysms. **Neurosurgery** 43:202–211, 1998; Discussion 211–212.
44. Vinuela F, Duckwiler G, Mawad M: Guglielmi detachable coil embolization of acute intracranial aneurysm: Perioperative anatomical and clinical outcome in 403 patients. **J Neurosurg** 86:475–482, 1997.
45. Vitaz TW, Gaskill-Shipley M, Tomsick T, Tew JM Jr: Utility, safety, and accuracy of intraoperative angiography in the surgical treatment of aneurysms and arteriovenous malformations. **Am J Neuroradiol** 20:1457–1461, 1999.

46. Weill A, Cognard C, Levy D, Robert G, Moret J: Giant aneurysms of the middle cerebral artery trifurcation treated with extracranial-intracranial arterial bypass and endovascular occlusion: Report of two cases. **J Neurosurg** 89:474–478, 1998.
47. Yasargil MG, Fox JL, Ray MW: The operative approach to aneurysms of the anterior communicating artery, in Krayenbuhl H (ed): *Advances and Technical Standards in Neurosurgery,* Vol. 2. New York, Springer-Verlag, 1975, pp 113–170.

CHAPTER

12

Present and Future Technical Developments on Aneurysm Embolization. Impact on Indications and Anatomic Results

FERNANDO VIÑUELA, M.D., YUICHI MURAYAMA, M.D.,
GARY R. DUCKWILER, M.D., Y. PIERRE GOBIN, M.D.

INTRODUCTION

The techniques of intracranial intravascular navigation have dramatically improved in the last 10 years. Pioneers such as Serbinenko, Debrun, Kerber, and others succeeded in overcoming the natural obstacle of the circle of Willis using microcatheters and balloons and, for the first time, navigated into intracranial arteries with a low technical morbidity (9, 22, 39). Their technical success launched the genesis of the modern interventional neuroradiology.

The intracranial navigation into arteries and veins of anterior and posterior circulations is now a standard procedure, and it is used in numerous functional (37) and/or therapeutic procedures. They include endovascular occlusion of congenital or acquired vascular diseases such as intracranial arteriovenous malformations (10, 44), arteriovenous fistulae (11), aneurysms (12), endovascular angioplasty occlusive diseases of brachycephalic and intracranial arteries (18, 46), and intraarterial chemotherapy of cerebral and head and neck vascular tumors (6).

The organization of stroke teams in neurovascular centers has also helped to develop appropriate standards of care for patients having a brain hemorrhagic or ischemic stroke. The interventional neuroradiologist is a very active member of this team and shares diagnostic and therapeutic challenges with vascular neurosurgeons, stroke neurologists, neurointensivists, and neuroanesthesiologists. The endovascular management (occlusion or angioplasty) of a vascular disease is only a small component of the therapeutic management of a patient having, for example, an acute subarachnoid hemorrhage, an intracerebral hematoma, or a cerebral infarct due to a thromboembolic complication.

These diseases are too complex and severe to be handled by an individual physician. One good example to the present multidisciplinary approach to cerebrovascular diseases is the modern therapeutic management of patients presenting with ruptured intracranial aneurysms. Neurosurgical and endovascular techniques of aneurysm occlusion must be complemented with the availability of modern neurointensive care and neuroimaging modalities to maximize clinical outcomes.

HISTORICAL PERSPECTIVES

The interventional neuroradiologist has been involved in the therapeutic management of intracranial aneurysms for more than 20 years. In the early phases of their experience, their role was limited to the embolization of intracranial nonsurgical, large, and giant aneurysm using the hunterian principle of occlusion of the parent artery using detachable balloons (12, 16). The next technical advancement included the capacity of selective catheterization and occlusion of an aneurysm using detachable balloons (17), regular coils (5), and liquid embolic agents (23, 40).

In 1991, Guglielmi et al. described the endovascular occlusion of intracranial aneurysms using a detachable platinum microcoil (14, 15). This endovascular device could be deposited and repositioned in the aneurysm as many times as necessary before being permanently detached. The GDC coil could be withdrawn from the aneurysm if it was inappropriate in size or shape. Today, the GDC technology is the gold standard for the endovascular occlusion of incidental and ruptured intracranial aneurysms (4, 24, 33, 42).

This technique was approved by the FDA in 1995, and today more than 45.000 patients have benefited from it worldwide.

In the early phases of its development, the GDC technology included a single microcatheter/microguidewire for aneurysm catheterization and no more than six types of GDC coils for aneurysm occlusion. The progressive addition of coated microcatheters and guidewires (sizes #10, #14, and #18) has facilitated the catheterization of aneurysms located in the circle of Willis or beyond (peripheral aneurysms). The present availability of more than 70 types of GDC coils (GDC coils #10 and 18, regular and soft GDC coils-standards, two- and three-dimensional coils) has also improved immediate and long-term anatomic and clinical outcomes.

ANATOMIC AND CLINICAL OUTCOMES AT UCLA: IMPACT OF TECHNICAL DEVELOPMENTS

The authors have treated 617 patients harboring 700 aneurysms using the GDC technology, from April 1990 to March 2000, at the UCLA Medical Center.

TABLE 12.1
Clinical Presentation
(617 Patients, 700 Aneurysms)

SAH-acute	301	48.7%
SAH-non-acute	75	12.1%
Incidental	168	27.2%
Mass effect	55	8.9%
Others	18	3%

Clinical Presentation

A total of 301 patients presented with an acute subarachnoid hemorrhage (SAH) (48.7%); 75 has a non-acute SAH (12.1%) (treatment performed after 15 days of the hemorrhagic episode), 168 patients had an incidental aneurysm (27.2%), and 55 presented with intracranial mass effect (8.9%) (*Table 12.1*).

Aneurysm Location

Four-hundred sixty-seven aneurysms were located in the anterior circulation (66%), and 233 were in the posterior circulation (34%).

The distribution of the most common aneurysms is detailed in *Table 12.2.*

In the early phase of our experience, we had a dominant referral pattern of posterior circulation aneurysms. This type of referral expressed the higher surgical morbimortality not infrequently related to this kind of aneurysm. After the FDA approval of the GDC technique, our referral pattern became similar to a standard neurosurgical practice, though there is still a higher incidence of posterior circulation aneurysms.

In the last 2 years, the three more common aneurysms treated with GDC at UCLA Medical Center have been carotid ophthalmic and parophthalmic, anterior cerebral and posterior communicating aneurysms.

TABLE 12.2
Most Common Aneurysms
(617 Patients, 700 Aneurysms)

Location	No.	Percentage (%)
Carotid-ophthalmic/paraophth.	198	28.3
Basilar tip	124	17.7
Anterior communicating	115	16.4
Posterior communicating	100	14.1
Middle cerebral	57	8.1
ICA bifurcation	22	3.1
PICA aneurysm	24	3.4

TABLE 12.3
Indication For GDC Embolization
(617 Patients, 700 Aneurysms)

Indication	No.	%
Anticipated surgical difficulty	319	51.7
Unsuccessful surgical exploration	88	4.2
Poor neurologic status	97	15.5
Patient refuses surgery	63	10.2
Poor medical status	50	8.4

The indications of the GDC technology at UCLA Medical Center are described on *Table 12.3.* Anticipated surgical difficulty was the most common indication (319 pts, 51.6%) followed by patient's poor neurologic status (97, 15.5%), unsuccessful surgical exploration (88 pts, 14.2%), and patient's poor medical condition (50 pts, 8.4%).

The degree of surgical difficulty was evaluated by the UCLA vascular neurosurgeon or by the referring neurosurgeon from the medical community.

Anatomic Results

The immediate and long-term anatomic results of the GDC technique are influenced by multiple factors. In our opinion the most important are anatomic characteristics of the aneurysm, hemodynamic control of the aneurysm inflow zone, and the biologic response elicited by the GDC technique when deposited in an aneurysm (*Table 12.4*).

ANATOMIC CHARACTERISTICS OF AN ANEURYSM

An aneurysm can be successfully and permanently occluded with GDC coils when a compact mesh of coils has been deposited in the body, and particularly across the neck of the aneurysm (*Fig. 12.1*). This is the

TABLE 12.4
Anatomic Results
(617 Patients, 700 Aneurysms)

		Residual	Residual	
Size	Complete	Small	Large	Attempt
		%		
Small aneurysm/small neck	89.3	9	—	1.7
Small and wide neck	59.2	32.3	1.5	7
Large	52.0	35.7	5.4	6.9
Giant	40.7	40.8	15.2	3.3

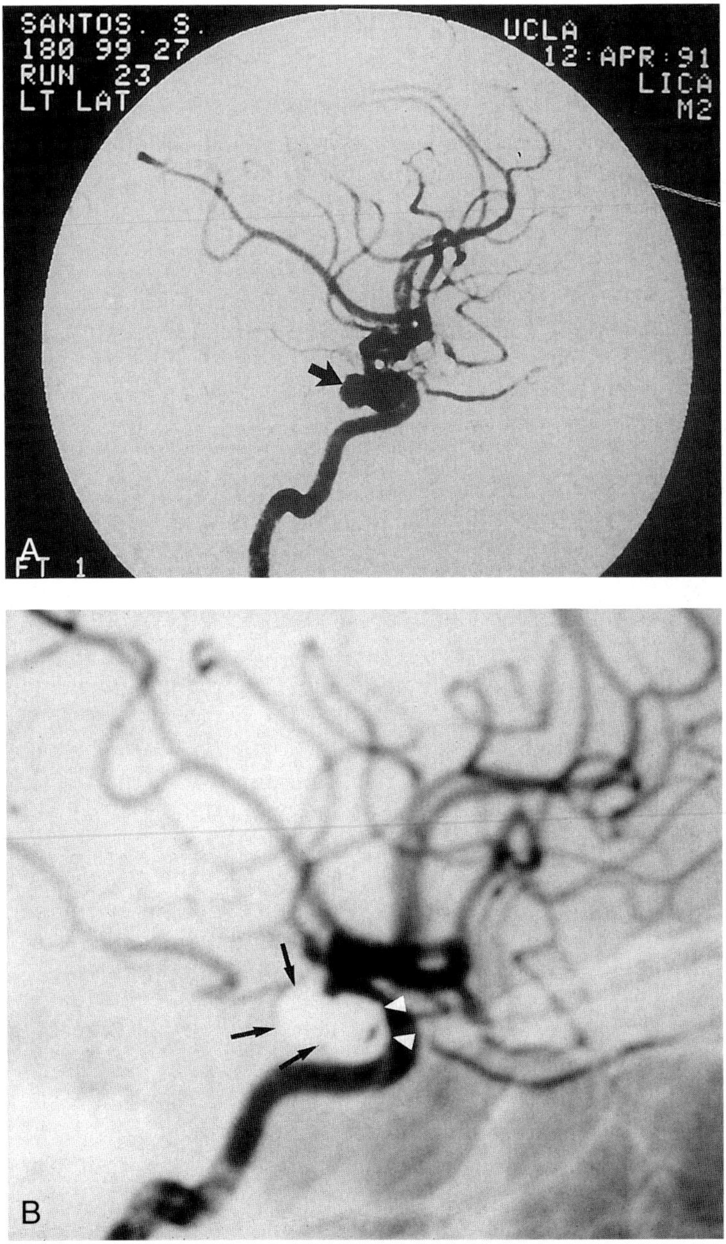

FIG. 12.1 Complete and permanent occlusion of aneurysm with GDC coils. (A) Lateral left carotid angiogram shows a bilobulated, saccular superior hypophyseal aneurysm. This aneurysm was incidentally found. (B) Seven years postembolization angiographic follow-up shows complete aneurysm occlusion. Notice the dense packing of the aneurysm by GDCs (*small arrows*). The aneurysm inflow zone (*white arrowheads*) remains totally obliterated.

main reason why the best anatomic results of our series are identified in small aneurysms with a small neck (89.3%). Our percentage of complete aneurysm occlusion dramatically dropped in small aneurysms with a wide neck and in large or giant aneurysms. In this kind of aneurysm, it is more difficult to obtain a dense aneurysm packing without increasing the risk of coil herniation into the parent artery.

Debrun et al. reported that the anatomic characteristics of an aneurysm were the most important factor related to the success or failure of its GDC embolization (8). Aneurysm neck size and its relationship to the body of the aneurysm are probably the most important factors, but parent artery hemodynamics, aneurysm location, original packing density, and the presence of an intraluminal thrombus are also significant factors (1).

In the last 2 years, the addition of the balloon-assisted technology (BAT), the use of GDC three-dimensional coils, and the deployment of intracranial microstents have improved anatomic results in those kind of aneurysms.

BAT was first used by Guglielmi et al. in 1992 (13) and later popularized and perfected by Moret et al. (32). This technique requires the inflation of a balloon across the neck of an aneurysm while deploying a GDC coil. The inflated balloon stabilizes the microcatheter and microcoil into the aneurysm, allowing the deployment of a denser mesh of GDC coils, particularly across its neck and inflow zone (part of the neck of the aneurysm where the arterial flow enters the aneurysm). The inflated balloon keeps the GDC coils in the aneurysm and protects the lumen of the parent artery. BAT, when performed by an experienced neurointerventional team, does not increase the technical morbidity of an aneurysm embolization (26, 34). We have found it particularly useful in large carotid-ophthalmic, superior hypophyseal, and mid-trunk basilar aneurysms (*Fig. 12.2*).

Tri-dimensional coils have been incorporated into the GDC armamentarium in the last year. They allow a better multiplanar anchorage and stabilization of the GDC coil in wide neck aneurysms. It has a higher resistance to mobilization and remodeling by the blood flow in the aneurysm inflow zone. In large or giant aneurysms, it may produce a compartmentalization of the aneurysm. This anatomic division of giant aneurysms can be useful in the anchoring of the GDC coil, but it can be also deleterious because it may not allow the microcatheter to move freely in the aneurysm.

Tri-dimensional GDC coils need to be used with care when treating ruptured intracranial aneurysms. They are more rigid than the standard/soft GDC coils, and they have a rotational movement during delivery that can be potentially dangerous in small acutely ruptured

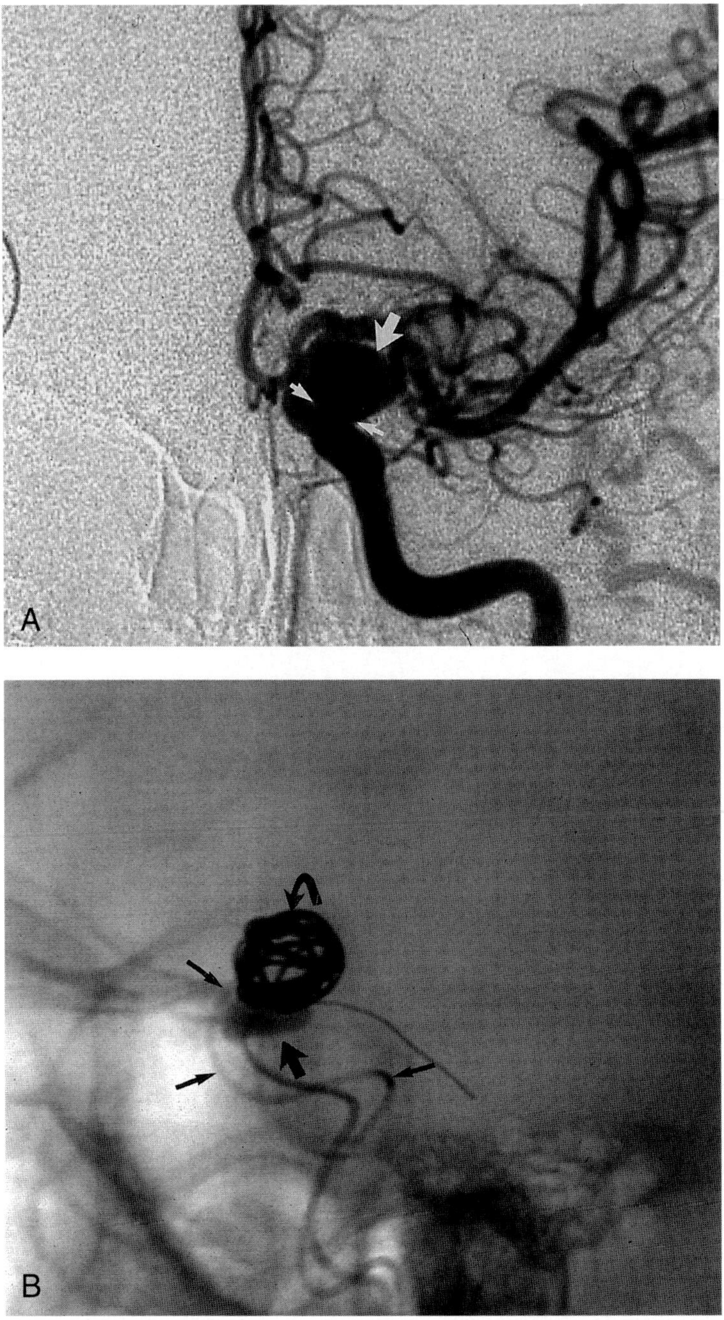

FIG. 12.2 Balloon-assisted technology. (A) AP view of left internal carotid angiogram shows a 10–mm aneurysm (*large arrow*) with a wide neck (*small arrows*). (B) A large tri-dimensional coil (*curved arrow*) has been deposited in the aneurysm. Notice an inflated ballon (*thick arrow*) blocking the neck of the aneurysm and the microcatheter (*small arrows*) inside the aneurysm.

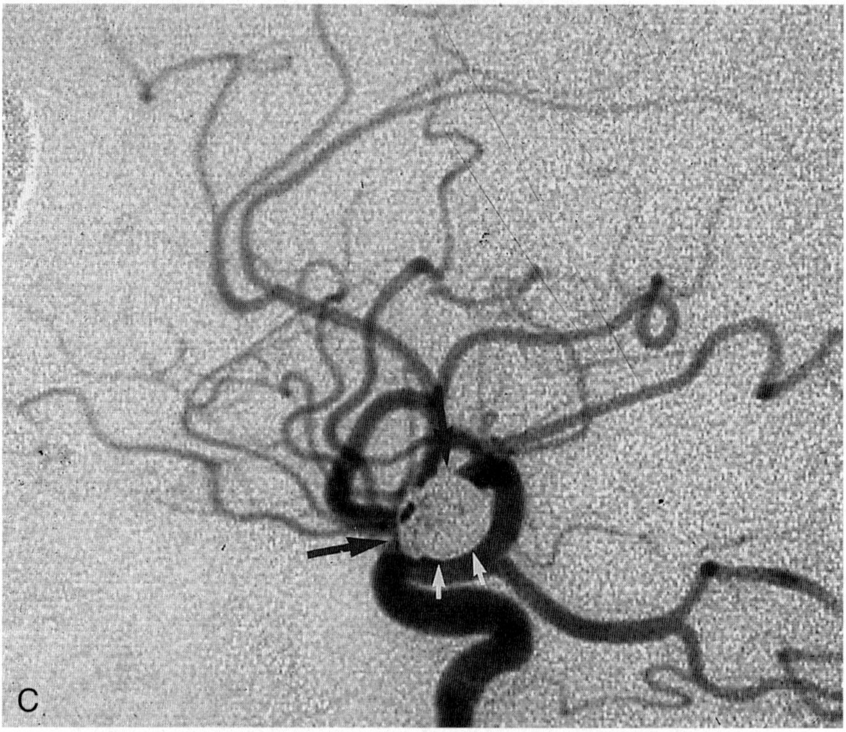

FIG. 12.2 Balloon-assisted technology. (C) Postembolization carotid angiogram demonstrated a complete obliteration of the aneurysm by a dense GDC packing (*black arrows*). Notice the smooth interface between the neck of the aneurysm and the parent artery (*white arrows*).

aneurysms. The clinical experience collected until now has been very positive, and their use has decreased the need of BAT.

INTRACRANIAL MICROSTENTS

Turjman et al. pioneered the utilization of a combination of microstents and GDC coils for the treatment of large and giant aneurysms (41). An increasing number of case reports have recently appeared in the neurointerventional literature, describing the deployment of microstents across the neck of large or giant aneurysms (19, 29, 31).

The deployment of a microstent creates an anatomic boundary separating the lumen of the normal artery from the aneurysm. After the microstent has been deployed, a microcatheter is positioned in the aneurysm through the struts of the stent, and the GDC coils are delivered until a dense coil packing has been obtained (*Fig. 12.3*).

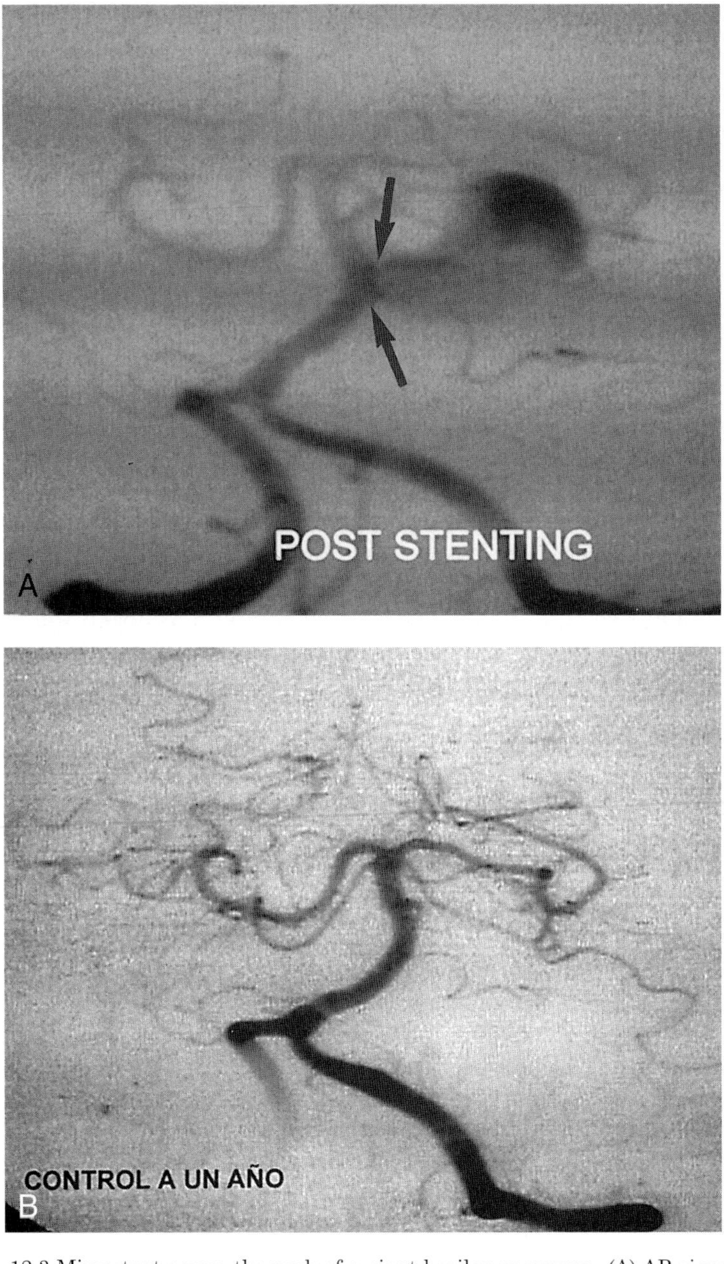

FIG. 12.3 Microstent across the neck of a giant basilar aneurysm. (A) AP view of left vertebral angiogram shows early filling of a giant basilar-anteroinferior cerebellar aneurysm. The neck of the aneurysm is relatively narrow (*arrows*), and a microstent was deployed across it. The patient presented with symptoms of posterior fossa mass effect. (B) One year angio follow-up shows a complete aneurysm occlusion and perfect preservation of the lumen of the basilar artery. The patient had a significant clinical improvement. (courtesy of Dr. Marco Zenteno).

Microstents are most useful for lateral aneurysms, and they are safer in aneurysms not associated with small perforating arteries. The deployment of a microstent in arteries such as the basilar artery or M1 portion of the middle cerebral artery carries a potential risk of occlusion of the ostium of a perforating artery.

Microstents used in the intracranial circulation are derived from the cardiology armamentarium. They are suitable to negotiate vascular turns of the cardiac circulation, but they are too rigid in many cases to negotiate the multiple and not unusually sharp turns of the intracranial circulation. Despite these present technical limitations, they are indeed a great help in those cases in which the microstent can be deployed across the neck of a large or giant aneurysm. The development of dedicated microstents to the intracranial circulation will allow a more universal and safer utilization of this very promising technique. The ideal neurovascular microstent needs to have an appropriate balance between softness and radial force to negotiate steep arterial curves. It must have a non-thrombogenic surface, and it must elicit a permanent neo-endothelial coverage with a mild or absent neo-intima hyperplasia.

HEMODYNAMIC CONTROL OF ANEURYSM INFLOW ZONE

The aneurysm inflow zone may be defined as the area of the neck of the aneurysm where the blood flow enters the aneurysmal sac. It is in this area where the blood flow changes its laminar characteristics to turbulent flow. In our experience, most recanalization of aneurysms embolized with GDC coils start in this region of the neck of the aneurysm. The water hammer effect of the blood flow is most intense in this region, and it needs to be controlled by an early and dense packing of GDC coils. This is more often achieved in small aneurysms with small necks and is more difficult in small aneurysms with a wide neck and in large and giant aneurysms. In our experience at the UCLA Medical Center, we have seen aneurysm recanalization in 6% of small aneurysms with a small neck, in 32% of aneurysms with a wide neck, in 35% of large aneurysms, and in 47% of giant aneurysms.

The utilization of the BAT and microstents has improved this hemodynamic control in the aneurysm inflow zone. We have used BAT in re-embolization of some recanalized aneurysms. It has provided an anatomic support for the safe delivery of GDC coils in residual necks and particularly for the dense packing of the aneurysm inflow zone. The delivery of a microstent may produce immediate hemodynamic changes observed in a rapid sequence cerebral angiography. Similar changes have been reported by Aenis et al. and Lieber et al. In computer simulation models of aneurysm embolization with coils and microstents (3, 27), the development of covered microstents will be the nal solution for a limited number of intracranial aneurysms (lateral aneurysms not associated with arterial perforators) (28).

BIOLOGIC RESPONSE TO THE GDC COIL DEPLOYMENT IN ANEURYSMS

Experimental analysis of the biologic response elicited by the deposit of GDC coils in aneurysms has been performed by Murayama et al. (35, 36). They reported that in swine the GDC coil elicits a mild and delayed in ammatory response, intermingled with areas of blood clot. The persistence of non-organized blood clots in aneurysms allows the blood ow to reposition the coils in the aneurysm in ow zone and produce an early aneurysm recanalization. An intense research is now underway to nd a biologic solution to this problem (7, 25, 35, 36). The next generation of GDC coils needs to have a bioactive surface capable of eliciting an intense intraneurysmal in ammatory response that will allow scar tissue formation in the body of the aneurysm and a denser neo-intima and neo-endothelial coverage of the aneurysmal neck (*Fig. 12.4*).

It is important to achieve this positive biologic response without increasing the thrombogenicity of the surface of the GDC coil. This positive biologic activity of surface-modi ed GDC coils has been achieved in animal models using ion implantation techniques (35, 36) or the addition cytokines/growth factors to the surface of the GDC coil (20, 21).

Technical Complications

The technical complications associated with the GDC technique at the UCLA Medical Center were aneurysm perforation (14 pts, 2%), parent artery occlusion (14 pts, 2%), cerebral embolization (15 pts, 2.1%), and arterial dissection in brachycephalic vessels (3 pts, 0.5%).

Aneurysm perforation is now rarely seen due to the utilization of a new generation of coated microcatheters and guidewires and soft GDC coils. It is more often observed in acutely ruptured aneurysms and seldom observed in incidental aneurysms. This complication can be fatal if it occurs in an unprotected aneurysm and sick patient. If it occurs when most of the aneurysm has been filled with GDC coils, it may produce only mild or moderate temporary neurologic deterioration (38, 45).

Parent artery occlusion is mostly related to untoward herniation of GDC coils into the parent artery. This complication can be minimized if an appropriate vascular mapping of the aneurysm is achieved. This information may be gathered by biplane standard digital angiogram

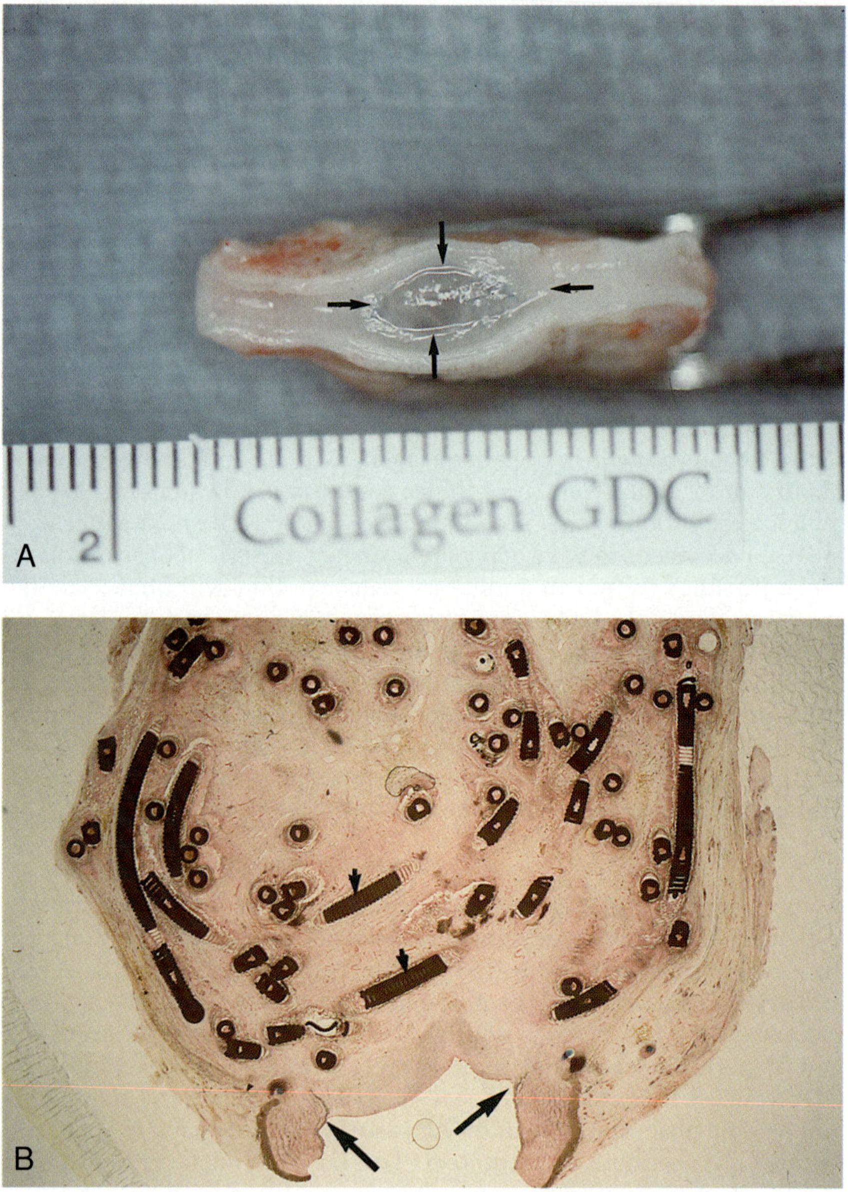

FIG. 12.4 Biological changes on GDC coils. (A) Macroscopic specimen of an experimental aneurysm 14 days postembolization with a GDC treated with ion implantation and collagen. The anatomic boundaries of the neck of the aneurysm are identi ed (*arrows*). Note a thick neo-intimal and neo-endothelial coverage of the neck of the aneurysm with a blurred vision of GDC coils within the aneurysm. (B) Histologic specimen of an aneurysm after 14 days of embolization with bioactive GDCs. The neck of the aneurysm has been identi ed (*arrows*). The coils (*small arrows*) are surrounded by a magna of -brous tissue, and a thick neo-intima is covering the neck of the aneurysm. Note it is made of the absence of non-organized clot in the aneurysm.

and more recently by three-dimensional CT, MRI, and digital angiography (2, 43).

Tri-dimensional imaging of an aneurysm and related vascular tree is particularly useful for vascular neurosurgeons and interventional neuroradiologists in middle cerebral and anterior communicating aneurysms as well as in large fusiform aneurysms. The tri-dimensional picture of giant and fusiform aneurysms shows at its best the relationship of the aneurysm with the ostium of normal arteries. It identi es those cases that will need a protective arterio-arterial bypass before surgical or endovascular trapping of the aneurysm (30) (*Fig. 12.5*).

Cerebral embolization was the most common technical complication of GDC technology. The utilization of per- and immediate postembolization systemic anticoagulation followed by a regime of aspirin/Ticlopidin for at least 3 months postembolization has dramatically de-

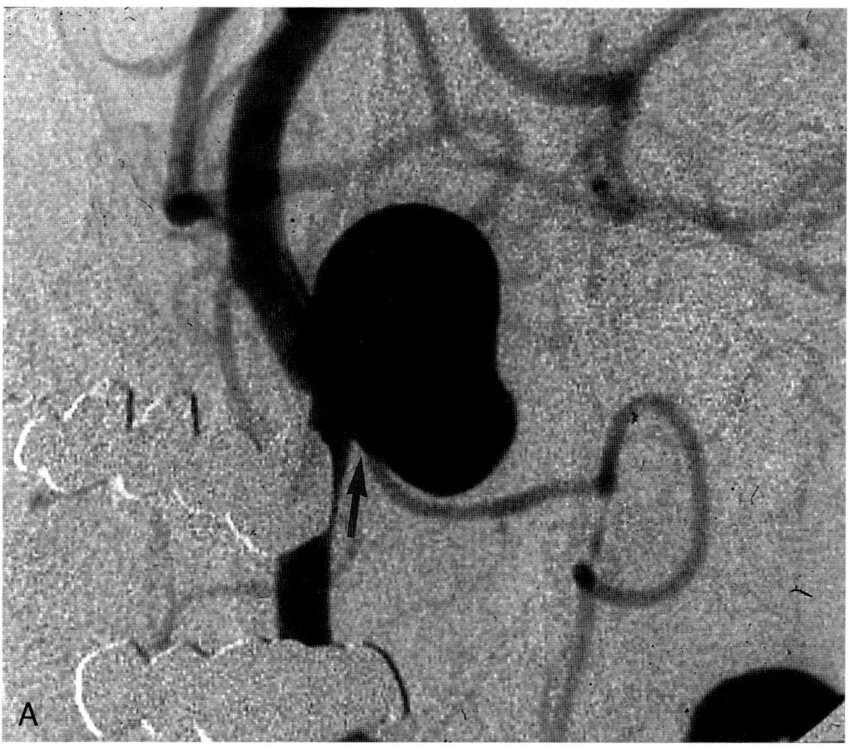

FIG. 12.5 Tri-dimensional evaluation of complex aneurysms. (A) Oblique view of left vertebral angiogram shows a large vertebro-PICA aneurysm. The ostium of the left PICA cannot be separated from the aneurysm (*arrow*).

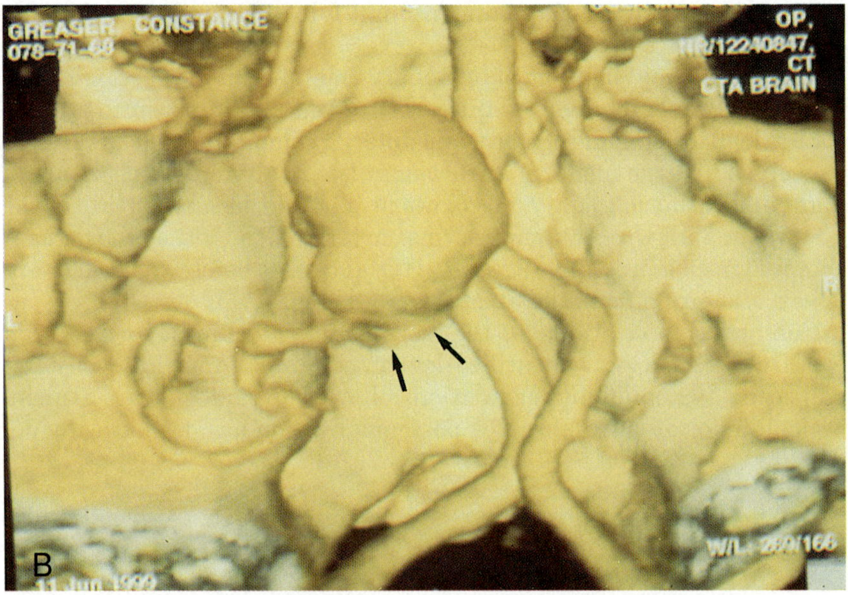

FIG. 12.5 Tri-dimensional evaluation of complex aneurysms. (B) Tri-dimensional CTA reconstruction of the vascular anatomy shows the involvement of the ostium of PICA by the inferior aspect of the aneurysm. (*straight arrows*). An occipital-PICA bypass preceded the GDC occlusion of the aneurysm. The patient remained neurologically intact after this combined therapeutic procedure.

creased untoward cerebral embolization in aneurysms treated with GDC. This is particularly valid in large aneurysms with a wide neck. Again, the appropriate visualization of the neck of the aneurysm during embolization decreases the chance of coil herniation into the parent artery. A GDC coil herniated into a normal artery may be silent, but it also may be the source of local thrombosis and distal embolic phenomena. This is particularly dangerous in small arteries such as anterior communicating artery, M1 portion of middle cerebral arteries, or P1 portion of posterior cerebral arteries.

Overall Immediate Clinical Outcome

The overall immediate morbidity of the 617 patients treated at UCLA was 6.4% and the peri-operative mortality was 1.7% (*Table 12.5*). In the anterior circulation (421 patients with 467 aneurysms), we observed a 5.2% morbidity and 1.3% mortality. In the posterior circulation (196 patients with 233 aneurysms), a 7.1% morbidity and 2.2% mortality was noted.

TABLE 12.5
Immediate Clinical Outcome
(617 Patients, 700 Aneurysms)

Outcome	No.	Percentage (%)
Intact	260	42.4
Unchanged	306	49.5
Deteriorated	40	6.4
Death	11	1.7

IMMEDIATE MORBIMORTALITY AND CLINICAL PRESENTATION

Patients presenting with acute SAH (301 pts) had a 9.4% morbidity and 3.7% mortality. Cases of non-acute SAH (75 pts) had 8.6% morbidity and 0% mortality, patients with incidental aneurysms (168 pts) showed 3.4% morbidity and 0.6% mortality and patients presenting with mass effect (55 pts) had 3.7% morbidity and 0% mortality. We explain the increased incidence of morbimortality in acutely ruptured aneurysms due to the increased severity of the primary disease plus the increased incidence of aneurysm perforation in this category of aneurysms.

IMMEDIATE MORBIMORTALITY AND ANEURYSM LOCATION

At difference with the neurosurgical experience, aneurysm location plays a minor role in the incidence of morbidity of the GDC technology (*Table 12.6*).

Most intracranial aneurysms can be safely catheterized with the present generation of microcatheters and guidewires. Extreme vascular tortuosity in the brachycephalic arteries and post-SAH arterial vasospasm may increase its technical difficulty. The anatomic characteristics of the aneurysm remain the most important factor when considering anatomic outcome and morbimortality. In our experience, wide neck anterior communicating aneurysms pointing upward and backward are the most dif-

TABLE 12.6
Morbimortality and Aneurysm Location
(617 Patients, 700 Aneurysms)

Type	Number	Morbidity (%)	Mortality (%)
Car. Ophth.	198 an.	2.4	0.5
Basilar tip	124 an.	5.1	1.8
ACom	115 an.	7.0	3.
PCom	100 an.	6.9	0
MCA	57 an.	6.0	2.0

ficult ones to treat with GDCs. The microcatheter tends to have an unstable position, and the GDC coil migrates downward into the anterior communicating artery. The BAT is difficult to use due to the small size of the anterior cerebral artery complex.

The presence of arterial vasospasm does not preclude the catheterization of an aneurysm distally located. In a limited number of cases, there is a need of performing angioplasty of the spastic artery to enter the ruptured aneurysm (*Fig. 12.6*). This maneuver does not appear to increase aneurysm re-rupture.

Long-Term Clinical Outcome

Long-term clinical outcome includes patients seen from 6 months to 8 years postembolization. We could not obtain telephone or direct con-

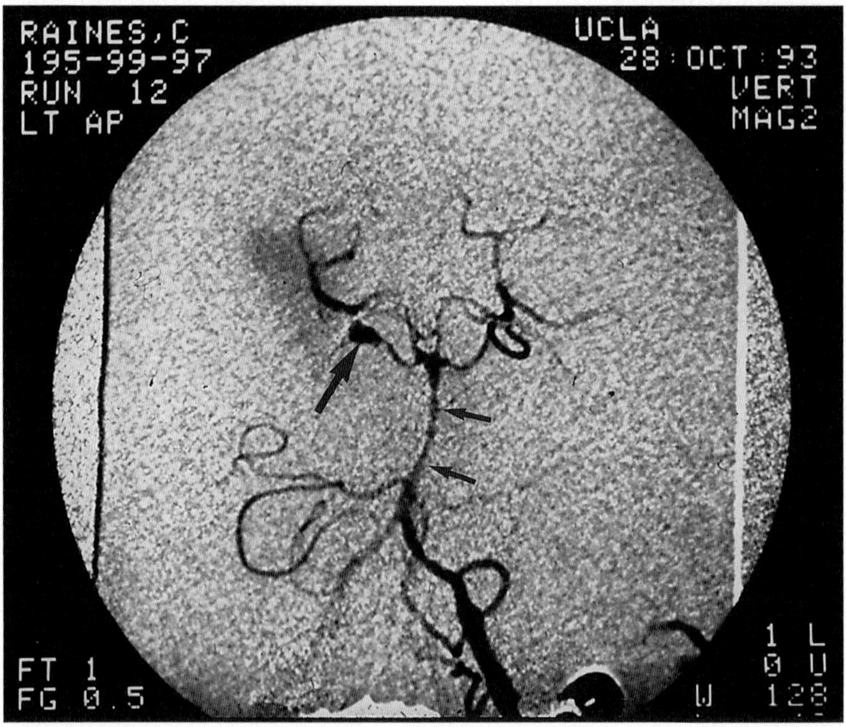

FIG. 12.6 GDC embolization and severe arterial vasospasm. (A) AP view of left vertebral angiogram shows a left fusiform superior cerebellar aneurysm. Notice a severe vasospasm involving the basilar artery trunk (*arrows*). The patient was a grade III in Hunt and Hess classification. Preembolization mechanical angioplasty and GDC occlusion of the aneurysm was performed.

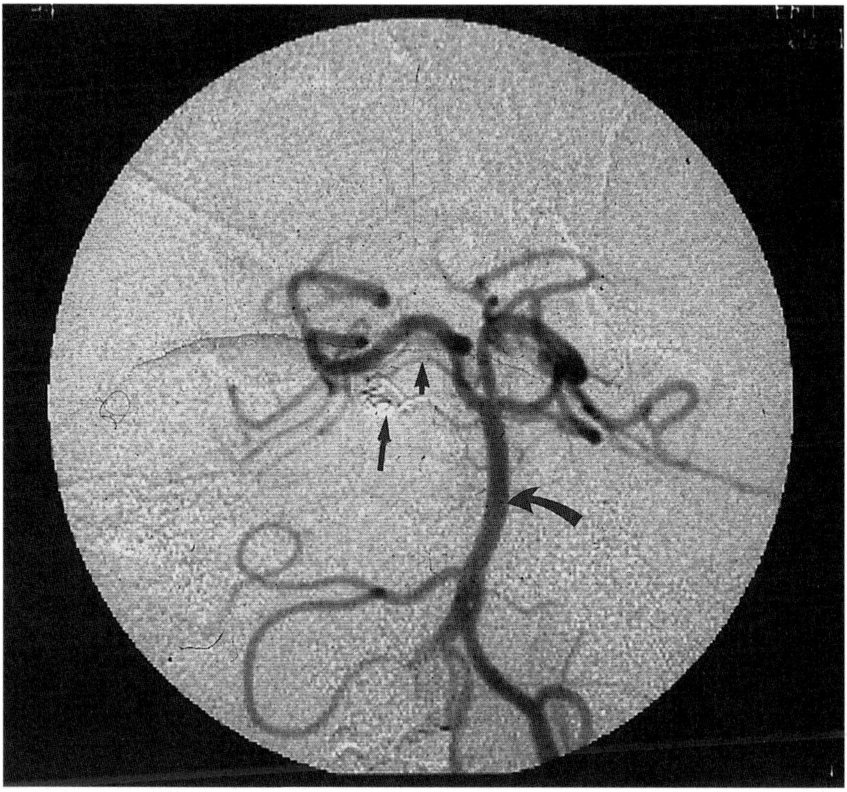

FIG. 12.6 GDC embolization and severe arterial vasospasm. (B) Three weeks postembolization vertebral angiogram shows a normal appearance of the basilar artery (*curved arrow*), a patent, small left superior cerebellar artery and GDC coils occluding the aneurysm, and a second left superior cerebellar artery. The patient had a complete neurologic recovery.

tact with 92 patients (14.9%). In total, 376 patients (61%) were neurologically intact, and 79 (12.6%) remained neurologically unchanged when compared with their clinical presentation. Thirty-nine patients (6.5%) had a neurologic deterioration, and 31 died (5%). Ten deaths were related to GDC procedural complications (1.7%), 13 were associated with the severity of the SAH, and eight patients died from unrelated causes (bacterial endocarditis, AIDS, ventriculitis, etc.).

Postembolization Aneurysm Rerupture

Eight patients presenting with acute SAH had a postembolization delayed aneurysm rerupture (8/376 pts, 2.1%). All cases showed a significant coil remodeling at the aneurysm inflow zone and exposure of the body of the aneurysm to the blood flow. In our experience, no cases of aneurysm rerupture were observed in aneurysms completely embolized or showing a stable neck remnant in long-term angiographic follow-up. The significance of a small neck remnant after incomplete GDC coiling is unknown. Thorough long-term angiographic and clinical follow-ups are needed to learn their natural history to be able to make valid therapeutic decisions. We have observed cases of **new** aneurysm rupture in giant aneurysms partially embolized with GDC coils (5 in 72 patients, 7%). This incidence of hemorrhage may be related to the natural history of the disease, but we cannot exclude a relationship with their incomplete occlusion by GDC coils. The presence of intra-aneurysmal thrombus and inadequate GDC packing permits the GDC coils to be pushed inward by the arterial blood flow with a concomitant high rate of aneurysm recanalization. The hemodynamic characteristics of this "new" aneurysm may be different from the original one, and it may change its natural history, favoring rupturing over size increase. The utilization of microstents, without or with GDC coils, may be the solution to a limited number of giant, saccular, or fusiform intracranial aneurysms. The involvement of large or perforating arteries in the body of these aneurysms remains an insoluble problem to the endovascular technique.

CONCLUSIONS

GDC is a safe alternative to the surgical clipping of ruptured or unruptured intracranial aneurysms. It may be applied in anterior or posterior circulation aneurysms, and it is more efficient in small aneurysms with a small neck. GDC can completely and permanently occlude an aneurysm when a tight packing of the aneurysm has been achieved. This is true not only for small aneurysms but also for large aneurysms when the aneurysm inflow zone has been tightly obliterated. This anatomic goal can now be more often achieved with the use of the balloon-assisted technology and microstents. The present generation of microstents needs to be technically improved to obtain safe and consistent anatomic results. The future development of biologically active microcoils may have a positive impact on the permanent anchoring of the coils with reduction of coil remodeling and aneurysm recanalization. Histologic results in animal models have shown that the early development of scar tissue in an aneurysm elicits a faster and more intense deposit of neo-intima and neo-endothelium across the neck of the aneurysm.

In contrast with neurosurgery, the Morbimortality related to GDC is not strongly influenced by the location of the aneurysm or the age of the patient. Anterior and posterior circulation aneurysms have similar technical complications, and their morbimortality are dictated by their anatomic characteristics and patient's neurologic status.

The utilization of GDC technique in giant intracranial aneurysms should be limited to inoperable cases. The relative low morbidity of this procedure is counterbalanced by its poor anatomic results. It may play a more positive role in association with neurosurgical techniques of arterio-arterial bypass and trapping.

REFERENCES

1. Adams WM, Laitt RG: Aneurysms remnants: **Neurointervencionist** 1:74–83, 2000.
2. Adams WM, Laitt RD, Jackson A: Time of flight 3D magnetic resonance angiography in the follow-up of coiled cerebral aneurysms. **Intervent Neuroradiol** 5:127–137, 1999.
3. Aenis M, Stancampiano AP, Wakhloo AK, Lieber BB: Modeling of flow in a straight stented and non-stented side wall aneurysms model. **J. Biomech Eng** 119:206–212, 1997.
4. Byrne JV, Molyneux AJ, Brennan RP, Renowden SA: Embolisation of recently ruptured intracranial aneurysms. **J Neurosurg Psychiatry** 59:616–20, 1995
5. Casasco AE, Aymard A, Gobin YP, Houdart E, Rogopoulos A, George B, Hodes JE, Cophignon J, Merland JJ: Selective endovascular treatment of 71 intracranial aneurysms with platinum coils. **J Neurosurg** 79:3–10, 1993.
6. Cloughesy TE, Gobin YP, Black K, Viñuela F, Taft F, Kadkhoda B, Kabbinavar F: Intraarterial carboplatin chemotherapy for brain tumors: A dose escalation study based on cerebral blood flow. **J. Neurooncol** 35:121–131, 1997.
7. Dawson RC, Shengelaia GG, Krisht AF, Bonner GB: Histologic effects of collagen-filled interlocking detachable coils in the ablation of experimental aneurysms in swine. **Am J Neuroradiol** 17:859–863, 1996.
8. Debrun GM, Aletich VA, Kehrli P, Misra M, Ausman JI, Charbel F: Selection of cerebral aneurysms for treatment using Guglielmi detachable coils: The Preliminary University of Illinois at Chicago experience. **Neurosurgery** 43:1281–1297, 1998.
9. Debrun G, Lacour P, Caron JO, Hurth M, Comoy J, Keravel Y: Inflatable and released balloon technique: Experimentation in dog. Application in man. **Neuroradiology** 9:267–271, 1975.
10. Debrun G, Vinuela F, Fox AJ, Drake CG: Embolization of cerebral arteriovenous malformations with bucrylate; Experience in 46 cases. **J Neurosurg** 56:615–627, 1982.
11. Debrun GM, Vinuela F, Fox AJ, Davis KR, Ahn HS: Indications fro treatment and classification of 132 carotid-cavernous fistulas. **Neurosurgery** 22:285–289, 1988.
12. Fox AJ, Vinuela F, Pelz DM, Peerless SJ, Ferguson GG, Drake CG, Deburn G: Use of detachable balloons for proximal artery occlusion in the treatment of unclippable aneurysms. **J Neurosurg** 66:40–46, 1987.
13. Guglielmi G, Vinuela F, Briganti F, Duckwiler G: Carotid-cavernous fistula caused by a ruptured intracavernous aneurysm: Endovascular treatment by electrothrombosis with detachable coils. **Neurosurgery** 31:591–596, 1992.
14. Guglielmi G, Vinuela F, Dion J, Duckwiler G: Electrothrombosis of saccular aneurysms via endovascular approach: Part 2. Preliminary clinical experience. **J Neurosurg** 75:8–14, 1991.

15. Guglielmi G, Vinuela F, Sepetka I, Macellari V: Electrothrombosis of saccular aneurysms via endovascular approach; Part I. Electrochemical basis, technique and experimental results. **J Neurosurg** 75:1–7, 1991.
16. Halbach VV, Hieshima GB, Higashida RT: Treatment of intracranial aneurysms by balloon embolization. **Semin Intervent Radiol** 4:261–268, 1987.
17. Hieshima GB, Higashida RT, Halbach VV, Cahan L, Goto K: Intravascular embolization of a carotid-ophthalmic aneurysm with preservation of the parent vessel. **Am J Neuroradiol** 7:916–918, 1986.
18. Higashida RT, Hieshima GB, Tsai FY, Halbach VV, Norman D, Newton TH: Transluminal angioplasty of the vertebral and basilar artery. **Am J Neuroradiol** 8:745–749, 1987.
19. Higashida RT, Smith W, Gress D, Urwin R, Dowd CJ, Balouse PA, Halback VV: Intravascular stent and endovascular coil placement for a ruptured fusiform aneurysm of the basilar artery. **J Neurosurg** 87:944–949, 1997.
20. Kalmes DF, Borland MK, Cloft HJ, Altes TA, Dion JE, Jensen ME, Hankins GR, Helm GA: In vitro proliferation and adhesion of basic fibroblast growth factor-producing fibroblasts on platinum coils. **Radiology** 206:237–243, 1998.
21. Kalmes DF, Williams AD, Cloft HJ, Lopes MB, Hankins GR, Helm GA: Platinum coil-mediated implantation of growth factor-secreting endovascular tissue grafts: An in vivo study. **Radiology** 207:519–523, 1999.
22. Kerber C.: Balloon catheter with a calibrated leak: A new system for superselective angiotherapy and occlusive catheter therapy. **Radiology** 120:547–549, 1976.
23. Kinugasa K, Mandai S, Terai, Y, Karnata I, Sugui K, Ohmoto T, Nishimoto A: Direct thrombosis of aneurysms with cellulose acetate polymer: Part II. Preliminary clinical experience **J Neurosurg** 77: 501–507, 1992.
24. Kuether TA, Nesbit GM, Barnwell SL: Clinical and angiographic outcomes with treatment data for patients with cerebral aneurysms treated with Guglielmi detachable coils: A single-center experience. **Neurosurgery** 43:1016–1025, 1998.
25. Kwan ESK, Heilman CB, Roth PA: Endovascular packing of carotid bifurcation aneurysms with polyester fiber-coated platinum coils in a rabbit model. **Am J Neuroradiol** 14:323–333, 1993.
26. Lefkowitz MA, Gobin YP, Akiba Y, Duckwiler GR, Murayama Y, Guglielmi G, Martin NA, Viñuela F: Balloon-assisted Guglielmi detachable coiling of wide-necked aneurysms: Part 2. Clinical results. **Neurosurgery** 45:531–538, 1999.
27. Lieber BB, Stancampiano AP, Wakhloo AK: Alteration of hemodynamics in aneurysm models by stenting: Influence of stent porosity. **Ann Biomed Eng** 25:460–469, 1997.
28. Link J, Feyerabend B, Grabener M, Linstedt U, Brossmann J, Thomsen H, Heller M: Dacron-covered stent-grafts for the percutaneous treatment of carotid aneurysms: Effectiveness and bio-compatibility. Experimental study in swine. **Radiology** 200:397–401, 1996.
29. Lylyk P, Ceratto R, Hurvitz R: Treatment of a vertebral dissecting aneurysm with stents and coils: Technical case report. **Neurosurgery** 43:385–388, 1998.
30. Martin N: Arterial bypass for the treatment of giant and fusiform intracranial aneurysms. **Techniques Neurosurg** 4:153–178, 1998.
31. Mericle RA, Lanzino G, Wakhloo AK, Guterman LR, Hopkins LN: Stenting and secondary coiling of intracranial internal carotid artery aneurysm: Technical case report. **Neurosurgery** 43:1229–1234, 1998.
32. Moret J, Cognard C, Weill A, Castaings L, Rey A: The "remodeling technique" in the treatment of wide neck intracranial aneurysms: Angiographic results and clinical follow-up in 56 cases. **Interv Neuroradiol** 3:21–35, 1997.

33. Moret J, Pierot L, Boulin A, Castaigns L, Rey A: Endovascular treatment of anterior communicating artery aneurysms using Guglielmi detachable coils. **Neuroradiology** 38:800–805, 1996.
34. Moret J, Ross IB, Weill A: The retrograde approach: A consideration for the endovascular treatment of aneurysms. **Am J Neuroradiol** 21:262–268, 2000.
35. Murayama Y, Vinuela F, Suzuki Y, Masoud TF, Gugliemi G, Iwaki M, Kamio M, Abe T: Ion implantation modified the surface of GDCs: An experimental study in swine aneurysms. **Intervent Neuroradiol** 3:156–161, 1997.
36. Murayama Y, Vinuela F, Suzuki Y, et al: Ion implantation and protein coating for detachable coils for endovascular treatment of cerebral aneurysms: Concepts and preliminary results in swine models. **Neurosurgery** 40:1233–1244, 1997.
37. Rauch RA, Vinuela F, Dion J, Duckwiler G, Amos EC, Jordan SE, Martin N, Jensen ME, Bentson J: Pre-embolization functional evaluation in brain AVMs: Part 2. The ability of superselective Amytal test to predict neurologic dysfunction before embolization. **Am J Neuroradiol** 13:309–314, 1992.
38. Richling B, Bavinzki G, Gross C, Gruber A, Killer M: Early clinical outcome of patients with ruptured cerebral aneurysms treated by endovascular (GDC) or microsurgical techniques: A single center experience. **Intervent Neuroradiol** 1:19–27, 1995.
39. Serbinenko FA: Balloon catheterization and occlusion of major cerebral vessels. **J Neurosurg** 41:125–145, 1974.
40. Szikora I, Guterman LR, Standard SC, Wakhloo AK, Hopkins LN: Endovascular treatment of experimental aneurysms with liquid polymers: The protective potential of stents. **Neurosurgery** 38:339–347, 1996.
41. Turjman F, Massoud TF, Ji C, Guglielmi G, Viñuela F, Robert J: Combined stent implantation and endosaccular coil placement for treatment of experimental wide-necked aneurysms: A feasibility study in swine. **Am J Neuroradiol** 15:1087–1090, 1994.
42. Vanninen R, Koivisto T, Saari T, Hernesniemi J, Vapalahti M: Ruptured intracranial aneurysms: Acute endovascular treatment with electrolytically detachable coils. A prospective randomized trial. **Radiology** 211:325–336, 1999.
43. Villablanca JP, Martin N, Jahan R, et al: Volume rendered helical CT angiography in detection and characterization of intracranial aneurysms. **J Neurosurg** (in press).
44. Vinuela F: Endovascular therapy of brain arteriovenous malformations. **Semin Intervent Radiol** 4:269–278, 1987.
45. Vinuela F, Duckwiler G, Mawad M: Guglielmi detachable coil embolization of acute intracranial aneurysm: Perioperative anatomical and clinical outcome in 403 patients. **J Neurosurg** 86:475–482, 1997.
46. Vitek JJ, Raymon BC, Oh SJ: Innominate artery angioplasty. **Am J Neuroradiol** 5:113–114, 1984.

CHAPTER

13

Arteriovenous Malformations: Indications for Stereotactic Radiosurgery

PHILIP E. STIEG, PH.D., M.D., R. M. FRIEDLANDER, M.D., J. S. LOEFFLER, E. ALEXANDER III, M.D.

INTRODUCTION

The treatment goal for all intracranial arteriovenous malformations (AVMs) is complete obliteration. Over the past several decades, multiple modalities have been developed and refined for AVM management and include microsurgery, endovascular surgery, and stereotactic radiosurgery.

Radiosurgery is a technique for delivering a high dose of single fraction radiation to a well-defined target (11). Cushing was the first to treat AVMs with ionizing radiation and suggested that it demonstrated considerable promise for cure (18). Since that time, there has been rapid expansion in imaging technology as well as megavoltage delivery systems (11). In addition, the development of proton beam radiation, heavy particle radiation (helium ions), the use of photons with the gamma knife, and most recently adaptations of linear accelerators have led to an increasing number of patients with AVMs treated with radiosurgery (8, 12, 13). With this accrual of technologic sophistication and longer follow-up, we are now able to more accurately assess the risks and benefits associated with radiosurgery.

Decision analysis schemes must be devised for the treatment of AVMs with the end result being complete obliteration achieved at a minimal complication rate. Unfortunately, most of the data in the radiosurgical literature are from non-randomized, retrospective studies, which is also true for microsurgical and endovascular reports. Given these limitations, we will attempt to review the indications for stereotactic radiosurgery as well as review the results from various institutions, including our own. Finally, the complications associated with this therapy will be evaluated, with the ultimate intention of providing a scheme for selecting the appropriate patients for treatment with radiosurgery.

TABLE 13.1
Volumetric Evaluation for AVMs

Diameter (cm)	Radius (cm)	Volume* (cc)
1	0.5	0.52
2	1	4.17
2.5	1.25	8.18
3	1.5	14.13
3.5	1.75	22.44
4	2	33.5
5	2.5	65.41

*Assuming purely spherical volumes.

INDICATIONS FOR STEREOTACTIC RADIOSURGERY

The Spetzler-Martin grading system for art eriovenous malformations was designed to preoperatively assess the surgical risks experienced in the treatment of these lesions (20). This system uses size, location, and venous drainage to predict surgical risk and can be used prospectively (5). Large, eloquently located AVMs carry the greatest risk for poor outcome. Similarly, the predominant limitation to stereotactic radiosurgery is lesion volume. The ideal treatment volumes for radiosurgery are between 0.1 and 10cc (3). The Spetzler-Martin grading scale uses maximum diameter. Therefore, volume conversions must be performed to integrate or compare the potential risks and benefits of radiosurgery versus microsurgery. Thus, assuming purely spherical volumes, the maximum diameter, which can be treated ideally with radiosurgery, is 2.75 cm (*Table 13.1*). When correlating those lesions that can be ideally treated with stereotactic radiosurgery to the Spetzler-Martin scale, it is observed that grade I–III lesions are most amenable to radiosurgery (*Fig. 13.1*). These AVM grades also have the lowest microsurgical morbidity (5).

The continued development of microsurgery, radiosurgery, and endovascular techniques has increased the debate regarding the appropriate lesions treated by each modality (19, 23). A single institution study suggests that smaller lesions were best managed with microsurgery; however, they referred to the ideal patient as 40 years in age, in excellent health, with an "operable" lesion (16). Comparison between radiosurgical and surgical series regarding the proportion of grade III–IV Spetzler-Martin AVMs is also quite similar (*Table 13.2*). However, deep-seated AVMs are more commonly treated by stereotactic radiosurgery (5, 7, 15). Thus, most cerebrovascular centers would agree that the most appropriate lesion for treatment with radiosurgery is small (volume less

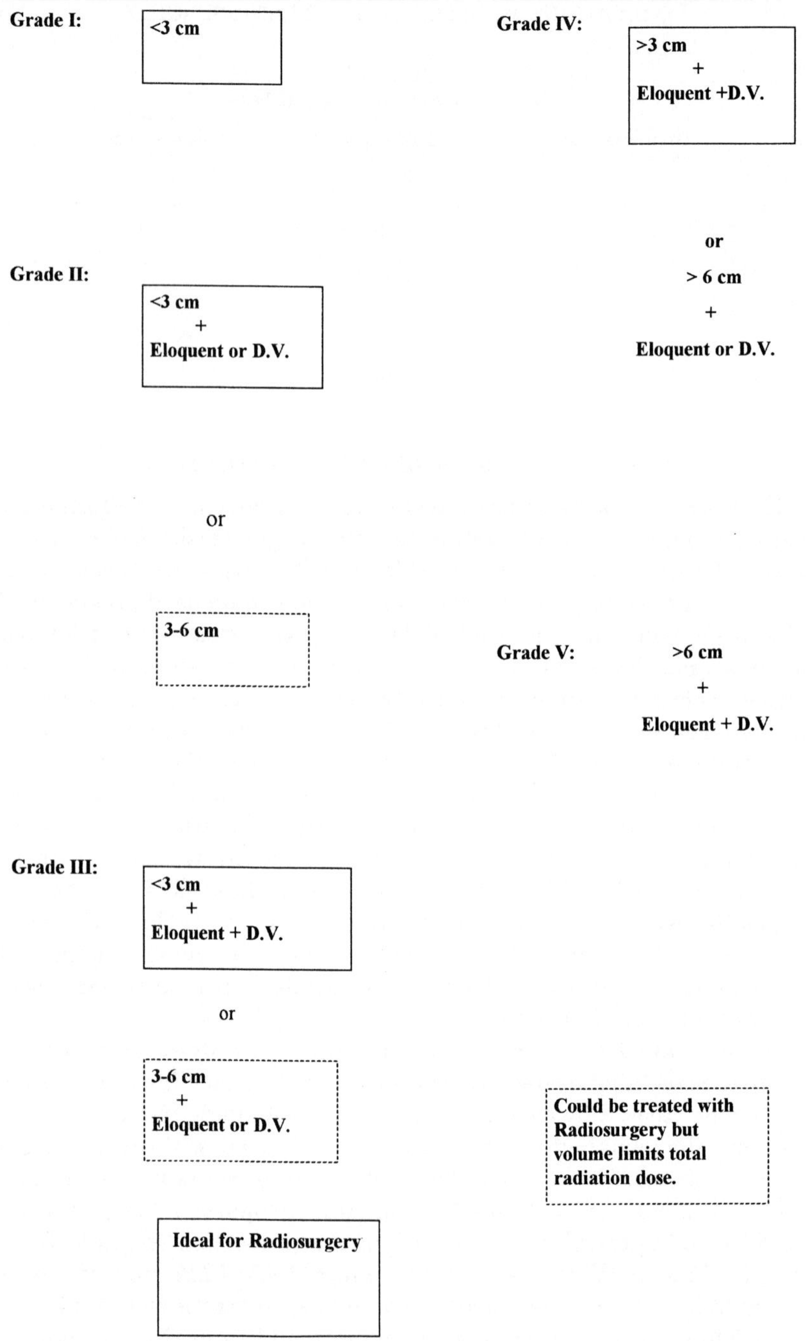

FIG. 13.1. Correlation between Spetzler-Martin grading system and AVMs ideally treated with radiosurgery.

TABLE 13.2
Comparison by Grade and Location between Radiosurgical and Surgical Series: Proportion of Patients Treated in Specific Series

	Radiosurgical Series Pollock et al (13–15)	Hamilton (5)	Heros (7)
		%	
Spetzler-Martin grade III–IV	58	67	69
Deep AVM	32	7	11

than 10cc) and located deep within the cerebral hemispheres or brain stem. Other small lesions must be considered individually and related to the success each institution has had with specific treatment modalities. Radiosurgery is less effective for larger (>10cc) lesions.

STEREOTACTIC RADIOSURGICAL RESULTS

The efficacy of stereotactic radiosurgery is relatively uniform when compared across institutions using varied techniques and energy sources. Despite the uniformity of results, comments regarding incomplete patient follow-up in large patient populations and the impact this has on the statistical data are concerning (6). The obliteration rate with the linear accelerator at the University of Florida is 79% for lesions with volumes less than 10cc (3). Lesions greater than 10cc in volume were obliterated in 47% of the cases. The total obliteration rate with the gamma knife at the University of Pittsburgh is also dependent upon volume. In 222 patients, the authors describe a 61% obliteration rate. However, hemispheric lesions with volumes less than or equal to 4cc were obliterated in 83% of the cases (14). These authors also suggested that radiosurgery for AVMs was most successful in lesions with smaller volumes, younger patients, hemispheric lesions with single draining veins, lesions with a compact nidus, and no previous history of embolization. Heavy particles were also extremely effective for lesions less than 4cc with a reported obliteration rate of 100% (21). However, lesions with diameters greater than 3.7 cm had only a 70% obliteration rate. In a total of 128 patients treated at the Brigham and Women's Hospital/Harvard Medical School, 76% of the lesions were totally obliterated at 3 years. In summary, the overall obliteration rate, with all radiosurgical modalities, is near 80% at 3 years with probable higher efficacy for smaller lesions.

POTENTIAL COMPLICATIONS

Transient and permanent complications may occur after stereotactic radiosurgery and include hemorrhage prior to obliteration, temporary radiation effects, radiation necrosis, and, rarely, secondary tumors. Specific anatomic factors that may increase the risk for hemorrhage during the time to obliteration include small AVM size, deep venous drainage, associated aneurysms within the nidus or along feeding arteries, higher feeding artery pressures, and increasing age. The evidence is mixed whether radiosurgery affects the risk of posttreatment bleeding. During the latency interval, the first year after treatment in which no angiographic change is expected, there is no evidence for any change in hemorrhage risk. There is anecdotal clinical evidence for an increased hemorrhage risk in large AVMs, which are not completely irradiated, and the obliteration is incomplete. In contrast, the data are controversial regarding completely irradiated AVMs in which the obliteration is incomplete. There may be a stable hemorrhage risk during the latency period with a possible decrease in bleeding as partial obliteration progresses. Subtotal obliteration with disappearance of the nidus and persistence of an early draining vein seems to be associated with decreased hemorrhage risk (23). Total AVM obliteration provides complete protection from subsequent hemorrhage.

There are also transient effects on normal brain tissue in response to radiation treatment including acute reactions, early delayed reactions, and late reactions (9, 17). Acute side effects related to radiosurgery are caused by worsening intracranial edema and can be treated with steroids. In addition, an exacerbation of electrochemical activity with resultant seizures has been reported in approximately 5% of patients (4, 22). Early delayed reactions to radiation typically appear several weeks to a few months after treatment and can usually be managed conservatively (1). Late delayed reactions or symptomatic radiation necrosis has been reported in up to 3% of patients treated with radiosurgery (4). Other factors, such as minimum dose to the periphery of the AVM and dose/volume relationships, have been used to predict potential complications; however, they have not been uniformly applied at all centers (2, 10).

EMBOLIZATION AND RADIOSURGERY

The combination of therapies including embolization and radiosurgery have been suggested as a means to decrease the total nidus volume. Unfortunately, embolization rarely reduces the overall volume of the lesion. Rather, it decreases the density within a fixed volume and therefore is of limited benefit in the overall treatment plan for larger arteriovenous malformations. Prospective, multicenter studies on the use of fractionated therapy for larger lesions are needed.

CONCLUSIONS

After thorough review of the literature, it is apparent that AVMs that are difficult to treat by surgery are also difficult for stereotactic radiosurgeons. Thus, a team of physicians, including microvascular surgeons, radiosurgeons, and endovascular surgeons, is needed to assess each case individually. Essentially, AVM volume and location are the central factors in selecting the most appropriate treatment modality. Recent advances in imaging technology have improved our ability to accurately identify the nidus. Hopefully, this will improve the long-term results with stereotactic radiosurgery. For large AVMs, the utility of pretreatment embolization remains unclear. Fractionated schemes for these lesions also need greater evaluation.

Relative risk and cost analyses will usually favor microsurgical excision for smaller lesions. However, there are clearly locations such as the thalamus, basal ganglia, and brain stem in which surgery carries a significantly higher risk. Careful analysis by a team of physicians specializing in these lesions will lead to the selection of the best treatment option for the individual patient in a complimentary rather that competitive fashion.

REFERENCES

1. Flickinger JC, Kondziolka D, Pollack BE, Maitz AH, Lundsford LD: Complications from arteriovenous malformation radiosurgery: Multivariant analysis and risk modeling. **Int J Radiat Oncol Biol Phys** 38:485–490, 1997.
2. Flickinger JC: An integrated logistic formula for prediction of complications from radiosurgery. **Int J Radiat Oncol Biol Phys** 17:879–885, 1989.
3. Friedman WA: Radiosurgery vs surgery for arteriovenous malformations: The case for radiosurgery. **Clin Neurosurg** 45:18–20, 1997.
4. Friedman WA, Bova FJ, Mendenhill WM: Linear accelerator radiosurgery for arteriovenous malformations: The relationship of size to outcome. **J Neurosurg** 82:180–189, 1995.
5. Hamilton MG, Spetzler RF: The prospective application of a grading system for arteriovenous malformations. **Neurosurgery** 34:2–7, 1994.
6. Heffez DS, Osterdock RJ, Alderute L, Grutsch J: The effect of incomplete patient follow-up on the reported results of AVM radiosurgery. **Surg Neurol** 49:373–384, 1998.
7. Heros RC, Korosue K, Diebold PM: Surgical excision of cerebral arteriovenous malformations: Late results. **Neurosurgery** 26:570–578, 1990.
8. Kjellberg RN, Hanamura T, Davis KR, Lyons S, Butler W, Adams R: Bragg-Peak proton beam therapy for arteriovenous malformation of the brain. **N Engl J Med** 309:269–274, 1983.
9. Lampert PW, Davis RL: Delayed effects of radiation on the human central nervous system: Early and late delayed reactions. **Neurology** 14:912–917, 1964.
10. Lax I, Karlsson B: Prediction of complications in gamma knife radiosurgery of arteriovenous malformations. **Acta Oncol** 35:49–55, 1996.

11. Leksell L: The stereotactic method and radiosurgery of the brain. **Acta Chirurg Scand** 102:316–319, 1951.
12. Loeffler JS, Eben AI, Siddon RL, Saunders WM, Coleman CN, Winston KR: Stereotactic radiosurgery for intracranial arteriovenous malformations using a standard linear accelerator. **Int J Radiat Oncol Biol Phys** 17:673–677, 1989.
13. Pollack BE: Stereotactic radiosurgery for arteriovenous malformations. **Neurosurg Clin North Am** 10:281–290, April 1999.
14. Pollock BE, Flickinger JC, Lunsford LD, Maitz A, Kondziolka D: Factors associated with successful arteriovenous malformation radiosurgery. **Neurosurgery** 42:1239–1247, 1998.
15. Pollock BE, Lunsford LD, Kondziolka D, Maitz A, Flickinger JC: Patient outcomes after stereotactic radiosurgery for "operable" arteriovenous malformations. **Neurosurgery** 34:1–8, 1994. Volume 34.
16. Porter PJ, Shin AY, Dtsky AS et al: Surgery vs radiosurgery for small, operable cerebral arteriovenous malformations: A clinical and cost comparison. **Neurosurgery** 41:751–766, 1997.
17. Sheline GE, Wara WM, Smith V: Therapeutic radiation and brain injury. **Int J Radiat Oncol Biol Phys** 6:1215–1228, 1980.
18. Shulder M, Black PM, Alexander E III, Loeffler JS: The influence of Harvey Cushing on neuroradiologic therapy. **Radiology** 201:671–674, 1996.
19. Sisty MB, Kater A, Stein BM: Microsurgery for sixty seven intracranial malformations less than 3 cm in diameter. **J Neurosurg** 79:653–660, 1993.
20. Spetzler RF, Martin NA: A proposed grading system for arteriovenous malformations. **J Neurosurg** 65:476–483, 1986.
21. Steinberg GK, Fabrikant JI, Marks MP, Levy RP, Frankel KA, Phillips MH, Shuer LM, Silverberg GD: Stereotactic heavy: Charged: Particle Bragg: Peak radiation for intracranial arteriovenous malformations. **N Engl J Med** 323:96–101, 1990.
22. Steiner L, Lindquist C, Adler J, Horner J, Albes W, Steiner M: Clinical outcome of radiosurgery for arteriovenous malformations. **J Neurosurg** 77:1–8, 1992.
23. Steiner L, Lindquist C, Cail W, Karlsson B, Steiner M: Microsurgery and radiosurgery in brain arteriovenous malformations. **J Neurosurg** 79:647–652, 1993.

CHAPTER

14

Extracranial Carotid Lesions That Should Be Managed with Angioplasty and Stenting

CHRISTOPHER M. LOFTUS, M.D., FACS

We should begin a discussion of carotid stenting versus carotid surgery with a review of the indications for carotid treatment in symptomatic or asymptomatic patients. For the purpose of this discussion, I will avoid the use of the term "carotid surgery" and rather say "carotid treatment," although it must be remembered that the cooperative trials that we will discuss here compared surgery versus medical therapy and did not include endovascular treatment as part of their randomization or outcomes-based paradigm.

I offer carotid treatment to asymptomatic patients with greater than or equal to 60% stenosis, based on the results of the ACAS trial. I am cognizant of the fact that a tangible benefit was not demonstrated for women in this trial, and I have explained this to female patients considering carotid reconstruction. For symptomatic patients, I rely on the combined and corroborating results of the NASCET, ECST, and VASST trials, which determined conclusively that surgery was of benefit for patients with linear angiographic stenosis of greater than or equal to 50%. Surgery is of higher benefit for patients with linear angiographic stenosis of greater than or equal to 70%. Patients with stenosis less than 50% should not be offered surgical and/or endovascular treatment and are best managed with optimal medical therapy.

There are a number of other situations in which I offer carotid treatment to patients. The first of these encompasses the group of patients with so-called "stump syndromes" in which an internal carotid occlusion has left behind a residual carotid stump at the takeoff of the internal carotid from the cervical carotid bifurcation. Under these circumstances, if the patient has ipsilateral transient ischemic-type symptoms, and if all other potential sources of embolic phenomena are excluded, I offer treatment, customarily consisting of surgical intervention with common to external carotid endarterectomy and ligation of the offending stump with a large Weck clip or with hand-sewn plication of the carotid stump. This is a low-risk procedure that has a very tangible benefit if done properly and in the proper patients.

I offer surgery to symptomatic patients with recurrent carotid artery stenosis so long as they understand the higher risk/benefit ration inherent in such treatment. Asymptomatic patients with recurrent and progressing high-grade stenosis may well be offered treatment also, but the risk/benefit ratio in this group is higher still, and careful thought needs to be given to how the patient should be counseled.

For patients with intraluminal thrombus, as I have published elsewhere, I propose delayed treatment after a period of anticoagulation to dissolve the thrombus and make for a safer treatment, whether surgery or endovascular. In point of fact, I have never offered endovascular treatment to such a patient, and all patients after anticoagulation have been surgically reconstructed with excellent results.

Surgery for patients with recent stroke is not delayed in my practice unless there is a decreased level of consciousness or a large space-occupying infarct evident on axial cerebral imaging. The old wisdom that 6 weeks should elapse to allow autoregulation to be re-established in the brain is, in my mind, putting the patient at high risk for recurrent embolic phenomena, and I do not delay surgery except when the above criteria are invoked. Likewise, patients who are heparinized because of recent ischemic phenomena are maintained on full heparinization up to and through the time of surgery, and this has not in my practice produced any untoward hemorrhagic consequences either in the neck or intracranially.

We must then ask ourselves, in considering the dilemma of whether to offer carotid patients surgical reconstruction versus endovascular stenting, whether there is an outcomes-based reason to choose endovascular over surgical treatment. If we are going to make a rational comparison with these two treatment strategies, we need to consider and take into account the standard complications reported in carotid surgery to allow us to evaluate both treatment strategies in an equal light.

Outcome analysis in carotid reconstruction and carotid endovascular treatment is divided in the following way. The first consideration is perioperative stroke, and this event is customarily stratified into major or minor stroke and likewise ipsilateral or all-stroke. The second category to be considered is that of wound complications, meaning primarily hematoma or wound infection. The third category is nerve injury, and the fourth category is medical complications, most commonly perioperative myocardial infarction.

If we look at the surgical results from randomized cooperative trials, we see that the complication rates are gratifyingly quite low. In the

ACAS trial, the perioperative stroke and death rate was 2.3%. In the VA symptomatic surgery trial (VAAST), the 30-day mortality was 1.9%, all referable to myocardial infarction. The perioperative stroke rate was 2.4%. The nerve injury rate was 3.8%, and the rate of nonfatal myocardial infarction was likewise 1.9%.

In evaluating the results of symptomatic cooperative trials, we look first at the NASCET trial (9) where the 30-day mortality was 0.6%. The perioperative major stroke and death rate was 2.1%. The all-stroke rate was 5.5%. The nerve injury rate, evaluated by independent examiners, was 7.6%, the wound hematoma rate was 5.5%, and the myocardial infarction rate was 0.9%. In the ECST symptomatic cooperative trial (7), it is very difficult to tease out the major stroke or death rate because the data are presented in several different manuscripts. However, it seems to be quite variable depending on the stratification of percent stenosis being considered. In the 0.9% surgery group, the major death or stroke rate was 2.3%. In the 30 to 49% group it was 8%. In the 50 to 69% group it was 7.9%, and in the 70 to 99% group it was 3.7%. In the VASST trial (6), the 30-day mortality was 3.3%, the perioperative stroke rate was 2.2%, the nerve injury rate was 5%, the wound hematoma rate was 5%, and the myocardial infarction rate was 2%.

If we look at the results, cooperative trials customarily represent fixed observation points and evaluation by nonbiased observers. Randomized trial data are often felt to be the most valid and the highest level of evidence data that we have available to make therapeutic judgements. If we look at the published results of individual skilled carotid surgeons, we come up with data that shed a bit more of a favorable light on carotid reconstruction. It is to be recalled, nonetheless, that essentially all the major cooperative trials demonstrated that carotid artery surgery was superior to medical therapy despite their higher complication rates as compared with the results of individual surgeons.

Returning to the individual surgeon's published results category, the data published by Spetzler (10) for carotid microsurgery show that in 200 cases the all-stroke rate was 1%, the mortality was 0.5%, the wound hematoma rate was 1.5%, and the nerve injury rate was 5%. The data presented by Findlay (1) in carotid microsurgery document an all-stroke rate of 1.7%, a wound hematoma rate of 3.3%, and a nerve injury rate of 5.1%. The data presented by Steiger (11), again considering carotid microsurgery, document a perioperative stroke rate of zero, a myocardial infarction rate of 2%, a mortality of 2%, and a nerve injury rate of 2%.

The data presented by Harbaugh (2) employing regional anesthesia with loupe-magnified carotid reconstruction show an all-stroke rate of

2.5% with an ipsilateral rate of 1.3% and a major stroke rate of 0.9%. Harbaugh's myocardial infarction rate is 1.3%. The wound hematoma rate is 2.1%, and the nerve injury rate is 3%.

Finally, my own data representing conventional loupe-magnified carotid reconstruction, under general anesthesia and with Hemashield patch angioplasty in the second half of the series, show an all-stroke rate of 1.8% with a major stroke rate of 0.72%. My mortality rate is 0.72%, and my wound hematoma rate is 0.4% (5).

If you look then at the data from leading surgeons published on an individual basis with their own observations of complications, we find that the all-stroke rate is customarily less than 2.6%, the nerve injury rate is less than 5.1%, the mortality is less than 2%, and the wound hematoma rate varies between a low of 0.35% and a high of 3.35%.

We must then ask ourselves this question: which carotid lesions do endovascular specialists propose for treatment with stenting as an alternative to open surgical carotid reconstruction? The first article we should consider is that by Theron et al., stenting patients with primary stenosis (12). This paper discusses a protection scheme in about half the patients with distal balloon protection being employed during the stenting procedure. In total, 259 patients were treated, of which 136 underwent cerebral protection and 123 did not. In the unprotected cases, the rate of carotid dissection was 5%, and the rate of embolization was 8%. In the protected cases, no dissection was reported, and the embolization rate is 1%. Some of these patients were not stented but merely had angioplasty. In these authors' experience, stenting reduced the restenosis rate from 16% to 4%, and the authors' conclusion was that all patients undergoing endovascular carotid treatment should be stented and should be treated with cerebral protective strategies during the stenting process.

The second endovascular manuscript to be considered is that of Yadav et al. (13), in which 126 arteries were treated, all stented. There were seven minor strokes, two major strokes, and one death in this series. The stroke and death rate was 7.9% with an ipsilateral major stroke risk of 1.6%. The restenosis rate was quoted at 4.9%; all of these patients were asymptomatic. Yadav concluded that it was feasible to stent high-risk carotid patients who were not considered to be surgical candidates.

Interesting data are reported by Lanzino et al. (4) regarding recurrent carotid stenosis, and we point out that these data are in the neurosurgical literature. Lanzino and collaborators treated 25 arteries for recurrent stenosis with percutaneous angioplasty alone in seven patients and placement of a stent in 18 patients. There were no major neurologic or cardiac events. Complications were limited to one TIA and one femoral pseudo aneurysm. Lanzino et al. demonstrated that 60% of angioplasty-alone patients restenosed, and only one stent patient restenosed. Accordingly, their recommendation was first that the stenting procedure without protective strategies was safe for recurrent carotid stenosis and that stenting was far superior to angioplasty alone in the treatment of restenotic carotid disease.

A contrary viewpoint is presented by Naylor et al. (8) in the United Kingdom, who conducted a randomized trial of angioplasty/stenting versus carotid surgery. In this trial, 23 patients were randomized who had greater than or equal to 70% carotid stenosis. Seventeen of these patients were treated, 10 of whom had carotid surgery with no complications. Seven patients underwent either angioplasty or stent, and five of these patients had a stroke. This trial was prematurely stopped because of an extremely negative outcome in the endovascular side and has been reported as strong evidence to suggest that carotid surgery is superior to endovascular carotid treatment.

Non-atheromatous lesions such as fibromuscular dysplasia have also been studied with endovascular treatment. Hasso et al. (3) report three cases, all of which were symptomatic, that were treated with angioplasty alone in which no complications were evident. This is an extremely small series, but it represents essentially the only experience in the literature regarding the endovascular treatment of fibromuscular dysplasia.

Diethrich et al. discussed primary stenting for carotid surgery in 110 patients, treating 117 arteries. There were seven strokes (two major) for a stroke rate of 6.4%. Three patients were converted from endovascular treatment to open carotid artery surgery, with a rate of 2.7% for conversion. There were two deaths, one cardiac and one stroke, for a mortality of 1.8%. The 30-day angiographic success rate was 89.1%, and there was an 89% patency rate at 7.6 months follow-up in this series.

If endovascular treatment is to be considered, we should likewise ask this question: which lesions are there that the surgeon does not want to operate on? This brings to mind the question of what constitutes a high-risk carotid operation. I would put high-risk patients in several categories. The first consists of patients who have predictably difficult operations. The second consists of patients who are at a high risk for medical complications. The third consists of patients who are at a high risk for intraoperative ischemia, and the fourth consists of patients who, for anatomic or other reasons, are at high risk for postoperative occlusion and/or stroke.

Considering the first category, predictably difficult operations would include anatomic variants such as a medially directed internal carotid artery, a long and high carotid plaque, a high carotid bifurcation, or other anatomic anomalies such as cervical carotid aneurysm, which would render an operation significantly more difficult. Predictably difficult operations also include carotid reoperation, operation upon carotids that have been previously irradiated for other reasons, and cases in which distal exposure will be extremely high in the region of C1 or C2 on a lateral angiogram.

In the second category, patients at high risk for medical complication, I would include patients with recent myocardial infarction, patients with unstable angina, diabetic patients (who in my experience are at high risk for postoperative occlusion), patients with severe pulmonary disease rendering general anesthesia a major risk, and patients who require preoperative anticoagulation.

In the third category, those at high risk for intraoperative ischemia, I would include patients with contralateral occlusion, although in my experience this does not appreciably increase the risk. Patients who will have difficult or impossible shunt placement have a high risk for intraoperative ischemia if a shunt is required. This includes patients who have a right angle bend distal to the carotid plaque and in whom this bend cannot be straightened out through operative exposure, or patients who have a large cervical aneurysm that precludes placement of a shunt. High risk for intraoperative ischemia also includes patients with difficult cervical carotid exposures, patients who are neurologically unstable with a fluctuating deficit, and patients who have a propagating thrombus in the cervical carotid artery distal to an area of high-grade stenosis but who continue to have antegrade flow beyond the region of the thrombus.

Patients at high risk for postoperative occlusion and/or stroke include the following categories. Diabetic patients, in my experience, have a higher risk than normal for a postoperative occlusion, patients who experience postoperative hypotension seem to have a higher risk for carotid occlusion, patients in whom a repair is done high up in the internal carotid artery with consequent narrowing of the internal carotid are at high risk for occlusion, and patients who are hypertensive who experience dysautoregulation-type headache following reconstruction of a tight stenosis are at high risk for postoperative intracerebral hemorrhage. In my experience, most of these complications are avoided by the use of the Hemashield patch graft, which I now employ in every case.

Let me point out then the cases that I take particular pleasure and pride in reconstructing surgically. These include primary stenosis, recurrent stenosis, irradiated carotids, cases with previous cervical irradiation or radical neck dissection, contralateral occlusion, high exposures, and perhaps the most enjoyable of all, cases that are turned down by other surgeons and referred for tertiary care center specialty attention. In my opinion, all of these cases can be satisfactorily addressed with reasonable surgical morbidity and mortality by an experienced carotid surgeon with a careful management approach.

Cases I might send for stenting include the following. Cases of carotid dissection, which we previously treated with anticoagulation alone, may well be managed by a careful cannulation of the vessel and crossing of the lesion followed by placement of a stent. This, in my mind, represents a very significant advance over any surgical treatment or over anticoagulation alone as a therapeutic strategy. Cases with high cervical carotid aneurysms, beyond the reach of the surgeon, are well treated by stenting across the mouth of the lesion. Cases in which extreme high exposures are required at the base of the skull may well be better treated by stenting than by surgical exposure, particularly when one considers the risk of cranial nerve injury. Patients who are medically unstable with recent myocardial infarction are probably better off treated with endovascular treatment than with surgery, which entails an increased risk from general anesthesia. Finally, cases of fibromuscular dysplasia, which I customarily do not treat with surgery, may well be rational cases for an endovascular stenting approach.

In conclusion, it is my opinion that the endovascular versus surgical debate for carotid artery therapy and/or asymptomatic patients will continue for certainly the next 5 to 10 years, and most likely both treatments will ultimately enjoy some degree of acceptance. I would reiterate that at the present time only carotid artery surgery is proven by level one evidence to be superior to medical therapy, and endovascular treatment stands where we stood with carotid artery surgery approximately 15 years ago, leaving us to accept only the results of individual practitioners rather than any randomized data. This will not forever be the case, and randomized data will be available for surgery versus endovascular treatment in major centers, where presumably the lowest morbidity and mortality can be obtained in each camp by skilled practitioners of the art.

Trained, skilled carotid artery surgeons offer an excellent treatment for stroke prevention in symptomatic or asymptomatic patients. There is no documentation in literature for the superiority of endovascular treatment at the present time. However, I am quick to point out that selected cases, as I mentioned in the body of this work, may be more appropriately treated with endovascular strategies, and I personally refer patients for such treatment under special circumstances as mentioned, such as medically unstable patients, very high cervical carotid exposures, carotid dissection, and/or fibromuscular dysplasia. Individual referral patterns will depend on the surgeon's comfort with high-risk patients. For surgeons with lesser carotid experience or whose morbidity and mortality data may not be quite satisfactory, endovascular referrals may be an appropriate strategy. For surgeons with a large degree of experience and a high degree of comfort in handling the challenge of complex carotid reconstruction cases, carotid surgery continues to represent the only therapy proven by randomized trials to be superior to medical treatment in specific and selected patients.

REFERENCES

1. Findlay JM: Carotid microendarterectomy. **Neurosurgery** 32:792–798, 1993.
2. Harbaugh RE: Carotid surgery under local anesthesia. **Tech Neurosurg** 3:25–33, 1997.
3. Hasso AN, Bird CR, Zinke DE, Thompson JR: Fibromuscular dysplasia of the internal carotid artery: Percutaneous transluminal angioplasty. **Am J Radiol** 136:955–960, 1980.
4. Lanzino G, Mericle RA, Lopes DK, Wakhloo AK, Guterman LR, Hopkins LN: Percutaneous transluminal angioplasty and stent placement for recurrent carotid artery stenosis. **J Neurosurg** 90:688–694, 1999.
5. Loftus CM, Kresowik TF: Anatomical basis and technique of carotid endarterectomy, in Loftus C, Kresowik T (eds): *Carotid Artery Surgery.* New York, Thieme Medical Publishers, 2000.
6. Mayberg MR, Wilson E, Yatsu F, et al: Carotid endarterectomy and prevention of cerebral ischemia in symptomatic carotid stenosis. **JAMA** 266:3289–3294, 1991.
7. MRC European Carotid Study Trialists: Interim results for symptomatic patients with severe (70–99%) or with mild (0–29%) carotid stenosis. **Lancet** 337:1235–1243, 1991.
8. Naylor AR, Bolia A, Abbott RJ, et al: Randomized study of carotid angioplasty and stenting versus carotid endarterectomy: A stopped trial. **J Vasc Surg** 28:326–334, 1998.
9. North American Symptomatic Carotid Endarterectomy Trial Collaborators: Beneficial effect of carotid endarterectomy in symptomatic patients with high grade stenosis. **N Engl J Med** 325:445–453, 1991.
10. Spetzler RF, Martin N, Hadley MN, Thompson R, Wilkinson E, Raudzens P: Microsurgical endarterectomy under barbiturate protection: a prospective study. **J Neurosurg** 51:147–150, 1986.
11. Steiger H, Schaffler L, Liechti S: Results of microsurgical carotid endarterectomy. **Acta Neurochir** 100:31–38, 1989.
12. Theron JG, Payelle GG, Coskun O, Huet HF, Guimaraens L: Carotid artery stenosis: Treatment with protected balloon angioplasty and stent placement. **Radiology** 201:627–636, 1996.
13. Yadav JS, Roubin GS, Iyer S, et al: Elective stenting of the extracranial carotid arteries. **Circulation** 95:376–381, 1997.

III

General Scientific Session III Pediatric Update for the General Neurosurgeon

CHAPTER

15

Pediatric Brain Tumors: A Contemporary Prospectus

TODD G. MAINPRIZE, M.D., MICHAEL D. TAYLOR, M.D.,
JAMES T. RUTKA, M.D., PH.D., F.R.C.S.(C.)

INTRODUCTION

In the pediatric population, CNS tumors are second only to leukemia in frequency and have shown a modest, but statistically significant, increase in recent years (19). CNS tumors currently account for 21.7% of all pediatric cancer. Although mortality rates for brain tumors have decreased 20% in children since 1975, the rates for other childhood cancers have decreased well over 50%, making brain tumors the number one cause of cancer death in children (88).

Despite these numbers, pediatric tumors are generally more favorable than their counterparts in the adult population. Many of the astrocytic tumors are low grade, and many of the higher grade malignancies respond better to treatment than in adults. Lesions like craniopharyngioma, cerebellar astrocytomas and focal brainstem gliomas can be cured by the neurosurgeon, underscoring the importance of surgical treatment in pediatric brain tumors.

MEDULLOBLASTOMA

Medulloblastoma (MB) is the most common malignant brain tumor of childhood, accounting for 20 to 25% of all pediatric brain tumors. Ten to fifteen percent of CNS tumors in patients under the age of 20 are MB, with a peak incidence between 5 and 7 years of age. MB of childhood arise most commonly in the vermis and constitute 30% of all posterior fossa tumors (128, 135). Although considered primarily a pediatric malignancy, MB may also occur in adults where they arise more commonly in the cerebellar hemispheres. Most series report a male to female predominance between 1.4 and 4.8:1 (12, 46, 159).

Some authors have suggested that the incidence of MB has decreased in recent times. A report by Thorne et al. demonstrated a decrease from 5.5 cases per million to 2.8 cases per million in the combined southwestern and northern regions of England (150). Another report from Japan did not show a decline in the incidence of MB in the region of Hokkaido (98). It is possible that this may reflect the lower incidence of MB in Japan (85). Although no detailed epidemiologic data are available for North America, it is the impression of the senior author that the number of patients being treated for MB has decreased. Although Thorne et al. suggest that improved maternal vitamin supplementation may be the cause of the decreasing incidence, no conclusive evidence has been presented, and the etiology of any true reduction in incidence is unknown (150).

Clinical Presentation

In the era of modern neuroimaging, patients commonly present with a relatively short history. Approximately 80% of patients have symptoms for less than 3 months at the time of diagnosis (106). MB most commonly arises in proximity to the fourth ventricle from the anterior or posterior medullary velum and obstructs CSF flow, leading to patients presenting with signs and symptoms of increased intracranial pressure. Headache, from high ICP, is the most common symptom and is present in over 90% of cases. The clinical syndrome progresses to more frequent headaches, lethargy, vomiting, and ataxia as the intracranial pressure rises. Headaches often occur in the morning, may waken the child, and are often relieved by vomiting. Some authors feel that vomiting without a preceding headache is more characteristic of an ependymoma because of their propensity to arise from the area postrema in the floor of the fourth ventricle. Papilledema is present in most of the patients at the time of diagnosis. Cerebellar signs are usually present late. Gait or truncal ataxia is present in 62% of patients but is usually mild. Limb ataxia or dysmetria, present in about 44%, may indicate a lateral hemispheric tumor and is more common in cerebellar astrocytomas (106). Cranial nerve palsies are often present. Abducens or trochlear nerve palsies are usually secondary to hydrocephalus, but a unilateral VIth nerve palsy with an ipsilateral lower motor neuron VIIth paralysis indicates brainstem invasion. Occasionally, patients have a head tilt secondary to impaction of the cerebellar tonsils through the foramen magnum with compression of C1 and C2 nerve roots with reflex nuchal muscle spasm. This may also occur secondary to tumor growth down through the foramen magnum. In the small percentage of patients without hydrocephalus, incoordination and ataxia are usually the presenting symptoms, possibly because the mass is more lateral and does not obstruct CSF flow. Hemorrhage into the tumor may lead to a presentation similar to subarachnoid hemorrhage or as acute obstructive hydrocephalus. Spontaneous tumor hemorrhage can be seen in both primary and recurrent tumors and is present in up to 5.6% of cases (106). In about 5% of cases, symptoms referable to drop metastasis such as spinal cord compression/cauda equina syndrome or seizures may bring a patient to clinical attention (128).

Pathology

The term MB was first coined in 1925 by Cushing and Bailey, who described 29 patients with similar tumors they believed to be a type of glioma (8). The cell of origin of the MB has remained controversial for the last 75 years. Cushing and Bailey believed that the "medulloblast," a pleuripotential embryonal cell that can differentiate into spongioblasts or neuroblasts, was the cell of origin. Currently, there are three main hypotheses regarding the histogenesis of MB. Some believe that the cells of the external granule cell layer become transformed into malignant cells as they migrate around the rhombic lip and proliferate to give rise to the internal granule cell layer (155). The second concept, originally put forth by Rourke in 1983 and further revised in 1994, suggests that the MB arises from a primitive neuroectodermal cell found in the subependymal region. Accordingly, this is the same cell suggested to give rise to PNETs throughout the CNS (124, 162). The third hypothesis suggests that, depending on the location and subtype of the MB, the cell of origin varies between the ventricular matrix cells and the external granular cells (80, 157).

Macroscopically, the neoplasm is pinkish gray and variable in its consistency. CSF dissemination is common in MB, occurring in 20 to 50% of cases, manifesting at operation as a whitish, thickened arachnoid ("sugar-coating") over the exposed cerebellum.

Several histologic variants of MB are recognized. The classic MB (80%) is composed of sheets of "small blue cells" (*Fig. 15.1A*). These are round to oval cells with hyperchromatic nuclei, scant cytoplasm, frequent mitoses, a high nuclear-cytoplasmic ratio, and neuroblastic rosettes. These Homer-Wright rosettes indicate neuroblastic differentiation and are present in about 40% of MB. The second most common variant is the desmoplastic MB (15%). This variant is rich in collagen and reticulin and characteristically has reticulin-free nodules that appear as "pale islands." It is generally thought that this variant occurs in an older population, is found more frequently in the lateral hemispheres, and may have a better prognosis. Other variants include large cell MB (worse prognosis), medullomyoblastoma, melanotic MB, and lipomatous MB (much more favorable prognosis) (54). Recently, atypical teratoid/rhabdoid (ATT/R) tumors have been better characterized

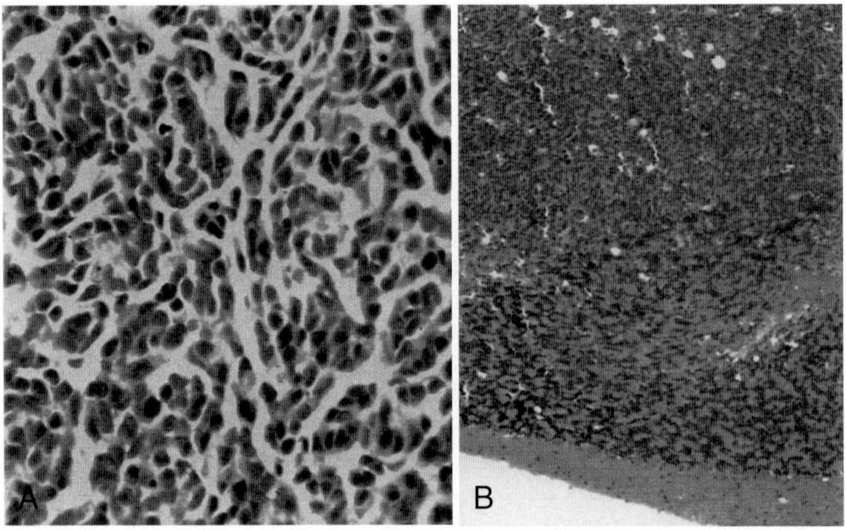

FIG. 15.1 (*A*) A high-power hematoxylin and eosin (H&E) stain of a human medulloblastoma demonstrating sheets of "small blue cells" and a high nuclear:cytoplasmic ratio. (*B*) A low-power H&E stain of a medulloblastoma-like tumor that developed in the cerebellum of a heterozygous *Patched* knock-out mouse.

and may represent another variant of MB diagnosed in young infants. ATT/R tumors resemble the large cell MB but have cells containing distinctive pink hyalinized cytoplasmic bodies that are desmin positive (125). Interestingly, many of these tumors have a deletion on chromosome 22q. Recently, a gene identified as hSNF5/INI1, which encodes a protein that aids in chromosomal remodeling, has been reported to be deleted in renal rhabdoid and brain tumors (14–16, 125, 127, 156). Due to the worse prognosis of these patients and the specific age group, some consider this a separate clinical and pathologic entity.

The MB can remain undifferentiated or differentiate into neuronal, glial, or ependymal lineages as shown by the immunohistochemical phenotype. Tumor cells with neuronal differentiation are often immunopositive for synaptophysin and neuron-specific intermediate filaments (neurofilaments). With glial differentiation, there is expression of glial fibrillary acid protein (GFAP). There may be immunopositivity for vimentin and nestin, both indicating a less differentiated state.

Certain pathologic findings have been shown to correlate with outcome. The literature has shown a lack of correlation between outcome and histologic features such as necrosis, nuclear atypia, vascular proliferation, and mitotic index (74). The desmoplastic variant of MB may have an improved survival, whereas the large cell MB is more aggressive. MBs that express GFAP have an increased 5-year survival from 30 to 82% (57). Tumors that express low amounts of the neurotrophin-3 receptor, TrkC, have a worse prognosis than those that expressed high levels (82, 138). Expression of rhodopsin and retinal S-antigen may herald a better prognosis (31, 89). Loss of heterozygosity at 17p has been correlated with a poor response to therapy as well as decreased survival in the "standard risk" group of patients (29).

Etiology

For the majority of cases of MB, the cause remains to be discovered. Many clues as to the molecular biology of MB have been obtained through studies of familial syndromes and cytogenetics.

Chromosomal analysis of tumor specimens has demonstrated several recurrent, consistent, cytogenetic abnormalities. The most common change, present in almost 50% of tumors, is a deletion of the short arm of chromosome 17 resulting in an isochromosome 17q (17). Although isochromosome 17q is the most common mechanism for loss of 17p (a region known to contain tumor suppressor genes), there are cases of unbalanced translocations and monosomy 17. Various alterations in chromosome 1 are also frequent and include deletions, translocations, duplications, and trisomy 1q (17). Other cytogenetic changes described include deletions in 9q, 6q, 10q, 11p, 11q, 16q, and 22q (13). These karyotypic abnormalities point to loci encoding possible genes important in the malignant transformation of MB.

Evans reported in 1993 that 6.4% of 173 consecutive patients with MB had evidence of a genetic syndrome or a congenital anomaly (43). Several inherited conditions predispose affected individuals to a high risk of developing MB. Gorlin's syndrome is an autosomal dominant disorder in which affected individuals have multiple basal cell carcinomas, jaw cysts, macrocephaly, rib abnormalities, dural calcifications, meningiomas, and MBs. Approximately 3 to 5% of patients with Gorlin's syndrome will develop an MB, often at a very young age (44). The gene mutated in Gorlin's syndrome families was identified as the human homolog of the *Drosophila melanogaster Patched* gene. The *Patched* gene is located on the long arm of chromosome 9, a locus frequently deleted in MB. Mutations in *Patched* have been subsequently demonstrated in sporadic MBs and mice with heterozygous for *Patched* develop MB-like lesions (*Fig. 15.1B*). The protein product of the *Patched* gene is the receptor for *Sonic Hedgehog* (*SHH*), an important morphogen and mitogen of the developing brain. *SHH* is a powerful mitogen for cells of the external granular cell layer of the cerebellum, consistent with a role in MB pathogenesis (58). Other downstream genes in this signaling pathway are currently being investigated as to a possible role in MB tumorogenesis. Concurrent neuroepithelial tumors (most commonly glioblastoma and MB) and multiple colorectal neoplasms occur in Turcot's syndrome. This is an autosomal dominant disorder that is divided in two groups, those with familial adenomatous poliposis (FAP) and those with hereditary non-polyposis colorectal carcinoma (HNPCC). The first variant is due to a mutation in the *APC* gene found on chromsome 5q21. These patients are at a 92-fold risk of developing an MB as compared with the general population (66). *APC* is part of the WNT signaling pathway, which, similar to the *SHH* pathway, is important in embryonic development. *APC* normally functions in conjunction with several other molecules of this pathway to degrade beta-catenin, an activator of transcription of various genes including c-myc and cyclin D1 (25, 77). Although no mutations in *APC* have been described in sporadic MB, a minority of tumors have mutations in beta-catenin (166). Other hereditary syndromes that lead to an increased risk of MB include Li-Fraumeni syndrome (p53 germline mutation, 17p) and Rubinstein-Taybi syndrome. Recently, our laboratory has found a family affected by posterior fossa brain tumors over multiple generations, including both ATT/R tumor and choroid plexus carcinoma (see "Choroid Plexus Tumors").

Radiologic Diagnosis

Classically, with non-contrast CT scans, the MB appears as a well circumscribed, hyperdense, vermian lesion displacing the fourth ventricle anteriorly that enhances homogeneously and densely with contrast administration. The hyperdensity of this lesion is thought to be secondary to the high nuclear-cytoplasmic ratio. Obstructive hydrocephalus is common. Approximately 15% of these tumors contain calcifications (18). "Atypical" CT features of MB that are nevertheless quite common include cystic changes (65%), isodensity on plain CT (3%), and absent contrast enhancement (3%) (101).

MRI has improved the ability to visualize the extent of the tumor and the distorted regional anatomy. Generally, the MB fills the fourth ventricle, is heterogeneously hypointense to white matter on T1-weighted image, but can be hypo-, iso-, or hyperintense to surrounding white matter with T2-weighted images. Gadolinium enhancement is less consistent than with CT enhancement and is usually moderately intense and heterogeneous, occasionally showing partial enhancement. These imaging characteristics are more diverse in older children and adults.

As up to 50% of patients have evidence of leptomeningeal spread of disease, full craniospinal imaging is mandatory in those suspected of harboring an MB. Initial cranial CT scan may detect up to 30% with CSF spread; however, gadolinium-enhanced MRI is more sensitive in discovering small lesions (*Fig. 15.2*) (18). Gadolinium-enhanced MRI has become the imaging modality of choice, replacing the CT-myelogram, as it is non-invasive and demonstrates small nodularity and pial sheeting. If preoperative spinal imaging was not possible, a postoperative MRI should be performed at least 2 weeks following surgery to allow the blood products in the CSF time to resolve. Postoperative MRI of the resection site is recommended within 48 hours after surgery to assess the amount of residual tumor at a time when imaging artifacts are minimal.

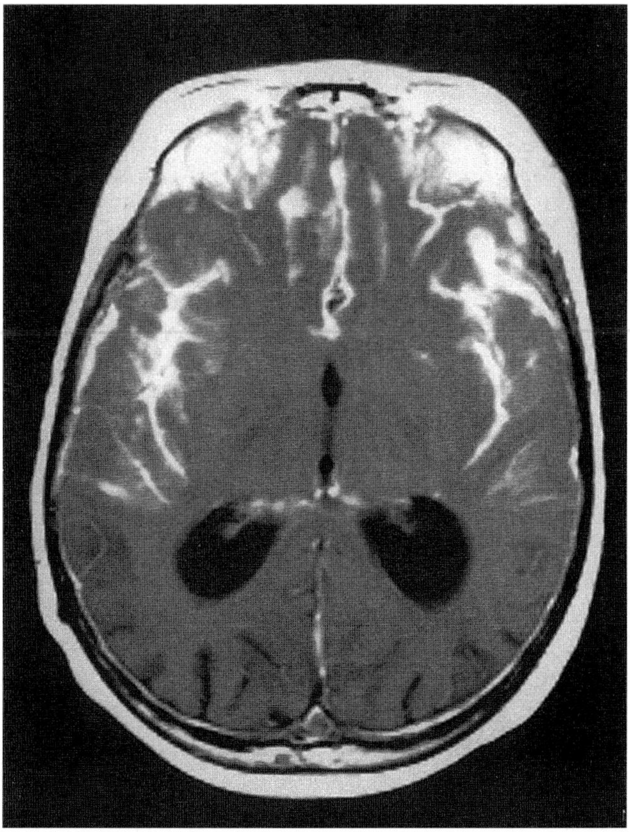

FIG. 15.2 An axial T1-weighted MRI with gadolinium contrast enhancement demonstrating diffuse CSF seeding in a recurrent medulloblastoma.

Surgical Management

MANAGEMENT OF HYDROCEPHALUS

The vast majority of patients with MB present with associated hydrocephalus. In the past, these patients would undergo a procedure for CSF diversion (VP shunt) prior to having the tumor tackled directly. In the experience of the senior author and others, preoperative CSF diversion is rarely needed except in the setting of acute hydrocephalus (most commonly secondary to intratumoral hemorrhage and sudden blockage of CSF ventricular outflow) (56, 128). In most cases, raised ICP is chronic and can be ameliorated with the use of steroids as a temporizing measure for 2 to 3 days. In addition, there are specific risks to shunting patients with an MB and hydrocephalus. With decompression of the ventricular system, an increased pressure differential between the supratentorial and infratentorial compartments may be created that may lead to tumor shifting and intratumoral hemorrhage, which may be associated with "upward herniation" and further brainstem compression.

Between 25 and 30% of postoperative MB patients become shunt dependent long-term (33). Several risk factors for postoperative shunt dependency include younger patients, larger residual tumor, large preoperative ventricles, aseptic meningitis, and open dura (10, 33). In the early period, they present with progressive symptoms of raised intracranial pressure or a psuedomeningocele. If the wound has not fully healed, a CSF leak may develop. Generally, both a pseudomeningocele and a CSF leak can be treated with repeat lumbar punctures or lumbar drain insertion; however, a small percentage of these patients will require permanent CSF diversion. Third ventriculostomy is becoming a more frequently performed procedure in these patients to avoid insertion of foreign material (28).

OPERATIVE MANAGEMENT

The goals of surgery include obtaining a tissue diagnosis, reestablish CSF circulation, and resect as much tumor as is safe. As there is a correlation between amount of tumor resection and outcome, maximally safe tumor extirpation should be attempted.

Patients are positioned prone on bolsters with pressure points well padded. In patients older than 4 years of age, rigid head fixation in pins is preferred. Between the ages of 2 and 4 years of age, rigid pin fixation can still be used, but with caution because of the thin skull. Children under the age of 2 should have their head placed on a padded horseshoe. Concorde position is useful in obtaining optimal access to tumors of the superior vermis and the tentorial hiatus.

A midline exposure is the best approach to vermian cerebellar lesions. The senior author prefers occipital craniotomies over craniectomies as they are no more difficult, produce better cosmetic results, and decrease postoperative pain. The dura is incised in a Y-shape fashion. Attention must be paid to both the occipital and circular sinuses. These venous structures can be taken without risk even though they are generally larger in infants and can bleed significantly unless proper consideration is given. Electrocautery is the best method to achieve hemostasis as hemostatic clips will lead to artifact on the postoperative MRI. Once the cerebellum is exposed, the neurosurgeon should inspect the region for evidence of leptomeningeal disease. The inferior vermis is split, and the cerebellum is gently retracted away from the tumor as a plane is developed between it and the normal tissue. When the fourth ventricle is entered, care should be taken to find the floor. If the floor is not involved with tumor, cottonoids are used to protect it from surgical manipulation. As up to 36% of MBs invade the brainstem, it is important to resect only the part of the tumor that projects beyond the floor to minimize postoperative neurologic deficits (106). If there is no evidence of brainstem invasion, then gross total resection should be attempted. The tumor margins should be inspected thoroughly before closure.

Both the Children's Cancer Study Group and the Pediatric Oncology Group recommend a postoperative MRI within the first 48 hours to assess the amount of residual tumor. Some advocate a second-look craniotomy if the amount of residual tumor is more than 1.5 cm^2, as this puts the patient into the "high-risk" group (see below). Approximately 80% of patients have resection of >90% of their tumor (6).

With improvements in neuro-anaesthesia and surgical techniques, operative mortality has decreased to about 1 to 2%. Surgical morbidity remains significant, as up to 41% of patients with MB will develop an increased neurologic deficit postoperatively with only 14% resolving completely. Cerebellar mutism occurs between 5 and 30% of patients. Although the pathophysiology is not fully known, it has been suggested to result from splitting the inferior vermis (42).

Staging and Risk Segregation

Patients are staged postoperatively according to the Chang Staging System based on tumor size (T) as well as presence and extent of metastases (M). The metastatic stage is more prognostic.

Based on patient age, size of residual tumor, and presence of metastases, patients are divided into two groups. Patients are considered low risk if they are older than 3 years of age, have a residual tumor of less than 1.5 cm^2, and have no evidence of tumor dissemination by cytology or imaging. On the other hand, high-risk patients are younger than 3, have residual tumor >1.5 cm^2, and have leptomeningeal spread.

Adjuvant Therapy

Of the patients originally described by Cushing and Bailey, the mean survival was 5.5 months. In 1953, full craniospinal radiation was demonstrated to increase the 5-year survival to approximately 50% (107). Since this time, radiation therapy (RT) has played a major role in the treatment of MB. Currently, patients older than 3 years of age receive 3500 Rads of craniospinal radiation and 5500 Rads to the posterior fossa (128). If metastases are present, a boost of radiation is given regionally to equal the dose given to the primary site (78).

To increase progression-free survival (PFS) and overall survival (OS), several trials used various combinations of chemotherapy as postirradiation adjuvant treatment. A phase III trial published by the Children's Cancer Group in 1991 helped to usher in the era of risk-stratified therapy. The 5-year PFS and OS for those treated with RT alone (50% and 65%, respectively) as compared with those receiving RT and chemotherapy (59% and 65%, respectively) was not statistically significant. However, a subgroup of patients with high-risk criteria had an improved outcome with combined RT and chemotherapy. Those given RT and chemotherapy had a 5-year PFS and OS of 46% and 57%, respectively, versus 0% and 19% 5-year PFS and OS, respectively, for those treated with radiation alone. As a consequence, it is now standard therapy for high-risk patients to receive postirradiation chemotherapy. At the HSC in Toronto, current chemotherapy consists of the ICE regimen: iphosphamide, carboplatinum, and etoposide.

Radiation therapy has been shown to have significant side-effects in long-term survivors, especially in children under the age of 3. During and after radiation therapy, IQ can drop 3.9 points per year (159). Furthermore, radiation can lead to endocrinopathies, moyamoya syndrome, and secondary radiation-induced malignancies. Currently, postoperative chemotherapy is given to patients under the age of 3 years to delay adjuvant radiation therapy, giving the immature brain time to develop (38).

In an attempt to minimize the sequelae of craniospinal radiation in standard-risk patients, the Children's Cancer Group and the Pediatric Oncology Group performed a randomized trial comparing the standard 3500 Rads to 2340 Rads. Unfortunately, the study had to be terminated within 16 months because of the increased incidence of leptomeningeal failure in the low-dose arm of the trial (32). Recently, a prospective study comparing standard-dose radiation with low-dose radiation and chemotherapy had to be closed because of poor patient enrollment (52).

Recurrent Medulloblastoma

Medulloblastoma most commonly recurs in the posterior fossa, but may recur in other sites of the neuroaxis such as the basal cisterns, the subfrontal subarachnoid space, ventricular system, spinal cord, or cauda equina. Systemic metastases have been reported in the bone, lymph nodes, lungs, and liver. Once MB recurs following radiation and chemotherapy, there is very little chance of prolonged remission. Autologous bone marrow transplantation is advocated in some centers permitting the use of higher dosages of chemotherapy than would otherwise be tolerated. Other centers are using radiosurgery to treat localized recurrences with a reported median survival of 10 months (161).

Attempts at surveillance in the hopes of detecting recurrences early have not proved to be of benefit, as most of the recurrences were missed (151).

Prognosis

Survival data between 1980 and 1989 were reviewed at the Hospital for Sick Children in Toronto. Of the 50 patients treated, 26 were considered low risk and 24 were high risk. The 5-year survival for the low-risk group was 70% as compared to 40% for the high-risk group. However, a non-randomized study published 5-year survival rates for high-risk patients in excess of 80% when given standard craniospinal radiation with adjuvant cisplatinum, CCNU, and vincristine. Patients with metastatic disease at the time of diagnosis had a 5-year PFS of 67% compared to 90% in those with local disease (103). This points to the possibility of improving outcomes in standard-risk patients by initially treating them with radiation and chemotherapy.

INTRACRANIAL EPENDYMOMAS

Ependymomas comprise between 2 and 6% of all intracranial neoplasms and between 5 and 10% of childhood brain tumors (112). They are the third most common primary brain tumor in children after MB and astrocytoma. The peak incidence is in the first 3 years of life, where ependymomas may account for up to 30% of tumors. There is a slight male prevalence with a male to female ratio of 1.4:1. The tumor is located infatentorially in 60 to 70% of cases, the vast majority being midline. This location is much more common in young children, the supratentorial compartment being involved more commonly in older children and adults. Half of the supratentorial tumors are found adjacent to the ventricular surface.

Ependymomas may spread via the CSF. There is considerable controversy in the literature regarding how common ependymomas disseminate throughout the spinal fluid compartment. An autopsy report found CSF seeding in 30% of cases (all from infratentorial tumors), whereas some large clinical studies have reported dissemination in 3 to 9% of cases (up to 23% in infratentorial tumors) (36, 113).

Clinical Features

Children present with a median 3-month history of symptoms prior to diagnosis. The presenting features depend on the location of the mass. Because of the propensity for this tumor to occur in the region of the fourth ventricle, patients present with symptoms of a midline posterior fossa lesion similar to those with MB (see "Medulloblastoma"). Headache secondary to obstructive hydrocephalus is usually an early finding, progressing to nausea, vomiting, and finally lethargy. Patients may have vomiting without antecedent headache or significantly raised ICP, as ependymal tumors can arise from the area postrema.

Ependymomas grow through the foramen of Lushka more frequently than MBs. Patients may present with a clinical syndrome referable to the cerebellopontine angle including facial paresis, hearing loss, and swallowing difficulties. Between 20 and 50% of children with ependymomas have extension of the tumor into the cervical subarachnoid space. Accordingly, these patients may present with neck pain, nuchal rigidity, head tilt, and torticollis.

Patients with tumors in the supratentorial compartment present with seizures, hemiparesis, speech difficulties, and cranial nerve deficits. Increased ICP with headaches, nausea, vomiting, and papilledema occur when the tumor reaches large sizes.

Pathology

Ependymomas are glial tumors that generally arise adjacent to the ventricles and are composed predominantly of neoplastic ependymal cells. The WHO defines two grades of ependymal tumors, the ependymomas (WHO grade II) and anaplastic ependymomas (WHO grade III).

Macroscopically, they are pinkish gray and have a soft consistency. They tend to be vascular, but not to the degree of MB. Ependymomas can be cystic or solid with or without foci of necrosis. They can be lobulated or even grossly papillary, resembling choroid plexus tumors. Unlike the other glial tumors, ependymomas are often well circumscribed and solid, tending to displace the brain instead of invading through the parenchyma.

Ependymomas are moderately cellular tumors. The nuclei are monotonous and uniform, moderately hyperchromatic, vary from round to oval, and have small but distinct nucleoli. The two most characteristic findings on light microscopy are perivascular pseudorosettes and ependymal rosettes (*Fig. 15.3*). Perivascular pseudorosettes consist of ependymomas cells arranged circumferentially around blood vessels with cytoplasmic projections toward the vessel creating a distinctive "nuclear-free zone" around vessels. The actual diameter of the pseudorosettes varies from tumor to tumor, but they are present in the vast majority. On the other hand, true ependymal rosettes are both difficult to find and are far less common.

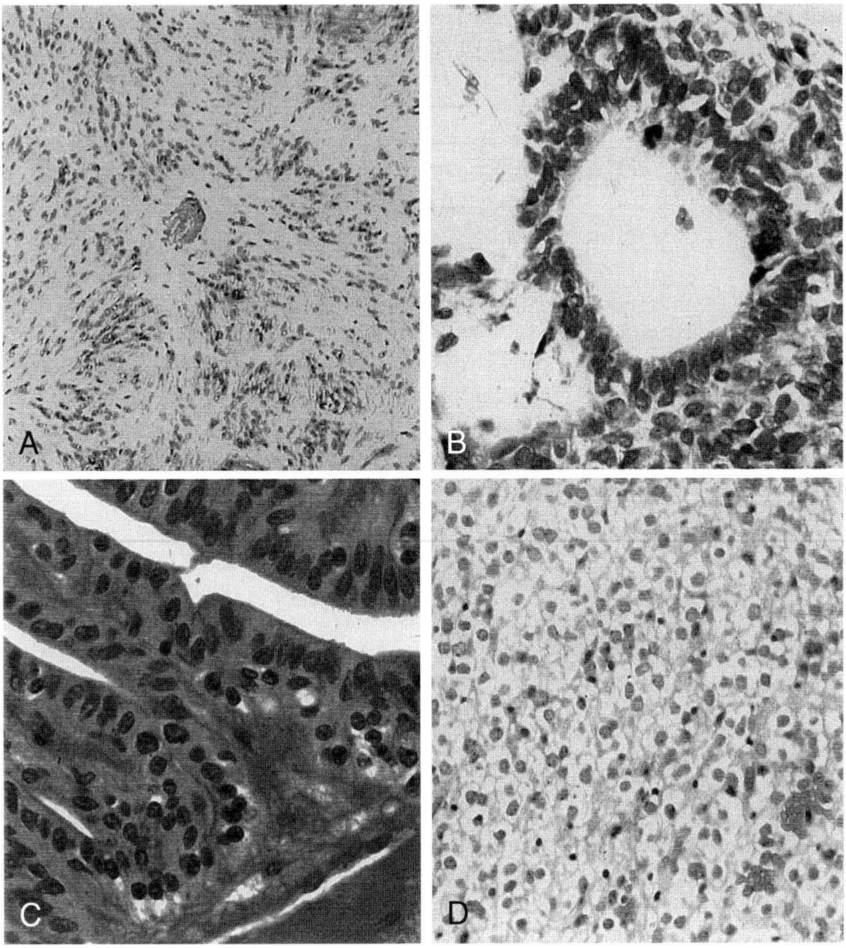

FIG. 15.3 (*A*) A medium-power H&E stain of a tanycytic ependymoma demonstrating perivascular pseudorosetting. This tumor can be confused histologically with an astrocytoma because of the elongated spindle shape of the cells. (*B*) A high-power H&E stain showing a true ependymal rosette. The cells arrange themselves in a circle with a ciliated luminal border. (*C*) Ependymomas can form a papillary architecture. (*D*) Clear cell ependymomas can histologically appear similar to oligodendrogliomas and central neurocytomas on H&E staining.

They consist of ependymal cells oriented circumferentially around a central canal. These lining cells may in fact be ciliated like the ventricular lining. Ultrastructurally, ependymomas have evidence of cilia, microvilli, and blepharoplasts at the apical surface and zonula adherens laterally.

Immunohistochemically, ependymomas are focally positive for GFAP, positive for S-100 antigen, and can stain positively for EMA at the luminal surface of the ependymal rosettes.

Four variants of ependymomas have been described: classic, papillary, tanycytic, and clear cell. There are no prognostic differences between the different histologic patterns, but they may resemble other tumors and must be kept in mind when formulating the differential diagnosis. The classic or cellular ependymomas is the most common. They typically are more cellular with fewer pseudorosettes and rare ependymal rosettes. Papillary ependymoma is a rare variant that morphologically resembles choroid plexus tumors (*Fig. 15.3*). Fronds of tissue are lined by epithelia-like ependymal cells and rest on a vascular core, but they lack a basement membrane. The clear cell ependymoma resembles both oligodendroglioma and central neurocytoma (*Fig. 15.3*). Immunohistochemistry for GFAP and synaptophsyin as well as electron microscopy can differentiate between these tumors. The tanycytic ependymoma is thought to arise from tanycytes. These tumors have a more astrocytic phenotype with elongated nuclei, long processes, and indistinct pseudorosettes. This can be a difficult diagnosis and may necessitate electron microscopy.

If significant nuclear pleomorphism, high cellular density, high proliferative index/mitotic rate, necrosis, and vascular endothelial proliferation are present, the diagnosis is anaplastic ependymomas (WHO grade III). Anaplastic ependymomas account for up to 25% of all intracranial ependymomas.

Etiology

A study in 1992 looking at the expression of large T-antigen from the polyoma virus SV40 demonstrated DNA sequences for the virus in 10 of 11 pediatric ependymomas. Furthermore, immunohistochemical analysis showed nuclear staining in three of six ependymomas investigated (11). Large T-antigen is an oncogenic protein produced by the SV40 virus that binds to and inactivates the tumor suppressor gene p53. It is hypothesized that expression of large T-antigen may in fact lead to neoplastic transformation. When hamsters were inoculated with SV40 virus, they developed ependymomas (83). The actual role that this protein plays in carcinogenesis in humans remains uncertain.

Ependymomas demonstrate complex and recurrent cytogenetic abnormalities. Chromosome 22 is most commonly affected (30%). Monosomy 22 is the most frequent change, although deletions and translocations of 22q have been documented. Several studies have shown mutations in the NF-2 gene, *merlin,* in sporadic ependymomas. A recent study reported that all the ependymomas with *merlin* mutations were spinal (40, 63). Losses of chromosome 17p have been found in 50%; however, mutations of the p53 tumor suppressor gene are rare, suggesting that undiscovered tumor suppressor genes may be present at this locus. Other chromosomes commonly involved in ependymomas are 6q, 9q, 10, and 13 (65, 117). Ependymomas have been reported in patients with Turcot's syndrome, multiple endocrine neoplasia, NF-2, and Li-Fraumeni syndrome (133).

Radiologic Diagnosis

CT findings of infratentorial ependymomas are variable. They are usually isodense on non-contrast CT scan with calcifications occurring in up to 50% of tumors. They are heterogeneous with cysts and necrotic areas appearing hypodense; evidence of hemorrhage can be seen in over 10%. Seventy percent of tumors demonstrate mild to moderate inhomogeneous contrast enhancement (101). Hydrocephalus is almost an invariable finding with fourth ventricular tumors.

MRI scans can help to differentiate between ependymomas and other glial tissues by location and morphology, not by signal differences. Typically, the tumor fills the fourth ventricle and may have a rim of peritumoral edema or CSF signal. They have a lobulated appearance and can extrude through the foramen of Luscka and Magandie into the cerebellopontine angle and cervical subarachnoid space. The MRI scan must extend down the cervical cord to adequately visualize the inferior extent of the tumor to aid in surgical planning. Vessels in this region may be encased up to 30% (152). The solid components of the tumor are hypo- to isointense compared to brain on a T1-weighted image and hyperintense on a T2-weighted image. Moderate inhomogeneous enhancement is seen with gadolinium injection. Supratentorial ependymomas generally are found intraparenchymally with abutment to the ventricular system. They are very difficult to differentiate from astrocytomas and commonly have ring-enhancing patterns.

As already discussed above, a postoperative MRI should be obtained within 48 hours after surgical resection.

Management

SURGERY

As with MB surgery, the goals of the operation are to establish a tissue diagnosis, to reestablish CSF flow, and to resect as much of the tumor as possible. Studies have shown that the extent of resection is a strong prognostic factor for both progression-free survival and overall survival.

For ependymomas originating in the fourth ventricle, a prone or Concorde position is used, even if there is extension into the cerebellopontine angle. If the tumor originates for the foramen of Luschka or the cerebellopontine angle, then a lateral decubitus position is favored. For fourth ventricular tumors, a midline suboccipital incision is used to gain exposure from the inion down to the posterior elements of the upper cervical spine. Preoperative radiologic imaging will aid in deciding the inferior extent of the incision. The tumor can usually be identified once the tonsils have been retracted gently. Although ependymomas are not truly encapsulated, they are often discrete and do not invade into the surrounding nervous tissue. The general approach is to debulk the core of the tumor and then to dissect the wall of the tumor from the adjacent normal tissue. A plane can be created between tumor and nervous tissue to the area of attachment. Care must be taken when removing the attachment, as it generally originates from the region of the obex and area postrema; if disturbed, it may lead to swallowing difficulties and sleep apnea. If there is attachment to the brainstem or the cerebellar peduncle, caution is exercised to avoid causing significant neurologic deficits. As the tumor exits the foramen of Luschka and enters the cerebellopontine and cervical subarachnoid spaces, various vessels such as PICA and the vertebral arteries may become encased, leading to significant postoperative complications if not recognized.

For tumors of the supratentorial compartment, craniotomy for the specific location is undertaken. Generally speaking, more complete resections can be achieved in the supratentorial compartment than in the infratentorial compartment.

As with MBs, an MRI scan should be obtained within 48 hours postoperatively to assess the residual tumor. Forman et al. recommend a second-look procedure for residual tumor that is potentially resectable (49).

Surgery alone has historically given 5-year survival rates of 17 to 27%. These studies represented all ranges of histologic grade and degree of postoperative resections. Studies have demonstrated that routine postoperative radiation may not be required for those tumors with radiologic evidence of gross total resection. A report published in 1990 showed that for intramedullary ependymomas, complete resection without radiation leads to a mean progression-free survival of 62 months (93). A study of eight supratentorial and two infratentorial ependymomas demonstrated a 48-month progression-free survival of 70%. The three relapses (one posterior fossa and three supratentorial ependymomas) went on to receive either further resection or further resection and radiotherapy (75). The role of surgery without radiation is currently uncertain, and many centers would treat all postoperative patients with a course of radiation therapy.

ADJUVANT THERAPY

Several studies have shown the benefit of radiation therapy in prolonging overall and progression-free survivals. For those patients older than 4 years of age, 5-year PFS are in the order of 45 to 60% (139, 146). A recently published retrospective review of 63 cases of ependymoma demonstrates a significant benefit to patients receiving postoperative radiation therapy. Progression-free survival for those not receiving radiation therapy was 0% in 5 years as compared to 45% for the irradiated group. The 5-year survival rates were also significantly higher for those receiving radiation (63% versus 23%) (126).

Because of the frequency with which ependymomas disseminate thorough the CSF space, studies were undertaken to see if prophylactic craniospinal irradiation would increase survival and progression-free survival. These studies have shown that craniospinal irradiation should only be pursued if there is dissemination at time of presentation (126).

Because of the toxicity of radiation to the developing brain, children under the age of 3 receive postoperative chemotherapy to delay the need for radiation. This is effective in up to 30 to 48% (38, 91).

Hyperfractionated radiotherapy is used to increase the dose of radiation and decrease the damage. Up to 80% 5-year PFS rates have been reported if the ependymoma is completely resected and followed by chemotherapy, suggesting that good control rates may be achieved with very radical treatment and combined therapies.

The role of chemotherapy in ependymoma for patients over the age of 3 is yet to be defined and will require large, multicentered trials (21).

Prognostic Factors

To stratify patients into treatment groups and ensure that those at high risk of recurring or progressing receive the most intensive therapies, studies have reported various prognostic factors in ependymomas. The age at presentation has been associated with a worse prognosis. Those younger than 3 years of age have 5-year PFS and overall survivals of 12 and 22%, respectively, compared with 60 and 75% rates in older children (113). This may have been a reflection of the overall tumor biology as younger patients have more anaplastic disease, which disseminates more commonly. Some reports find an association with poorer survival and disseminated disease at the time of presentation, whereas others have not found this correlation (113, 119). The location of the tumor as a prognostic factor has long been a point of debate with reports indicating a correlation with better survival for supratentorial compartments, infratentorial compartments, or for neither. Histologic grade has been associated with worse prognosis; however, this is not a universal finding (113, 119). Those with symptoms for less than 1 month tend to fair worse that those with symptoms greater than 1 month (33% versus 64% 5-year survival) (113).

The most significant factor correlating with survival is the extent of the surgical resection. Those with residual tumor have 5-year PFS and overall survival of 8.9% and 22%, respectively. If there is complete resection as seen radiologically, these numbers improve to 68% and 80%, respectively, underscoring the need to fully resect these tumors when able (113). Up to 30% of intracranial ependymomas can be completely resected (39).

Recurrence

The vast majority of ependymomas recur locally; however, there may be a component of leptomeningeal dissemination that precludes any attempt at a second local resection. For this reason, complete preoperative neuroradiologic studies with contrast enhancement should be performed. Patients with recurrences very rarely have long-term control. Treatment options include further surgery, radiosurgery, and chemotherapy. The role of surveillance imaging has not been elucidated for ependymomas, and several centers perform scans at regular intervals.

CEREBELLAR ASTROCYTOMA

Cerebellar astrocytomas occur in the pediatric population much more commonly than in adults. They comprise about 15% of CNS tumors in this population and are responsible for 25 to 30% of childhood posterior fossa tumors. Of all cerebellar astrocytomas, 70% occur in children. There is a peak incidence at 6 to 8 years of life, with a mean age of 7.3 years and a slight male predominance (1).

Histologically, benign pilocytic astrocytomas generally comprise about 80% of these tumors, with diffuse fibrillary astrocytomas accounting for the remaining 20% (67, 104). The pilocytic astrocytoma occur in a younger age group, are more commonly cystic in nature, and have a better outcome.

Clinical Presentation

Patients generally have symptoms between 5 and 9 months before diagnosis, but this is decreasing with improved neuroimaging. Because of the slow growing nature of cerebellar astrocytomas, the duration of symptoms before diagnosis is longer than with ependymomas and MBs.

As with the other cerebellar tumors described, astrocytomas most commonly present with symptoms and signs of hydrocephalus (>75%). Cerebellar ataxia and gait disturbances occur more often in cerebellar astrocytomas than in MB and ependymoma presumably because they occur more commonly in the lateral hemispheres than the vermis. The cerebellar syndrome occurs in 69% of these patients (108). Papilledema is found in up to 69%. Other signs such as cranial nerve palsies, nystagmus, pyramidal signs, and macrocephaly are comparable to MB as described above.

Pathology

On gross examination, these tumors vary from solid to cystic. Classically, cerebellar astrocytomas are discrete, cystic, well-circumscribed tumors with a mural nodule. The cyst contains clear yellowish fluid representing old blood products. The tumor can be solid in nature without cystic components, and these are most commonly found in the midline of the cerebellum. Not uncommonly, the tumor grows through the leptomeninges and spreads along the CSF space; however, this is not a negative prognostic factor.

Microscopically, cerebellar astrocytomas can be pilocytic (80%) or fibrillary (20%). In the past, a distinction was made between pilocytic and fibrillary histological subtypes, all are now considered low-grade astrocytomas amenable to complete surgical extirpation.

Etiology

Although patients with NF-1 have a propensity to develop pilocytic astrocytomas, these are generally located in the optic pathway and not the cerebellum. Karyotypic analyses have not revealed any distinct or repetitive cytogenetic abnormalities, although there are reports of 17q deletions. Contrary to expected findings, the NF-1 gene is actually overexpressed when studied in sporadic pilocytic astrocytomas (111). Only 1 in 34 tumors examined had a *p53* mutation, implying that it does not play a significant role in transformation of this tumor (87).

Radiologic Features

On non-contrast CT scan, the typical benign cerebellar pilocytic astrocytoma is a round, well-demarcated cystic lesion with a hypo- to isodense mural nodule (*Fig. 15.4*). The cystic fluid is commonly hyperdense to CSF because of the high protein content. Small hyperdense foci of calcifications are present in about 10%. The mural nodule enhances homogeneously and intensely. There is usually no enhancement from the cyst wall, as this is composed of compressed glial tissue and not neo-

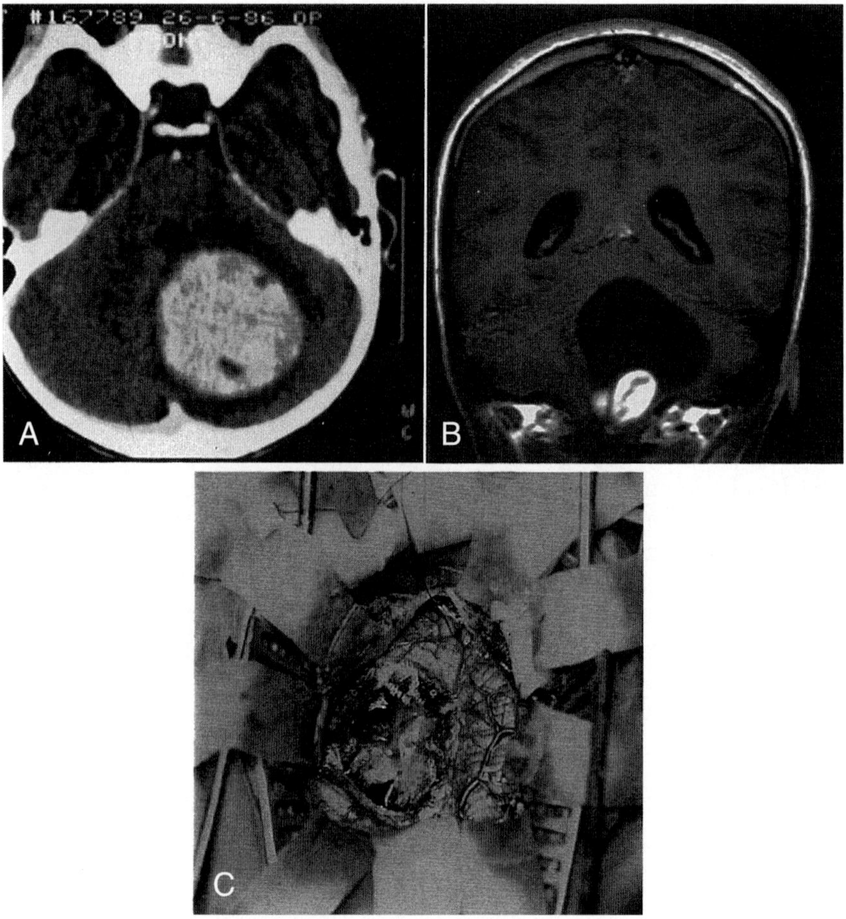

FIG. 15.4 (*A*) An axial CT scan with contrast showing a large, well-demarcated, solid, homogeneously enhancing pilocytic astrocytoma in the left cerebellar hemisphere. Two small cystic areas are seen. (*B*) Another cerebellar astrocytoma with a more characteristic appearance on a T1-weighted MRI with contrast. There is a large cyst with a non-enhancing wall and a mural nodule that strongly takes up gadolinium. (*C*) An intraoperative photo of the tumor from panel A.

plastic cells, although this is not a consistent finding. About 30% of cerebellar astrocytomas demonstrate these classic findings, and between 32 and 56% are solid tumors, which more often indicates a diffuse histology (73, 134). The solid tumors are more frequently found in the vermis and the cystic variety in the hemispheres. On MRI scan, the tumor appears hypo- to isointense to surrounding brain on the T1-weighted image and hyperintense on the T2-wieghted image (*Fig. 15.4*). The mural nodule enhances strongly but inhomogeneously with gadolinium (101). Brain stem invasion is noted in 10 to 48% of cases (1, 108, 134).

Postoperative imaging should be obtained within 48 hours postoperatively to assess surgical resection, as this is more reliable than the surgeon's impression intraoperatively (97).

Management

Complete surgical extirpation of benign pilocytic astrocytomas carries 5-year survival rates in the range of 90 to 100%, highlighting the importance of total resection. In a recent review of these tumors at Sick Children's Hospital in Toronto, 61 of 66 tumors were completely resected. Brainstem invasion limited total removal in the remaining five patients (1). As pilocytic astrocytomas do not invade the surrounding tissue, there is typically a pseudoplane that can be discerned separating it from normal tissue, allowing for gentle dissection off of the brainstem. On the other hand, this is rarely possible for diffuse astrocytomas (134). If the postoperative CT/MRI reveals a significant residual tumor nodule that is accessible, a second operation should be considered as residual tumor has been reported to grow back in 30 to 100% of cases (134, 144). Postoperative radiation therapy for residual tumor should be reserved for unresectable lesions involving the cerebellar peduncles or brainstem. An observational approach can be taken because of the slow growth potential, propensity to recur locally, good long-term survival in partial resections, and the rarity of malignant degeneration, especially in absence of radiation (108). This also avoids the intellectual risks associated with radiation therapy, as these patients generally live many years. The role of more focused radiation such as stereotactic radiosurgery and stereotactic radiotherapy remains to be clarified.

In the rare instance of a malignant cerebellar astrocytoma, attempts at gross, total resection should be continued if possible (84). Postoperative imaging of the craniospinal axis and CSF sampling is obtained to determine CSF spread. Generally, craniospinal radiation with adjuvant chemotherapy is advocated in cases where there is CSF dissemination.

Recurrence

Recurrences for pilocytic tumors are local and can occur many years after the original operation. Most do not progress; however, malignant degeneration has been reported (34, 136). Recurrences are generally treated with reoperation. If the tumor has dedifferentiated or has recurred quickly, then radiation and chemotherapy should be considered.

Prognostic Factors

For low-grade cerebellar astrocytomas, several factors have been correlated with worse prognosis. One study showed a relative risk of 8.9 for tumor recurrence in those without radiologic evidence of complete resection (108). All five subtotally resected tumors recurred between 1 and 8 years at Sick Children's Hospital in Toronto (1). Some studies correlate brainstem invasion with worse prognosis, but this is most likely related to the resectablity of these tumors. Although characteristic features of malignancy in fibrillary astrocytomas harbor significantly worse prognoses, there is disagreement regarding the importance of pilocytic and low-grade fibrillary designations in predicting recurrence.

BRAIN STEM GLIOMAS

Tumors of the brain stem, defined as the region of the neuraxis extending from the diencephalon to the cervical spinal cord, account for 10 to 20% of all pediatric tumors and up to 30% of posterior fossa tumors. In the past, neoplasms in this area were generally considered as a single disease entity with an extremely poor prognosis, which did not warrant surgical intervention. During the early 1980s, several reports in the literature identified these tumors as heterogeneous in terms of clinical, histologic, and biologic features. As such, several different subgroups have been recognized, which carries different therapeutic and prognostic implications (71, 92, 145). These tumors are classified by location in the brain stem and their focal or diffuse growth pattern.

Focal Brain Stem Gliomas

These tumors comprise 5 to 10% of all brain stem gliomas and can occur in any location but are most commonly found in the midbrain and medulla. They are usually less than 2 cm in diameter and are well circumscribed on neuroimaging, lacking features of diffuse invasion.

Periaqueductal or tectal tumors of children have recently been better defined in terms of presentation and natural history. The mean age at presentation is 10 years with complaints of increasing headaches and clinical features of increased intracranial pressure from late-onset hydrocephalus. As focal neurologic deficits are rare, symptoms are usually present for several months before a diagnosis is made. As these tumors are exceedingly small, they are frequently not identified on CT scan alone (115), and patients presenting with late-onset hydrocephalus should have an MRI to rule out a low-grade brain stem tumor (143). On MRI scan, these tumors appear focal, non-infiltrating with increased signal on T2-weighted image and diffuse enhancement with gadolinium administration. Due to the indolent nature of these lesions, current management centers on CSF diversion for the obstructive hydrocephalus and yearly imaging follow-up. A review of six patients from the Hospital for Sick Children highlights the favorable prognosis for these tumors. All six patients presented with symptoms and signs of raised intracranial pressure from aqueductal stenosis from a tectal tumor, and all six were treated with CSF diversion. None of the patients had radiation therapy. None of the patients had neurologic deficits referable to the brain stem at diagnosis, and all remain clinically and radiologically stable in the follow-up period ranging from 8 months to 17 years (92). In a recent report, two patients with tectal tumors treated with endoscopic third ventriculostomy alone have shown radiologic evidence of spontaneous involution (7).

Surgery is the treatment of choice for accessible focal brainstem tumors in other locations. Before endeavoring to remove these neoplasms, complete neuroimaging should be obtained to define the optimum surgical corridor. The radiologic characteristics of the tumor should be carefully assessed for features correlating with benign or malignant behavior such as peritumoral edema, heterogeneous enhancement, and less defined tumor edge as these indicate a poorer local control with surgery. Gross total resection of benign, focal brain stem tumors have up to a 94% 5-year survival compared with a 52% 5-year survival for partial resections. There was no benefit shown with surgery if the tumor was histologically malignant. Benign tumors with gross total resection should not be treated with adjuvant postoperative radiotherapy (110).

For surgically inaccessible lesions, symptomatic focal lesions, or those found to be high grade, treatment options include conventional radiotherapy, hyperfractionated radiotherapy, or stereotactic radiotherapy (50).

Dorsal Exophytic Brain Stem Tumors

Comprising about 20% of brain stem tumors, dorsally exophytic gliomas arise from the floor of the fourth ventricle and may grow to a large size filling the confines of the ventricle. These tumors are slow growing, and patients usually present more insidiously with longer duration of symptoms. As with most lesions that grow in the fourth ventricle, children present with headaches and ataxia. Papilledema is usually present.

Imaging of these patients demonstrates obstructive hydrocephalus. On CT scans, these lesions are iso- to hypodense and may enhance brightly with contrast administration highlighting cystic components. By MRI, the tumor is hypointense on the T1-weighted image and hyperintense on the T2-weighted image. Gadolinium can cause homogeneous, bright enhancement of the tumor. Extension laterally through the pia instead of through the ependymal may be a feature of a more high-grade lesion.

The vast majority of these tumors are low grade. In a series from the Hospital for Sick Children, 13 of 16 tumors were low-grade astrocytomas, 2 of 16 gangliogliomas and 1 of 16 were anaplastic astrocytomas. This is in agreement with a series reported by Pollack et al., finding 16 of 18 are low-grade astrocytomas,1 of 16 ganglioglioma, and 1 of 16 anaplastic astrocytomas (114).

Surgery is the treatment of choice for dorsally exophytic brain stem tumors. These can be approached via the midline. As the tumor is generally large and fills the fourth ventricle, it frequently spreads the cerebellar tonsils and is visible once the dura is opened. The vermis may have to be split a variable distance to fully access the sessile attachment to the floor of the fourth ventricle. The goal is to achieve maximal subtotal resection without damaging surrounding structures. Electrophysiologic monitoring of cranial nerves VI and VII may assist in the safety of removal. The ultrasonic aspirator is useful in shaving the tumor flush with the floor of the ventricle. As there is no sharp demarcation of the tumor/parenchyma interface, care must be taken not to follow the tumor into the brain stem, leading to unnecessary neurologic deficits. This generally requires leaving a thin layer of tumor tissue on the floor of the fourth ventricle.

The prognosis is excellent in most patients following surgery alone. The follow-up of Hoffman's origin series describing this entity reports 17 of 18 patients alive after a mean of 9.2 years. The only death was attributed to a shunt malfunction. Routine postoperative radiation is not indicated. Recurrences should be treated operatively when possible with the consideration of radiation if significant tumor is left or the lesion is inoperable. Radiotherapy is also considered for patients with high grade lesions or with early recurrence (50).

Cervicomedullary Tumors

Cervicomedullary tumors comprise 5 to 10% of brain stem tumors. They are generally thought of in two distinct groups, those whose epicenter is in the medulla and grow caudally and those who begin in the cervical cord and grow rostrally. It is rare for these tumors to extend past the pontomedullary junction. The majority of these tumors are slow growing with extremely slow neurologic progression. Signs and symptoms are present for up to 1 year in 80% of patients (120).

Presenting manifestations of this tumor is a reflection of the primary location of the mass. Tumors arising in the medulla usually lead to frequent respiratory tract infections, dysphagia, dysarthria, nausea, vomiting, and sleep apnea. Those with tumors in the cervical region generally present with neck pain and torticollis (129). About half of these patients will have motor and sensory dysfunction. Hydrocephalus is an uncommon finding.

CT scans are of limited use in cervicomedullary tumors because of the bony artifact from the foramen magnum. MRI is the diagnostic modality of choice as it allows for multiplanar imaging and better defines the extent of the tumor. Tumors originating in the medulla generally do not extend past the pontomedullary junction but may have a significant dorsal exophytic component. Those that arise from the cervical cord generally extend rostrally until its growth is impeded by the pyramidal decussations and forms a bulge on the dorsal aspect of the medulla.

Pathologically, these tumors are most commonly benign with 80 to 88% being low-grade gliomas (41, 120). Higher grade lesions can exist (up to 20%) and have a more invasive phenotype.

Surgery is considered the initial treatment of choice in view of the indolent nature of the majority of these tumors. Cervicomedullary tumors may be approached via a suboccipital craniotomy and upper cervical laminectomy (*Fig. 15.5*). MRI imaging is important to help define the caudal extent of the exposure. An ultrasound probe is helpful to define the extent of the tumor prior to opening the dura. Following dural opening, a midline myelotomy is performed, as much of the cervical extension is intra-axial. An aggressive resection of tumor can be performed in the cervical region; however, a subtotal resection is usually carried out in the medullary region to avoid significant neurologic deficits. Somatosensory and motor-evoked potentials are essential for safe removal of the tumor.

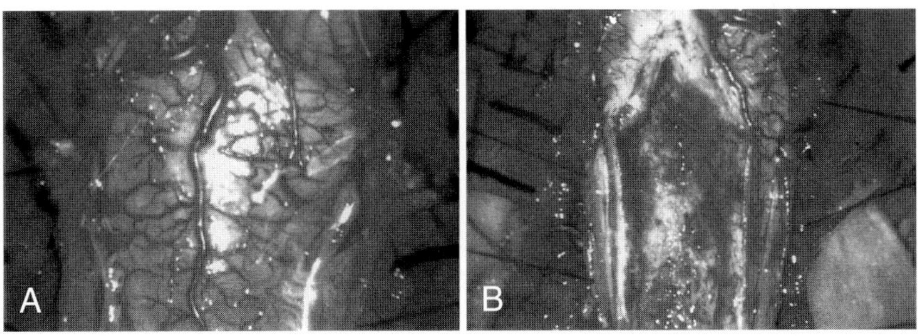

FIG. 15.5 (*A*) The cervicomedullary junction is swollen beneath the posterior spinal artery from a large low-grade astrocytoma. (*B*) A postoperative photo showing gross total removal of the lesion.

For patients with typical low-grade gliomas, postoperative radiotherapy is not required, as there is good long-term control with surgery alone. Total survival and progression-free survival have been reported in up to 100% and 70% of patients, respectively (120). High-grade tumors are generally treated as diffuse intrinsic brain stem tumors with radiation therapy and chemotherapy.

Diffuse Intrinsic Pontine Glioma

Diffuse intrinsic pontine gliomas (DIPG) account for the majority of brain stem neoplasms. They arise within the pons causing diffuse enlargement. Historically, this tumor is the reason for the nihilistic approach to brain stem tumors, and unfortunately the prognosis has not changed significantly in the past two decades.

Children usually present between the ages of 6 to 10 with a very short duration of symptoms, typically weeks to months. Progressive cranial nerve palsies (often bilateral reflecting the diffuse nature), pyramidal tract signs, and ataxia are the common manifestations, with hydrocephalus occurring late in the disease. Radiologically, DIPGs are hypodense on non-contrast CT scan and expand the pons. Rarely, there is focal uptake of contrast. MRI allows for better delineation and extent of the tumor. The mass is hypointense on the T1-weighted image and hyperintense on the T2-weighted image (*Fig. 15.6*). Gadolinium enhancement is variable.

The prognosis for these children is dismal, with a 2-year survival of less than 20%. As the survival rate is so poor, the natural history is known so well, and the radiologic features are so characteristic, a biopsy is generally not recommended. As these tumors are invariably malignant; radiation and/or chemotherapy are given after diagnostic imaging. Conventional radiotherapy offered to this group usually consists of 54 Gy total dose over 30 fractions. Approximately 75% of children will have some type of clinical improvement. However, this response is short-lived. Patients relapse in about 5 to 6 months with a mean survival of just under 1 year. Higher dose radiation as well as hyperfractionated radiotherapy have not proven to extend survival. As of yet, chemotherapy has not been shown to significantly improve survival. Accordingly, new chemotherapy protocols are being attempted.

CRANIOPHARYNGIOMA

Craniopharyngiomas are one of the most challenging tumors that neurosurgeons treat. Although benign histologically, the location in which these neoplasms reside may preclude complete surgical extirpation. All treatment modalities to date may be associated with signifi-

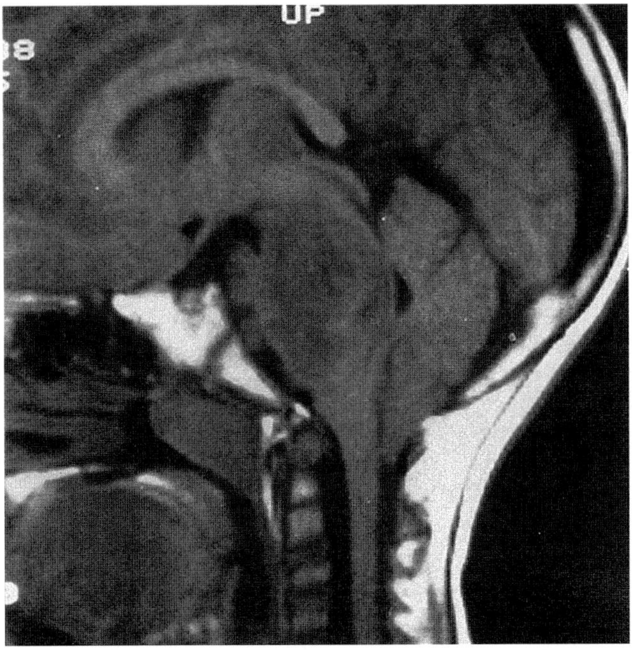

FIG. 15.6 A saggital T1-weighted MRI showing the characteristically hypointense, swollen pons of a patient with a diffuse pontine glioma.

cant morbidity, as these tumors are often attached to the hypothalamus, pituitary stalk, and the optic nerves/chiasm. As such, much controversy exists over the optimal treatment.

Although craniopharyngiomas are the most common non-neuroepithelial intracranial pediatric tumor, they comprise only 1 to 4.5% of all intracranial tumors and 5 to 10% of those in the pediatric population. This translates to less than 2 cases per million population per year (23). The age distribution is bimodal, with the majority of pediatric cases presenting between 5 and 10 years of age. Another peak appears between the ages of 40 and 45 years (2, 30). There does not seem to be any racial or sex predisposition.

Clinical Presentation

The clinical presentation of craniopharyngiomas is protean due to the various structures that may be affected in these patients. Although adults present with visual failure most commonly, this accounts for only 20 to 30% of children who seem to better tolerate gradual loss of vision. A decline in school performance, frequent bumping in to objects, and sitting close to the television are common scenarios indicating possible visual loss.

Children present far more commonly with headaches and signs of increased intracranial pressure as the tumor slowly grows to obstruct the Foramen of Monroe and leads to hydrocephalus. As such, children with craniopharyngioma most frequently present with non-specific nausea, vomiting, and gait disturbance. Papilledema is present in 40% of cases (60).

Impingement on the pituitary stalk and hypothalamus can lead to various endocrinopathies and neuropsychologic problems. Endocrinopathies are more common in children than adults and occur in over 50% of cases. These children usually present with clinical stigmata due to deficiencies in growth hormone (75%) and LH/FSH (40%). Diabetes insipidus is found in approximately 17% and is usually partial. If there is significant compression of the pituitary stalk, children may rarely present with galactorrhea and hyperprolactinemia. Hypothalamic disorders such as central hyperphagia, precocious puberty, and hyperthermia may rarely be seen. Abulia, flattened affect, loss of interest, and declining cognitive abilities are attributed to involvement of the basal forebrain and the septal area (105, 163).

Pathology

Craniopharyngiomas are a benign epithelial tumor arising in the sellar region with a variable cystic component. They are midline tumors that arise from the pituitary stalk or the tuber cinereum (68). Depending on the site of attachment, the growth pattern of the tumor varies, having direct implications for surgical removal. Craniopharyngiomas arising from the pituitary stalk tend to grow toward the sella and may extend laterally. Those that arise from the tuber cinereum generally grow into the third ventricle, invaginating and inverting the normal hypothalamus. As such, approximately one-third of craniopharyngiomas are retrochiasmatic and push the pituitary stalk forward and the optic chiasm forward and upward. The compression of the hypothalamus into the third ventricle makes this class of craniopharyngiomas less amenable to safe complete resection (*Fig. 15.7*). Another one-third are subchiasmatic and distort the pituitary stalk backward and stretch the optic chiasm straight upward. Approximately 20% are prechiasmatic and grow to a significant size in the frontal lobes (105). This growth pattern is less commonly attached to the hypothalamus and is more easily accessible surgically, lending themselves better to complete extirpation (*Fig. 15.7*). Craniopharyngiomas are uncommonly found intraventricularly, intrasellarly, intrasphenoidally, and in the nasopharynx.

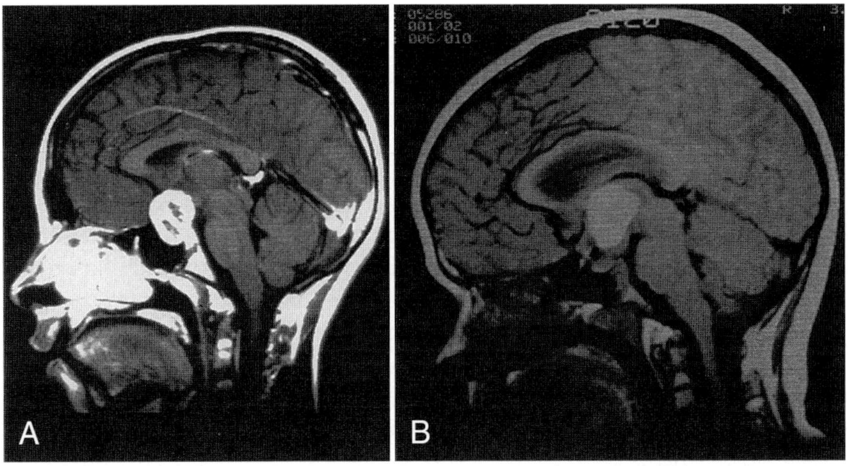

FIG. 15.7 (*A*) A T1-weighted MRI with contrast of a prechiasmatic craniopharyngioma. Note the minimal hypothalamic involvement as compared with the MRI on the right. (*B*) A T1-weighted MRI with contrast of a postaxial craniopharyngioma highlighting the extension into the third ventricle.

There are two histologic variants of craniopharyngioma, the classical adamantinomatous and the papillary types. Immunohistochemically, craniopharyngiomas stain positive for keratin. Estrogen and progesterone receptor expression has been described.

There are very few histologic features that correlate with progression-free survival. As to be expected in benign tumors, the proliferative index is low and does not correlate with recurrence. The most significant factor predicting recurrence is the extent of the surgical resection.

The molecular etiology of craniopharyngioma remains to be elucidated. Except for a single report of craniopharyngiomas occurring in consanguineous twins, there are no hereditary tumor syndromes that have a propensity for craniopharyngiomas (20). There have been case reports of craniopharyngiomas containing complex cytogenetic abnormalities in chromosomes 2 and 12; however, the significance of this is unknown as other reports find a normal karyotype in this tumor (20, 59, 62, 79).

Radiologic Features

Although no longer used, craniopharyngiomas are one of the rare tumors that can be seen on plain radiographs due to the bony changes in the sella and clinoid processes and intracranial calcifications. In the current era, CT and MRI scans play a major role in the diagnosis and surgical planning of these tumors. Both modalities are important, as each demonstrates different anatomic and pathologic features that are important to the management of the patient. Non-contrast CT scans show a cystic-appearing lobulated mass in the sellar/supersellar region. There are calcifications in the rim or in the solid component of the tumor in almost 90% of cases. The cystic component is hypodense but is usually slightly higher in attenuation than CSF because of the high protein content. CT scans are important to classify the relative cystic-to-solid composition, as the high protein content can confuse this determination on an MRI scan. Predominantly solid tumors have less than a 30% cystic component, whereas predominantly cystic tumors have less than a 30% solid component. The CT scan allows for better assessment of the surrounding bony architecture and the amount of calcifications present.

Typically, on an MRI scan, the tumor has a very heterogenous signal. The cystic fluid is usually hypointense on the T1-weighted image, but the signal may be increased in intensity, depending on the concentration of protein, cholesterol, and blood breakdown products (4). There is strong but heterogeneous enhancement with contrast administration. The MRI scan is better than CT in determining the interface between the tumor and the surrounding neural tissue, and the multi-planar capabilities permit improved visualization of the extent of involvement of the third ventricle, the polar extensions of the tumor, and the vascular involvement, all of which are important in management.

Management

Craniopharyngiomas require not only complete neuroradiologic assessment but preoperative endocrinologic and neuropsychological evaluations as well. GH and LH/FSH are the most common hormones to be involved, but knowledge of the ACTH and TSH status is much more useful in the preoperative and operative phases. All should be treated as corticosteroid deficient and receive preoperative doses. Thyroid replacement, either orally or intravenously, should be initiated immediately if the patient is found to be deficient.

The patient's preoperative visual status should be documented by detailed visual acuity and visual field tests. Because of the neurobehavioural problems associated with this tumor and with its therapy, neuropsychological assessments before treatment are useful if the clinical situation permits.

Successful removal of craniopharyngiomas with low morbidity and mortality can be achieved in centers that have experience with these lesions. Mortality rates in the era of microneurosurgery have been quoted between 1 and 2% for the primary operation (45, 70, 72). Complete surgical removal, with neuroradiologic confirmation, gives the patient the best chance at cure or long-term tumor control. With proper preoperative planning, complete surgical resection can be achieved in 60 to 90% of cases, but attempts at complete removal must be altered if tumor characteristics found at the time of operation unduly increase the risk of damage to the surrounding structures. The most common intraoperative findings that lead to a subtotal resection were adherence to the hypothalamus and vessels (45%), obstructed view (21%), and major calcifications (14%). As such, the retrochiasmatic tumors lend themselves less frequently to complete removal as compared to the prechiasmatic or sellar lesions. Patients with total removal have long-term progression-free survival over 85% at 5 years and 80% at 10 years. One report indicates that 79% of patients treated with the intent of complete removal were independent and without impairment at the time of the last follow-up (mean 64 months) (45, 70, 72).

Subtotal resection without radiation therapy leads to much poorer tumor control and survival. The recurrence rate approaches 75%, with 10-year survival around 25%. If these patients are given radiotherapy following subtotal resection, the recurrence rates at 5 and 10 years approaches that of complete resection (69, 116, 118). Currently, there is controversy about the role of complete resection versus planned subtotal resection followed by radiotherapy, the rationale being that planned subtotal resection will have less morbidity and mortality due to less manipulation of the hypothalamus and surrounding structures. Radiation therapy carries with it significant morbidity. Visual failure, dementia, vascular damage, hypopituitarism, and radiation-induced second malignancies have all been reported.

Predominantly cystic craniopharyngiomas have been successfully treated with stereotactic intracavitary brachytherapy or bleomycin injections. Both radioactive phosphorus and bleomycin poorly penetrate the wall of the cyst, requiring an absence of a thick solid tumor component. Reports have indicated cyst control of over 90% with complete resolution in up to 30% (26, 154). Cyst progression and new cyst formation still occur at a significant rate. Although intracavitary therapy is relatively safe, there are complications such as worsening endocrine function, visual deterioration, occlusive cerebrovasculopathy, and death (130, 132). Intracavitary therapy is a reasonable alternative to repeat surgery for recurrent cystic lesions, especially for the purpose of delaying postoperative radiation in young children.

The role of stereotactic radiosurgery in the treatment of primary and recurrent craniopharyngiomas is still being evaluated. Most of the reports have a short follow-up period, making solid treatment recommendations difficult. However, as the technology evolves and the ability to more accurately focus radiation in this eloquent area of the brain improves, there may be a role for radiosurgery in certain cases.

CHOROID PLEXUS TUMORS

Neoplasms of the choroid plexus make up less than 1% of all intracranial neoplasms but are considerably more common in the pediatric age group, where they comprise up to 3% of brain tumors (102, 109, 131). Among children less than 12 months of age, between 10 and 20% of neoplasms originate in the choroid plexus. About two-thirds of choroid plexus tumors are diagnosed as papillomas (CPP), with the remaining one-third being choroid plexus carcinomas (CPC) (109). Most choroid plexus tumors of childhood occur in the lateral ventricles, whereas adult tumors tend to occur in the fourth ventricle. Both age groups show rare examples of third ventricular and cerebellopontine angle tumors (22, 51, 148). The median duration of symptoms at the time of presentation in children with choroid plexus tumors is about 1 month. The median age at presentation in children quoted in the literature varies from 12 to 26 months (102, 109). Currently, some choroid plexus tumors are being diagnosed antenatally on prenatal ultrasound examinations (140). Most choroid plexus tumors are sporadic in nature, but associations with rare familial syndromes and viral infections have been suggested in exceptional cases (see below).

Etiology

Two familial syndromes have been reported to predispose to choroid plexus tumors, the Li-Fraumeni syndrome and the Aicardi syndrome. The Li-Fraumeni syndrome (LFS) is usually due to a germline mutation in the tumor suppressor gene *p53*. Several families with germline *p53* mutations have been shown to have an increased incidence of malignancy that includes choroid plexus tumors. Mutations in codon 248 of *p53* have been reported by some authors as predisposing to a high risk of choroid plexus tumors (158). Oncogenesis in individuals with germline *p53* mutations is thought to occur with the deletion or mutation of the remaining wild-type *p53* allele (so called loss of heterozygosity). Some choroid plexus tumors from individuals with LFS retain the wild-type allele at a DNA level, suggesting that alternative routes exist to disable the second allele such as infection with SV40 virus (see below) (137). The Aicardi syndrome is a rare, X-linked disorder that includes infantile spasms, callosal agenesis, chorioretinal lacunae, periventricular and cortical heterotopias, microphthalmia, optic disk coloboma, and choroid plexus tumors. These patients have severe developmental delay and only 40% survival at 15 years. There are numerous reports of choroid plexus tumors in individuals with the Aicardi syndrome (3, 5, 64, 99, 121, 123). The Aicardi gene has been mapped to chromosome Xp22.3. Another X-linked syndrome, Hypomelanosis of Ito consisting of hypopigmented lesions and psychomotor retardation, has also been reported in association with choroid plexus papilloma (142, 147, 164). Constitutional duplication of chromosome 9p results in a phenotype that can include hyperplasia of the choroid plexus and/or CPP (100). Extra copies of chromosome 9 have also been found in sporadic choroid plexus tumors (100). Our laboratory has recently discovered a family with a germline mutation of the tumor suppressor gene *hSNF5* on chromosome 22q11.2 that is afflicted with posterior fossa tumors of infancy, including medulloblastoma and choroid plexus carcinoma (149). The *hSNF5* gene is involved in control of the structure of DNA by remodeling nucleosomes and has been shown to be a key tumor suppressor gene in rhabdoid tumors (156). A number of abnormal karyotypes have been reported from cases of CPP and CPC, but consistent changes are lacking other than hyperdiploidy/hyperhaploidy (37, 94, 122). Transgenic mice that overexpress the large T antigen protein from the SV40 virus develop tumors of the choroid plexus, and expression of the SV40 large T antigen is found within human choroid plexus tumors (9, 86, 90, 141, 165). SV40 large T binds to and inactivates two well-characterized tumor suppressor genes, *p53* and *pRb* (the product of the Retinoblastoma tumor suppressor gene). SV40 large T antigen protein from human brain tumors has been shown to bind to *p53* and *pRb in vivo,* suggesting that it may inactivate these tumor suppressor genes in human tumors. Polio vaccine distributed last century was contaminated with SV40 virus, as such many individuals have been exposed to SV40 (26, 47, 48). Although SV40 large T antigen has been found in choroid plexus tumors, whether or not it has a causal role in oncogenesis is not yet clear.

Clinical Presentation

Like all intracranial neoplasms, the presentation depends on the location of the tumor and the age of the patient. The typical infant presenting with a lateral ventricular CPP will present with signs and symptoms of intracranial hypertension (enlarging head circumference, vomiting, sunsetting eyes, lethargy, developmental delay). Focal signs do occur but are less common in children due to the predominant occurrence of tumors in the lateral ventricles.

Intracranial hypertension can be secondary to tumor mass or hydrocephalus. Hydrocephalus in patients with choroid plexus tumors has received a great deal of attention in the literature over the years, especially when one considers the low incidence of this tumor (24, 27, 35, 55). This intense interest is due to the ability of CPP and CPC to produce, and perhaps even overproduce, cerebrospinal fluid (CSF) (24, 95, 96). Children with choroid plexus tumors and external ventricular drains have been noted to produce in excess of 800 ml of CSF per day (109). It is hypothesized that this overproduction of CSF overwhelms the arachnoid granulations, resulting in hydrocephalus. If overproduction of CSF was the sole cause of hydrocephalus in these patients, surgical resection should cure the hydrocephalus by removing the mass, reconstituting the CSF pathways and eliminating excess CSF production. In many children, this is indeed the case, but many children do require ventriculoperitoneal shunting post gross total resection. Many theories for this phenomena have been suggested including tumor, blood, and protein obstructing various levels of the CSF pathway.

Radiologic Feature

CT scans of choroid plexus tumors reveal a hyperdense mass, usually within the lateral ventricle that enhances diffusely with contrast. Hydrocephalus is usually, but not universally, present. Calcification can be seen in about 10% of cases (109). Intratumoral cysts and necrosis may be seen in some patients. On MRI, tumors are isointense to gray matter on T1- and T2-weighted images and enhance diffusely with administration of gadolinium (102). MR may show large serpentine flow voids within these tumors consistent with their well known vascularity. In cases of CPC, contrast enhancement is typically heterogeneous, and invasion of the brain with surrounding edema is apparent. Angiography reveals an intense tumor blush with feeding vessels coming from the choroidal branches of the posterior cerebral artery.

Pathology

Grossly, choroid plexus neoplasms appear as pink-gray pedunculated neoplasms with a cauliflower-like surface (53). They may have areas of calcification, hemorrhage, and cystic change internally (162). CPPs are usually well delineated from brain as opposed to CPCs, which often invade the brain substance. Most metastases from CPC occur along the CSF axis, but rare hematologic metastases have been described (53). Metastases are not often seen at presentation of CPC patients (only 1 in 13 cases in one recent series) (109). Histologically, the tumor appears as a simple columnar or cuboidal epithelium sitting on a basement membrane (reviewed in Ref. 53). True papillae with a fibrovascular core are seen. Nuclei are regular and oval with few or no mitoses being seen in a case of CPP. CPCs make up about one-third of choroid plexus neoplasms in childhood, and most CPCs occur in childhood (109). Features of a CPC as opposed to a CPP include multilayered sheets and solid nests of anaplastic cells, cellular and nuclei pleomorphisms, and frequent mitotic figures (53) (*Fig. 15.8*).

Normal choroid plexus, CPP, and often CPC exhibit cytoplasmic staining with antibodies to cytokeratin, vimentin, transthyretin, and S-100 (reviewed in Ref. 53). Choroid plexus, CPP, and CPC may also show immunopositivity for the neuronal marker synaptophysin; this may be useful in the differentiation of metastatic adenocarcinoma and CPC (81). MIB-1 labeling of normal choroid plexus (0.02% to 0.06%), CPP (3.7 %), and CPC (14%) may provide some evidence as to the degree of malignancy in a given case (153).

Management

The treatment of a CPP is surgical with complete resection resulting in a cure in most cases (109). Failure to obtain a complete resection can result in later recurrence.

Surgery is also the mainstay of treatment for CPC but should be used after doses of chemotherapy to diminish the vascularity of the tumor and to enhance the extent of surgical resection. Radiotherapy may be

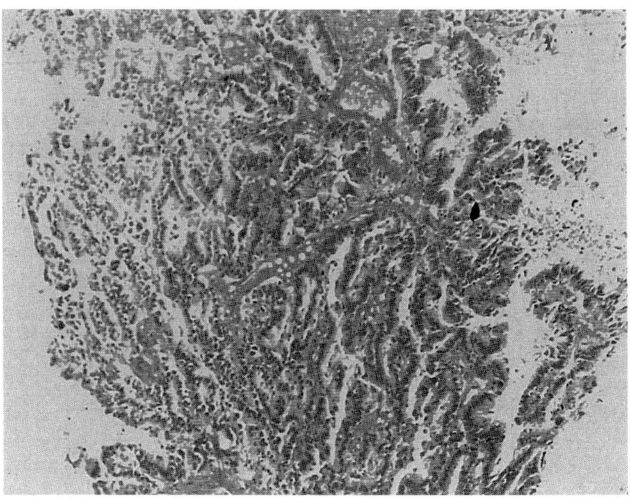

FIG. 15.8 A medium-power H&E stain of a choroid plexus carcinoma. Notice the progression from a more benign, papillary architecture on the left where the cells are well separated to the more compact and aggressive nature of the cells on the right.

of benefit to patients with CPC after surgical resection and chemotherapy (160). A number of different chemotherapy regimes have been tried with varying success in cases of CPC (reviewed in Ref. 61). The prognosis in cases of CPC with a recent series of 13 cases reports a 40% 5-year survival (109).

REFERENCES

1. Abdollahzadeh M, Hoffman, HJ, Blazer SI, Becker LE, Humphreys RP, Drake JM, Rutka JT: Benign cerebellar astrocytoma in childhood: Experience at the Hospital for Sick Children 1980–1992. **Childs Nerv Syst** 10:380–383, 1994.
2. Adamson TE, Wiestler OD, Kleihues P,Yasargil MG: Correlation of clinical and pathological features in surgically treated craniopharyngiomas. **J Neurosurg** 73:12–17, 1990.
3. Aguiar MD, Cavalcanti M, Barbosa H, Vilela SL, Mendonca JL, Horta E: Aicardi syndrome and choroid plexus papilloma: A rare association. Case report. **Arq Neuropsiquiatr** 54:313–317, 1996.
4. Ahmadi J, Destian S, Apuzzo ML, Segall HD, Zee CS: Cystic fluid in craniopharyngiomas: MR imaging and quantitative analysis. **Radiology** 182:783–785, 1992.
5. Aicardi J, Garcia J, Lepintre J, Chevrie JJ, Thieffry S: Papillomas of the choroid plexus in children. **Arch Fr Pediatr** 25:673–686, 1968.
6. Albright AL, Wisoff JH, Zeltzer PM, Boyett JM, Rorke LB, Stanley P: Effects of medulloblastoma resections on outcome in children: A report from the Children's Cancer Group. **Neurosurgery** 38:265–271, 1996.
7. Alkhani AM, Boop FA, Rutka JT: Involution of enhancing intrinsic tectal tumors after endoscopic third ventriculostomy. Report of two cases. **J Neurosurg** 91:863–866, 1999.
8. Bailey P, Cushing H: Medulloblastoma cerebelli: A common type of mid-cerebellar glioma of childhood. **Arch Neurol Psychiatr** 14:192–224, 1925.
9. Becker LE, Narayan O, Johnson RT: Studies of human papovavirus tumor antigen in experimental and human cerebral neoplasms. **Can J Neurol Sci** 3:105–109, 1976.
10. Berger M, Magrassi L, Geyer R: Medulloblastoma and primitive neuroectodermal tumors, in Kaye A, Laws E (eds): *Brain Tumors.* Edinburgh, Churchill, 1995, pp 561–574.
11. Bergsagel DJ, Finegold MJ, Butel JS, Kupsky WJ, Garcea RL: DNA sequences similar to those of simian virus 40 in ependymomas and choroid plexus tumors of childhood. **N Engl J Med** 326:988–993, 1992.
12. Berry MP, Jenkin RD, Keen CW, Nair BD, Simpson WJ: Radiation treatment for medulloblastoma: A 21-year review. **J Neurosurg** 55:43–51, 1981.
13. Bhattacharjee MB, Armstrong DD, Vogel H, Cooley LD: Cytogenetic analysis of 120 primary pediatric brain tumors and literature review. **Cancer Genet Cytogenet** 97:39–53, 1997.
14. Biegel JA, Allen CS, Kawasaki K, Shimizu N, Budarf ML, Bell CJ: Narrowing the critical region for a rhabdoid tumor locus in 22q11. **Genes Chromosom Cancer** 16:94–105, 1996.
15. Biegel JA, Burk CD, Parmiter AH, Emanuel BS: Molecular analysis of a partial deletion of 22q in a central nervous system rhabdoid tumor. **Genes Chromosom Cancer** 5:104–108, 1992.
16. Biegel JA, Zhou JY, Rorke LB, Stenstrom C, Wainwright LM, Fogelgren B: Germ-line

and acquired mutations of INI1 in atypical teratoid and rhabdoid tumors. **Cancer Res** 59:74–79, 1999.
17. Bigner SH, Mark J, Friedman HS, Biegel JA, Bigner DD: Structural chromosomal abnormalities in human medulloblastoma. **Cancer Genet Cytogenet** 30:91–101, 1988.
18. Blaser SI, Harwood-Nash DC: Neuroradiology of pediatric posterior fossa medulloblastoma. **J Neurooncol** 29:23–34, 1996.
19. Bleyer WA: Epidemiologic impact of children with brain tumors. **Childs Nerv Syst** 15:758–763, 1999.
20. Boch AL, van Effenterre R, Kujas M: Craniopharyngiomas in two consanguineous siblings: Case report. **Neurosurgery** 41:1185–1187, 1997.
21. Bouffet E, Foreman N: Chemotherapy for intracranial ependymomas. **Childs Nerv Syst** 15:563–570, 1999.
22. Broad RW, Allen PB: Third ventricle choroid plexus carcinoma. **Can J Neurol Sci** 11:461–465, 1984.
23. Bunin GR, Surawicz TS, Witman PA, Preston-Martin S, Davis F, Bruner JM: The descriptive epidemiology of craniopharyngioma [see comments]. **J Neurosurg** 89:547–551, 1998.
24. Buxton N, Punt J: Choroid plexus papilloma producing symptoms by secretion of cerebrospinal fluid. **Pediatr Neurosurg** 27:108–111, 1997.
25. Cadigan KM, Nusse R: Wnt signaling: A common theme in animal development. **Genes Dev** 11:3286–3305, 1997.
26. Cavalheiro S, Sparapani FV, Franco JO, da Silva MC, Braga FM: Use of bleomycin in intratumoral chemotherapy for cystic craniopharyngioma: Case report [see comments]. **J Neurosurg** 84:124–126, 1996.
27. Ceddia A, Di Rocco C, Carlucci A: Hypersecretive congenital hydrocephalus due to choroid plexus villous hypertrophy associated with controlateral papilloma. **Minerva Pediatr** 45:363–367, 1993.
28. Cinalli G, Salazar C, Mallucci C, Yada JZ, Zerah M, Sainte-Rose C: The role of endoscopic third ventriculostomy in the management of shunt malfunction. **Neurosurgery** 43:1323–1327, 1998; Discussion 1327–1329.
29. Cogen PH, McDonald JD: Tumor suppressor genes and medulloblastoma. **J Neurooncol** 29:103–112, 1996.
30. Crotty TB, Scheithauer BW, Young WF, Jr, Davis DH, Shaw EG, Miller GM, et al: Papillary craniopharyngioma: A clinicopathological study of 48 cases. **J Neurosurg** 83:206–214, 1995.
31. Czerwionka M, Korf HW, Hoffmann O, Busch H, Schachenmayr W: Differentiation in medulloblastomas: Correlation between the immunocytochemical demonstration of photoreceptor markers (S-antigen, rod-opsin) and the survival rate in 66 patients. **Acta Neuropathol** 78:629–636, 1989.
32. Deutsch M, Thomas PR, Krischer J, Boyett JM, Albright L, Aronin P, et al: Results of a prospective randomized trial comparing standard dose neuraxis irradiation (3,600 cGy/20) with reduced neuraxis irradiation (2,340 cGy/13) in patients with low-stage medulloblastoma: A combined children's cancer group-pediatric oncology group study. **Pediatr Neurosurg** 24:167–176, 1996.
33. Dias MS, Albright AL: Management of hydrocephalus complicating childhood posterior fossa tumors. **Pediatr Neurosci** 15:283–289, 1989.
34. Dirks PB, Jay V, Becker LE, Drake JM, Humphreys RP, Hoffman HJ, Rutka JT: Development of anaplastic changes in low-grade astrocytomas of childhood. **Neurosurgery** 34:68–78, 1994.

35. Di Rocco C, Iannelli A: Poor outcome of bilateral congenital choroid plexus papillomas with extreme hydrocephalus. **Eur Neurol** 37:33–37, 1997.
36. Dohrmann G: Ependymomas, in Wilkins R, Rengachary S (eds): *Neurosurgery.* New York, McGraw-Hill, 1996, pp 1195–1200.
37. Donovan MJ, Yunis EJ, DeGirolami U, Fletcher JA, Schofield DE: Chromosome aberrations in choroid plexus papillomas. **Genes Chromosom Cancer** 11:267–270, 1994.
38. Duffner PK, Horowitz ME, Krischer JP, Friedman HS, Burger PC, Cohen ME, Sanford RA, Mulhern RK, James HE, Freeman CR: Postoperative chemotherapy and delayed radiation in children less than three years of age with malignant brain tumors [see comments]. **N Engl J Med** 328:1725–1731, 1993.
39. Duncan J III, Hoffman H: Intracranial ependymomas, in Kaye A, Laws E (eds.): *Brain Tumors.* Edinburgh, Churchill-Livingstone, 1995, pp 493–504.
40. Ebert C, von Haken M, Meyer-Puttlitz B, Wiestler OD, Reifenberger G, Pietsch T, von Deimling A: Molecular genetic analysis of ependymal tumors: NF2 mutations and chromosome 22q loss occur preferentially in intramedullary spinal ependymomas. **Am J Pathol** 155:627–632, 1999.
41. Epstein F,Wisoff J: Intra-axial tumors of the cervicomedullary junction. **J Neurosurg** 67:483–487, 1987.
42. Ersahin Y: Is splitting of the vermis responsible for cerebellar mutism? [letter; comment]. **Pediatr Neurosurg** 28:328, 1998.
43. Evans G, Burnell L, Campbell R, Gattamaneni HR, Birch J: Congenital anomalies and genetic syndromes in 173 cases of medulloblastoma. **Med Pediatr Oncol** 21:433–434, 1993.
44. Evans DG, Farndon PA, Burnell LD, Gattamaneni HR, Birch JM: The incidence of Gorlin syndrome in 173 consecutive cases of medulloblastoma. **Br J Cancer** 64:959–961, 1991.
45. Fahlbusch R, Honegger J, Paulus W, Huk W, Buchfelder M: Surgical treatment of craniopharyngiomas: Experience with 168 patients. **J Neurosurg** 90:237–250, 1990.
46. Farwell JR, Dohrmann GJ, Flannery JT: Medulloblastoma in childhood: An epidemiological study. **J Neurosurg** 61:657–664, 1984.
47. Farwell JR, Dohrmann GJ, Marrett LD, Meigs JW: Effect of SV40 virus-contaminated polio vaccine on the incidence and type of CNS neoplasms in children: A population-based study. **Trans Am Neurol Assoc** 104:261–264, 1979.
48. Fisher SG, Weber L, Carbone M: Cancer risk associated with simian virus 40 contaminated polio vaccine. **Anticancer Res** 19:2173–180, 1999.
49. Foreman NK, Love S, Gill SS, Coakham HB: Second-look surgery for incompletely resected fourth ventricle ependymomas: Technical case report. **Neurosurgery** 40:856–860, 1997; Discussion 860.
50. Freeman CR, Farmer JP: Pediatric brain stem gliomas: A review. **Int J Radiat Oncol Biol Phys** 40:265–271, 1998.
51. Furuya K, Sasaki T, Saito N, Atsuchi M, Kirino T: Primary large choroid plexus papillomas in the cerebellopontine angle: Radiological manifestations and surgical management. **Acta Neurochir** 135:144–149, 1995.
52. Gajjar A, Kuhl J, Epelman S, Bailey C, Allen J: Chemotherapy of medulloblastoma. **Childs Nerv Syst** 15:554–562, 1999.
53. Gaudio RM, Tacconi L, Rossi ML: Pathology of choroid plexus papillomas: A review. **Clin Neurol Neurosurg** 100:165–186, 1998.
54. Giangaspero F, Bigner S, Giordana M, Kleihues P, Trojanowski J: Medulloblastoma, Kleihues P, Cavenee W (eds): *Tumours of the Nervous System.* Lyon, International Agency for Research on Cancer, 1997, pp 96–103.

55. Go KG: The normal and pathological physiology of brain water. **Adv Tech Stand Neurosurg** 23:47–142, 1997.
56. Goel A: Whither preoperative shunts for posterior fossa tumours? **Br J Neurosurg** 7:395–399, 1993.
57. Goldberg-Stern H, Gadoth N, Stern S, Cohen IJ, Zaizov R, Sandbank U: The prognostic significance of glial fibrillary acidic protein staining in medulloblastoma. **Cancer** 68:568–573, 1991.
58. Goodrich LV, Scott MP: Hedgehog and patched in neural development and disease. **Neuron** 21:1243–1257, 1998.
59. Gorski GK, McMorrow LE, Donaldson MH, Freed M: Multiple chromosomal abnormalities in a case of craniopharyngioma [letter]. **Cancer Genet Cytogenet** 60:212–213, 1992.
60. Graham PH, Gattamaneni HR, Birch JM: Paediatric craniopharyngiomas: A regional review. **Br J Neurosurg** 6:187–193, 1992.
61. Greenberg ML: Chemotherapy of choroid plexus carcinoma. **Childs Nerv Syst** 15:571–577, 1999.
62. Griffin CA, Long PP, Carson BS, Brem H: Chromosome abnormalities in low-grade central nervous system tumors. **Cancer Genet Cytogenet** 60:67–73, 1992.
63. Gutmann DH, Giordano MJ, Fishback AS, Guha A: Loss of merlin expression in sporadic meningiomas, ependymomas and schwannomas. **Neurology** 49:267–270, 1997.
64. Hamano K, Matsubara T, Shibata S, Hirano C, Ito Z, Ase Y, et al: Aicardi syndrome accompanied by auditory disturbance and multiple brain tumors. **Brain Dev** 13:438–441, 1991.
65. Hamilton RL, Pollack IF: The molecular biology of ependymomas. **Brain Pathol** 7:807–822, 1997.
66. Hamilton SR, Liu B, Parsons RE, Papadopoulos N, Jen J, Powell SM, Krush AJ, Berk T, Cohen Z, Tetu B: The molecular basis of Turcot's syndrome [see comments]. **N Engl J Med** 332:839–847, 1995.
67. Hayostek CJ, Shaw EG, Scheithauer B, O'Fallon JR, Weiland TL, Schomberg PJ, Kelly PJ, Hu TC: Astrocytomas of the cerebellum: A comparative clinicopathologic study of pilocytic and diffuse astrocytomas. **Cancer** 72:856–869, 1993.
68. Hayward R: The present and future management of childhood craniopharyngioma. **Childs Nerv Syst** 15:764–769, 1999.
69. Hetelekidis S, Barnes PD, Tao ML, Fischer EG, Schneider L, Scott RM, et al: 20-year experience in childhood craniopharyngioma [see comments]. **Int J Radiat Oncol Biol Phys** 27:189–195, 1993.
70. Hoffman HJ: Surgical management of craniopharyngioma. **Pediatr Neurosurg** 21:44–49, 1994.
71. Hoffman HJ, Becker L, Craven MA: A clinically and pathologically distinct group of benign brain stem gliomas. **Neurosurgery** 7:243–248, 1980.
72. Hoffman HJ, De Silva M, Humphreys RP, Drake JM, Smith ML, Blaser SI: Aggressive surgical management of craniopharyngiomas in children. **J Neurosurg** 76:47–52, 1992.
73. Hoffman PL, Snell LD, Bhave SV, Tabakoff B: Ethanol inhibition of NMDA receptor function in primary cultures of rat cerebellar granule cells and cerebral cortical cells. **Alcohol Suppl** 2:199–204, 1994.
74. Hubbard JL, Scheithauer BW, Kispert DB, Carpenter SM, Wick MR, Laws ER Jr: Adult cerebellar medulloblastomas: The pathological, radiographic, and clinical disease spectrum. **J Neurosurg** 70:536–544, 1989.
75. Hukin J, Epstein F, Lefton D, Allen J: Treatment of intracranial ependymoma by surgery alone. **Pediatr Neurosurg** 29:40–45, 1998.

76. Innis MD: Simian virus 40-contaminated polio vaccine and cancer rates [letter; comment]. **JAMA** 280:1481–1482, 1998.
77. Jankowski JA, Bruton R, Shepherd N, Sanders DS: Cadherin and catenin biology represent a global mechanism for epithelial cancer progression. **Mol Pathol** 50:289–290, 1997.
78. Jenkin D: The radiation treatment of medulloblastoma. **J Neurooncol** 29:45–54, 1996.
79. Karnes PS, Tran TN, Cui MY, Raffel C, Gilles FH, Barranger JA, Ying KL: Cytogenetic analysis of 39 pediatric central nervous system tumors. **Cancer Genet Cytogenet** 59:12–19, 1992.
80. Katsetos CD, Burger PC: Medulloblastoma. **Semin Diagn Pathol** 11:85–97, 1994.
81. Kepes JJ, Collins J: Choroid plexus epithelium (normal and neoplastic) expresses synaptophysin: A potentially useful aid in differentiating carcinoma of the choroid plexus from metastatic papillary carcinomas. **J Neuropathol Exp Neurol** 58:398–401, 1999.
82. Kim JY, Sutton ME, Lu DJ, Cho TA, Goumnerova LC, Goritchenko L, Kaufman JR, Lam KK, Billet AL, Tarbell NJ, Wu J, Allen JC, Stiles CD, Segal RA, Pomeroy SL: Activation of neurotrophin-3 receptor TrkC induces apoptosis in medulloblastomas. **Cancer Res** 59:711–719, 1999.
83. Kirchstein RL, Rabson AS, O'Conor GT: Ependymomas produced in Syrian hamsters by adenovirus 7, strain E46 ("hybrid" of adenovirus 7 and SV40). **Proc Soc Exp Biol Med** 120:484–487, 1965.
84. Kulkarni AV, Becker LE, Jay V, Armstrong DC, Drake JM: Primary cerebellar glioblastomas multiforme in children: Report of four cases. **J Neurosurg** 90:546–550, 1999.
85. Kuratsu J, Ushio Y: Epidemiological study of primary intracranial tumors in childhood: A population-based survey in Kumamoto Prefecture, Japan. **Pediatr Neurosurg** 25:240–246, 1996; Discussion 247.
86. Lafond RE, Giammalvo JT, Norkin LC: Relationship between expression of epidermal growth factor and simian virus 40 T antigen in a line of transgenic mice. **Transgenic Res** 4:306–314, 1995.
87. Lang FF, Miller DC, Pisharody S, Koslow M, Newcomb EW: High frequency of p53 protein accumulation without p53 gene mutation in human juvenile pilocytic, low grade and anaplastic astrocytomas. **Oncogene** 9:949–954, 1994.
88. Linet MS, Ries LA, Smith MA, Tarone RE, Devesa SS: Cancer surveillance series: Recent trends in childhood cancer incidence and mortality in the United States. **J Natl Cancer Inst** 91:1051–1058, 1999.
89. Maraziotis T, Perentes E, Karamitopoulou E, Nakagawa Y, Gessaga EC, Probst A, Frankforter A: Neuron-associated class III beta-tubulin isotype, retinal S-antigen, synaptophysin, and glial fibrillary acidic protein in human medulloblastomas: A clinicopathological analysis of 36 cases. **Acta Neuropathol** 84:355–363, 1992.
90. Marks JR, Lin J, Hinds P, Miller D, Levine AJ: Cellular gene expression in papillomas of the choroid plexus from transgenic mice that express the simian virus 40 large T antigen. **J Virol** 63:790–797, 1989.
91. Mason WP, Goldman S, Yates AJ, Boyett J, Li H, Finlay JL: Survival following intensive chemotherapy with bone marrow reconstitution for children with recurrent intracranial ependymoma: a report of the Children's Cancer Group [see comments]. **J Neurooncol** 37:135–143, 1998.
92. May PL, Blaser SI, Hoffman HJ, Humphreys RP, Harwood-Nash DC: Benign intrinsic tectal "tumors" in children. **J Neurosurg** 74:867–871, 1991.
93. McCormick PC, Torres R, Post KD, Stein BM: Intramedullary ependymoma of the spinal cord. **J Neurosurg** 72:523–532, 1990.

94. Mertens F, Heim S, Mandahl N, Mitelman F, Brun A, Stromblad LG, Kullendorff CM, Donner M: Recurrent chromosomal imbalances in choroid plexus tumors [letter]. **Cancer Genet Cytogenet** 80:83–84, 1995.
95. Milhorat TH, Hammock MK, Chien T, Davis DA: Normal rate of cerebrospinal fluid formation five years after bilateral choroid plexectomy: Case report. **J Neurosurg** 44:735–739, 1976.
96. Milhorat TH, Hammock MK, Davis DA, Fenstermacher JD: Choroid plexus papilloma: I. Proof of cerebrospinal fluid overproduction. **Childs Brain** 2:273–289, 1976.
97. Morreale VM, Ebersold MJ, Quast LM, Parisi JE: Cerebellar astrocytoma: Experience with 54 cases surgically treated at the Mayo Clinic, Rochester, Minnesota, from 1978 to 1990. **J Neurosurg** 87:257–261, 1997.
98. Nishi M, Miyake H, Takeda T, Hatae Y: Epidemiology of childhood brain tumors in Japan. **Int J Oncol** 15:721–725, 1999.
99. Nishimura S, Tanaka T, Takakura H, Tachibana H, Takashima S, Takeshita K, Shimizu M: Aicardi syndrome: an unusual association of neoplastic or cystic lesions. **No To Hattatsu** 18:217–222, 1986.
100. Norman MG, Harrison KJ, Poskitt KJ, Kalousek DK: Duplication of 9P and hyperplasia of the choroid plexus: A pathologic, radiologic, and molecular cytogenetics study. **Pediatr Pathol Lab Med** 15:109–120, 1995.
101. Osborne A: *Diagnostic Neuroradiology.* St. Louis, Mosby, 1994, p 936.
102. Packer RJ, Perilongo G, Johnson D, Sutton LN, Vezina G, Zimmerman RA, Ryan J, Reaman G, Schut L: Choroid plexus carcinoma of childhood. **Cancer** 69:580–585, 1992.
103. Packer RJ, Sutton LN, Elterman R, Lange B, Goldwein J, Nicholson HS, Mulne L, Boyett J, D'Angio G, Wechsler-Jentzsen K: Outcome for children with medulloblastoma treated with radiation and cisplatin, CCNU, and vincristine chemotherapy. **J Neurosurg** 81:690–698, 1994.
104. Palma L, Russo A,Celli P: Prognosis of the so-called "diffuse" cerebellar astrocytoma. **Neurosurgery** 15:315–317, 1984.
105. Pang D: Craniopharyngiomas, in Rengachary S, Wilkins R (eds): *Principles of Neurosurgery.* Hong Kong, Mosby-Wolfe, 1994.
106. Park TS, Hoffman HJ, Hendrick EB, Humphreys RP, Becker LE: Medulloblastoma: Clinical presentation and management. Experience at the hospital for sick children, Toronto, 1950–1980. **J Neurosurg** 58:543–552, 1983.
107. Patterson E, Farr R: Cerebellar medulloblastoma: Treatment by irradiation of the whole central neurvous system. **Acta Radiol** 39:323–336, 1953.
108. Pencalet P, Maixner W, Sainte-Rose C, Lellouch-Tubiana A, Cinalli G, Zerah M, Pierre-Kahn A, Hoppe-Hirsch E, Bourgeois M, Renier D: Benign cerebellar astrocytomas in children. **J Neurosurg** 90:265–273, 1999.
109. Pencalet P, Sainte-Rose C, Lellouch-Tubiana A, Kalifa C, Brunelle F, Sgouros S, Meyer P, Cinalli G, Zerah M, Pierre-Kahn A: Papillomas and carcinomas of the choroid plexus in children. **J Neurosurg** 88:521–528, 1998.
110. Pierre-Kahn A, Hirsch JF, Vinchon M, Payan C, Sainte-Rose C, Renier D, Lelouch-Tubiana A, Fermanian J: Surgical management of brain-stem tumors in children: Results and statistical analysis of 75 cases [see comments]. **J Neurosurg** 79:845–852, 1993.
111. Platten M, Giordano MJ, Dirven CM, Gutmann DH, Louis DN: Up-regulation of specific NF 1 gene transcripts in sporadic pilocytic astrocytomas. **Am J Pathol** 149:621–627, 1996.
112. Pollack IF: Brain tumors in children [see comments]. **N Engl J Med** 331: 1500–1507, 1994.
113. Pollack IF, Gerszten PC, Martinez AJ, Lo KH, Shultz B, Albright AL, Janosky J,

Deutsch MF: Intracranial ependymomas of childhood: Long-term outcome and prognostic factors. **Neurosurgery** 37:655–666, 1995; Discussion 666–667.
114. Pollack IF, Hoffman HJ, Humphreys RP, Becker L: The long-term outcome after surgical treatment of dorsally exophytic brain-stem gliomas. **J Neurosurg** 78:859–863, 1993.
115. Raffel C, Hudgins R, Edwards MS: Symptomatic hydrocephalus: Initial findings in brainstem gliomas not detected on computed tomographic scans. **Pediatrics** 82:733–737, 1988.
116. Rajan B, Ashley S, Gorman C, Jose CC, Horwich A, Bloom HJ, Marsh H, Brada M: Craniopharyngioma: A long-term results following limited surgery and radiotherapy. **Radiother Oncol** 26:1–10, 1993.
117. Reardon DA, Entrekin RE, Sublett J, Ragsdale S, Li H, Boyett J, Kepner JL: Chromosome arm 6q loss is the most common recurrent autosomal alteration detected in primary pediatric ependymoma. **Genes Chromosom Cancer** 24:230–237, 1999.
118. Regine WF, Mohiuddin M, Kramer S: Long-term results of pediatric and adult craniopharyngiomas treated with combined surgery and radiation. **Radiother Oncol** 27:13–21, 1993.
119. Rezai AR, Woo HH, Lee M, Cohen H, Zagzag D, Epstein FJ: Disseminated ependymomas of the central nervous system. **J Neurosurg** 85:618–624, 1996.
120. Robertson PL, Allen JC, Abbott IR, Miller DC, Fidel J, Epstein FJ: Cervicomedullary tumors in children: A distinct subset of brainstem gliomas. **Neurology** 44:1798–1803, 1994.
121. Robinow M, Johnson GF, Minella PA: Aicardi syndrome, papilloma of the choroid plexus, cleft lip, and cleft of the posterior palate. **J Pediatr** 104:404–405, 1984.
122. Roland B, Pinto A: Hyperdiploid karyotype in a choroid plexus papilloma. **Cancer Genet Cytogenet** 90:130–131, 1996.
123. Roland EH, Flodmark O, Hill A: Neurosonographic features of Aicardi's syndrome. **J Child Neurol** 4:307–310, 1989.
124. Rorke LB: The cerebellar medulloblastoma and its relationship to primitive neuroectodermal tumors. **J Neuropathol Exp Neurol** 42:1–15, 1983.
125. Rorke LB, Packer RJ, Biegel JA: Central nervous system atypical teratoid/rhabdoid tumors of infancy and childhood: Definition of an entity. **J Neurosurg** 85:56–65, 1996.
126. Rousseau P, Habrand JL, Sarrazin D, Kalifa C, Terrier-Lacombe MJ, Rekacewicz C, Rey A: Treatment of intracranial ependymomas of children: Review of a 15-year experience. **Int J Radiat Oncol Biol Phys** 28:381–386, 1994.
127. Rousseau-Merck MF, Versteege I, Legrand I, Couturier J, Mairal A, Delattre O, Aurias A: hSNF5/INI1 inactivation is mainly associated with homozygous deletions and mitotic recombinations in rhabdoid tumors. **Cancer Res** 59:3152–3156, 1999.
128. Rutka JT: Medulloblastoma. **Clin Neurosurg** 44:571–585, 1997.
129. Rutka J, Hoffman H, Duncan J: Astrocytomas of the posterior fossa, in Cohen A (ed): *Surgical Disorders of the Fourth Ventricle.* Cambridge, MA, Blackwell Science, 1996, pp 147–160.
130. Sagoh M, Murakami H, Hirose Y, Mayanagi K: Occlusive cerebrovasculopathy after internal radiation and bleomycin therapy for craniopharyngioma: Case report. *Neurol Med Chir (Tokyo)* 37:920–923, 1997.
131. Sarkar C, Sharma MC, Gaikwad S, Sharma C, Singh VP: Choroid plexus papilloma: A clinicopathological study of 23 cases. **Surg Neurol** 52:37–39, 1999.
132. Savas A, Erdem A, Tun K, Kanpolat Y: Fatal toxic effect of bleomycin on brain tissue after intracystic chemotherapy for a craniopharyngioma: Case report. **Neurosurgery** 46:213–216, 2000; Discussion 216–217.
133. Schiffer D, Wiestler O: Ependymoma, in Kleihues P, Cavenee W (ed): *Tumours of the Nervous System.* Lyon, International Agency for Research on Cancer, 1997, pp 50–53.

134. Schneider JH Jr, Raffel C, McComb JG: Benign cerebellar astrocytomas of childhood. **Neurosurgery** 30:58–62, 1992; Discussion 62–63.
135. Schut L, Bruce D, Sutton L: Medulloblastomas, in Wilkins R, Rengachary S (eds): *Neurosurgery.* New York, McGraw-Hill, 1996, pp 1177–1181.
136. Schwartz AM, Ghatak NR: Malignant transformation of benign cerebellar astrocytoma. **Cancer** 65:333–336, 1990.
137. Sedlacek Z, Kodet R, Seemanova E, Vodvarka P, Wilgenbus P, Mares J, Poustka A, Goetz P: Two Li-Fraumeni syndrome families with novel germline p53 mutations: Loss of the wild-type p53 allele in only 50% of tumours. **Br J Cancer** 77:1034–1039, 1998.
138. Segal RA, Goumnerova LC, Kwon YK, Stiles CD, Pomeroy SL: Expression of the neurotrophin receptor TrkC is linked to a favorable outcome in medulloblastoma. **Proc Natl Acad Sci USA** 91:12867–12871, 1994.
139. Shaw EG, Evans RG, Scheithauer BW, Ilstrup DM, Earle JD: Postoperative radiotherapy of intracranial ependymoma in pediatric and adult patients. **Int J Radiat Oncol Biol Phys** 13:1457–1462, 1987.
140. Sherer DM, Onyeije CI: Prenatal ultrasonographic diagnosis of fetal intracranial tumors: A review. **Am J Perinatol** 15:319–328, 1998.
141. Shibata MA, Maroulakou IG, Jorcyk CL, Gold LG, Ward JM, Green JE: p53-independent apoptosis during mammary tumor progression in C3(1)/SV40 large T antigen transgenic mice: Suppression of apoptosis during the transition from preneoplasia to carcinoma. **Cancer Res** 56:2998–3003, 1996.
142. Steichen-Gersdorf E, Trawoger R, Duba HC, Mayr U, Felber S, Utermann G: Hypomelanosis of Ito in a girl with plexus papilloma and translocation (X;17). **Hum Genet** 90:611–613, 1993.
143. Steinbok P, Boyd MC: Periaqueductal tumor as a cause of late-onset aqueductal stenosis. **Childs Nerv Syst** 3:170–174, 1987.
144. Steinbok P, Mutat A: Cerebellar astrocytomas, in Albright A, Pollack I, Adelson P (eds): *Principles and Practice of Pediatric Neurosurgery.* New York, Thieme, 1999, pp 641–662.
145. Stroink AR, Hoffman HJ, Hendrick EB, Humphreys RP, Davidson G: Transependymal benign dorsally exophytic brain stem gliomas in childhood: Diagnosis and treatment recommendations. **Neurosurgery** 20:439–444, 1987.
146. Sutton L, Goldwein J, Schwartz D: Ependymomas, in Albright A, Pollack I, Adelson P (eds): *Principles and Practice of Pediatric Neurosurgery.* New York, Thieme, 1999, pp 609–628.
147. Sybert VP, Pagon RA: Hypomelanosis of Ito in a girl with plexus papilloma and translocation (X;17) [letter]. **Hum Genet** 93:227, 1994.
148. Talacchi A, De Micheli E, Lombardo C, Turazzi S, Bricolo A: Choroid plexus papilloma of the cerebellopontine angle: A twelve patient series. **Surg Neurol** 51:621–629, 1999.
149. Taylor M, Gokgoz N, Andrulis I, Mainprize T, Drake J, Rutka J: Familial posterior fossa brain tumors of infancy secondary to a germline mutation of the hSNF5 gene. **Am J Hum Genet** 66:1403–1406, 2000.
150. Thorne RN, Pearson AD, Nicoll JA, Coakham HB, Oakhill A, Mott MG, Foreman NK: Decline in incidence of medulloblastoma in children [see comments]. **Cancer** 74:3240–3244, 1994.
151. Torres CF, Rebsamen S, Silber JH, Sutton LN, Bilaniuk LT, Zimmerman RA, Golowein JW, Phillips PC, Lange BJ: Surveillance scanning of children with medulloblastoma [see comments]. **N Engl J Med** 330:892–895, 1994.
152. Tortori-Donati P, Fondelli MP, Cama A, Garre ML, Rossi A, Andreussi L: Ependy-

momas of the posterior cranial fossa: CT and MRI findings. **Neuroradiology** 37:238–243, 1995.

153. Vajtai I, Varga Z, Aguzzi A: MIB-1 immunoreactivity reveals different labelling in low-grade and in malignant epithelial neoplasms of the choroid plexus. **Histopathology** 29:147–151, 1996.
154. Van den Berge JH, Blaauw G, Breeman WA, Rahmy A, Wijngaarde R: Intracavitary brachytherapy of cystic craniopharyngiomas [see comments]. **J Neurosurg** 77:545–550, 1992.
155. Vandenberg SR, Herman MM, Rubinstein LJ: Embryonal central neuroepithelial tumors: Current concepts and future challenges. **Cancer Metastas Rev** 5:343–365, 1987.
156. Versteege I, Sevenet N, Lange J, Rousseau-Merck MF, Ambros P, Handgretinger R, Aurias A, Delattre O: Truncating mutations of hSNF5/INI1 in aggressive paediatric cancer. **Nature** 394:203–206, 1998.
157. Vinores SA, Herman MM, Katsetos CD, May EE, Frankfurter A: Neuron-associated class III beta-tubulin, tau, and MAP2 in the D-283 Med cell line and in primary explants of human medulloblastoma. **Histochem J** 26:678–685, 1994.
158. Vital A, Bringuier PP, Huang H, San Galli F, Rivel J, Ansoborlo S, Cazauran JM, Taillandier L, Kleihues P, Ohgaki H: Astrocytomas and choroid plexus tumors in two families with identical p53 germline mutations. **J Neuropathol Exp Neurol** 57:1061–1069, 1998.
159. Walter AW, Mulhern RK, Gajjar A, Heideman RL, Reardon D, Sanford RA, Xiong X, Kun LE: Survival and deurodevelopmental outcome of young children with medulloblastoma at St Jude Children's Research Hospital. **J Clin Oncol** 17:3720–3728, 1999.
160. Wolff JE, Sajedi M, Coppes MJ, Anderson RA, Egeler RM: Radiation therapy and survival in choroid plexus carcinoma [letter]. **Lancet** 353:2126, 1999.
161. Woo C, Stea B, Lulu B, Hamilton A, Cassady JR: The use of stereotactic radiosurgical boost in the treatment of medulloblastomas. **Int J Radiat Oncol Biol Phys** 37:761–764, 1997.
162. Yachnis AT, Rorke LB, Trojanowski JQ: Cerebellar dysplasias in humans: Development and possible relationship to glial and primitive neuroectodermal tumors of the cerebellar vermis. **J Neuropathol Exp Neurol** 53:61–71, 1994.
163. Yasargil MG, Curcic M, Kis M, Siegenthaler G, Teddy PJ, Roth P: Total removal of craniopharyngiomas: Approaches and long-term results in 144 patients. **J Neurosurg** 73:3–11, 1990.
164. Zajac V, Kirchhoff T, Levy ER, Horsley SW, Miller A, Steichen-Gersdorf E, Monaco AP: Characterisation of X;17(q12;p13) translocation breakpoints in a female patient with hypomelanosis of Ito and choroid plexus papilloma. **Eur J Hum Genet** 5:61–68, 1997.
165. Zhen HN, Zhang X, Bu XY, Zhang ZW, Huang WJ, Zhang P, Liang JW, Wang XL: Expression of the simian virus 40 large tumor antigen (Tag) and formation of tag-p53 and tag-pRb complexes in human brain tumors. **Cancer** 86:2124–2132, 1999.
166. Zurawel RH, Chiappa SA, Allen C, Raffel C: Sporadic medulloblastomas contain oncogenic beta-catenin mutations. **Cancer Res** 58:896–899, 1998.

CHAPTER

16

Update on Craniofacial Surgery: The Differential Diagnosis of Lambdoid Synostosis/Posterior Plagiocephaly

RICHARD G. ELLENBOGEN, M.D., JOSEPH S. GRUSS, M.D., MICHAEL L. CUNNINGHAM, M.D., PH.D.

INTRODUCTION

The cosmetic abnormality of the posterior skull consisting of flattening of the parietal and occipital bones is called posterior plagiocephaly. The term plagiocephaly is derived from the Greek language: *plagios* = slant, twisted, or oblique and *kephale* = head (49). Posterior plagiocephaly can occur as a result of fusion of the lambdoid suture, i.e., with synostosis, or can occur without synostosis of the lambdoid sutture. When a child has posterior plagiocephaly for any reason, the result is a flattening of the affected occipitoparietal region (47). The word plagiocephaly in modern day literature has been used to denote a deformed, flattened skull without focusing on a specific etiology. This has led to ambiguity both in the literature and in medical practice. This ambiguity has turned out to be pertinent because each of the major causes of posterior plagiocephaly requires a different treatment.

Lambdoid synostosis/posterior plagiocephaly, of all the various craniofacial deformities, has been the one most mired in controversy in the last decade. There is disagreement among surgeons in its incidence, diagnosis, and treatment. Unfortunately, the difference of opinion among clinicians is being analyzed and critiqued in a public forum, especially the lay press, as well as in academic circles. It has peaked the interest of the journalist to the point that disputes surrounding the indications for performing surgery on a misshapened skull have been elevated to front page news (35). The treatment of posterior plagiocephaly is a controversial subject for many reasons. There is disagreement on whether an operation for correction of the cosmetic deformity is warranted. And, if surgery is indicated, is it performed too often? The answers to this point of contention are elusive. The evidence to date suggests that craniosynostosis, as a disease process, is pathologically heterogenous. That is, as Cohen argues, several different mechanisms can cause the same cosmetic skull base defect (7). In posterior plagiocephaly, this is clearly true and has lead to confusion in diagnosis and subsequent treatment.

In this chapter, we will review both classic and current thoughts on the etiology, diagnosis, imaging, and indications for surgery of lambdoid synostosis/posterior plagiocephaly.

ETIOLOGY

The term lambdoid synostosis is reserved for use when premature fusion of one or both of the lambdoid sutures has been proven by clinical, radiologic, and/or pathologic evidence. When both lambdoid sutures are involved, as they are in only 15% of the patients with lambdoid synostosis, the skull deformity can be severe and is best described by the bifrontal bone prominence, a flattened parieto-occiput and elevation of the vertex of the skull, *turribrachycephy* (25, 37, 47). Genetic transmission of the lambdoid synostosis trait within a family has been only rarely reported (14).

Bruneteau and Mullikan eloquently delineated three major causes of (frontal) plagiocephaly: (a) *synostotic,* a premature (unilateral or bilateral) closure of a suture, (b) *compensatory,* that is, compensatory growth ipsilateral or contralateral to a fused suture, and (c) *deformational,* a "non-synostotic" asymmetry resulting from external compressive forces in utero, during delivery, or postnatally (2). In a subsequent paper, Hansen and Mulliken used a similar analysis for posterior plagiocephaly. They separated posterior plagiocephaly into two distinct categories: (a) "*synostotic* occipital plagiocephaly" and (b) "deformational occipital plagiocephaly"; i.e., *non-synostotic* posterior plagiocephaly (18). The term "postural" plagiocephaly has been used by some clinicians because of its apropos descriptive adjective, which indicates a deformation due to intrauterine compression, torticollis, or postnatal sleeping position (17). Marsh and Vannier applied the precise term, *plagiocephaly without synostosis* for non-synostotic posterior flattening of the head. These aforementioned terms have clinical implications because they serve to differentiate patients with plagiocephaly without synostosis, who rarely need surgery, from those who benefit from surgery, true lambdoid synostosis.

Non-synostotic plagiocephaly is the most common type of head deformation occurring in anywhere from 5 to 48% of healthy neonates (18). The deformational forces that can cause non-synostotic posterior plagiocephaly are diverse. For example, a mild form called "molding" occurs presumably from passing the soft distensible fetal head through the birth canal in a normal vaginal delivery. It is hypothesized that compression of the head, in utero, combined with cranial growth restriction caused by the rigid pelvic inlet appears to be contributory (8, 18). There is convincing evidence supporting the hypothesis that compression and restriction can cause deformational plagiocephaly. This evidence consists of reports of an association between head shape and fetal position, uterine anomalies, multiple pregnancies, and vertex presentation (9, 32, 52). Severely plagiocephalic children appear to engage the pelvic structures much earlier than do normocephalic children. Seventy-three percent of deformational frontal plagiocephaly are left-sided (2, 50). This correlates nicely with the incidence (85%) of vertex presentations that are left occipital anterior position.

Another factor associated with plagiocephaly is torticollis. Torticollis is defined as a head tilt to the abnormal side. Torticollis is often seen in non-synostotic plagiocephaly. Torticollis and deformational non-synostotic plagiocephaly occur together 1 in every 300 live births (10). We have noted torticollis in both our patients with posterior as well as frontal plagiocephaly. It is hypothesized that intrauterine compression during pregnancy can cause foreshortening of the sternocleidomastoid muscle (9, 10). Torticollis is deemed responsible for the associated head asymmetry. This makes teleologic sense if torticollis causes a child to position his head on his affected occiput. However, an alternative explanation is that the torticollis is merely casually related to the skull asymmetry. That is, both the torticollis and head asymmetry are a result of an intrauterine process and not "cause and effect".

There are forms of plagiocephaly that are associated with severe torticollis such as the Klippel-Feil syndrome and the craniocervicofacial complex (15, 38). There is even a small group of children who have "craniofacial scoliosis" composed of torticollis and synostosis whose plagiocephaly recurs following surgical correction (12). The pathophysiology of these unusual syndromes is unclear.

The vast majority of children with posterior plagiocephaly associated with torticollis will experience improvement in their skull shape by treatment of the underlying sternocleidomastoid muscle shortening. The treatment of the torticollis makes it easier to prevent the children from sleeping on their flattened occiput. If the spine x-rays are normal, the child undergoes regular stretching exercises performed by the parents under the direction of a physician or physical therapist. This mild form of torticollis rarely requires muscle division.

We have not noted the high incidence of extraocular muscle dysfunction in posterior plagiocephaly, which has been reported in frontal plagiocephaly from coronal synostosis (16). "Ocular torticollis," or more accurately head tilt to the normal side from strabismus, is reported in approximately 50% of the children with synostotic plagiocephaly (mostly frontal). This head tilt may result from an imbalance of the superior and inferior oblique muscles (33, 40). The child attempts to correct diplopia from his strabismus by tilting his head toward the normal side (33). This is not true torticollis, thus the imprecise term, "ocular torticollis."

The most common form of posterior plagiocephaly we see in our clinics is non-synostotic. An infant in whom we postulate the occciput progressively worsens from sleeping on it or an infant who suffers intrauterine compression and restriction of the malleable skull are both illustrative examples. The infant whose skull is distorted from sleeping on one side of the head usually suffers only a mild deformity that may not worsen, can be covered by hair, and will potentially improve as the child grows, rolls over, or begins to walk.

Regardless, the posterior deformity can progress, despite efforts to change the position of the infant's head during sleep. If there is an open lambdoid suture, some surgeons believe a "functional" suture abnormality exists in which bone growth from that suture is slow or halted; that is, simply not normal (31, 47). The concept of a "functional suture" abnormality is not, however, universally embraced (21).

Posterior plagiocephaly without synostosis is being diagnosed more frequently by primary care physicians. Many institutions, including our own, have noted a marked increase in the number of infants referred for evaluation of posterior plagiocephaly (26). A logical hypothesis for this may be the increasingly common practice of placing an infant in the supine instead of the prone position when sleeping. The American Academy of Pediatrics has recommended that infants be placed on their backs or sides during sleep to reduce the risk of sudden infant death syndrome (SIDS) (43). This relatively recent practice is being continued based upon mounting evidence that SIDS occurs less frequently in infants who sleep in the supine position compared to those who sleep in the prone position. In addition, pediatricians are more actively pursing craniofacial deformities at the insistence of their surgical colleagues, regardless of how mild, and are referring them earlier to specialized centers (41).

It is unlikely to conceive that there has been an increase in the synostotic component of posterior plagiocephaly. The reported incidence of radiologically confirmed lambdoid synostosis in the literature from established craniofacial centers varies from extremely infrequent to common (24). Thus, an accurate incidence of lambdoid synostosis is difficult to define. Several surgeons report an unusually high incidence of lambdoid synostosis in their series on craniosynostosis, ranging from 18.5 to 21% (24, 31, 34). Other surgeons feel that many of the previous series with a high incidence of lambdoid synostosis were mistakenly composed of patients with posterior plagiocephaly without synostosis. They support this postulate with detailed high-resolution CT analysis of cranial morphology, which serves to differentiate the non-synostotic from the synostotic skulls (21, 29). In Shillito and Matson's Boston Children's Hospital series of 519 children with craniosynostosis reported in 1968, only 12 children had lambdoid synostosis for an incidence of 2.3% (42). We also believe that the incidence of true isolated lambdoid synostosis is low. In our practice, premature unilateral lambdoid suture closure is a rare cause of posterior plagiocephaly and seen only four times in five years (1991 to 1994) in 130 patients with craniosynostosis for an incidence of 3.1% (21) This corresponds more closely to incidence in the series of Matson and Shillito (30).

However, it is possible that since we only recently began to carefully analyze the craniofacial anomaly of posterior pagiocephaly, a spectrum of this disease may exist. Jimenez et al. diagnosed lambdoid synostosis in patients with significant asterion stenosis by three-dimensional CT and histologic analysis in patients who otherwise had open lambdoid sutures (24). Vander Kolk and Carson's histologic studies in humans demonstrated a microscopic fibrous bridge across functionally fused sutures (47). Burke et al. used the neonatal rabbit craniosynostosis model to support their microspicule hypothesis (3). This hypothesis states that bony microspicules normally bridge a suture. A spicule that fails to fracture from normal mechanical forces results in more bone formation, resulting in a sutural fusion. This hypothesis may explain the evolution of the fused suture process. If this process of fusion is discovered in progression or occurs to varying degrees, the findings may explain the spectrum of the severity of the disease.

PATIENT SELECTION AND DIFFERENTIAL DIAGNOSIS

Proper patient selection for treatment is one of the most difficult aspects of caring for these patients and their parents. Our approach to patient selection is one based on an algorithm that has evolved over the past 10 years. Regardless of proposed etiology, all patients seen with posterior plagiocephaly undergo a thorough examination. Tulasne and Tessier stated in 1981 that plagiocephaly is best analyzed by physical exam as opposed to making decisions based solely on x-ray (45). We have headed their prudent advice. Our patients are examined in multiple visits to the craniofacial clinic over a period of several months to evaluate progression of the deformity.

In addition, our patients may undergo a cervical spine x-ray series. Any child with torticollis undergoes cervical spine x-rays to rule out any congenital or vertebral anomalies. If an infant has a moderate to severe deformity, we order a high-resolution, three-dimensional reconstructed CT scan of the head using commercially available Medical 3D software (1 to 3–mm axial cuts). This study can define the morphology of the underlying brain, the degree of skull base abnormality, and the contour the cranium (See Radiology section). We grade the occipital deformity as mild, moderate, or severe. Mild deformities can be observed, often requiring no further work-up or treatment.

A true lambdoid suture synostosis may be palpable as an external raised ridge. There is often a mastoid bulge on the affected side with contralateral occipital parietal bossing. Conversely, the patients with non-synostotic plagiocephaly do not have these findings.

Children with moderate to severe posterior plagiocephaly of any cause may exhibit displacement of the ipsilateral ear, compensatory bulging of the frontal bone, and posterior bossing. When viewed from the vertex, the shape of the skull in a child with unilambdoid synostosis, may resemble a trapezoid. In a child with non-synostotic, posterior plagiocephaly, the head shape resembles a parallelogram. The most compelling and complete differential diagnosis of non-synostotic posterior plagiocephaly versus true lambdoid synostosis was published by Huang et al. from Children's Hospital Medical Center in Seattle, Washington (21). In the parallelogram-shaped skull of a child with positional molding, or non-synostotic plagiocephaly, one can see ipsilateral frontal bossing, anterior displacement of the ipsilateral ear, ipsilateral occipitoparietal flattening without ridging of the lambdoid suture, and contralateral occipital bossing. In true unilambdoid synostosis, the trapezoid-shaped head is composed of contralateral frontal bossing, posterior displacement of the ipsilateral ear, ipsilateral lambdoid suture ridging with occipitomastoid bossing, ipsilateral occipitoparietal flattening, and contralateral parietal bossing (21). Frontal plagiocephaly with or without coronal synostosis is occasionally confused with posterior plagiocephaly. Frontal plagiocephaly without synostosis can appear similar to posterior plagiocephaly without synostosis since both are characterized by parallelogram-shaped skulls. Since both usually improve with conservative measures, the differential diagnosis may be of academic interest and be best differentiated by the history, i.e., determining the nature, vectors, and direction of the compressive force. Frontal plagiocephaly with coronal synostosis is more easily differentiated from posterior plagiocephaly. Coronal synostosis is best characterized by a more trapezoid-shaped skull, anteriorsuperior deviation of the ipsilateral ear, ipsilateral elevation of the orbit, and lesser sphenoid wing (harlequin eye), and deviation of the nasal root to the affected side (see *Table 16.1* and *Fig. 16.3*).

Our first recommendation to the parents of children who have a non-synostotic etiology for their posterior flattening is to change the child's

TABLE 16.1
Pertinent Features and Differential Diagnosis of Plagiocephaly based on [1,20]

Finding	Posterior Plagiocephaly without Synostosis	Unilambdoid Synostosis	UniCoronal Synostosis
Ipsilateral ear position	Anterior-inferior	Posterior	Anterior-superior
Flattening	Ipsilateral occipitoparietal	Ipsilateral occipitoparietal	Ipsilateral frontal, with orbital rim elevation
Vertex view	Parallelogram	Trapezoid	Trapezoid
Suture	No lambdoid fusion, may have fibrous union, no ridging	Lambdoid fusion, ridging	Coronal fusion, ridging
Bossing	Ipsilateral frontal, contralateral occipital	Contralateral parietal, ipsilateral mastoid	Contralateral frontal
Skull base (three-dimensional)	No tilt, no mid-line deviation	Tilt, posterior fossa deviation off midline	Anterior fossa deviation off midline

position in the crib. Since SIDS is still an overriding concern, the infant is best placed in a more lateral position or supine with the head turned to the unaffected side of the occiput during sleep. This can often be easier said than done. More often than not, the child is in a crib set against a wall. The child sleeps on the affected side of the occiput to see or hear when the parent enters the baby's room. A simple first step is to ask the parents to turn the crib 180 degrees so that the child is forced to lie on the unaffected side to see or hear the parents. The American Academy of Pediatrics guidelines do not preclude placing an awake baby in the prone position if he has posterior skull deformity. Of course, it should be reiterated that sleeping babies should not be place prone.

In selected patients we try helmet therapy, with the goal of contouring the head to a more normal shape. Helmet or band therapy is labor intensive and requires the services of a skilled orthotics department. Many craniofacial clinics have reported remarkable success with helmets and bands, a technique that was first proposed by Clarren in 1979 (5, 28, 39). Levy et al. (28), have conducted a study of operative versus non-operative treatment of non-synostotic posterior plagiocephaly. They concluded that non-operative treatment with a molded headband provided equivalently satisfactory cosmetic results when compared to operative treatment.

There has been an evolution of thinking on this subject based, in part, on the recent careful radiologic and clinical studies performed by many investigators (2, 6, 18, 21, 29). McComb has markedly changed his perspective and states that he currently manages posterior plagiocephaly patients with headbands, patients who in the past may have undergone surgical remoldings (35). Even though parents may not be uniformly compliant with helmets or bands, especially when faced with an uncomfortable, fussy infant, frequent head turning has also achieved a moderate amount of success. Turk also reported good results of conservative therapy for posterior plagiocephaly by employing frequent head turning or helmet therapy (46).

We recommend surgical therapy for posterior plagiocephaly only in infants with a progressive and severe cosmetic deformity. Worsening of the condition must be demonstrated over the period of several months that we follow the patient prior to surgery. Furthermore, the parents must be convinced that it is a cosmetic deformity that cannot be hidden by hair and one that they feel will negatively impact the child's psychological development. We dispel any misconceptions by the parents concerning a need to treat generalized increased intracranial pressure (ICP) or predicted developmental delay from an unusual brain contour, unless there is more than one suture affected (31). We emphasize performing the surgical procedure to treat the cosmetic aspects of the posterior deformity.

Radiologic and Pathologic Considerations

The lambdoid sutures are a paired structure that turns into the sagittal suture superiorly and the parietomastoid and occipitomastoid sutures inferiorly and laterally. Posterior skull growth is influenced by growth of the occipital and parietal bones in conjunction with their adjacent sutures in the skull base. Plain x-rays may show an absent or sclerotic suture (30) (Fig. 16.3).

The CT scans of children with posterior plagiocephaly have been reported to show cerebrospinal fluid collections in the frontal region, diminished subarachnoid space on the affected side, and digital markings, thumbprinting (or thinning) of the bone. Chadduck et al., in 1992, described the presence of prominent subarachnoid spaces in 10 of 14 patients with posterior plagiocephaly (4). Since that time, others have commented on the presence of prominent subarachnoid spaces, especially in areas of compensatory bulging (47). Two theories have been advanced to explain this finding, a hydrodynamic theory and one that implicates impaired CSF absorption (1, 19). However, there are no studies that accurately measure the intracranial pressure in the children with lambdoid synostosis to confirm these theories. In our clinics, we commonly see these prominent CSF spaces and thinning of the posterior bone in children with posterior plagiocephaly. Neurosurgeons have noted thinning of the skull adjacent to a single prematurely closed suture for nearly three decades but have been reluctant to attribute generalized central nervous system delay to it (30). In none of the children with posterior plagiocephaly and prominent CSF collections or bone thinning have we found typical parenchymal cortical changes or any other radiologic changes consistent with raised intracranial pressure, and we are reluctant at this time to implicate anything more significant than a local phenomenon. This is not the case when more than one suture is involved. Bilateral involvement of the lambdoid suture, which is uncommon, can cause decreased skull growth and raised intracranial pressure, both which respond to surgical decompression (25).

The plain x-ray and bone window CT diagnosis of synostosis is supported by elevation, sclerosis, fusion of a suture, or change in obliquity of the suture from its normal overlapping appearance. The high-resolution three-dimensional CT, including three-dimensional osseous surface reformations, can demonstrate complete synostosis of a suture and asymmetry of the skull base and vault (i.e., craniofacial dysmorphology (29) (*Fig. 16.1*). The three-dimensional CT scan must be evaluated care-

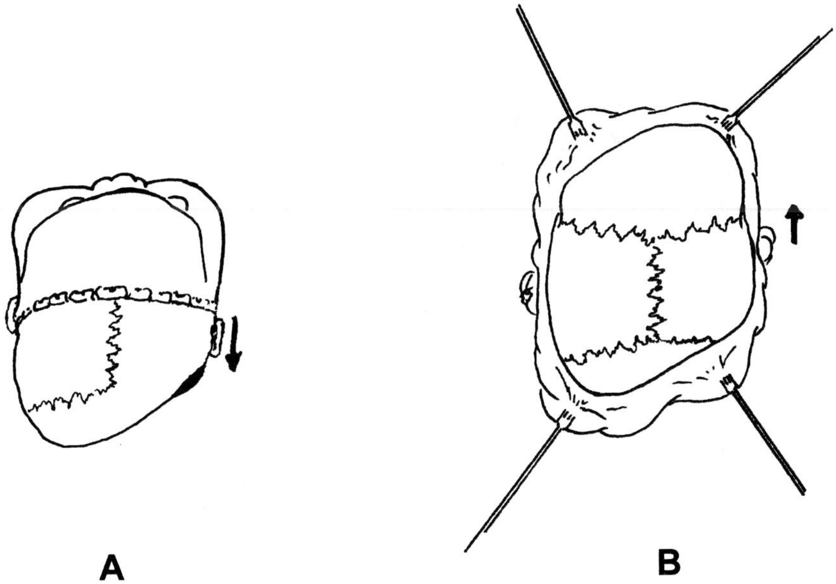

FIG. 16.1 This schematic highlights the differences between posterior plagiocephaly from lambdoid synostosis (*A*) and posterior plagiocephaly from non-sysnostotic (*B*) positional molding. In *A,* note the absent right lambdoid suture, the ipsilateral mastoid bossing, the ipsilateral ear pushed back, and the contralateral parietal bossing. The head is shaped like a trapezoid. In *B,* note the lambdoid suture is open despite the flattened occiput. The ipsilateral ear is pushed forward, and there is ipsilateral frontal bossing and contralateral occipital bossing. The head shape resembles a parallelogram. This type of patient can usually be managed with non-surgical therapy such as a helmet, band, or observation.

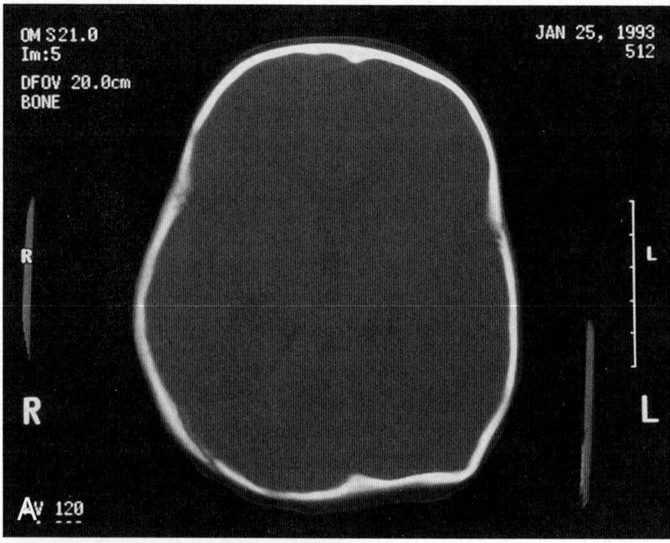

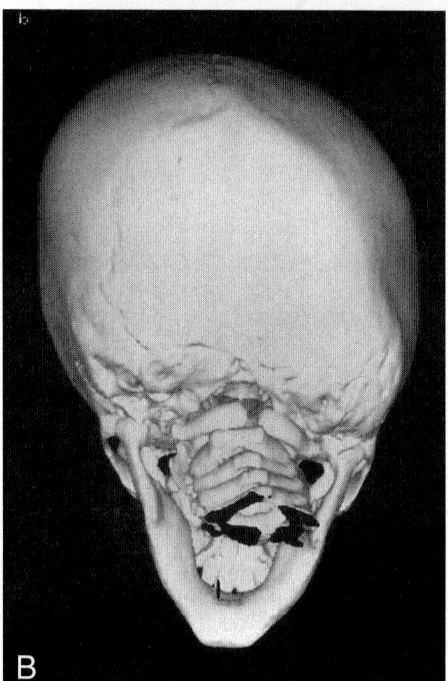

FIG. 16.2 Imaging of a 6-month-old child with left unilambdoid synostosis. (*A*) CT scan, bone window. Note the stenotic left lambdoid suture with a heaped-up margin. (*B*) Three-dimensional CT scan demonstrating stenosis of left lambdoid suture with ridging of the suture and a normal contralateral right lambdoid suture. Note the contralateral parietal bossing. The three-dimensional CT scan can be misleading, as rotations of these images can cause an open suture to disappear or appear fused. In this patient, all views of this fused suture correlated with the other x-ray and physical findings.

fully (*Fig. 16.2*). Slight rotations in the images can cause an open lambdoid suture to disappear or appear fused. The suture morphology must be analyzed in concert with the cranial vault pathology to include ear position, anterior posterior angulation, and skull base deformations (29). In this fashion, Lo et al. were able to accurately differentiate posterior plagiocephaly without synostosis, unilambdoid synostosis, and coronal synostosis based solely on three-dimensional CT endocranial base morphology data (29). Specifically, patients with unilambdoid synostosis had deviation off the anterior posterior midline predominantly in the posterior fossa. The anterior fossa was normal, there was minor asymmetry of the middle fossa, and there was compression of the flattened posterior side with expansion of the contralateral posterior side. Plagiocephaly without synostosis demonstrated minimal deviation off the anterior posterior midline, despite the parallelogram skewing. There was expansion and ventral displacement of the ipsilateral anterior hemi-fossa compartment, a symmetric middle fossa, and ventral

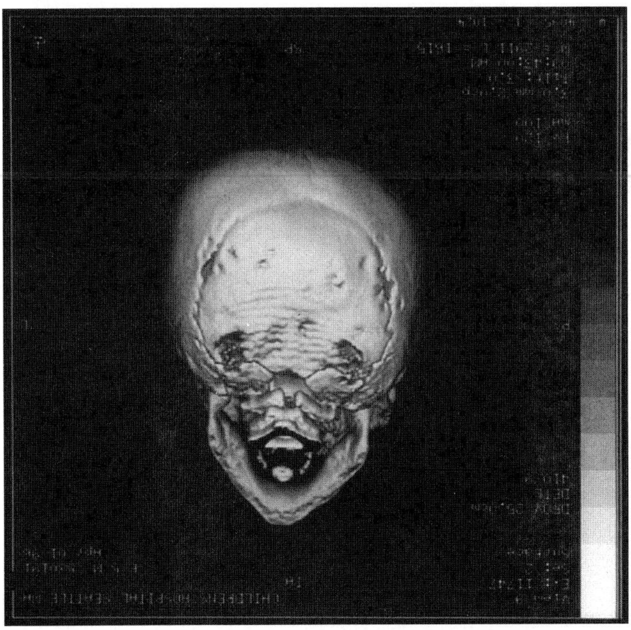

FIG. 16.3 In contrast, this figure demonstrates a three-dimensional CT on a 5-month-old child referred to us for evaluation of a severely flattened posterior occciput, "rule out" bilateral lambdoid synostosis. This child has posterior plagiocephaly without synostosis. Note both lambdoid sutures are open.

displacement of the ipsilateral posterior hemi-fossa on the flattened side (29).

We use the exam in concordance with the photographs, x-rays, and high resolution three-dimensional CT to help guide us in an accurate diagnosis and subsequent treatment options (*Figs. 16.3* and *16.4*).

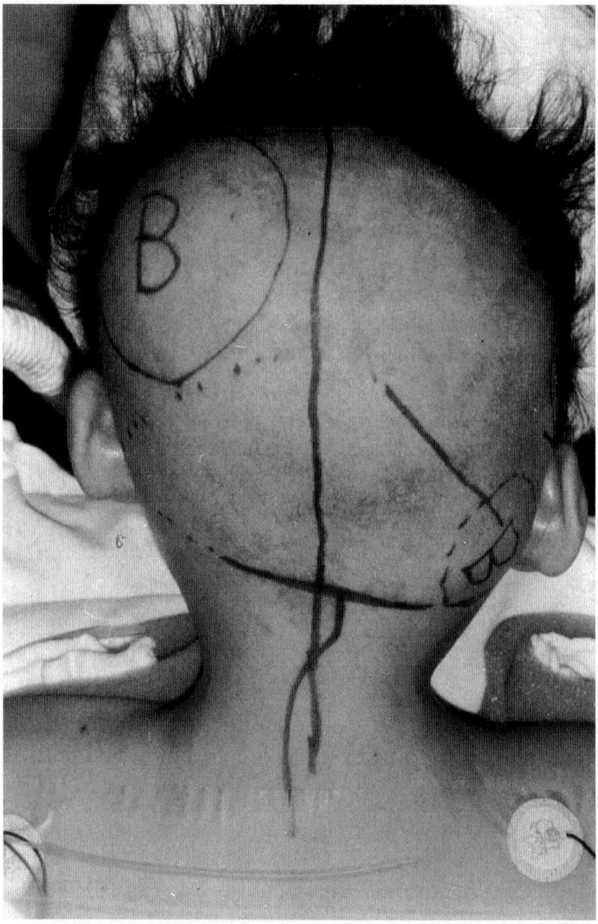

FIG. 16.4 Photograph of an 8-month-old child with progressive posterior plagiocephaly from right unilambdoid synostosis. Preoperatively, the three-dimensional CT scan and examination supported lambdoid synostosis; the child's head was trapezoid shaped when viewed from the vertex. Note the posterior displacement of the ipsilateral ear, right ipsilateral mastoid bossing, contralateral parietal bossing, and head tilt. Parents are informed that the compensatory changes seen in the forehead will improve with time. The ear position will improve but will not be perfectly symmetrical.

SURGICAL TREATMENT

An infant with lambdoid synostosis often has a cosmetic deformity that is not mild and will progress. Also, the small number of patients with posterior plagiocephaly without synostosis whose cosmetic deformity worsens despite adequate non-surgical therapy are candidates for surgery. Such patients undergo surgery between 6 and 12 months of age. Unlike patients with sagittal suture synostosis who undergo surgery earlier (6 weeks to 6 months of age), we prefer to operate only after confirming the progressive nature of the posterior deformity. Parents are counseled that there is no evidence to support operating upon a single suture stenosis/plagiocephaly to prevent intellectual impairment or developmental delay.

Historically, craniosynostosis has been treated by a variety of techniques to include subtemporal decompression, craniectomy, creation of artificial sutures, and morcellation of the entire skull (30). In the 1940 to 1980s, unilambdoid synostosis was often treated by strip craniectomy of the lambdoid suture with placement of a sialastic strip to prevent suture re-stenosis (34, 42). This technique was performed on very young children, 6 to 12 weeks old. When performed on children at such a young age, this type of limited surgery seemed to achieve success. This technique fell out of favor, as it did not treat the skull base deformity associated with this disease, completely correct the asymmetry, or achieve uniform success in older children. In the last decade, a more aggressive posture has been taken by craniofacial surgeons. Pershing, in 1988, proposed bilateral treatment of the occipital bone with barrel staves of the posterior fossa to treat the skull base deformity (37).

There are many different variations on a technique that is primarily a bilateral craniotomy with reshaping of the entire occiput and portion of the skull base (11, 21, 23, 24, 27, 31, 37, 44, 47). We favor the bilateral pariteal-occipital craniotomy followed by occipital barrel staves down to the level of the posterior fossa. We hold the bones in place with suture and rigid fixation consisting of absorbable screws and plates.

SUMMARY

There has been an evolution of thought on the diagnosis and treatment of posterior plagiocephaly. Synostotic posterior plagiocephaly (lambdoid synostosis) can be diagnosed and differentiated from non-synostotic posterior plagiocephaly (positional molding) based on specific cosmetic and radiologic criteria. The advent of high-resolution three-dimensional CT analysis of cranial morphology combined with meticulous clinical studies of the two major causes of posterior plagiocephaly has added much to our understanding of this skull deformity.

Children with lambdoid synostosis have a trapezoid-shaped skull with posterior displacement of their ipsilateral ear, ipsilateral mastoid bossing, contralateral occipital bossing, and a fused lambdoid suture that appears as a ridge. Children with posterior plagiocephaly without lambdoid synostosis have a characteristic parallelogram-shaped skull with anterior displacement of the ipsilateral ear and ipsilateral frontal bossing. This subject is surrounded in controversy because many of the children in the past thought to have lambdoid synostosis probably did not, based in part on the aforementioned specific criteria. This is an important point, as most patients with posterior plagiocephaly without synostosis will improve without surgery.

One should thus be appropriately conservative in the selection of patients for surgery. The majority of infants evaluated at craniofacial clinics presumably have posterior plagiocephaly without synostosis and can be successfully treated with frequent head turning, helmet, or band therapy. Patients with clinically and radiologically proven synostotic posterior plagiocephaly and a severe deformity should undergo craniofacial surgery. The technique of biparieto-occipital craniotomy is safe, simple, and delivers a good cosmetic result. Our postoperative photographic evaluations have shown an immediate, aesthetically pleasing change in the contour of the occiput, which tends to improve with time.

REFERENCES

1. Boop F: The subarachnoid spaces in craniosynostosis. **J Neurosurg** 30:867–871, 1992.
2. Bruneteau RM, John B: Frontal plagiocephaly: Synostotic, compensational, or deformational. **J Plast Reconstr Surg** 89:21–31, 1992.
3. Burke MJ, Winston KR, Williams R: Normal sutural fusion and the etiology of single suture craniosynostosis: The microspicule hypothesis. **Pediatr Neurosurg** 22: 241–2427, 1995.
4. Chadduck W, Chadduck JB, Boop FA: The subarachnoid spaces in craniosynostosis. **Neurosurgery** 30:867–871, 1992.
5. Clarren SK: Plagiocephaly and torticollis: Etiology, natural history, and helmet treatment. **J Pediatr** 98:92, 1981.
6. Cohen MJ: Perspectives on craniofacial asymmetry: V. The craniosynostoses. **Int J Oral Maxillofac Surg** 24:191–194, 1995.
7. Cohen MMJ: The Etiology of Craniosynostosis, in E. M. T. Pershing and JA Jane (eds). **Scientific Foundations and Surgical Treatment of Craniosynostosis,** Baltimore, Williams and Wilkins, 1989, pp 9–20.
8. Danby PM: Plagiocephaly in some 10-year-old children. **Arch Dis Child** 37:500, 1962.
9. Dunn P: Congenital postural deformities. **Br Med Bull** 32:71, 1976.
10. Dunn PM: Congenital sternocmastoid torticollis: An intrauterine postural deformity (abstract). **Arch Dis Child** 49:824, 1974.
11. Ellenbogen RG, Mayer MH: Surgical management of posterior plagiocephaly, in Ren-

ganchary WA (ed): **Surgical Atlas,** Chicago, The American Association of Neurological Surgeons, 1996 Vol. 5, Pp.43–55.
12. Fearon JaMI: Cranioscoliosis. **Plast Reconstr Surg** 92:202, 1993.
13. Francel PC, Bell A, Jane JA: Operative positioning for patients undergoing repair of craniosynostosis. **Neurosurgery** 35:304–306; Discussion 306, 1994.
14. Fryburg J, Hwang V, Lin KY: Recurrent lambdoid synostosis within two families. **Am J Med Genet** 58:262–266, 1995.
15. Gorlin RJ, Cohen MM Jr., Levin LS: **Syndrome of the Head and Neck,** ed 3, New York, NY Oxford University Press, 1990.
16. Gosain A, Steele MA, McCarthy JG, Thorne CH: A prospective study of the relationship between strabismus and head posture in patients with frontal plagiocephaly. **Plast Reconstr Surg** 97:881–891, 1996.
17. Haberkern CM, Smith DW, Jones KL: The "breech head" and its relevance. **Am J Dis Child** 133:154, 1979.
18. Hansen JB: Frontal plagiocephaly: Diagnosis and treatment. **Clin Plast Surg 21:**543–553, 1994.
19. Hassler W, Zetner J: Radical osteoclastic craniectomy in sagittal synostosis. **Neurosurgery** 27:539, 1990.
20. Hinton DR, Becker LE, Muakkassa KF, Hoffman HJ: Lambdoid synostosis: 1. The lambdoid suture: Normal development and pathology of synostosis **J Neurosurg** 61:333, 1984.
21. Huang MH, Gruss JS, Clarren SK, Mouradian WE, Cunningham ML, Roberts TS, Loeser JD, Cornell CJ: The differential diagnosis of posterior plagiocephaly: True lambdoid synostosis versus positional molding. **Plast Reconstr Surg** 98:765–774, 1996.
22. Jimenez DF, Barone CM: Intraoperative autologous blood transfusion in the surgical correction of craniosynostosis. **Neurosurgery** 37:1075–1079, 1995.
23. Jimenez DF, Barone CM: The Sunrise Technique: The correction of occipital plagiocephaly using bandeau occipital plate and radial osteotomies. **Pediatr Neurosurg** 22:162–165, 1995.
24. Jimenez DF, Barone CM, Argamaso RV, Goodrich JT, Shprintzen RJ: Asterion region synostosis. **Cleft Palate Craniofac J** 31:136–141, 1994.
25. Kaiser G: The clinical significance of bilateral synostosis of the lambdoid suture and the usefulness of its treatment. **Childs Brain** 11:87–98, 1984.
26. Kane AA, Mitchell LE, Craven KP, Marsh JL: Observations on a recent increase in plagiocephaly without synostosis. **Pediatrics** 97(6 Pt. 1)877–885, 1996.
27. Keating RT: Lambdoid plagiocephaly. **Contemp Neurosurg** 18:1–6, 1996.
28. Levy M, McComb JG, Wells K, et al: Comparison of operative versus nonoperative treatment of functional lambdoid synostosis. Annual Meeting of the Joint Section on Pediatric Neurosurgery of the AANS and CNS, December 6–9, 1994.
29. Lo LJ, Marsh JL, Pilgram TK, Vannier MW: Plagiocephaly: differential diagnosis based on endocranial morphology. **Plast Reconstr Surg** 97:282–291, 1996.
30. Matson, DD. **Neurosurgery of Infancy and Childhood,** ed. 2. Springfield, IL. Charles C. Thomas, 1969.
31. McComb JG: Treatment of functional lambdoid synostosis. **Neurosurg Clin North Am** 2:665–672, 1991.
32. Miller M, Dunne PM, Smith DW: Uterine malformation and fetal deformation. **J Paediatr** 94:387, 1979.
33. Morax S: Oculomotor disorders in craniofacial malformations, in Caronni E. (ed): **Craniofacial Surgery.** Boston, Little, Brown, 1985, p 97.

34. Muakkassa KF, Hoffman HJ, Hinton DR, Hendrick EB, Humphreys RP, Ash J: Lambdoid synostosis. Part 2: Review of cases managed at The Hospital for Sick Children, 1972–1982. **J Neurosurgery** 61:340–347, 1984.
35. Ortega B: Unkind cut: Some physicians do unnecessary surgery on heads of infants. Wall Street J:5, 1996.
36. Park T, Broaddus WC, Harris M, Pershing JA, Jane JA: Vaccum-stiffened beenbag for cranial remolding procedures in modified prone position. Technical note. **J Neurosurg** 71:623–625, 1989.
37. Persing JA, Delashaw, Johnny B, Jane, JA, Edgerton, MT: Lambdoid synostosis: Surgical considerations. **J Plast Reconstr Surg** 81:852–860, 1988.
38. Poole M, Briggs M: The cranio-facio-cervical scoliosis complex. **Br J Plast Surg** 43:670, 1990.
39. Ripley CE, Pomatto J, Beals SP, Joganic EF, Manwaring KH, Moss SE: Treatment of positional plagiocephaly with dynamic orthotic cranioplasty. **J Craniofac Surg** 5:150–159, 1994.
40. Robb R, Boger WP: Vertical strabismus associated with plagiocephaly. **J Pediatr Ophthalmol Strabismus** 20:58, 1983.
41. Shillito J, Jr: A plea for early operation for craniosynostosis. **Surg Neurol** 37:182–188, 1992.
42. Shillito J, Jr., Matson D.D: Craniosynostosis: A review of 519 surgical patients. **Pediatrics** 41:829, 1968.
43. SIDS ATFolPa: Positioning and SIDS. **Pediatrics** 89:1120, 1992.
44. Thaller SR, Hoyt J, Broggan J: Surgical correction of unilateral lambdoid synostosis: Occipital rotation flap. **J Craniofac Surg** 3:12–17, 1992.
45. Tulasne JF, Tessier P: Analysis and late treatment of plagiocephaly: Unilateral coronal synostosis. **Scand J Plast Reconstr Surg** 15:257, 1981.
46. Turk A, McCarthy JG, Thorne CHM, Wisoff JH: The "back to sleep" campaign and deformational plagiocephaly: Is there cause for concern? **J Craniofac Surg** 7:12, 1996.
47. Vander Kolk CA, Carson, BS: Lambdoid synostosis, in Vander Kolk CA (ed): **Clinics in Plastic Surgery: Craniofacial Surgery.** Philadelphia, W.B. Saunders Company, 1994, pp 575–584.
48. Vander Kolk CA, Carson, BS., Robertson, BC, Manson, PN: The occipital bar and internal osteotomies in the treatment of lambdoid synostosis. **J Craniofac Surg** 4:112–118, 1993.
49. Virchow R: Uber den cretinismus, namentlich in franken, und uber pathologische schadelformen. **Verh Phys Med Ges Wurtburg** 2:230, 1851.
50. Watson G: Relation between side of plagiocephaly, dislocation of hip, scoliosis, bat ears and sternomastoid tumors. **Arch Dis Child** 46:203, 1971.
51. Wynne-Davis R: Infantile idiopathic scoliosis: Causative factors, particularly in the 1st 6 months of life. **J Bone Joint Surg** 578:138, 1975.

CHAPTER

17

Pediatric Trauma Made Simple

P. DAVID ADELSON, M.D.

INTRODUCTION

Despite the explosive growth of multiple preventative programs including ThinkFirst, ThinkFirst for Kids, National Safe Kids Campaign, etc., trauma remains the leading cause of death and disability in children (3). Head trauma or traumatic brain injury (TBI) is the major comorbid factor leading to mortality and major morbidity in this population (39). TBI accounts for over 50% of the deaths in the pediatric population, which is five times that of the next leading cause, leukemia, and 18 times that of brain tumors. There continues on a yearly basis to be over 150,000 new head injuries in children with two peak periods of incidence (39, 53). The first is in early childhood (less than 5 years of age) and the second in mid to late adolescence. The more severely injured children suffer the highest morbidity and mortality, with a mortality rate up to 30 to 50% with the vast majority of survivors left with permanent disabilities. Specific mechanisms of injury in children are often unique to the individual age groups. For children ages 5 to 15, biking and recreational sports are the more common mechanisms of injury. In mid to late adolescence, motor vehicle-related injuries are the most common, and, with regard to mortality, motor vehicle collisions make up the largest percentage of deaths in all groups. In the younger age group, those less than 4 years of age, the most common mechanisms of injury include falls and motor vehicle-related injuries, though of concern is the high incidence of child abuse or non-accidental trauma. Child abuse in this group, as a mechanism of injury, represents, in some series, upward of two-thirds of the severe TBI (33, 36, 39).

Children in general tend to suffer more diffuse-type primary injuries compared to focal injuries in adults, whereas skull fractures are variable in children and less commonly associated with hematomas as is found in adult patients. Children more frequently suffer from diffuse cerebral swelling and intracranial hypertension, which, as a result, leads to less surgical interventions and a higher incidence of primary critical care management. Typical findings at autopsy in children with diffuse severe brain injuries and swelling include vascular congestion or axonal injury as well as ischemic neurodamage or infarction (24, 25). In addition, whereas most injured children will suffer only a mild or moderate TBI (85–90%), it has become increasingly recognized that these children also can suffer significant cognitive deficits that can permanently impact on concentration, complex thinking, decision-making capability, and/or motor impairments that impact not only on their day-to-day life but on their future scholastic and vocational achievements.

The economic burden to our society secondary to TBI in children continues to expand not only because of the increasing costs for medical expenses and rehabilitation in the acute setting (22) but also in lost productivity time of these children and their families throughout their affected lives. Further expenses are expected to accrue in the future as more and more children with acquired disabilities require further and extended services throughout their lifetimes. Given the scope of this problem within the pediatric population and in neurosurgery in general, it is important for the neurosurgical practitioner to attain the basic concepts of neurotrauma care as it relates to both adults and children acutely. It is important to begin to appreciate some of the unique aspects in children that may affect their care. It is believed that a meticulous approach to these acutely ill patients may have the greatest impact on their outcome both in the short term as well as in the long term. Although it cannot be claimed that children are a completely different "breed" and need to be absolutely treated differently than adult trauma patients similarly injured, there are truly unique differences that play a role in the perspective of the treating physician in their management in the acute setting as well as throughout the recovery period. The purpose of this review is to provide a few basic concepts that will assist in understanding the perspective of treating children with head injuries and facilitate the optimization not only of acute care but long-term issues as well.

UNIQUENESS OF PEDIATRIC TBI

Prior to the discussion of treatment in children, it is important to understand what is believed to make children unique from the adult patient. There are multiple differences that exist between the pediatric, immature brain compared to the adult, mature brain; differences at all levels that include not only the basic anatomic make-up of the brain but some of the basic physiologic functional mechanisms. These differences impact not only on the brain's primary response to injury but the secondary response as well.

Anatomically, children have a different water content of the brain, myelination, and cerebral blood volume. As well, they have a different head mass and neck musculature. This leads to differences in the biomechanics of the brain and its susceptibility to injury, shearing, hemorrhage, etc. (1). Physiologic differences in cerebral blood flow and metabolism lead to differences in oxygen content, demands for O_2, and decreased susceptibility to injury with hypoxia and/or hypotension from a traumatic event. Other differences include autoregulatory mechanisms and receptor expression, all of which may be differentially altered compared to the adult. In the first five years of life, the brain is undergoing hypertrophy and significant myelination. There is a significant dendritic arborization and the onset of synaptogenesis that occurs through young childhood. This is also a time in which the critical periods of development are occurring, laying down the foundation for more complex functions. Injury during these different periods leads to different structural differences and impact on the timing and implementation of the specific critical periods and developmental phases. This results in varied and differing levels of recovery and outcome in these patients that still remain to be defined.

CONCEPTS OF PRIMARY VERSUS SECONDARY INJURY

Often, there is a significant amount of confusion in regard to the concepts and terms used in regard to "primary" versus "secondary" injury. This arises because of the different terminology and definitions used throughout the literature over the past few years. The "primary" injury is defined as that damage that occurs as a direct result of the mechanism of injury. To date, other than prevention and safety devices, such as helmets, airbags, etc., there are no other ways to eliminate or lessen the damage incurred from the primary injury. The "secondary" injury is the physiologic and/or biochemical cascade of events that occur as a result of the primary injury, such as excitotoxicity, lipid peroxidation from free radicals, etc.

The secondary injury has been the focus of the aggressive management and novel therapeutic interventions for TBI. This secondary injury is sometimes confused with a "second" injury, which is an added insult to the primary injury that is defined as an event that contributes or worsens the secondary injury. An example of this would be hypoxia at the scene following a motor vehicle collision. A second insult/injury can occur later (e.g., in the ICU), again a hypoxic episode that leads to further injury and a secondary cascade of events (3).

INITIAL ASSESSMENT AND MANAGEMENT

Similar to adults', the leading contributors in children of morbidity and mortality, which are, in essence, second insults following TBI, include: 1) hypoxia, 2) hypotension, 3) systemic injury, and/or 4) intracranial hypertension. Based on these observations, the approach to the assessment and management of traumatized patients must therefore address and aggressively treat these "second" injuries to lessen their impact on outcome. The initial stabilization and care of the patient takes place as acutely as possible, and the "ABCs" (airway, breathing, and circulation) of initial trauma management are carefully managed and monitored. Most important, these concepts are not solely at the time of the initial resuscitation but must be adhered to throughout the acute hospital course, particularly in the early treatment phase in the ICU setting to ensure against iatrogenic second injury. The maintenance of adequate oxygenation, ventilation, and systemic perfusion, as well as the optimization of the cerebral perfusion in the injured patients is a minimum standard to which the practitioner must strive. Realize, too, that differences exist for "adequacy" for each of these basic parameters in children based on age and size. Clearly, the optimal management in these patients is through the individualization of therapy.

ABCs

Control of the "airway" and adequate ventilation ("breathing") are the first priorities in the management of any traumatized and head-injured patient, child or adult. As previously noted, it is of paramount importance to maintain oxygenation and prevent hypoxemia (O_2 saturation > 93%), as even moderate reductions in PaO_2 may contribute to a second neural injury (21). Whereas moderate levels of hypoxia in experimental models does not produce pathologic effects in the normal brain, hypoxia in association with the traumatically injured brain induces further and significant damage (21). In addition, initially normocarbia or only slight hyperventilation ($PaCO_2$ 35–38 mmHg) should be maintained because hypercarbia and hypocarbia cause arteriolar vasodilation and constriction, respectively, which may further contribute to second injuries.

Adequate systemic perfusion or "circulation" resulting in adequate cerebral perfusion remains the goal in the treatment of patients with severe TBI. In children, blood pressure is maintained normal to slightly elevated for age and is continuously monitored. Often following trauma, besides the head injuries, there can be extensive extracranial injuries that produce shock or hypotension from hemorrhage. Young children (<4 years) in particular have a higher incidence of hypotension compared to other age groups (8, 39). Treatment should include volume expansion followed by pressors as necessary in these instances to maintain perfusion and hemodynamic stability.

Initial Neurologic Assessment

The initial examination or primary survey in the ED and neurologic assessment are simultaneously obtained to provide a baseline functional status. It minimally consists of the Glasgow Coma Score (GCS); cranial and cranial nerve exam; and motor, sensory, and reflex exams. Many have found the GCS to not adequately assess young children and infants. For that reason, modifications to the GCS that are age-appropriate have been proposed and are presently being tested in a clinical trial. Lacerations and signs of skull fractures can usually be discovered during the primary survey, whereas basilar skull fractures and other intracranial damage may be suspected if otorrhea, rhinorrhea, or Battle's sign or Raccoon's eyes are discovered.

Radiologic Assessment

In the initial evaluation and resuscitation of the pediatric patient, in conjunction with the standard series of evaluative plain trauma films, a lateral C-spine x-ray is obtained. Clearance of the cervical spine in children, though, still requires the completion of the standard three views (anterior- posterior, lateral, and open-mouth) that adequately visualize C-1 through T-1. Questions of abnormalities or instability require further assessment with further views of the C-spine or CT scan. Normal x-rays, though, do not provide *clinical clearance* due to the higher incidence of ligamentous injury in children compared to adults. Clinical clearance, though, requires the patient to perform a full range of motion on exam when cleared to do so from the other injuries.

Plain skull x-rays are probably not useful in the age of CT, though if one suspects a skull fracture, the resultant anatomic study via CT is more definitive for both bone and underlying parenchymal injury. If a skull film shows a fracture, a CT will often be obtained to ensure no extra-axial collections of blood. At times, where there is concern about sedating the young child for the radiologic study, especially if they are neurologically normal, a skull x-ray may be helpful if there is a scalp hematoma and the underlying skull cannot adequately be palpated (6). The decision to obtain a CT in these patients should be based on the above criteria for severity even if they are a GCS of 14 or 15 and have a normal neurologic and a plain x-ray exam.

Following stabilization, a CT scan of the head is obtained in any child who has an altered level of consciousness (GCS $\leq$ 13), focal neurologic signs, or preceding any surgical intervention such as laparotomy or open reduction of fracture when anesthesia will preclude assessment of the mental status for any length of time. A CT is particularly important if the history revealed a loss of consciousness, a severe accident or mechanism of injury, a seizure, or a deformation of the scalp/skull on exam. Intracranial hypertension still may occur with a normal CT (35, 36, 45), and therefore the total assessment of the severely head-injured patient is necessary. If other injuries demand immediate intervention prior to CT, intraoperative ICP monitoring may be required during the procedure to prevent undiagnosed intracranial hypertension. Obviously, significant mass lesions require operative intervention prior to monitoring.

Other radiologic methods can be used in children to provide further information as to the acute cerebral function in the traumatized patient. Increasingly, stable Xenon-CT (XeCT), which is coupled to the CT scan, can be used to define the functional correlates to the anatomic abnormalities (27, 55). Measurement of the metabolic and/or pressure autoregulation of CBF (through the manipulation of $PaCO_2$ and blood pressure) can be achieved in the clinical setting, which may help guide clinical care. The radioactive ^{133}Xe method also provides a regional assessment of cerebral blood flow and is a useful adjunct as it can be performed at the bedside with serial studies obtained with little manipulation of the patient. Positron emission tomography and magnetic resonance imaging have been used, but not widely, in the acute setting.

The measurement of jugular venous saturation has also been used following head injury to assess cerebral perfusion and metabolism. In children, jugular venous information has been used in a few centers to assess the metabolic changes (9, 47), though the usefulness of this modality and efficacy in pediatric severe TBI remain to be investigated fully.

TREATMENT OF PEDIATRIC TRAUMATIC BRAIN INJURY

In the past 20 years, mortality from head injury in children has declined due at least in part to appropriate and aggressive management (5, 44). Because primary brain injury following trauma is not believed to be amenable to treatment, the goal of conventional therapeutic interventions has been to prevent second injuries and interrupt the "secondary" response. As was noted earlier, since mortality following the initial TBI is believed due most often as a result of second insults such as 1) systemic deterioration and/or hypotension, 2) prolonged hypoxemia, and 3) uncontrolled intracranial hypertension—all which may be treatable events, the goals of acute head injury management are to 1) prevent secondary neuronal damage to an already compromised nervous system and 2) attempt to create an environment conducive to functional recovery. "Aggressive" management is, therefore, not so much an invasive protocol but a compulsive adherence to detail acutely. This includes maintaining adequate blood pressure (mean arterial pressure

[MAP]) and cerebral perfusion pressure (CPP) by aggressively treating raised intracranial pressure (ICP), oxygenation, and ventilation. Because after TBI there may be a loss of the normal autoregulatory mechanisms, therapeutic modalities may need to be tailored to provide the optimal oxygenation and perfusion to the injured brain in the acute period after injury.

ICP MANAGEMENT

Intracranial hypertension contributes significantly to mortality in over half the patients with a severe TBI (42). Increased ICP occurs as a result of brain swelling, an increasing mass lesion, or cerebrospinal fluid (CSF) accumulation (hydrocephalus). Intracranial hypertension ultimately impedes cerebral perfusion and causes secondary ischemia. The treatment of the head-injured child as in the adult depends on the maintenance of adequate CPP. Whereas at present, "adequate" CPP does not ensure adequate cerebral perfusion in focally injured regions of the brain in children and optimal parameters have yet to be determined, both ICP and CPP at this time should be used to guide efficacy of therapy. Optimal perfusion must therefore be assessed and tailored to the individual patients. In reality, the normal initial treatment of an ICP of 20 mmHg in the adult is too high for the infant due to a normally lower CPP and MAP. For infants, we treat ICP elevations of 15 mmHg and, in young children, ICP elevations of 17 to 18 mmHg, again individualizing to the situation.

First Tier Therapies

ICP MONITOR/CSF DRAINAGE

The continuous monitoring of ICP is recommended for all adult patients with Glasgow Coma Scores (GCS) $\leq$8, though the guidelines for its use in children are still being developed (Thomas Luerrsen, personal communication). While conclusive data are lacking for the use of ICP monitoring in severely head-injured infants and young children, and not a "standard of care" in their management, its use has widely increased due to its efficacy in guiding acute care. ICP monitoring 1) aids in the early detection of intracranial mass lesions, 2) can determine the efficacy of therapies, which themselves may be potentially harmful, 3) can reduce ICP by CSF drainage and thus improve CPP (provided a ventricular catheter is used), and 4) helps in determining prognosis. Continuous ICP monitoring can be accomplished by available online systems using either an indwelling ventriculostomy (EVD) or a fiberoptic or strain gauge-type ICP monitor. The EVD remains the gold standard following trauma as it can be used to measure ICP and to therapeutically drain CSF either continuously or intermittently during periods of increased ICP.

HEAD POSITION AND SEDATION

Elevation of the head of the bed to 15 to 30° and maintaining the head in a neutral position have commonly been used to facilitate adequate cerebral venous drainage (and possibly CSF drainage) by avoiding jugular venous compression. This results in optimizing cerebral venous pressure, cerebral blood volume, and a lower ICP. Moving the head from 0° to 30° has been shown to decrease ICP and MAP significantly, though it has no effect on CPP or CBF. Elevation to 60° has been shown to negatively impact on CBF in the adult (20). It remains unclear the optimal height in children and again should be tailored based on MAP, ICP, and CBF as available.

Sedation and/or paralysis are often used in the initial treatment of severely head-injured patients, since it may reduce the noxious stimulation of intubation, suctioning, patient agitation, and asynchronous ventilation that can increase ICP, particularly as will occur in the frightened, injured child. Sedation and paralysis can be carefully titrated once ICP monitoring has been established using short-acting medications; narcotics and benzodiazepines along with a nondepolarizing muscle relaxant are generally recommended for intermittent or continuous use. In this way, intermittent exams can still be obtained.

CONTROLLED VENTILATION

The use of controlled ventilation has long been a modality for the treatment of intracranial hypertension and is based on the known cerebrovascular response to changes in $PaCO_2$. Bruce et al. (13, 14) initially suggested that intracranial hypertension in children could be effectively treated almost exclusively with vigorous hyperventilation. Random and "blind" hyperventilation recently has come into question as a therapeutic intervention because it tended to worsen outcome in adults with severe TBI (44). The limited therapeutic effect, in conjunction with a concern of decreasing perfusion in the early period after injury, has prompted the use of moderate hyperventilation ($PaCO_2 \geq 35$ Torr), which may aid ICP management without inducing ischemia (11, 44). Most of these studies though, again, were done solely in adults and did not address age-related differences (44, 50).

Besides assessing and controlling $PaCO_2$, the maintenance of good cerebral oxygenation is also necessary for the prevention of second insults. Hypoxemia ($PaO_2 < 75$ mmHg by arterial blood gas analysis or oxygen saturation $< 94\%$) early after injury contributes to poor outcome (18, 36). Optimally, adequate oxygenation should be maintained throughout the acute course from the field through discharge.

MEAN ARTERIAL PRESSURE

Early after TBI, hypotension (systolic blood pressure < 90 mmHg [adult]) is associated with increased mortality and morbidity (15, 23, 46). Contemporary management of the infant or child with severe TBI includes maintenance of an adequate perfusion. This can usually be achieved with normotension or mild systemic hypertension, though this differs again by the age and size of the child. Since cerebral injury may be complicated by either partial or complete loss of pressure autoregulation, significant systemic hypertension may contribute to hyperemia and cerebral swelling and should, in general, be avoided. In some cases, a higher systemic pressure may be necessary to maintain adequate perfusion to compromised brain regions, though careful monitoring of ICP and CBF is necessary to determine the impact of blood pressure manipulation. Because of the uniqueness of children and age and size variances for the optimal CPP, the issue of optimal MAP in children is even that much more complex. It is becoming clear that, in the future, management of the TBI patient will need to be tailored and titrated individually so as not to iatrogenically worsen an already compromised brain. Hypotension (SBP ≤ 50 percentile for age, ranging from 55–65 mmHg for infants and 80–85 mmHg for adolescents) should be aggressively managed with fluids and, if necessary, using pressor support with dopamine, neosynephrine, or other agents as indicated to optimize and maintain adequate CPP.

Second Tier Therapy

OSMOTIC AND LOOP DIURETICS

Mannitol has been shown to attenuate intracranial hypertension, which is believed to occur as a result of two separate mechanisms. Upon infusion, mannitol decreases blood viscosity, which can potentiate pressure and/or metabolic autoregulation of the intact brain and reduce ICP. Mannitol also acts by reducing the extravascular volume through increasing the serum osmolality, thereby reducing brain edema. Mannitol may also affect CBF by increasing CBF and CBV, which may contribute to its overall therapeutic effect, though this has been controversial. Bruce et al. (14) dismissed the use of mannitol to treat ICP in children due to its tendency to increase CBF in patients after injury. Muizelaar et al. (43) disagreed, indicating that since mannitol potentiated autoregulatory mechanisms, its use was particularly useful in the acute setting. We have found mannitol to be particularly useful in the management of children with severe TBI. It can be given at 4 to 6-hour intervals or as necessary to maintain an "optimal" ICP. Its use is limited by the serum osmolality and resistance to the effect of infusion with the loss of efficacy occurring as soon as 24 hours. Different methods have been used to enhance and lengthen the time of efficacy. We initiate therapy at a dose of 0.25 g/kg and escalate to 0.5 then 1.0 g/kg once dosing has little effect. Furosemide can also be used acutely and in conjunction with mannitol to reduce the intravascular volume that initially follows the mannitol infusion. Because both fluid volume and Na^+ is excreted, serum osmolality may also be aided with the use of furosemide. Recent studies have also shown the possible efficacy of hypertonic saline after severe TBI. Though it has been used predominantly in adults, this adjunct to therapy may also be useful in children. Studies as to safety and efficacy have yet to be performed in the pediatric population.

Third Tier Therapy

BARBITURATES

Barbiturates, particularly pentobarbital, have long been known to be neuroprotective through multiple mechanisms. These include reducing cerebral metabolic demands, free radical inhibition, and alterations in vascular tone (41). By reducing the metabolic requirements of the brain, ischemic levels of CBF may be tolerated for longer periods, and CBF is decreased with subsequent decreases in CBV and potentially ICP. This has remained a somewhat controversial therapy in head injury and has not been used extensively except as a last resort. Early use, though, may have more beneficial effects prior to the actual development of malignant intracranial hypertension. The standard level of "barbiturate coma" is achieved when there is 10 to 20 seconds of burst suppression of cortical activity monitored by bedside EEG. This therapeutic goal may be limited by systemic hypotension because of myocardial depression; as a result, the patient may require pressor and fluid support to attain the desired level of cerebral suppression. Recent data suggest that "coma" levels of barbiturates may not be necessary to achieve the therapeutic effect of decreased metabolism and ICP (41). As a result, lower doses (e.g., 5 mg/kg every 4–6 hours) may adequately reduce metabolism and CBF to have beneficial effects and have less systemic complication. Therapy can be escalated to a continuous infusion if lesser therapy fails. Therapy is often continued for 48 to 96 hours or longer, depending on the cerebral hemodynamics, though longer periods may be necessary with prolonged intracranial hypertension.

Adjunctive Therapies

ANTICONVULSANTS

Anticonvulsants are often administered to patients with severe head injury to prevent early posttraumatic seizures, particularly if there is a penetrating or parenchymal injury noted on the initial CT scan. The incidence of seizures within the first week after TBI is 4 to 25% and can be upward of 70% in infants. The concern in the acute period is that seizures can increase ICP through multiple mechanisms by increasing metabolic demand, valsalva effects, release of excitotoxic neurotransmitters or other metabolites, and passively via systemic effects such as hypoxemia or hypertension. It also has generally been believed that the prevention of seizures in the early acute period will decrease the chance of the development of chronic epilepsy in children (7). Prophylactic treatment should be considered and is recommended acutely in the severely injured child (52). Therapy often continues for 10 days to 2 weeks (51) and can be extended depending on the cerebral injury, the extent and frequency of posttraumatic seizures, and/or EEG findings.

STEROIDS

Extensive literature in the use of steroids for head injury exists, though none have shown conclusively that corticosteroids improve outcome in severely head-injured adults (11). Though no study specifically addresses the use of steroids in children, many of the studies have included children, and steroids did not seem to contribute significantly to overall improvement in outcome in the pediatric population. At this time, their routine use in children is therefore not recommended.

TEMPERATURE MANIPULATION

The use of hypothermia to treat TBI in humans was first reported during the 1950s (29, 34, 49). Numerous reports have shown that outcome could be improved by cooling patients at various times up to 10 days after injury, even with different levels of hypothermia (34). Hendrick (29) reported on the specific benefit of hypothermia in children following TBI also as early as the 1950s and noted that there was improved outcome following treatment. Interestingly, because of the lack of scientific methodology in this study, the widespread use of this modality has been limited. Recent reports from the adult clinical trial of 48 hours of moderate hypothermia have not been as definitive. Despite the limited positive findings in this adult study, clinical trials are underway in children to determine the safety and efficacy in this group. Due to the differences in response to TBI in children, specifically the development of diffuse swelling, hypothermia may be particularly efficacious in this group.

OUTCOME

The overall mortality and morbidity in children is generally less than in adults (28,39). There are multiple factors that contribute to outcome following TBI, particularly in children. These include the mechanism of injury, the age of the child at time of injury, the severity of the injury, and the extent of the secondary injury (39). Though children, in general, survive severe TBI more often than adults, there is a clear distinction in mortality comparing young, middle, and older children (39). Younger children (less than 4 years of age) along with mid-to-late adolescents have a higher mortality rate compared to school-age children (39). The reason for this difference may be due in part to the differing mechanisms of injury within the different age subgroups. During the middle childhood school age years, since they more often suffer recreational injuries, there are more focal and less severe injuries compared to the young and adolescent children. In contrast, adolescents and older children tend to have high impact injuries secondary to motor vehicle collisions. Children in the younger age groups more likely suffer from diffuse injuries and from multiple insults. The true mortality rate as a result of a particular mechanism of injury at each age range has not been accurately assessed.

Though children as a group will more likely have a good functional recovery than adults (26), the final functional outcome of children at different ages depends not only on the recovery potential of the brain at the time of injury but the stage of neural development. Acquiring new information and interpreting incoming stimuli (19) are some of the primary functions of the developing brain. Disruption during development is believed to impede on the normal processing of new information and, thus, impact on the child's ability to acquire new and higher functions. This includes the ability to retain previously learned material as well as the processing of new information. Preschool age children have been found by most authors to be most sensitive to severe injuries (12, 32, 38, 40). More specifically, whereas some have reported that under 2 years of age is a critical age (10, 40), others have used ≤4 years as the critical age for predicting a poor long-term outcome (2, 32).

Deficits in Recovery

Often following TBI, and particularly severe injury, numerous aspects of neurologic and neuropsychologic function can be disrupted. These include intellect (full scale and performance IQ), attention/concentration, memory (spatial and verbal), language (syntax, location, linguistic ability), visuomotor skills, achievement and academic performance, and motor function (4, 19, 30, 31, 37, 54). Other types of morbidity include posttraumatic seizures, speech and gait abnormalities, hearing and visual changes, and cranial nerve dysfunction (19, 31, 32). The majority of children following TBI will have a dramatic recovery in their cognitive and other functions in the first 12 months following their head injury, but only about 20% attain a "good" outcome after severe TBI (19). For this reason, patients even with mild or moderate injuries who have returned to normal activities and school are often followed at 6 months and 1 year after injury to ensure that they have maintained their academic abilities and performance (16, 19). Though most studies of cognitive performance have been performed in children with severe TBI, in one study, Ewings-Cobb et al. (19) observed that there was a 20% difference in IQ between severely injured children and those with mild head injuries at time of recovery. Suffice it to say that following severe TBI, intellectual impairment may be significant and persistent and may affect many or all modalities of intelligence function. Many of these patients are eventually diagnosed with attention deficit disorders, and it is this group of children that has been treated chronically with medication trials to address persistent processing dysfunction.

Emotional behavioral changes and even exaggeration of pre-existing behavioral problems can occur following severe TBI in children. Even following mild and moderate TBI, behavioral problems are often magnified in the posttraumatic recovery period (48). Other chronic problems, typically behavioral, following severe TBI include changes in temperament, increased irritability, temper outbursts and impulsivity, aggressive behavior, hyperactivity, and problems with interpersonal social adaption and are common. In the mild to moderate injured child, these changes tend to resolve, but after severe TBI, behavioral problems often are magnified and persistent.

Special Problem: Child Abuse

As mentioned earlier, child abuse has become increasingly recognized as a major mechanism of injury in the infant and young child. Victims of non-accidental trauma or abuse, whether due to shaking or direct trauma to the head or other parts of the body, often suffer poor outcomes resulting in either death or severe permanent disability. There are many reasons that are believed to contribute to these poor outcomes, but at present the most likely include a delay in reporting of the injury by the perpetrator and/or family, or because the child suffers repeated injuries. From a physician perspective, clearly when the history does not match up with the extent of injury, it is important and now a legal requirement to report these kinds of concerns. This has significantly benefited the physician in that responsibility of investigation, support, and advocacy have been legislatively mandated, which allows the physician to focus on the care and treatment of these injured children. In these instances, these children should be treated, for the most part, as necessary for their TBI with adjunctive tests to determine the complete extent of injuries. These would include an ophthalmologic consultation and examination for the potential retinal hemorrhages as well as a skeletal survey to identify indications of previous fractures, either acute or chronic. (For an excellent review of this topic, see Duhaime et al. [17]).

SUMMARY

At present, similar to the adult, conventional management in the child following TBI appropriately attempts to lessen the second insults that occur after the injury and the effects of the secondary physiologic events. Many of the treatment modalities used for the child after severe TBI have been extrapolated from the adult data, as there is little literature that primarily involves children. Though children as a group overall have a better outcome than adults, there are many factors that influence prognosis in the pediatric population. The age at injury, mechanism of injury, injury severity, multiple trauma, second insults, and/or the extent of secondary injury can all impact on the final outcome. It is clear that many of the poor outcomes observed are best prevented by preventing either the initial impact or the second insults that typically occur following TBI. Interestingly, very young and preschool children have worse outcomes both in mortality and long-term disability than older children and adolescents. The deficits observed are often persistent and severe in the long term even with aggressive management. Continued aggressive intervention to prevent secondary injury and, in the future, mechanistically targeted therapeutic modalities in the acute setting will hopefully improve the mortality rates and functional recovery in these children.

REFERENCES

1. Adams JH, Graham DI, Murray LS, Scott G: Diffuse axonal injury due to non-missile head injury in humans: An analysis of 45 cases. **Ann Neurol** 12:557–563, 1982.
2. Alberico AM, Ward JD, Choi SC, Marmarou A, Young HE: Outcome after severe head injury: Relationship to mass lesions, diffuse injury, and ICP course in pediatric and adult patients. **J Neurosurg** 67:648–656, 1987.
3. Aldrich EF, Eisenberg HM, Saydjari C, et al: Diffuse brain swelling in severely head-injured children: A report from the NIH Traumatic Coma Data Bank. **J Neurosurg** 76:450–454, 1992.
4. Bawden HN, Knights RM, Winogron HW: Speeded performance following head injury in children. **J Clin Exp Neuropsychol** 7:39–54, 1985.

5. Becker DP, Miller JD, Word JD, et al: The outcome from severe head injury with early diagnosis and intensive management. **J Neurosurg** 56:26–32, 1982.
6. Bell, RS, Loop JW: The utility and futility of radiographic skull examination for trauma. **N Engl J Med** 284:236–239, 1971.
7. Ben Ari Y: Limbic sizure and brain damage produced by Kainic acid: Mechanisms and relevance to human temporal lobe epilepsy. **Neuroscience** 14:375–403, 1985.
8. Berger MS, Pitts LH, Lovely M, et al: Outcome from severe head injury in children and adolescents. **J Neurosurg** 62:194–199, 1985.
9. Beyda DH: Time course of cerebral blood flow and metabolism in pediatric head trauma. **Crit Care Med** 24:A134, 1996.
10. Boyer MG, Edwards P: Outcome 1 to 3 years after severe traumatic brain injury in children and adolescents. **Injury** 22:315–320, 1991.
11. Brain Trauma Foundation, The American Association of Neurological Surgeons, The Joint Section on Neurotrauma and Critical Care. *Guidelines for the Management of Severe Head Injury,* 1995.
12. Brink JD, Garrett AL, Hale WR, et al: Recovery of motor and intellectual function in children sustaining severe head injuries. **Dev Med Child Neurol** 12:565–571, 1970.
13. Bruce DA, Alavi A, Bilaniuk LT, et al: Diffuse cerebral swelling following head injuries in children: The syndrome of "malignant brain edema." **J Neurosurg** 54:170–178, 1981.
14. Bruce DA, Raphaely RC, Goldberg AI, et al: Pathophysiology, treatment, and outcome following severe head injury in children. **Childs Brain** 5:174–191, 1979.
15. Chestnut RM, Marshall LF, Klauber MR, et al: The role of secondary brain injury in determining outcome from severe head injury. **J Trauma** 34:216–222, 1993.
16. Choi SC, Barnes TY, Bullock R, et al: Temporal profile of outcomes in severe head injury. **J Neurosurg** 81:169–173, 1994.
17. Duhaime A-C, Christian CW, Rorke LB, Zimmerman RA: Non-accidental head injury in infants: The "Shaken Baby Syndrome." **N Engl J Med** 338:1822, 1998.
18. Eisenberg HM, Gary HE, Jr, Aldrich EF: Initial CT findings in 753 patients with severe head injury: A report from the NIH Traumatic Coma Data Bank. **J Neurosurg** 73:688–698, 1990.
19. Ewing-Cobbs L, Miner ME, Fletcher JM, et al: Intellectual, motor, and language sequelae following closed head injury in infants and preschoolers. **J Pediatr Psychol** 14:531–547, 1989.
20. Feldman Z, Kanter MJ, Robertson CS, et al: Effect of head elevation on intracranial pressure, cerebral perfusion pressure, and cerebral blood flow in head-injured patients. **J Neurosurg** 76:207–211, 1992.
21. Forbes MT, Hendrich KS, Schiding JK, et al: Perfusion-weighted MRI assessment of cerebral blood flow and CO_2 reactivity after controlled cortical impact in rats. **J Neurotrauma** 12:988, 1995.
22. Frankowski RF, Annegers JF, Whitman S: Epidemiological and descriptive studies: Part 1. The descriptive epidemiology of head trauma in the United States, in Becker DP, Povlishock JT (eds): *Central Nervous System Trauma Status Report-1985.* Bethesda, National Institute of Health, NINCDS, 1985, pp 33–43.
23. Gaab MR, Seegers K, Smedema RJ, et al: A comparative analysis of THAM (Tris-buffer) in traumatic brain oedema. **Acta Neurochir Suppl** 51:320–323, 1990.
24. Graham DI, Ford I, Adams J, et al: Fatal head injury in children. **J Clin Pathol** 42:18–22, 1988.
25. Graham DI, Lawrence AE, Adams JH, et al: Brain damage in fatal non-missile head injury without high intracranial pressure. **J Clin Pathol** 41:34–37, 1988.
26. Gross CR, Wolf C, Kunitz SC, et al: Pilot Traumatic Coma Data Bank: A profile of

head injuries in children, in Dacey RG, Jr, et al (eds): *Trauma of the Central Nervous System.* New York, Raven Press, 1985, pp 19–26.

27. Gur D, Yonas H, Good WF: Local cerebral blood flow by Xenon-enchanced CT: Current status, potential improvements and future directions. **Cerebrovasc Brain Metab Rev** 1:68–86, 1989.
28. Guyer B, Ellers B: Childhood injuries in the United States: Mortality, morbidity, and cost. **Am J Dis Child** 144:649–652, 1990.
29. Hendrick EB: The use of hypothermia in severe head injuries in childhood. **Arch Surg** 79:362–364, 1959.
30. Kaufmann PM, Fletcher JM, Levin HS: Attentional disturbance after pediatric closed head injury. **J Child Neurol** 8:348–353, 1993.
31. Klonoff H, Low MD, Clark C: Head injuries in children: A prospective five year follow-up. **J Neurol Neurosurg Psychiatry** 40:1211–1219, 1977.
32. Koskiniemi M, Kyykka T, Nybo T, et al: Long-term outcome after severe brain injury in preschoolers is worse than expected. **Arch Pediatr Adolesc Med** 149:249–254, 1995.
33. Kraus JF, Fife D, Conroy C: Pediatric brain injuries: The nature, clinical course, and early outcomes in a defined United States' population. **Pediatrics** 79:501–507, 1987.
34. Lazorthes G, Campan L: Hypothermia in the treatment of craniocerebral traumatism. **J Neurosurg** 15:162–167, 1958.
35. Levin HS: Neurobehavioral recovery. **J Neurotrauma** 9:S539–S373, 1992.
36. Levin HS, Aldrich EF, Saydjari C, et al: Severe head injury in children: Experience of the Traumatic Coma Data Bank. **Neurosurgery** 31:435–444, 1992.
37. Levin HS, Culhane KA, Fletcher JM, et al: Dissociation between delayed alternation and memory after pediatric head injury: Relationship to MRI findings. *J Child Neurol* 9:81–89, 1994.
38. Levin HS, Eisenberg HM, Wigg NR, et al: Memory and intellectual ability after head injury in children and adolescents. **Neurosurgery** 11:668–673, 1982.
39. Luerssen TG, Klauber MR, Marshall LF: Outcome from head injury related to patient's age: A longitudinal prospective study of adult and pediatric head injury. **J Neurosurg** 68:409–416, 1988.
40. Mahoney WJ, D'Souza BJ, Haller A, et al: Long-term outcome of children with severe head trauma and prolonged coma. **Pediatrics** 71:756–762, 1983.
41. Marshall LF, Smith RW, Shapiro HM: The outcome with aggressive treatment in severe head injuries. **J Neurosurg** 50:26–30, 1979.
42. Miller LP, Johnson AE, Gelhard RE, Insel TR: The ontogeny of excitatory amino acid receptors in the rat forebrain: II. Kainic acid receptors. **Neuroscience** 35:45–51, 1990.
43. Muizelaar JP, Marmarou A, DeSalles AAF, et al: Cerebral blood flow and metabolism in severely head-injured children. Part 1: Relationship with GCS score, outcome, ICP, and PVI. **J Neurosurg** 71:63–71, 1989.
44. Muizelaar JP, Marmarou A, Ward JD, et al: Adverse effects of prolonged hyperventilation in patients with severe head injury: A randomized clinical trial. **J Neurosurg** 75:731–739, 1991.
45. O'Sullivan MG, Statham PF, Jones PA, et al: Role of intracranial pressure monitoring in severely head-injured patients without signs of intracranial hypertension on initial computerized tomography. **J Neurosurg** 80:46–50, 1994.
46. Pigula FA, Wald SL, Shackford SR, et al: The effect of hypotension and hypoxia on children with severe head injuries. **J Pediatr Surg** 28:310–314, 1993; discussion 315- 316.

47. Robertson CS, Constant CF, Narayan RK, et al: Cerebral blood flow, $AVDO_2$, and neurologic outcome in head-injured patients. **J Neurotrauma** 9:S349–S358, 1992.
48. Rutter M, Chadwick O, Shaffer D: Head injury, in Rutter M (ed): *Developmental Neuropsychiatry.* New York, Guilford Press, 1983, pp 83–111.
49. Sedzimir CB: Therapeutic hypothermia in cases of head injury. **J Neurosurg** 16:407–414, 1959.
50. Stringer A, Hasso AN, Thompson JR, et al: Hyperventilation-induced cerebral ischemia in patients with acute brain lesions: Demonstration by Xenon-enhanced CT. **Am J Neurosurg Res** 14:475–484, 1993.
51. Temkin NR, Dikmen SS, Wilensky AJ, et al: A randomized, double-blind study of phenytoin for the prevention of post-traumatic seizures. **N Engl J Med** 323:497–502, 1990.
52. Temkin NR, Dikmen SS, Winn HR: Posttraumatic seizures. **Neurosurg Clin North Am** 2:425–435, 1991.
53. Wegman WE: Annual summary of vital statistics-1981. **Pediatrics** 75:835–843, 1982.
54. Winogron HW, Knights RM, Bawden HN: Neuropsychological deficits following head injury in children. **J Clin Neuropsychol** 6:269–286, 1984.
55. Yonas H, Gur D, Claassen D, et al: Stable Xenon-enhanced CT measurement of CBF in reversible focal ischemia in baboons. **J Neurosurg** 73:266–273, 1990.

CHAPTER

18

Cerebrospinal Fluid Shunt Technology

J. M. DRAKE, F.R.C.S.C., J. R. W. KESTLE, F.R.C.S.C., S. TULI, M.D.

INTRODUCTION

Since the invention of the first implantable shunt valve by Nulsen and Spitz (12) almost 50 years ago, there has been a remarkable number of ingenious modifications and new designs of shunt equipment to treat pediatric hydrocephalus. These developments were in response to the immediately evident high shunt failure rate. These designs included anti-siphon devices (15), on-off devices, gravity-actuated changes in opening pressure, and even externally adjustable valves, some with electromagnetic programmers (16) (*Fig. 18.1*). Aside from the introduction of the silicone elastomer material, there has in fact been little clinical impact on the treatment with patients with shunts. Moreover, there has been a recognition of the unexpected complications-cor pulmonale (11) and shunt nephritis (19) from cardiac shunts, bowel erosion from spring-coiled catheters (1), obstruction of anti-siphon devices by capsule formation (3), and tonsilar herniation by lumboperitoneal shunts (2). In fact, each new shunt equipment design has in many cases brought along its own unique set of complications.

Interpretation of the results of new shunt hardware was often hampered by the design of the studies. They often contained small retrospective series of patients, loosely defined inclusion criteria, poor definition of outcome events, short follow-up, and inappropriate statistical analysis. These studies were often conducted by enthusiasts of the devices who had vested interests in the outcome, including financial incentives. Early enthusiastic reports were often followed by less enthusiastic ones, often about unexpected complications.

PROSPECTIVE RANDOMIZED TRIALS OF CSF SHUNT VALVE DESIGN

Pediatric Shunt Design Trial

With the recent advances in valve design, aimed at reducing shunt overdrainage in the upright position, there were again reports of improved outcome in slightly improved but nevertheless significantly

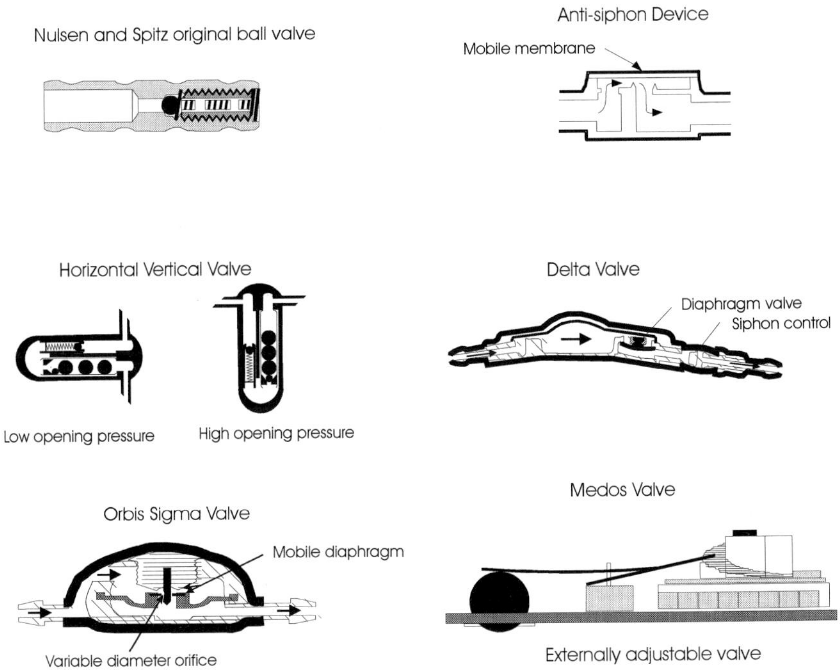

FIG. 18.1 Schematic diagrams of a number of valve designs starting with the original Nulsen and Spitz valve developed in the early 1950s (12). The designs reflect the progress valve development including antisiphon devices, gravity-actuated valves, and ultimately an externally adjustable valve. Unfortunately, the increased complexity and sophistication has not to date resulted in improved efficacy.

flawed clinical series (8, 18). It was at this point that the Pediatric Hydrocephalus Treatment and Evaluation Group decided to launch a carefully controlled prospective randomized trial on the Orbis Sigma valve (NMT, Boston, MA) (18), a flow-limiting device, and the Delta valve (Medtronic PS Medical, Goletta, CA) (8), a siphon control device, compared to standard differential pressure valves. The trial was well organized and multicentered, the blinded data were collected centrally, and the primary outcome event was clearly defined and blindly adjudicated (4). An adequate number of patients was recruited and followed. There was no difference in shunt failure rates between the three types of valve design at an average follow-up of 2 years (5) (*Fig. 18.2*). The patients were subsequently followed for an additional 3 years, and no obvious changes from the initial analysis were noted (9).

In this trial, shunt failure occurred at an exponential rate for the first year and then leveled off. Overall, the one-year failure rate was 40%,

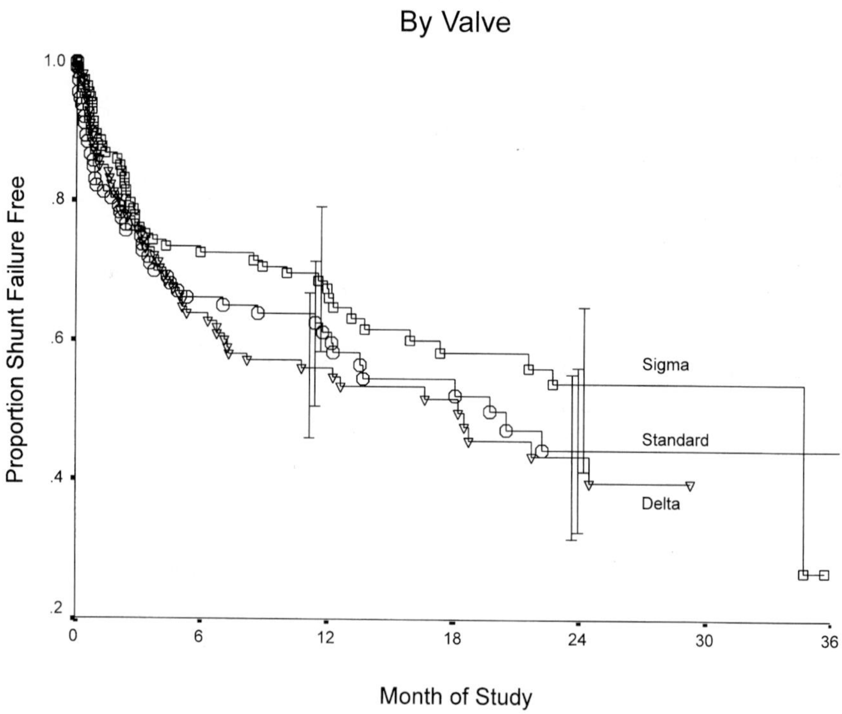

FIG. 18.2 Results of the prospective randomized trial of valve design comparing the Delta valve, the Orbis Sigma valve, and "standard" valves. There is no difference in complication free shunt survival between the three groups. From Ref. 5 with permission.

and the two-year failure rate was 50%, remarkably similar to what had been reported before, and upon which the trial estimates for sample size had been based. The commonest cause of shunt failure was obstruction (31.4%) followed by infection (8.1%), overdrainage (3.5%), and loculated ventricles (0.6%).

SECONDARY OUTCOMES

A number of other extremely interesting findings emerged from the data collected, which, though not part of the primary outcome, nevertheless shed some light on the state of treatment of pediatric hydrocephalus at the time. The secondary outcome measures of type of shunt failure and site of shunt obstruction indicated that the Delta valve, which was designed to prevent subdural collections, actually had the highest number (5). The Orbis-Sigma valve had very few obstructions of the ventricular catheter (the commonest site of shunt obstruction) but a higher number of valve failures, as though the site of obstruction had been moved downstream.

The trial received considerable attention, as well as some criticism. Some claimed that the valves were never designed for small children, that the wrong "level" of Delta valve was used, and that the results would have been different in older children. In fact, these valves were being implanted in enormous numbers of children at the time of the study; the number of overdrainage complications was similar in children over age 2; and inspection of the shunt survival curves for different standard valve opening pressures, or different Delta valve "levels," indicated that it likely had little effect. Since three very different valve designs had no apparent effect, the trial authors felt it was unlikely that small differences in valve design would have had much effect.

POST HOC ANALYSIS

There was a great deal of data collected during the trial that could be examined, particularly to explore whether previously held suppositions were possibly correct or could more appropriately be put to a subsequent clinical trial. There was no apparent difference in outcome according to whether the burr hole was frontal or occipital, whether the ventricular catheter was placed with assistance (ultrasound, endoscopy, or x-ray), the training level of the surgeon, or whether the hair was clipped, shaved, or left alone.

Perhaps the most interesting follow-up information was on the analysis of the considerable imaging data that had been collected. Each patient had up to six follow-up radiologic images. Excluding the images taken at the time of shunt failure, each image was analyzed for the size of the ventricles, the position of the tip of the ventricular catheter within the ventricle (frontal, occipital, or body), and the catheter tip environment (surrounded by CSF, touching ventricular wall, surrounded by slit ventricle). Ventricular size was measured using a modified Evan's ratio, which was an average of the frontal and occipital horn width divided by the maximum biparietal diameter. This ratio had been shown to be an accurate and reliable estimate of ventricular volume in pediatric patients (10, 13).

The ventricular size declined at an exponential rate reaching a minimum plateau at 1 year. Remarkably, there was no difference in ventricular size among the three valves (22) (*Fig. 18.3*). This was extremely interesting because the valves behave quite differently on bench testing. It had also been previously reported in a retrospective review with historical controls that the Orbis-Sigma valve in particular kept the ventricles enlarged (17). The newer valves had been designed with cer-

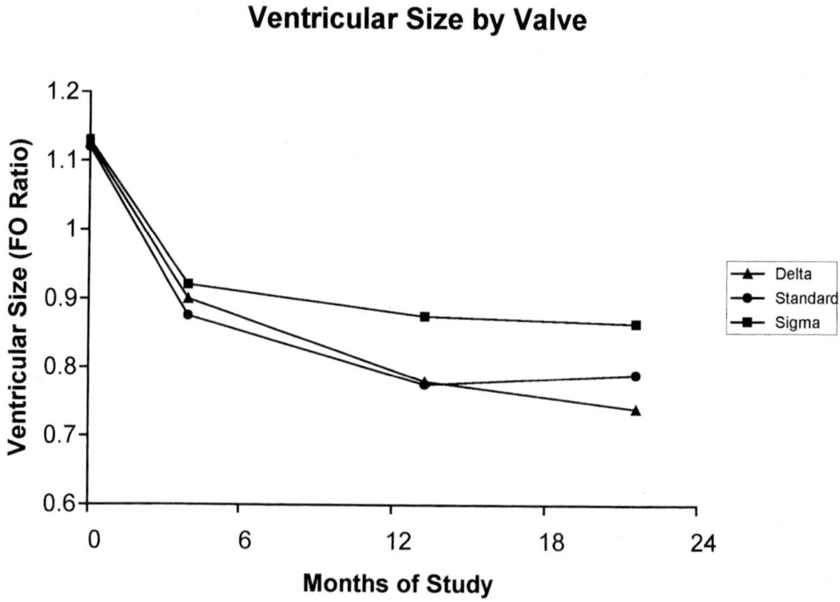

FIG. 18.3 Ventricular size as a function of time post shunt implantation from image data from the shunt design trial. There is no difference in ventricular size among the three valves, which have very different pressure/flow characteristics. From Ref. 22 with permission.

tain assumptions made about the brain's mechanical properties and the response to shunt implantation. These models are based on the limited knowledge of CSF production and pressure changes seen over very brief time periods (7). These ventricle size measurements from this study suggest that the current biomechanical models are woefully inadequate and must address much larger time scales-on the order of a year. A follow-up baseline study for a newly shunted patient, to determine ventricular size when the patient is well, should also be carried out at approximately 1 year after implantation.

The position of the ventricular catheter and the amount of CSF surrounding it also appeared to have an effect on shunt failure (22) (*Table 18.1*). By multivariate analysis, having a catheter in the occipital horn had a hazard ratio of .45 compared to catheters in the body of the ventricle. Ventricular catheters surrounded by CSF had a hazard ratio of .21 compared to those in a slit ventricle. The position and environment of the ventricular catheter tip accounted for fully three-quarters of the variability of the multivariate model, indicating that they are likely very significant risk factors. Maintaining a catheter tip surrounded by

TABLE 18.1
Independent Predictors of Cerebrospinal Fluid Shunt Malfunction

Predictors		Hazard Ratio	95% CI	*P* Value	R^2
Etiology	Myelomeningocele	1.78	1.18–2.67	0.006	0.037
	Head Injury	4.56	1.07–19.39	0.04	0.018
Ventricular size		2.33[1]	1.08–5.00	0.03	0.025
Ventricular catheter location	Occipital	0.45	0.28–0.74	0.001	0.052
	Frontal	0.60	0.39–0.91	0.02	0.033
Ventricular catheter environment	CSF	0.21	0.094–0.45	0.0001	0.13
	Touching Brain	0.33	0.21–0.51	0.0001	0.16

[1]HR of 2.33 refers to an increase in the risk of shunt malfunction for every unit increase in the ventricular size (as per the modified Evans' ratio).

CSF in an expanded occipital horn might significantly reduce shunt failure. Whereas this might seem like common sense, this is really the first time this has been demonstrated using prospectively collected data analyzed by multivariate methods. It should be added that there are many "common sense" solutions to shunt failure, such as using "more physiologic valves," which have not proved to have treatment value.

Other factors that might affect shunt failure were included in image data analysis. Etiology, namely myelomeningocele, also increased the risk of shunt failure. Although this is not a modifiable risk factor, identification of high risk groups is important to target those who might benefit the most from treatment changes.

The Medos Programmable Valve Randomized Trial

A subsequent prospective randomized trial comparing the Medos valve (Johnson & Johnson, Randalph MA), a programmable differential pressure valve, to all other valves also found no difference in reoperation rate for shunt failure (14). The trial was somewhat different in that it included pediatric and adult patients undergoing a first shunt insertion or valve revision. Nevertheless, the 2-year shunt survival rates for the patients for the first shunt insertion were 52% in the Medos group and 50% in the control group, remarkably similar to the previous randomized valve design study. Although the valve was frequently reprogrammed (66% of the patients) and this was felt to avert an operation in 61 patients, the overall reoperation rate was the same in the control group. Only four valves required explantation because of an inability to reprogram.

REPEATED SHUNT FAILURE

In the Medos trial referred to above, patients having a subsequent shunt operation including a valve revision fared slightly worse than the first implantation group, with 2-year survival rates of 43% in both groups. The issue of repeated shunt failure, particularly in the same patient, is a complex one. We enrolled a cohort of patients over 10 years into a hydrocephalus data base. Each patient was then followed for up to 10 years for any episodes of shunt failure to determine what if any were risk factors (21). The data were then analyzed by multivariable time to event analysis.

There were 1183 shunt failures in 839 patients. Failure time from the first shunt procedure was an important predictor for second and third failures so that if an individual patient failed early, they were likely to fail early again-and this was not a particular effect of infection. Age of less than 40 weeks' gestation at time of first shunt implantation had a hazard ratio of 2.49 (95% CI, 1.68–3.68) for the first failure and remained high for subsequent failures. Age of 40 weeks to 1 year (at the time of the initial surgery) also proved to be an important predictor of first malfunctions (HR = 1.77, 95% CI = 1.29–2.44). The etiology of hydrocephalus was significantly associated with the risk of initial failure and, to a lesser extent, later failures. Concurrent other surgical procedures were associated with an increased risk of failure (*Table 18.2*).

It was also interesting to note what did not appear to carry any risk for first or subsequent failures: valve design (standard/flow regulated), distal catheter design (slit/open ended), antibiotic prophylaxis, emergency/ASA class, burr hole site (frontal/occipital), burr hole side (left/right), duration of surgery, or preadmission stay. Although it was disappointing that easily modifiable factors were not important, nevertheless it identified patients at high risk. It also suggests that there is a process initiated by shunt failure, perhaps an inflammatory response, that leads to further shunt failure.

CONCLUSION

What should be our treatment goals over the next decade as we enter the next millennium? It seems eminently reasonable that neurosurgeons could achieve a 1-year failure rate of 5% including an infection rate of 1%. How can this be achieved? It seems clear that this will require a cooperative multifaceted approach. There is much about the complex interactions between the hydrocephalic patient and the shunt, which are not well understood. Better mathematical models would allow simulations of the response of the hydrocephalic patient to be carried out more accurately and over a much longer time scale. These mod-

TABLE 18.2

Hazard Ratios, 95% Confidence Interval, and P Values for the First Three Failure Groups

	Failure Groups								
	1st			2nd			3rd		
Risk Factors	Hazard Ratio	95% C.I.	*P* Value	Hazard Ratio	95% C.I.	*P* Value	Hazard Ratio	95% C.I.	*P* Value
Gap time of previous failure				1.72	1.28–2.30	<0.001	1.50	1.05–2.16	0.027
Age*									
Less than 40 weeks	2.49	1.68–3.68	<0.001	1.59	0.93–2.74	0.096	1.71	1.05–2.79	0.032
40 weeks to 1 year	1.77	1.29–2.44	<0.001	1.33	0.84–2.11	0.22	0.90	0.57–1.42	0.65
Etiology**								Not significant	
Aqueductal stenosis	1.83	1.13–2.96	0.01	0.77	0.36–1.64	0.50			
IVH	1.78	1.18–2.68	0.006	1.85	1.03–3.33	0.039			
Postmeninigitic	2.08	1.26–3.44	0.004	2.32	1.19–4.54	0.014			
Myelomeningocele	1.95	1.34–2.85	0.001	1.10	0.63–1.92	0.74			
Posttraumatic	2.80	1.39–5.64	<0.004	1.86	0.67–5.18	0.23			
Tumor	2.33	1.48–3.68	<0.001	2.34	1.22–4.48	0.01			
Other	1.56	1.03–2.35	0.03	1.31	0.72–2.39	0.38			
Ventriculoperitoneal vs. other shunt types	0.69	0.50–0.95	0.92		Not significant			Not significant	
Concurrent surgery	1.44	1.06–1.94	0.02		Not significant		1.89	1.01–3.53	0.047

*Corrected for gestation; age greater than 1 year is chosen as the reference category.

**Congenital is the reference category.

els are not easy to develop, as there is little known about even the normal mechanical parameters of the brain. Animal models of shunt failure would also allow the mechanisms of particularly proximal catheter occlusion to be dissected, including possible reactive mechanisms induced by repetitive trauma. Ongoing clinical trials are also extremely important; hypotheses such as placing a ventricular catheter in an expanded occipital horn need to be tested by prospective studies, as is currently being done with endoscopic placement of ventricular catheters.

The search for new shunt designs and new materials should continue. No one should conclude that shunt valve designs are not important. Whereas the shunt design trials have been negative to date, valves have important effects that just have not as yet been translated into improved outcome. The search for alternative treatment strategies should also continue, i.e., endoscopic third ventriculostomy, but should be subjected to the same scrutiny as the clinical trials in CSF shunts (20).

REFERENCES

1. Adeloye A: Protrusion of ventriculo peritoneal shunt through the anus: Report of two cases. **East Afr Med J** 74:337–339, 1997.
2. Chumas PD, Armstrong DC, Drake JM, Kulkarni AV, Hoffman HJ, Humphreys RP, Rutka JT, Hendrick EB: Tonsillar herniation: The rule rather than the exception after lumboperitoneal shunting in the pediatric population. **J Neurosurg** 78:568–573, 1993.
3. Drake JM, da Silva MC, Rutka JT: Functional obstruction of an antisiphon device by raised tissue capsule pressure. **Neurosurgery** 32:137–139, 1993.
4. Drake JM, Kestle J: Rationale and methodology of the multicenter pediatric cerebrospinal fluid shunt design trial. **Childs Nerv Syst** 12:434–447, 1996.
5. Drake JM, Kestle J, Milner R, Cinalli G, Boop F, Piatt J, Jr., Haines S, Schiff SJ, Cochrane DD, Steinbok P, MacNeil N: Randomized trial of cerebropsinal fluid shunt valve design in pediatric hydrocephalus. **Neurosurgery** 43:294–305, 1998.
6. Drake JM, Sainte-Rose C: *The Shunt Book*. New York, Blackwell Scientific, 1995, p 1.
7. Drake JM, Tenti G, Sivaloganathan S: Computer modeling of siphoning for CSF shunt design evaluation. **Pediatr Neurosurg** 21:6–15, 1994.
8. Horton D, Pollay M: Fluid flow performance of a new siphon-control device for ventricular shunts. **J Neurosurg** 72:926–932, 1990.
9. Kestle JRW, Drake JM, Group PHTE: Long-term follow-up from the shunt design trial. **Childs Nerv Syst** 15:426, 1999 (abstr.).
10. Kulkarni A, Drake J, Armstrong DC, Dirks P: Measurement of ventricular size: Reliability of the frontal and occiptial horn ratio compared to subjective assessment. **Pediatr Neurosurg** 31:65–70, 1999.
11. Ladouceur D, Giroux M: Echocardiographic detection of intracardiac thrombi complicating ventriculo-atrial shunt: Report of two cases. **Pediatr Neurosurg** 20:68–72, 1994.
12. Nulsen FE, Spitz EB: Treatment of hydrocephalus by direct shunt form ventricle to jugular vein. **Surg Forum** 399–403, 1952.
13. O'Hayon BB, Drake JM, Ossip MG, Tuli S, Clarke M: Frontal and occipital horn ra-

tio: A linear estimate of ventricular size for multiple imaging modalities in pediatric hydrocephalus. **Pediatr Neurosurg** 29:245–249, 1998.
14. Pollack IF, Albright AL, Adelson PD: A randomized, controlled study of a programmable shunt valve versus a conventional valve for patients with hydrocephalus. Hakim-Medos Investigator Group. **Neurosurgery** 45:1399–1408, 1999.
15. Portnoy HD, Schulte RR, Fox JL, Croissant PD, Tripp L: Anti-siphon and reversible occlusion valves for shunting in hydrocephalus and preventing post-shunt subdural hematomas. **J Neurosurg** 38:729–738, 1973.
16. Reinprecht A, Dietrich W, Bertalanffy A, Czech T: The Medos Hakim programmable valve in the treatment of pediatric hydrocephalus. **Childs Nerv Syst** 13:588–593, 1997; Discussion 593–594.
17. Sainte-Rose C: Shunt obstruction: A preventable complication? **Pediatr Neurosurg** 19:156–164, 1993.
18. Sainte-Rose C, Hooven MD, Hirsch JF: A new approach to the treatment of hydrocephalus. **J Neurosurg** 66:213–226, 1987.
19. Searle M, Lee HA: Ventriculo-atrial shunt nephritis. **Postgrad Med J** 58:566–569, 1982.
20. Tuli S, Alshail E, Drake J: Third ventriculostomy versus cerebrospinal fluid shunt as a first procedure in pediatric hydrocephalus. **Pediatr Neurosurg** 30:11–15, 1999.
21. Tuli S, Drake JM, Lawless J, Wigg M, Lamberti-Pasculli M: Risk factors for repeated cerebrospinal shunt failures in pediatric hydrocephalus. **Neurosurgery** (in press).
22. Tuli S, O'Hayon B, Drake JM, Kestle JRW: Change in ventricular size and effect of ventricular catheter placement in pediatric shunted hydrocephalus. **Neurosurgery** (in press).

CHAPTER

19

Congenital Malformations of the Central Nervous System

DAVID G. MCLONE, M.D., PH.D.

Congenital malformations of the central nervous system (CNS) are too numerous to consider in depth in this paper. Therefore, malformations will be grouped under three categories: 1) Cerebral malformations, 2) Cerebellar malformations, and 3) Spinal cord malformations. A single entity from each group will be discussed in some detail.

CEREBRAL MALFORMATIONS

Cerebral malformations include migrational disorders (lissencephaly, pachygyria, and microgyria) and disgenetic disorders (holoprosencephaly, agencies of the corpus callosum, schizencephaly, and hydranencephaly). Hydrocephalus is a sign of an underlying malformation, such as aqueductal stenosis.

Encephaloceles represent about 10 to 20% of craniospinal dysraphism (34, 47). This would be about 0.8 to 4/10,000 live births (37, 54, 74, 80). The actual incidence is much higher but the fetal loss is at least 70% (20, 73). There is an obvious racial and reginal difference in the number and location of the encephaloceles. In Southeast Asia, the nasofrontal encephaloceles, also called sincipital, are nine times more common than posterior encephaloceles (12, 82). In white Australians, only 2.2% of encephaloceles are sincipital, while in Aboriginals 50% are sincipital (74). In North America, the frequency of encephaloceles is much less, and 66 to 95% are occipital (11, 34, 74).

The vast majority of encephaloceles are sporadic, with only a small number the result of aberrant tissue bands or frontonasal dysplasia (15). An encephalocele has been reported in a child with Vaters syndrome, and occipital encephaloceles are known to occur in children with myelomeningoceles and dermoids (65, 72). The incidence does not increase with advancing maternal age or in the second twin (72).

Several theories have been used to explain the cause of encephaloceles. A common theory is that they are part of the spectrum of neural tube defects (76). This is unlike since encephaloceles almost always contain neural elements that originate after neurulation is completed. They have little in common with anencephaly, being closed or skin covered. The atretic encephalocele differs from other encephaloceles in that it usually contains primitive elements and has an attachment to the tectal area, mesencephalon, and probably occurs during late neurulation. It is an example of abnormal disjunction of neuroectoderm from superficial ectoderm and similar to the myelomeningocele manque of the spinal cord. Overdistension of the neural tube or fetal hydrocephalus, which causes a blow-out of the developing brain, is another theory, but again there is little evidence to support this (23, 24, 59). Another possibility is that a developmental failure in ossification of the skull allows the underlying tissue to herniate out of the intracranial compartment (16, 39, 80). However, this theory does not take into account that the encephalocele occurs prior to ossification of the skull, and herniation only rarely occurs at the normal fontanel. In our laboratory we have been able to create encephaloceles in fetal mice by disrupting the mesenchyme over the brain during the embryonic period (26). This may explain the vertex encephaloceles. I am aware of one newborn child with an encephalocele in a very unusual location, far lateral on the cerebral hemisphere, that had a known cranial puncture during an amniocentesis early in the second trimester. However, it is possible that encephaloceles have different etiologies that are related to the location of the encephalocele.

Encephaloceles have been illustrated in medieval art and archaic sculpture (40). The first medical report appeared in the 16th century (19). During the last half of this century, an aggressive approach aimed at cosmetic repair of the sincipital encephalocele has been developed. In the last decade, skull base surgery has developed techniques that make repair of even large basal encephaloceles possible. The large vertex encephaloceles still pose difficult ethical problems for the family and pediatric neurosurgeon.

All encephaloceles are obvious skin-covered, usually midline protuberances from the skull of varying size, except for the basal encephalocele, which may not be apparent at birth. The skin covering is usually intact, but may be ulcerated, bleeding, or leaking cerebrospinal fluid (CSF) at birth. Basal encephaloceles can present with airway obstruction but often are discovered at a later examination of the child or because of recurrent meningitis. Hydrocephalus may be present and cranial nerves may be involved, but usually the child's neurological examination is remarkably normal.

Computed tomographic (CT) scanning is of value in determining the relationship of the encephalocele to the osseous structure of the skull base (Figure 19.1). Basal and sincipital encephaloceles required a de-

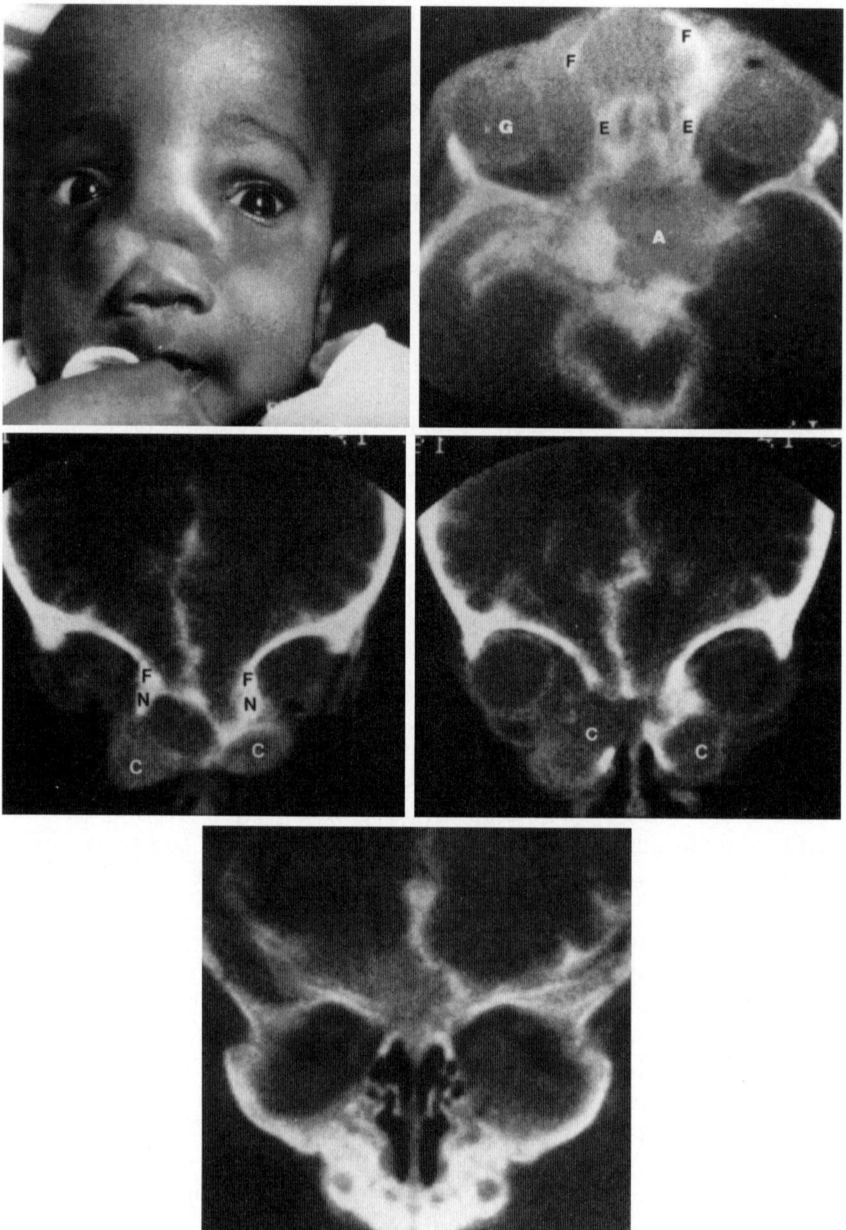

FIG. 19.1 A child with a frontal encephalocele. The CT scan shows the relationship of the globes (G), the ethmoids (E), and the frontal bones (F). A portion of the frontal lobe extends through the base (A). The cele (C) is anterior and below the frontal (F) bones.

tailed understanding of their relationships to surrounding structures in order to plan repair of the encephalocele and cosmetic reconstruction of the face and skull base. Three dimensional CT reconstructions of the skull are attractive but not essential.

Magnetic resonance imaging (MRI) and magnetic resonance angiograph (MRA) have greatly enhanced our ability to determine the anatomy of the cranial defect, the relationships to surrounding structures and contents (including which portion) and the amount of brain tissue found in the encephalocele (Figure 19.2). This allowed not only planning of the procedure but some insight into the likely functional outcome for the child. Knowing the relation of major vascular structure (both arterial and venous) especially venous sinuses is critical to limiting blood loss and preserving the vascular supply to the brain not involved in the encephalocele.

Basal and sincipital encephaloceles contain varying amounts of one or both frontal lobes. The anterior and third ventricle may extend into the encephalocele (44, 81). Abnormalities of the cortex, thalamus, hypothalamus, commissures, optic pathways, brain stem, and aqueduct

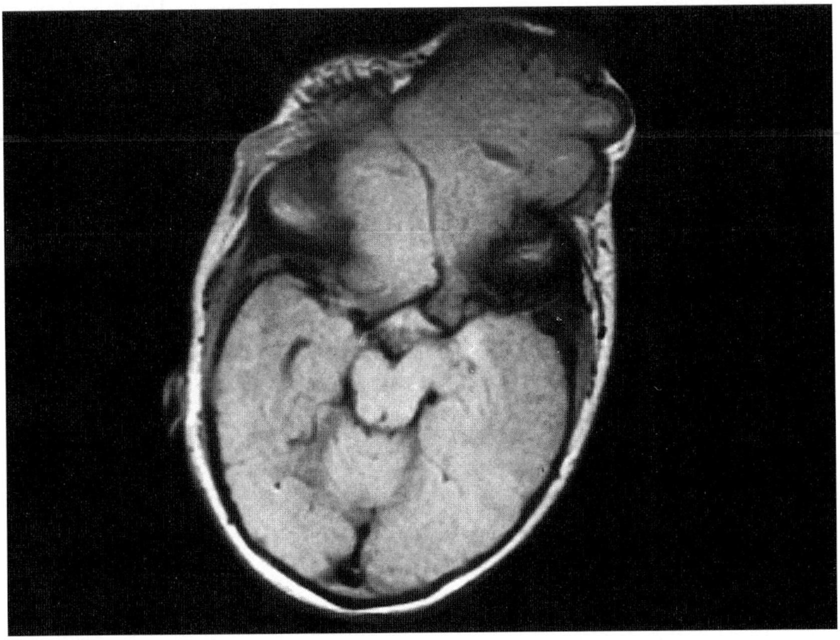

FIG. 19.2 An MRI shows a child with a large anterior encephalocele that contains major portions of both frontal lobes.

have been described (79, 81). Amazingly, large anterior encephaloceles have a much better prognosis for intellectual development and are less likely to develop hydrocephalus than occipital encephaloceles.

Parietal encephaloceles may contain part or all of one or both cerebral hemispheres. Many of these children are intellectually delayed and unfortunately some are profoundly delayed. When only a portion of one hemisphere is involved, the outlook for intellectual development is much better. Since these encephaloceles alter the CSF pathways, hydrocephalus is often present.

The atretic encephalocele is different from the other encephaloceles since it is a neurulation disjunction defect that alters the brain little (Figure 19.3). It contains none of the normal brain and only rarely is associated with hydrocephalus. The tissue within the extra cranial portion is usually disorganized glial elements and connective tissue. We have seen one child with hydrocephalus and a dermoid tumor of the fourth ventricle. The galenic venous system and straight sinus are abnormal and join the sagittal sinus at the encephalocele.

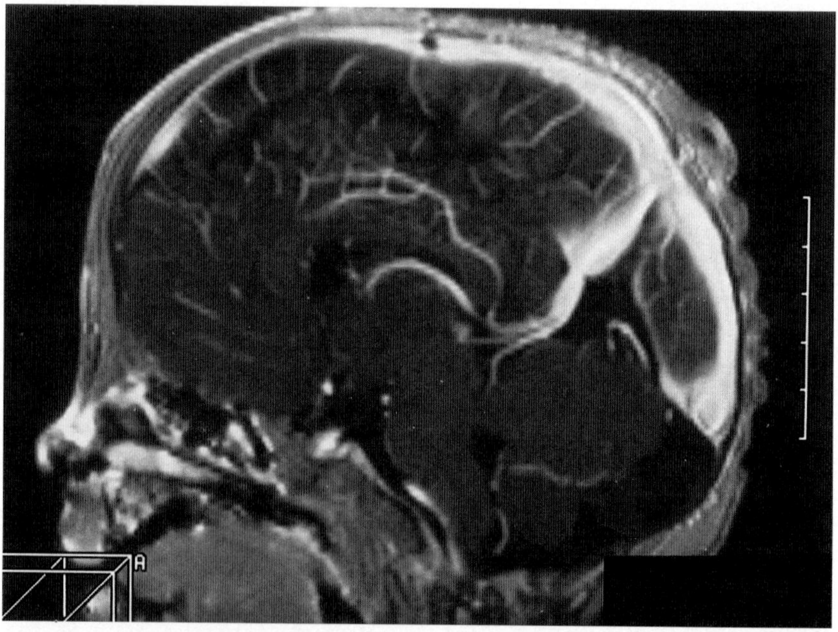

FIG. 19.3 An MRI shows a child with an atretic encephalocele. Note, as is usually the case, the straight sinus does not pass into the tentorium but enters the sagittal sinus at the encephalocele.

Occipital encephaloceles will contain brain tissue in about 80% of cases (54). The cerebellum may be partly or completely within the cyst (Figure 19.4). Cerebellar aplasia, absence, and, inversion occur (22, 45). Alterations in the CSF pathways frequently result in hydrocephalus. Lateral, third, and fourth ventricles can be within the encephalocele. The size and development of the brain stem is often abnormal. Encephaloceles have been reported in children with Chiari and Dandy-Walker malformations (33, 49).

The goal of surgical repair of encephaloceles is to reconstitute the integrity of the skull, resect as little neural tissue as possible, and achieve an acceptable cosmetic result. Only in rare cases is it reasonable to attempt to return the extracranial contents of the encephalocele to the intracranial compartment. In most cases, the tissue within the encephalocele is quite abnormal and unlikely to be functional, and the volume often exceeds the limits the intracranial compartment will accept without major reconstruction of the skull. Since encephaloceles are

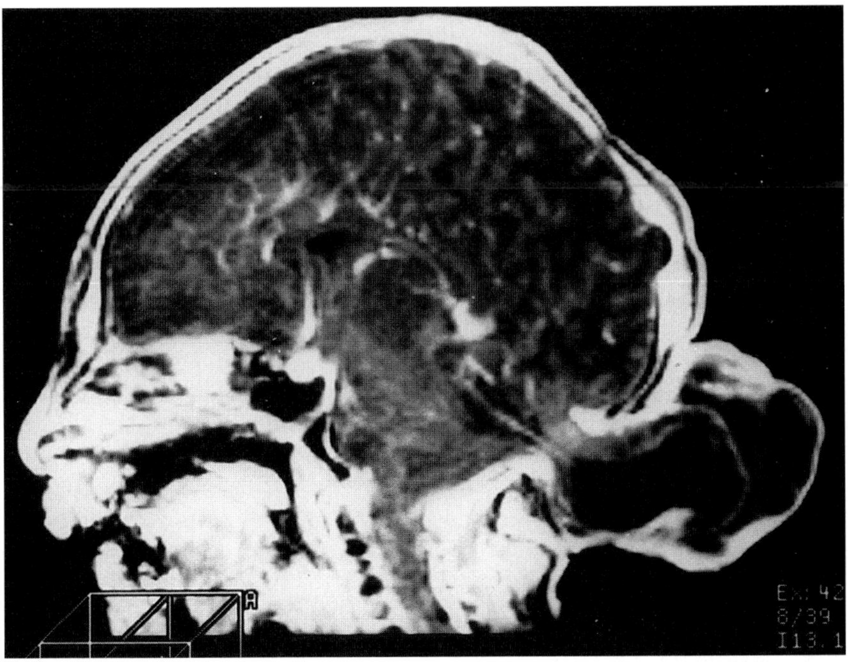

FIG. 19.4 An occipital encephalocele contains portions of both the occipital lobes and cerebellum. As in this case, portions of a deformed brain stem may also be in the encephalocele.

usually midline lesions, they are in close proximity to major vascular structures, and in the case of basal encephaloceles, the anterior cranial nerves are also at risk. Repair of the dura mater is an important part of the repair. As these lesions are almost always skin covered, closure of the skin is rarely a problem. Small cranial defects need not be repaired and whenever possible, large openings are best repaired with split bone grafts from the child's own skull.

Repair of these lesions in an infant requires special expertise on the part of the operating team. The infant has a small blood volume, cools rapidly, and has an immature circulatory and respiratory system. Obviously, a detailed discussion with the parents of risks, benefits, and likely outcome must be provided by an individual informed about the current state of the art. Matson recommended operative treatment for all patients with encephaloceles except those who are terminal. He emphasized that ease of care and diminution of parental psychic trauma are also considerations (47). Others have suggested that patients with microcephaly and large amounts of brain within the encephalocele may have a poor prognosis and should not have operative treatment (28, 80).

Basal Encephaloceles

It is often advisable to utilize otolaryngologist and/or plastic surgeons in a team approach to sincipital and basal encephaloceles. The involvement of the orbits, midface, skull base, and palate make the team approach advantageous. Timing of the operative correction varies. Meningitis, visual impairment, or airway obstruction warrant immediate repair. Some physicians believe that waiting beyond the third month significantly improves outcome and carries little risk. Others argue that repair of the encephalocele allows the resumption of normal facial growth and advocate that repair be done early during the period of rapid brain growth (12, 31, 66). There is also disagreement as to whether a one-stage repair is indicated. Arguments against a one-stage repair in a small child include blood loss, possible anterior facial growth impairment from early repair, and regression in growth due to the orbital correction.

Both the basal and sincipital encephaloceles can be approached by the same position and scalp incision. The head is placed in a brow up position. The hair need not be shaved. A "stealth" incision behind the hairline at about the level of the coronal suture provides adequate exposure and the best cosmetic result. The incision should be carried low enough to allow the scalp to be reflected anteriorly down to the level of the brow. The dissection of the scalp is carried through the loose areolar tissue plan and the pericranium is left intact. The pericranium is used as a vascular flap at closure to cover the dural repair and bone grafts.

In basal encephaloceles, a unilateral or bifrontal craniotomy from the coronal suture to the orbit is used to expose the floor of the anterior fossa. An intra and extradural approach is usually required to visualize the cranial nerves and vascular structures at the base of the brain. Brain tissue within the encephalocele is resected and the dura closed primarily or with a pericranial graft. The cranial base defect can be covered with a split portion of the bone flap, or in the case of the infant, a full thickness portion of the craniotomy bone flap. The vascularized pericranium is used as a flap to cover the repair. The plastic surgeon determines the time of the palatal repair.

Complications include infection, CSF leaks, and rarely, hydrocephalus. The overall mortality in infancy is as high as 50% (86).

Sincipital Encephaloceles

The positioning and skin approach is essentially the same for sincipital encephaloceles as for basal encephaloceles. The craniotomy varies depending on the size of the lesion and the need for an intradural approach. Recent experience with sincipital encephaloceles has demonstrated that a smaller nasal frontal craniotomy with an extradural repair and reconstruction of the nasal area is possible (35).

Complications include infection, CSF leaks, and lachrymal duct occlusion. The mortality rate is 7 to 20% (54, 80, 84).

Parietal Encephaloceles

These lesions are often quite large and sessile. A surgical clamp is useful to grasp and suspend the apex of the sac at a point where the skin is more normal. This allows preparation and draping of the encephalocele without traction on the brain stem. The skin incision is made on normal skin high enough on the encephalocele to insure adequate skin for closure.

Blunt dissection is used to separate the skin from the dura mater down to the level of the neck of the encephalocele. The bony margins of the skull defect are then identified and the intracranial dura is freed at the edges of the opening. It is essential to keep in mind that the superior sagittal sinus is usually involved in these lesions and care must be taken not to injure the sinus. A preoperative MRA gives useful information about the related vascular structures.

The sac is opened near the dome, CSF is drained, and cultures are taken. Dissection of the encephalocele is carried out from the apex toward the neck, taking care to identify and close vascular structure prior to transecting. It is possible that vessels may pass out of the intracranial compartment and reenter to supply functional brain structures. Once the blood supply has been eliminated, the abnormal tissue is transected at the neck of the encephalocele level with the bony opening. The dura mater is then trimmed and closed in a water tight manner. Small cranial defects need not be repaired but larger defects can be covered with a graft from adjacent parietal bone. Skin closure is accomplished by trimming the edges to allow a cosmetic repair without tension.

Occipital Encephaloceles

Encephaloceles located in the occipital area often involve the sinuses and torcula. Lesions below the torcula can contain cerebellum and occasionally brain stem. Again, imaging studies, such as MRI and MRA, offer the best opportunity to understand the anatomy and avoid surprises during repair. Undue traction or injury of the brain stem may result in postoperative inability for the child to breathe, and require prolonged intubation.

The surgical management is otherwise essentially the same for occipital as for parietal encephaloceles. A good dural closure is important since hydrocephalus commonly develops and CSF leaks can be avoided.

The overall mortality has been reported as high as 25 to 60% for parietal and occipital encephaloceles (43, 54, 74).

Atretic Encephaloceles

As stated previously, this lesion differs in the contents of the extracranial sac and probably in mechanism of development. The operative repair usually involves removal of the mass and closure of the skin. Only rarely will there be a need to deal with an intradural lesion. Preoperative imaging clearly shows the vascular changes typical of the atretic encephalocele.

Outcome

Intellectual development varies with the size and location of the lesions. The risk of intellectual delay increases based on location of the encephalocele from anterior to posterior. This does not include atretic encephaloceles, which appear not to influence intellectual development. Anterior encephaloceles are compatible with normal intelligence in 60+% of the children, with 15 to 20% mildly impaired and 20 to 35% severely impaired (7, 45, 74).

CEREBELLAR MALFORMATIONS

Cerebellar malformations include the four Chiari malformations and the Dandy Walker malformation. Again, hydrocephalus is often an accompanying sign of the underlying malformation.

Chiari II Malformation

The Chiari malformation makes the child with spina bifida different from all of the other children seen in our myelomeningocele clinic. The child with traumatic paraplegia or the child with a lipoma usually has problems restricted to the bladder and bowel or weakness in the lower extremities. These conditions should not be minimized and they are indeed significant problems in society. However, the Chiari malformation inflicts additional significant problems to the child. The Chiari malformation will kill 15 to 20% of the children before they reach the age of 20. It will render some 25% of the children dependent, and 90% of them will have hydrocephalus and all of the associated complications and revisions. Almost all of these children have abnormal respiratory problems and abnormal blood gasses. Vocal cord paralysis is present in one-third of the children. They have gastric reflux, apnea and poor swallowing, and learning disabilities. The more we study these children, the more we find that the majority of them have some degree of Attention Deficit Disorder (ADD).

For years, people from different disciplines, such as pathologists and anatomists, have attempted to link the myelomeningocele to this hindbrain malformation (3, 41, 60, 61). A variety of theories have been postulated, the simplest of which states that since the spinal cord is tethered at the bottom, it pulls the hindbrain out of the back of the skull (41). Other researchers postulate that the embryo has hydrocephalus, the hydrocephalus blows open the back so that the back actually reopens instead of never closing, and the force of the hydrocephalus pushes the posterior fossa content down into the upper cervical spine (60, 61).

Despite this pan cerebral abnormality, it is amazing that many of the children in our series of 100 (followed since 1975) have normal intelligence and normal participation in society. In addition, we anticipate independence in a high percentage of these children (51, 53). As is commonly accepted, in a Chiari malformation, a portion of the cerebellum, usually the vermis but also the tonsils, are herniated through the foramen magnum down into the cervical spine (Figure 19.5). What is often missed, however, is that there is also upward herniation (13, 14). The cerebellum is herniating upward out of the posterior fossa into the middle fossa (Figure 19.6). This is in fact a pan cephalic abnormality of the skull and brain. Lükenschadel of the skull, polymicrogyria, and ectopic gray mater exists. Dysgenesis and in some cases agenesis of the corpus callosum is present. The massa intermedia located in the third ventricle is huge. The tentorium is almost absent. There is an extremely small posterior fossa, and in some children, almost no posterior fossa. There is scalping at the base of the skull and a very enlarged foramen magnum. In spite of this grossly deformed brain, it generates normal intelligence and is compatible with independent living in the majority of these children. MRI shows these deformities clearly. What is the un-

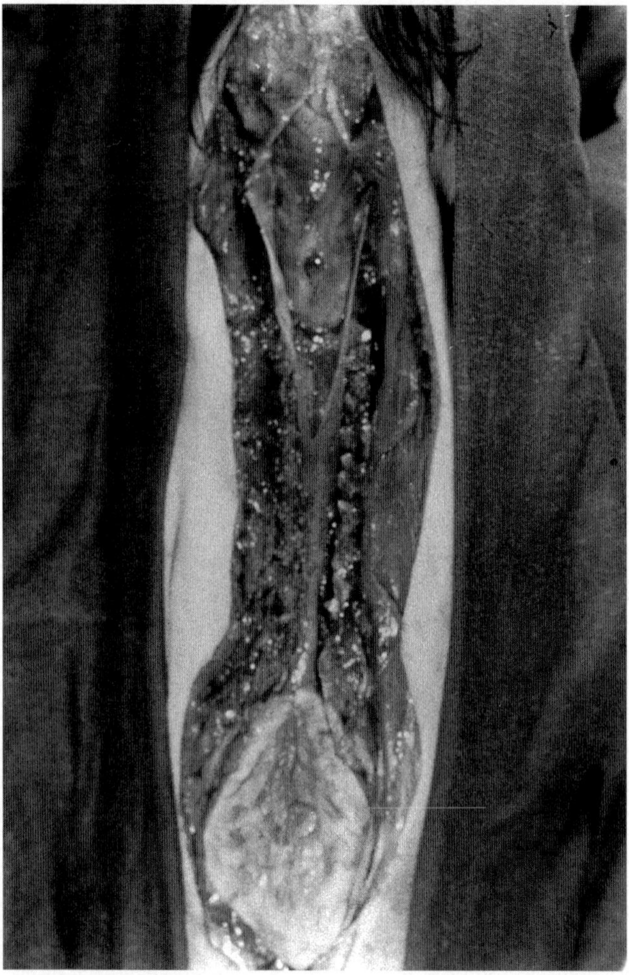

FIG. 19.5 An autopsy of an infant shows the cerebellar vermis and tonsils are herniated with the brain stem into the cervical canal. There is a kink of the brain stem. Note the large myelomeningocele in the lumbar spine.

derlying cause of the pan cephalic deformity? Is it related to the myelomeningocele or is there some genetic defect that causes disorganization of the head end of the embryo? A genetic defect is a possibility, but it would have to effect all of the germ layers since we know that the skull and nervous system are abnormal.

The splotch mouse in our laboratory develops at the lumbosacral junction (52). The scanning electron microscope shows that the myelo-

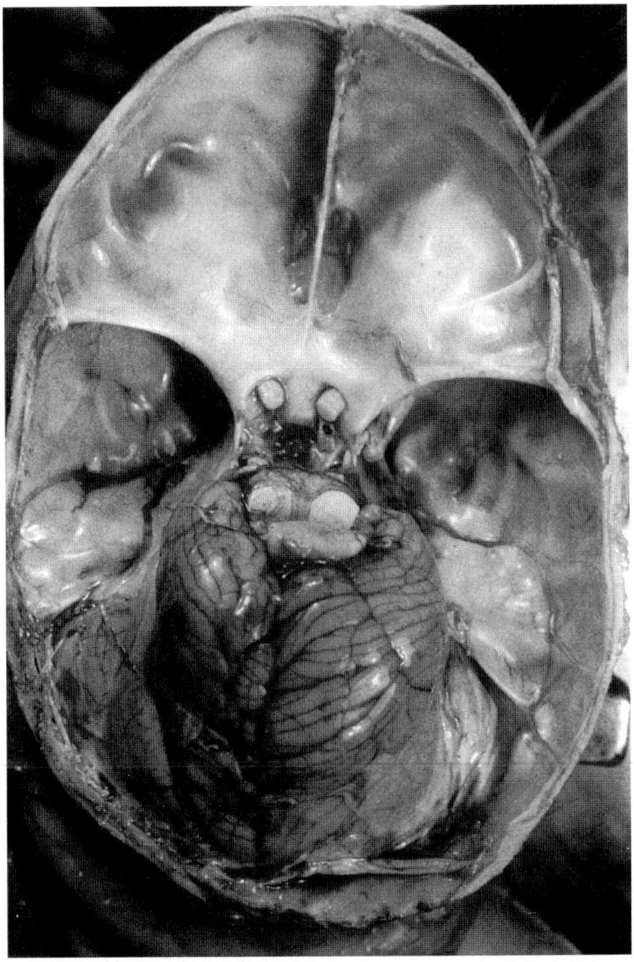

FIG. 19.6 A short tentorium with the cerebellum herniating into the middle fossa is typical of the Chiari II malformation.

meningocele is identical to the human neural tube defect. On occasion, instead of developing a myelomeningocele (as can happen in a human), the mouse will develop anencephaly. This mouse, at least anatomically, is an excellent example of what occurs in the human. The defect in this mouse is in the PAX3 gene. The PAX3 gene is a transcription factor, and is a gene that generates a protein that goes back into the nucleus and turns on and off a whole cascade of events which lead to neurulation. We took this information and in our clinic began to look for children who had the potential for a PAX3 defect (i.e., the HUP2 gene in humans).

Theories for the cause of this malformation have been advanced by many researchers. One theory accepted by the majority is Padget's theory (60). Padget's theory states that hydrocephalus is needed as the generator of the force to push the brain down into the brain stem. The difficulty with this theory is that not only is a downward herniation present, upward herniation is also present; therefore, it is unlikely that hydrocephalus is the generating force. Figure 19.7 is an example of a mid-trimester spontaneous aborted fetus. This fetus has a marked Chiari malformation in the posterior fossa and absolutely no hydrocephalus. Osaka looked at a whole group of aborted fetuses and showed quite clearly that the Chiari malformation was present in aborted fetus, in spite of the fact that there was no evidence of hydrocephalus (58). The Chiari malformation precedes hydrocephalus and we will clearly demonstrate that hydrocephalus is the result of the Chiari malformation, not the cause (53).

An interesting experiment was performed by Desmond and Schoenwolf in which they looked at developing chick embryo and showed that

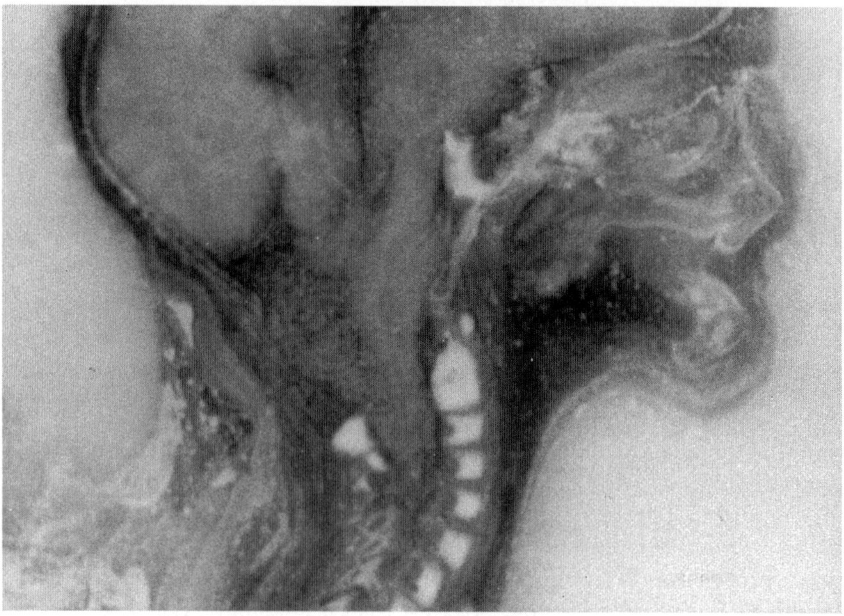

FIG. 19.7 Mid trimester fetus with a myelomeningocele and severe Chiari II malformation without hydrocephalus.

this hollow neural tube, the myelocele, goes from the head end of the embryo all the way to the posterior portion (17). Dye studies demonstrated that the neural tube closes from the cervical portion through the sacral portion spontaneously. This is called occlusion and occurs both in chickens and in mammals, including humans. There is a period of time, at about 48 hours, in which the central canal is occluded. Schoenwolf vented the fluid out of the cephalic portion (70). This caused the developing cerebral hemispheres to be markedly deformed. The distended ventricular system was essential for normal development of the hemispheres. It was the scaffolding that supported the normal development of the cerebral hemisphere. Had Schoenwolf looked in the posterior fossa, he would have seen that his embryos were developing a Chiari malformation.

In our laboratory, we performed this same experiment. We looked in the posterior fossa of the chick and showed that there were early Chiari malformations. This occlusion is a critical event that occurs and allows the cerebral hemispheres to distend. However, if there is an open myelomeningocele, when occlusion is over, after about 48 hours, the neural tube reopens, all of the fluid runs out through the open myelomeningocele, and the cerebral hemispheres are decompressed. At day 34 of the human embryo, the posterior fossa contains no cerebellum. There is a large amount of room in the posterior fossa due to cavity distended by the fluid. Surrounding the posterior fossa on either side is cartilage. The posterior fossa is already determined and solid, and is already in a cartilaginous box. What determines the size of this box is the distending force, which occurs during and after occlusion. If that force is lost, the posterior fossa is small. Not only are there cerebral deformities from the collapse of the mantle, but there is also a very small posterior fossa that leads to the Chiari malformation. The decompression of the embryonic ventricles during primary neurulation leads to the Chiari malformation. The neural tube is left open so that the fluid can pass out and decompress the head of the embryo. In the embryo, the telencephalic hemispheres are beginning to develop, and as seen in the embryo with a myelomeningocele, everything is collapsed (Figure 8A & 8B). In a normal embryo without a myelomeningocele, there is lots of space in the posterior fossa. Only the choroid plexus is present. The cerebellum will balloon into and fill in the spaces. In the mouse embryo with a myelomeningocele, there is no room for the anticipated cerebellum, which results in herniation of the contents of the posterior fossa into the upper cervical spine. Therefore, even before the cerebellum is developed, there are signs of herniation. The critical step is the loss of this volumetric expansion that the embryo needs to anticipate the development of the elements in the posterior fossa (Figure 9).

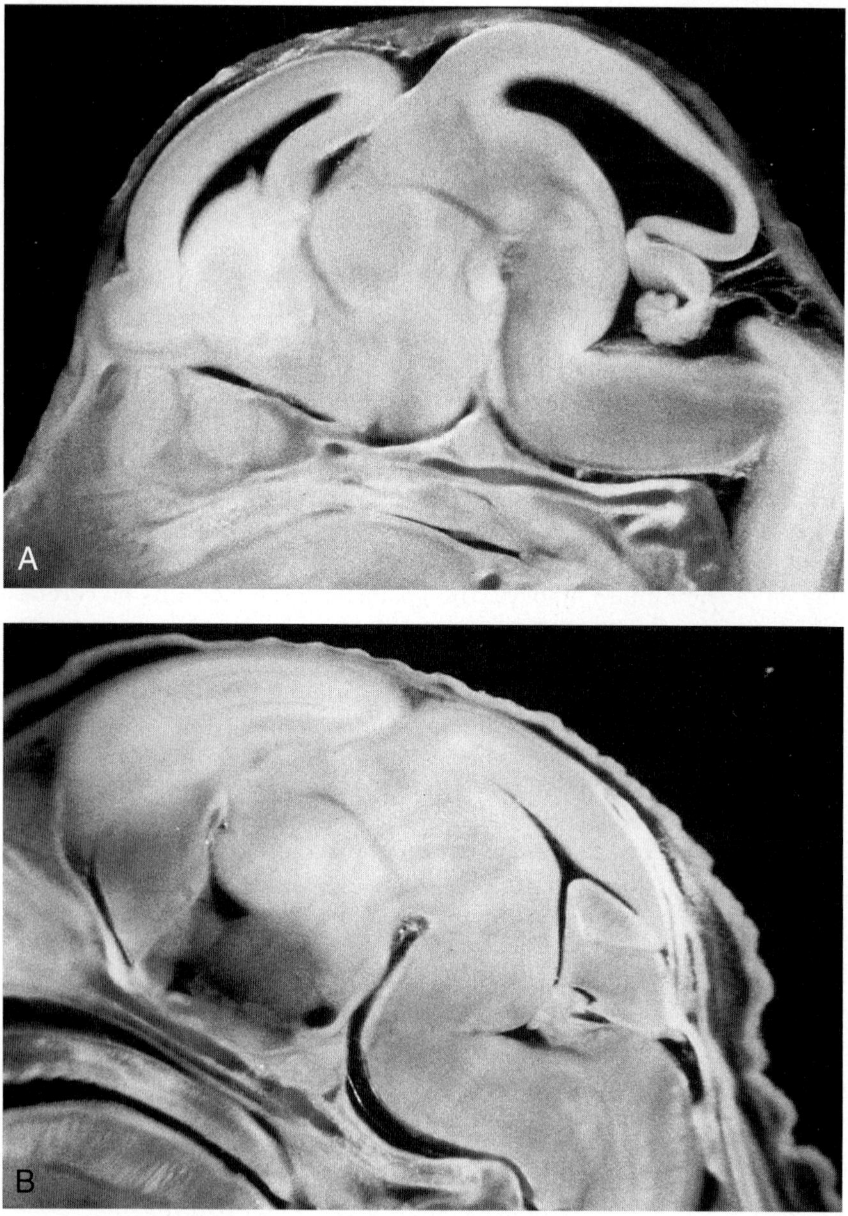

FIG. 19.8 (A) Shows the normal mouse embryonic hindbrain with a large fluid-filled space in the posterior fossa. (B) Mouse embryo with an open neural tube defect shows closure of these spaces.

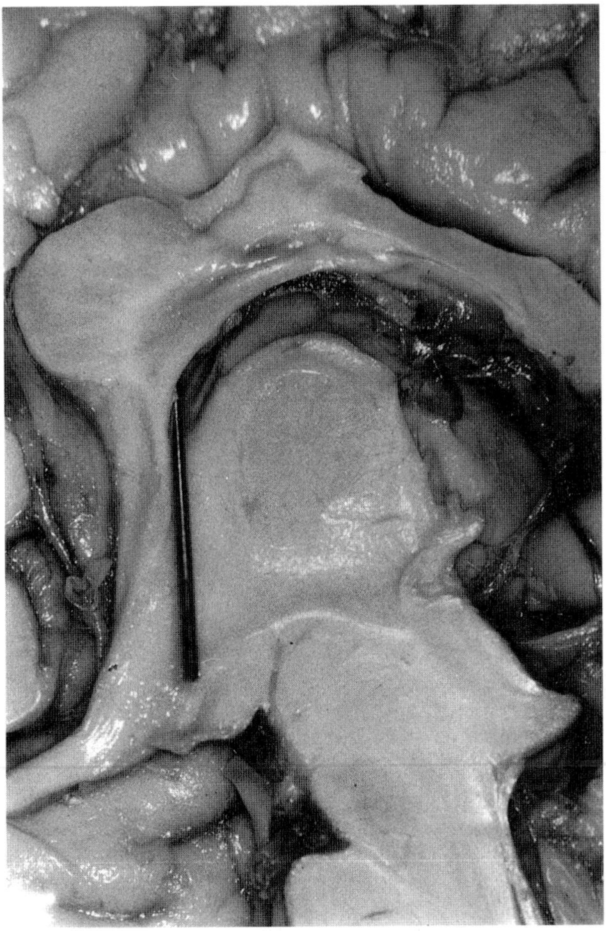

FIG. 19.9 Sagittal view of the 3rd ventricle demonstrates the extremely small area of the floor of the 3rd ventricle. A ventriculoscope shows the problem of selecting the site for a ventriculostomy

Overcrowding in the posterior fossa can make it impossible for the embryo to develop a subarachnoid space. The result is hydrocephalus. The severity of this compaction will determine the severity and how rapidly the hydrocephalus will progress. Since everything falls in on itself, instead of having a large third ventricle with a tiny massa intermedia, a big massa intermedia develops along with a small third ventricle, which makes it difficult in the newborn to determine where the surgeon can perform a third ventriculostomy to treat the hydrocephalus.

In the normal skull, the normal skull plate, the parietal plate, and the collagen bundles are streaming out as the brain expands, as if on the surface of a balloon. In the child with a myelomeningocele, because of a collapse of the mantle, the collagen bundles are generated at the center of the plate; however, they turn back on themselves because they are not pulled out. This leads to Lükenschadel of the skull. When an ultrasound is performed on the fetus, the frontal plates are caved in instead of being rounded externally. The myelomeningocele is linked to the formation of the Chiari malformation, since it is the myelomeningocele that allows escape of the embryonic CSF and decompression of the embryonic vesicles. This leads to the Chiari II malformation. In a child with a lipoma, a Chiari malformation does not develop because the lipoma plugs the hole and prevents the escape of fluid.

Surgical Management

Surgical management of a Chiari malformation is complicated by the presence of hydrocephalus. The initial treatment of manifestations of the Chiari II malformation in the neonate is directed at the hydrocephalus. Ventriculoperitoneal shunting is usually the only choice. Rarely the anatomy of the small 3rd ventricular floor in the Chiari II will permit a safe ventriculostomy. If shunting fails to improve the hindbrain function, decompression can be carried out. The outlook for neonates with apnea and/or stridor present from birth is not good even with decompression. The onset of stridor and apnea late in the neonatal period or later in childhood is more likely to respond to decompression. It is important to stress here that deterioration of any function in an individual with a myelomeningocele and hydrocephalus is the result of a *shunt malfunction* until proven otherwise. A shunt malfunction can mimic all other causes of deterioration in these patients. Exacerbations of hindbrain and upper extremity symptoms are especially likely to be due to a shunt malfunction in the patient with an enlarged 4th ventricle. Decompression of the Chiari II in the face of a shunt malfunction is a disaster from which few will recover.

Hydromyelia is commonly present in individuals with a Chiari II malformation. Again, this is often a manifestation of a shunt malfunction. It is essential to determine that the shunt is working optimally. Once the shunt has been determined to be working optimally, one can turn to other causes of deterioration in the patient with a myelomeningocele. In the Chiari I malformation, the most common cause of scoliosis is hydromyelia, while in the Chiari II, it is by far the tethered spinal cord. I have always been impressed with the finding of significant hydromyelia in a child with spina bifida who on repeat examination at long-term follow up is neurologically stable. On the other hand, the child with scoliosis usually does not have hydromyelia and responds to untethering of the spinal cord. Decompression of the Chiari II is often not successful in treating the hydromyelia. We have often used hydromyelia cavity to pleural space shunts successfully in these cases. It is unclear what the significance of segmental hydromyelia is in the children with spina bifida. Our experience with fenestration or shunting the segmental hydromyelic cavity has not resulted in improvement of the patients.

Decompression of the Chiari II malformation has often been referred to as "posterior fossa" decompression. This is almost never the case. Usually the foramen magnum is large and does not compress the cerebellum. It is also very important to be aware that the transverse sinus and torcula are located at the edge of the foramen magnum. Opening the dura mater into the posterior fossa may result in sinus hemorrhage that is difficult to manage. The cerebellum usually rests on the arch of C1. The cerebellar vermis, tonsils, and brain stem are compressed by the cervical lamina. This compression continues as far down as the lower extent of the cerebellar elements. Therefore, this is a dorsal or posterior cervical decompression that must be carried down beyond the level of lowest cerebellar extent. It is important to keep the lateral extent of the laminectomy medial to the articular processes to prevent deformity of the cervical spine. We have always opened the dura and placed a graft. Bony decompression only has been used, but we feel this is not adequate to insure decompression. In addition to decompression, fenestration of the 4th ventricle and/or cysts may be necessary. Routine fenestration has not been part of our standard decompression.

Complications have been few. CSF leakage is rare because an optimally functioning shunt has been established prior to the decompression. Instability of the cervical spine has not occurred. Over the years a few decompressions have required reoperation due to regrowth of the bone posterior to the Chiari elements. This is usually a single plate of bone, not regrowth of the lamina.

SPINAL CORD MALFORMATIONS

Spinal cord malformations include defects in embryogenesis involving both primary and secondary neurulation. These include split cord malformations (diastematomyelis), myelomeningoceles, myelocystoceles, dermal sinus tracts, myelomeningocele manque, and lipomas of the spinal cord.

Spinal Cord Lipomas

Spinal lipomas represent the most common of the lesions embraced by the term occult spinal dysraphism. Spinal lipomas are a developmental malformation that occurs in approximately one in 4,000 births

(8, 71). The precise prevalence, however, is unknown. Various forms of spinal lipoma are recognized. It is important that these are appropriately distinguished since there are practical implications with regard to clinical evaluation, surgical appraisal, and long-term prognosis that accompany each of these types (38, 63).

Tethering of the lipoma to the adjacent tissues results in mechanical stresses across the spinal cord, risking progressive and frequently irreversible neurological disability as well as secondary orthopedic and sphincteric disturbance. It is, in an attempt to prevent these consequences of mechanical tethering, that surgical intervention is undertaken.

Spinal lipomas are broadly classified into three categories. Although the classification is based upon anatomical site, there are other important distinctions with regard to embryogenesis, prognosis, and mechanism of producing neurological damage. Distinguishing between the three types of lipoma is usually straightforward; however, scant regard is often given to the differences in the literature. Specifically, lipomas of the conus and those of the filum terminale are frequently considered as a single entity, an assumption that is not justified on the basis of studies of long-term follow up of these children (38, 64).

Lipomas of the conus represent the largest single group of spinal lipomas and comprise approximately 75% of lumbosacral lipomas (38, 64). The dura is deficient dorsally in over 90% of cases, and in this instance, the lipoma is in continuity with the subcutaneous fat through a defect in the posterior vertebral elements and thoracolumbar fascia. The transition from intact to bifid lumbar vertebrae is often gradual, and in the region of the transition, a thick fibrovascular band commonly completes the dorsal neural arch. This itself frequently is responsible for significant spinal compression and tethering. Segmentation anomalies of the sacrum commonly coexist with these lesions.

Lipomas limited to the filum terminale account for between 13% and 26% of the largest series of lumbosacral lipomas (Figure 10) (38). In contrast to lipomas of the conus, these lesions are commonly truly occult with no external stigmata of dysraphism. In 50% of the patients reported, the overlying skin was entirely normal (64). Since the advent of MRI, a number of lipomas of the filum terminale have been diagnosed incidentally. These lesions are usually completely intradural, and the filum is thickened and may be asymmetric or even duplicated in its dural attachment.

Fat within the filum is found in as many as 90% of cases of the tight filum terminale syndrome and has been identified in 88% of cases of imperforate anus (50, 64).

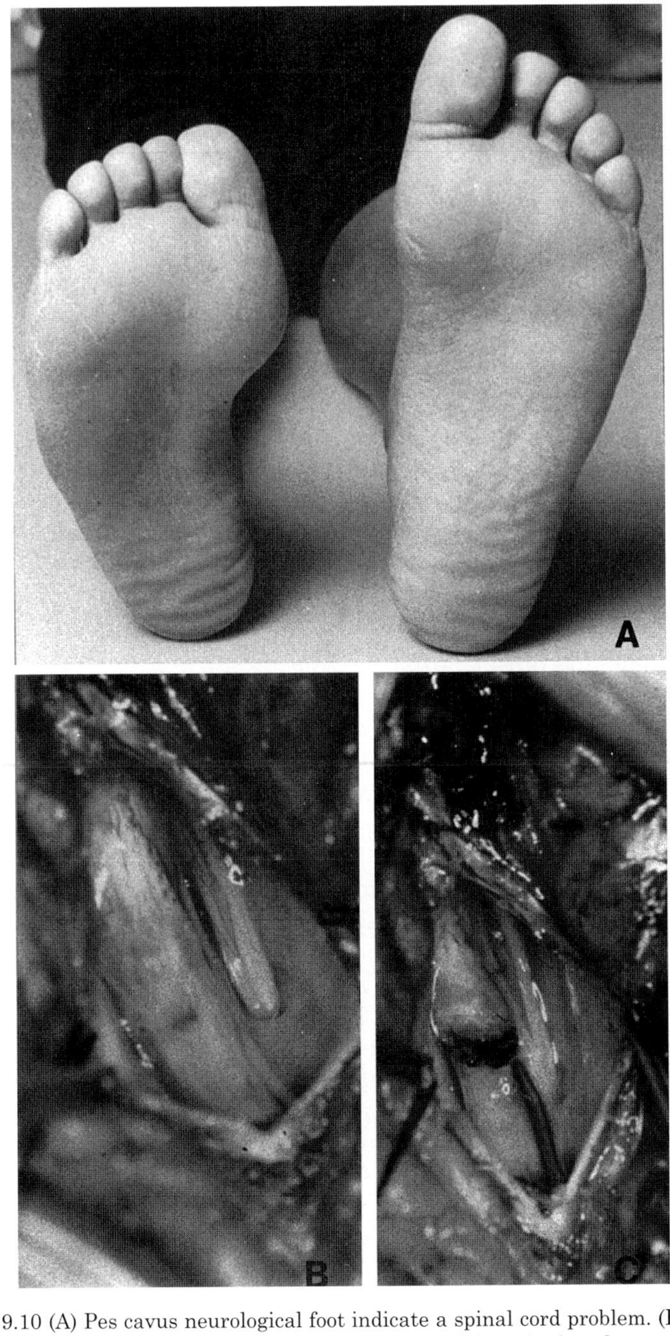

FIG. 19.10 (A) Pes cavus neurological foot indicate a spinal cord problem. (B) Lipoma of the filum at surgery. (C) After resection and release of the spinal cord.

Embryogenesis of Spinal Lipomas

Comprehension of the theories of embryogenesis of spinal lipomas requires a knowledge of normal human spinal cord embryology. There are two basic phases to spinal cord formation—primary neurulation and secondary neurulation.

McLone and Naidich recently advanced a theory of pathogenesis for lipomeningocele that embraces both the currently held view of spinal cord embryogenesis and the surgical anatomy of these lesions (57). They proposed that the process of disjunction, whereby the closed neural tube detaches from the cutaneous ectoderm, occurs prematurely. Consequently, the folding neuroectoderm remains cleft dorsally, which allows the paraxial mesenchyme access to the prospective lumen of the neural tube. The ingrowth of mesenchyme prevents further closure of the neural tube and results in the state of partial dorsal myeloschisis that is evident in lipomyelomeningocele. This theory necessitates differential effects of each ectodermal surface on the maturation of the mesenchyme to which it is exposed. The "luminal" surface of the ectoderm induces the mesenchymal cells to differentiate along a path resulting in adipocyte formation, while the outer surface of the incompletely closed neural tube causes the mesenchyme to form the piaarachnoid and dura (10, 62).

The surgical anatomy can be easily reconciled with this model. The lipoma is contiguous with the neural tissue since there is no intervening meningeal layer. It extends dorsally through the dysraphic lumbosacral vertebrae into the subcutaneous tissue. The meningeal layers will only become apparent at the margins of the lipoma, ipso facto the subarachnoid space will also lie ventral and will not contain lipoma. The lipoma is thus extradural, and its relationship to the meninges and the nerve roots can be compared with that seen in myeloceles and meningomyeloceles. Lipoma is certainly able to extend within the central canal of the spinal cord and even herniate through the parenchyma of the spinal cord; however, even in this instance, the lipoma would be invested by pia and would not truly lie in the subarachnoid space.

The neural tube formed as a result of primary neurulation extends only as far as the site of the former neurenteric canal and this corresponds to the second sacral segment. It is evident, therefore, that a defect in primary neurulation cannot account for lipomas of the filum terminale. Situated in the tail bud, between the caudal end of the neural tube and the cloaca (the end of the primitive hind gut), is an aggregation of cells known as the caudal cell mass. It is from this collection of cells that the terminal spinal cord (beyond S2) and filum terminale will develop. This process is termed secondary neurulation or retrogressive differentiation.

In view of the proximity of the cloaca and urogenital structures to the caudal cell mass, it is important to be aware that more extensive perineal deformities may coexist with abnormalities of the filum and conus. The constellation of anomalies that can occur include the Currarino syndrome, Vaters syndrome, caudal regression syndrome, and imperforate anus (18).

The fat content of spinal lipomas consists of mature adipocytes with no atypical cellular features. However, these cells most commonly lie in a densely fibrous connective tissue stroma (77). Striated muscle, epithelial derivatives, bone, and neural tissue may also be found within these lipomas. Metabolic features of the adipocytes within lumbosacral lipomas failed to demonstrate any differences when compared to normal adipose tissue (83). These lipomas are part of the body fat pool and as such, may increase along with other fat deposits during periods of fat deposition. Growth of spinal lipomas may be seen in sequential imaging and lipomas have occasionally recurred after resection (25, 82). Malignant transformation in a lumbosacral lipoma is exceedingly rare, while the appearance of malignant teratoma in association with lipomeningocele has been recognized (1, 29).

Despite the term occult, cutaneous stigmata of the dysraphic state are present in the majority of patients. Although a subcutaneous lipoma is the most common sign, a variety of lesions, frequently occurring in combination, can be found (Figure 19.11). Additional malformations of the perineal region may also be present, including imperforate anus, abnormal genitalia, and extrophy (27, 63, 69).

The deranged neural anatomy of the terminal spinal cord and cauda equina that occurs with lipomeningocele is reflected in the neuromuscular connections of the lower limbs. Imbalance between agonist and antagonist muscle groups ensues and predisposes the child to joint deformity. The constellation of musculoskeletal abnormalities that results is referred to as the neuroorthopedic syndrome and is seen in between one-third and one-half of patients at initial presentation (9, 64). The syndrome is seen in its most florid form in the context of open myelomeningocele.

The deformities include club feet (most commonly of equinovarus variety asymmetric leg length) trophic ulceration, hip subluxation, and scoliosis of the spine (42). These problems, although frequently necessitating specialist orthopedic treatment, should be considered as secondary to the problem of tethering of the spinal cord. In the older child, gait change, weakness, deformity, and pain may be the presenting symptoms of the neuroorthopedic syndrome and should alert the physician to the possibility of retethering (67). New onset hip subluxation,

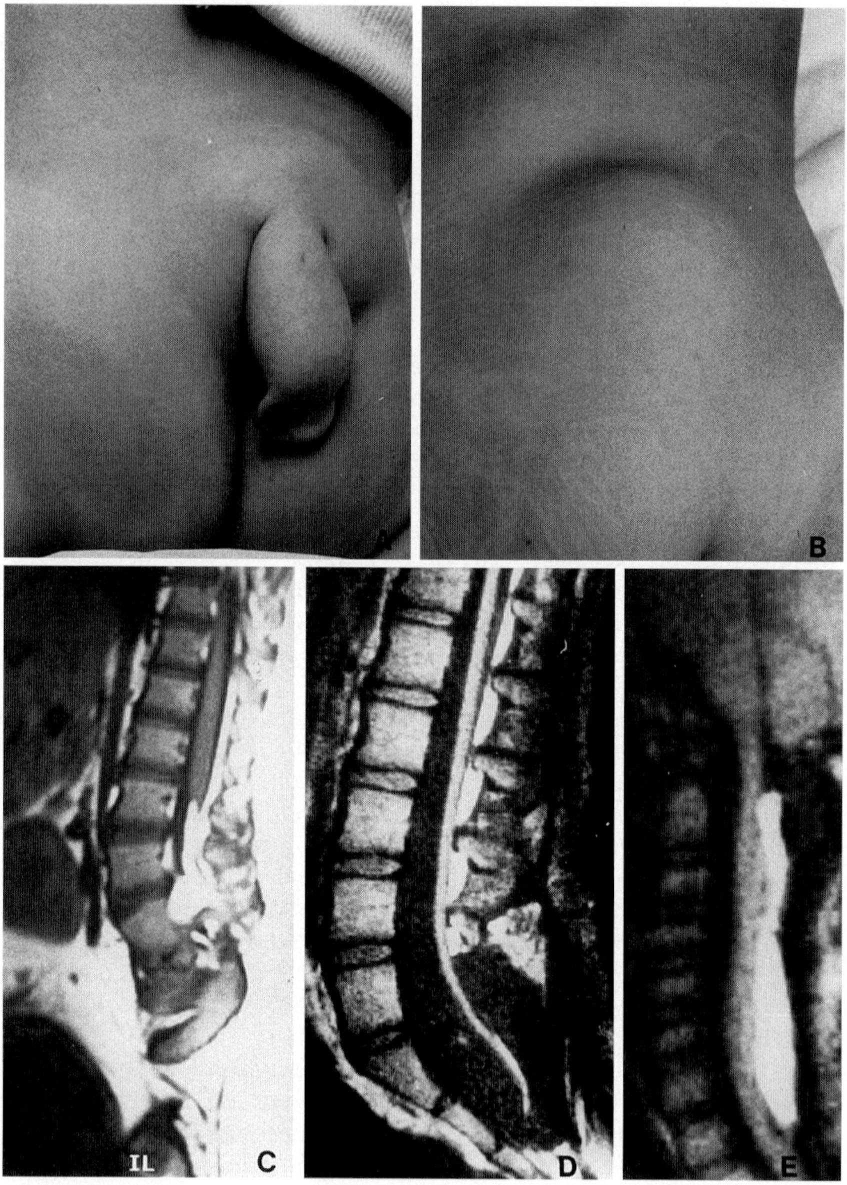

FIG. 19.11 (A and B) Subcutaneous lipomas; (A) an apendage; (B) a double lipoma. (C–E) MRIs of a lipoma C sacral agenesis; (D) Postoperative after removal and untethering; (E) Postoperative Cervicle Lipoma.

asymmetric lower limb weakness, or increased rate of progression of scoliosis are of particular significance.

It is well documented that spinal cord tethering is an important etiological factor in the development of scoliosis. Scoliosis accompanies spinal lipoma in roughly 10% of cases (38, 64, 67). Spinal radiographs should be part of the routine follow up in these children. The scoliosis seen in association with spinal cord tethering usually lacks the rotational deformity that is seen in association with vertebral body anomalies. Importantly, many of these skeletal changes can be stabilized or even improved by timely untethering of the spinal cord (38, 62).

The innervation of the lower urinary tract and the bladder and bowel sphincters is also threatened in the child with tethering of the spinal cord by lipomatous malformations. Repeated urinary tract infections, abnormal voiding pattern, frank incontinence of urine, and fecal soiling are common symptoms. In addition to the practical difficulties and social implications of incontinence, there is a more serious threat to the upper renal tracts and long-term renal function. Although in the infant a detailed urological assessment may be limited, careful history, physical examination, and urodynamic measurements will reveal urological abnormalities in approximately one-third and two-thirds of children under 1 year of age. The most common urodynamic abnormalities revealed by cystometrogram and sphincter electromyogram (EMG) include flaccid bladder, detrusor sphincter dyssynergia, and detrusor hyperreflexia.

Abnormal urodynamic tests may be the only feature neurological impairment. Unfortunately, a number of infants elude early detection only to present with incontinence later in childhood. Moreover, in children who have previously undergone primary surgery for resection of lipomeningocele, urological manifestations are among the most common changes that may herald the onset of retethering of the spinal cord. Hence, there is a need for continued surveillance of this population of patients (67).

Untethering of the spinal cord has been shown to have a beneficial effect on urodynamic function, both at initial presentation and in the instance of retethering, with some patients returning to normal urinary function (2, 38, 42, 62, 64). The urological benefits of untethering are, however, more evident in the young child (less than 18 months). Worsening urological function may also occur as a result of surgical untethering. This is a greater risk for the child with lipoma of the conus than with lipoma of the filum terminale (38, 64).

However, a number of authors caution that urological outcome is much more favorable in younger children (less than 18 months) who show a degree of reversibility in neuro-urological deficit that appears to lessen with age (21, 36). Early aggressive treatment of the tethering is therefore advocated in an attempt to avert permanent urological damage.

Pain and sensory disturbance infrequently accompany tethering of the spinal cord; however, they are less commonly reported in the child than in older patients. The symptoms are frequently nonspecific, with sensory loss often failing to follow a dermatomal distribution. Similarly, pain is often poorly localized without true radicular features. Sometimes pain is limited to the perineal region. Motor impairment is a more frequent manifestation. An integral part of clinical evaluation should be regular documentation of muscle strength so that a baseline examination can be established and allow for the early detection of motor problems.

Plain radiographs will demonstrate bifid spinous processes and a widened spinal canal in the majority of cases of lumbosacral lipoma. Associated sacral and vertebral anomalies, such as hemivertebrae, may also be visualized. Interpretation may be particularly difficult in the newborn and plain films are not part of the routine evaluation of these cases.

In the infant, spinal ultrasound can be of help in the initial assessment of the asymptomatic child with cutaneous stigmata of dysraphism (56). The lipomatous tissue is highly echogenic and permits the position and extent of the lipoma to be readily seen.

CT scan, following intrathecal contrast provides excellent resolution in the axial plane, and demonstrates the relationship between the subarachnoid space, the lipoma, and the placode and associated nerve roots. MRI avoids the radiation exposure and the need for lumbar puncture and is the current mainstay of neuroimaging of lumbosacral lipomas. Fat has a short relaxation time on T1 weighted sequences, and results in high signal. Imaging in the sagittal and axial planes will delineate the extent of the lipoma and confirm its relationship to surrounding structures. Associated pathologies, such as diastematomyelia and hydromyelia, may also be revealed.

The ventral subarachnoid space is usually well visualized, and differentiation between lipomyelocele and lipomeningocele is usually evident. The conus lies in an abnormally low position, while at the level of the lipoma, the spinal chord is displaced posteriorly. Dorsally, the subarachnoid space is obliterated at the liponeural junction. The lipoma is continuous with the subcutaneous fat, although thin stalks of fat may not be well demonstrated.

On occasion, the lipoma is seen to extend upwards beyond the limits of the spina bifida lying dorsal to the spinal cord. Extension into the central canal of the spinal cord may also be present.

Although extremely sensitive as an initial diagnostic modality for lumbosacral lipoma, MRI has been found to be less useful in the post operative setting (Figure 19.11). Despite surgically satisfactory untethering procedures, the caudal and posterior position of the conus is often little changed (85). Scanning in the prone position and the use of phase contrast MRI have been suggested as means of assessing the mobility of the lower spinal cord (6). To date, these techniques have not been widely used and the diagnosis of the tethered spinal cord remains foremost a clinical one.

Two processes may explain the emergence of neurological symptoms and signs in the infant with lumbosacral lipoma. Failure to develop continence and normal lower extremity function could simply be a reflection of a basic disorder in the neuroarchitecture of the terminal spinal cord consequent upon the underlying embryopathy. In this event, surgery would not necessarily be expected to have a beneficial effect on the natural history of the condition. The late deterioration of individuals, with loss of an established neurological function and the undoubted improvement in symptoms that may result from untethering procedures, suggests however that mechanical factors play some significant part in the natural history of these conditions.

Direct compression as a result of the lipoma acting as a space-occupying lesion has been advanced as a mechanism for deterioration. Indeed, this has been observed where the lipoma has an intramedullary component, hence the need to ensure this component is addressed at the time of surgery. Repeated injury to the lower spinal cord caused by a water hammer effect, trauma being transmitted from the subcutaneous component through the lipoma, is also reputed to occur.

The onset of new symptoms commonly coincides with a period of intense physical exercise or rapid physical growth (5, 29). Under normal circumstances, the spinal cord moves relative to the vertebral canal throughout the range of spinal movements. Anchoring of the spinal cord by a thickened filum or lumbar lipoma compromises these movements and may result in repeated traction injury to the spinal cord. At the time of surgery, the blood vessels on the nerve roots and over the surface of the spinal cord are often thin and attenuated. Following untethering, these vessels relax and become dilated. Similarly, disappointing results have been obtained when trying to use Somata Sensory Evoked Potentials to detect early onset tethering.

The aim of surgical treatment of spinal lipomas is to untether the spinal cord in order to prevent progressive orthopedic deformity, neurological damage, and preserve sphincter function. It is important to make certain distinctions when discussing the management and evaluating the outcome of lumbosacral lipoma surgery. First, isolated lipomas of the filum must be distinguished from lipomas of the conus medullaris, and second, the patient presenting with symptoms needs to be distinguished from the child with lipoma in whom there appears to have been no neurologic, orthopedic, or urologic impairment.

Surgery to resect a lipoma of the filum represents a much less formidable challenge than untethering a lipoma of the conus. In the majority of patients with filar lipomas, the thecal sac is intact and the dissection of the lipomatous filum from the rest of the cauda equina is straightforward. Resection of filum lipomas carries a much smaller risk of deterioration. By contrast, surgery of the conus lipoma has a much greater risk of inflicting a neurological insult. Similarly, the incidence of local wound complications is smaller in the filar lipoma group. This latter observation probably reflects a greater ease of achieving dural closure with this particular pathology.

For both types of lipoma, most series would concur with the need to operate on the symptomatic patient (32, 38, 64). The majority of patients presenting with symptoms will either improve or stabilize following surgical intervention. The risks of the surgical procedure are thus considered acceptable in the context of evolving symptomatology. It must be emphasized, however, that once symptoms are apparent, the results of surgery in terms of recovering deficits are variable. In the case of lipomas of the filum with preoperative symptoms, improvement or stabilization of symptoms can be anticipated for over half of patients (38, 64).

With regard to lipomas of the conus presenting with symptoms, return to normal function occurred in 12.6% of our series, while 13.8% showed some improvement, 50.6% remained stable, and 23% were identified as having deteriorated at long-term follow up when compared to their status at presentation (38).

Certain features may be instrumental in determining outcome. Most authors have suggested that a more favorable outcome is seen in younger children, although Pierre-Khan found no significant age-related benefit (62, 64). Sphincter deficits appear to be the most refractory to good functional recovery following untethering. Once neurogenic bladder dysfunction has occurred, return to normal is unlikely to be seen in more than 20% of cases (63). For motor function, too, a reversal of a preoperative deficit is seen in less than half of patients (30). In short, surgery for the symptomatic individual will stabilize a deficit more commonly than it will reverse one. Thus, the important question is whether surgery performed before the onset of symptoms can be performed safely and prevent the onset of symptoms.

Only 3% of asymptomatic patients in our series were over the age of

1 year. Furthermore, documentation of disease progression has been noted within individuals coming to surgery who were previously neurologically normal (38, 68, 69). In a review of 177 patients with lipomyelomeningocele, 37% were neurologically intact at presentation. Progressive neurological deterioration, which showed a logarithmic relationship to increasing age, was found in this group (46). In our series the figure is even higher, with approximately 60% of children thought to be normal at birth showing evidence of the neuroorthopedic syndrome at time of presentation (mean age 2.1 years) (38). Finally, in children who had solely cosmetic procedures to remove the subcutaneous lipoma, a high rate of emergence of deficits has been observed (84). In the United States today, pediatricians, neonatologists, and pediatric surgeons essentially refer all children with cutaneous lesions over the lumbosacral spine for evaluation. Thus, few escape detection.

As has already been noted, once symptoms supervene, surgical untethering will reverse deficits in only a small number of cases. This is particularly so for sphincter disturbance and orthopedic foot deformities, but true of motor and sensory deficits as well. It is only in the asymptomatic patients that superior long-term maintenance of sphincter function is seen following surgery (38, 36).

The risks of surgical intervention appear to be lower in the more recently reported series (78). A less aggressive removal of the subcutaneous component of the lipoma has been proposed as one factor. Use of the laser has also been reported to have had a beneficial impact on the frequency of retethering.

Untethering of the spinal cord should be undertaken in all symptomatic individuals. The morbidity of resection of lipomas of the filum is sufficiently low to recommend this even for asymptomatic children. It is the author's opinion that surgery, prior to the onset of symptoms, offers the best protection against long-term deterioration, and therefore, also strongly recommend prophylactic spinal cord untethering.

REFERENCES

1. Aoki N: Rapid growth of intraspinal lipoma demonstrated by magnetic resonance imaging. *Surg Neurol* 34(2):107, 1990.
2. Atala A, Bauer SB, Dyro FM, et al.: Bladder functional changes resulting from lipomyelomeningocele repair. *J Urol* 148(2 Pt 2):592, 1992.
3. Barry A, Patten BM, Stewart BH: Possible factors in the development of the Arnold-Chiari malformation: J Neurosurg 14:285–301, 1957.
4. Basset RC: The neurologic deficit associated with lipomas of the cauda equina. *Ann Surg* 131:109, 1950.
5. Breig A: Overstretching of and circumscribed pathological tension in the spinal cord: A basic cause of symptoms in cord disorders. *J Biomechanics* 3(1):7, 1970.

6. Brophy JD, Sutton LN, Zimmerman RA, et al.: Magnetic resonance imaging of lipomyelomeningocele and tethered cord. *Neurosurgery* 25(3):336, 1989.
7. Brown MS, Sheridan-Pereira M: Outlook for a child with a cephalocele. *Pediatrics* 90:914–919, 1992.
8. Bruce DA, Schut L: Spinal lipomas in infancy and childhood. *Childs Brain* 5(3):192, 1979.
9. Byrne RW, Hayes EA, George TM, et al.: Operative resection of 100 spinal lipomas in infants less than 1 year of age. *Ped Neurosurg* 23(4):182, 1995.
10. Chapman PH: Congenital intraspinal lipomas: Anatomic considerations and surgical treatment. *Childs Brain* 9(1):37, 1982.
11. Chapman PH, Swearingen B, Caviness VS: Subtorcular occipital encephaloceles. *J Neurosurg* 71:375–381, 1989.
12. Charoonsmith, TSC: Frontoethmoidal encephalomeningocele with special refrence to plastic reconstruction. *Clin Plast Surg* 1:27–47, 1974.
13. Chiari H: Uber Veranderungen des Kleinhirns infolge von Hydrocephalie des Grosshirns. *Dt med Wschr* 17:1172, 1891.
14. Chiari H: Uber Veranderungen des Kleinhirns, der Pons und der Medulla oblongata infolge von congenitaler Hydrocephalie des Grosshirns. *Denkschr Akad Wiss* 63:71, 1895.
15. Cohen MM, Lemire RJ: Syndromes with cephaloceles. *Teratology* 25:161–172, 1982.
16. David DJ, Sheffield L, Simpson DA et al.: Fronto-ethmoidal meningoencephaloceles morphology and treatment. *Br J Plast Surg* 37:271–284, 1984.
17. Desmond ME, Schoenwolf G: Timing and positioning of occlusion of the spinal neurocele in the chick embryo. J Comp Neurol 235(4):479, 1985.
18. Ehni G, Love JG: Intraspinal lipomas: Report of cases, review of the literature, and clinical and pathological study. *Arch Neurol Psychiatry* 53:1, 1945.
19. Emery JL, Kalhan SC: The pathology of exencephalus. *Dev Med Child Neurol* 22:51–64, 1970.
20. Field B: The child with an encephalocele. *Med J Aust* i:700–703, 1974.
21. Foster LS, Kogan BA, Cogen PH, et al.: Bladder function in patients with lipomyelomeningocele. *J Urol* 143(5):984, 1990.
22. Friede RL: Uncommon syndromes of cerebellar vermis aplasia. II. Tecto-cerebellar dysraphia with occipital encephalocele. *Dev Med Child Neurol* 20:764–772, 1978.
23. Gardner WJ: Diastematomyelia and Klippelfeil syndrome. Relationship to hydrocephalus, syringomyelia, meningocele, meningomyelocele, and iniencephalus. *Cleve Clin Q* 31:19–44, 1964.
24. Gardner WJ: Hydrodynamic mechanism of syringomyelia: Its relationship to myelocele. *J Neurol Neurosurg Psychiatry* 8:247–259, 1965.
25. Giudicelli Y, Pierre-Kahn A, Bourdeaux AM, et al.: Are the metabolic characteristics of congenital intraspinal lipoma cells identical to, or different from normal adipocytes? *Childs Nerv Syst* 2(6):290, 1986.
26. Gluckman TJ, George TM, McLone DG: Postneurulation rapid brain growth represents a critical time for encephalocele formation: A chick model. *Ped Neurosurg* 25:130–136, 1996.
27. Greene WB, Dias LS, Lindseth RE, et al.: Musculoskeletal problems in association with cloacal exstrophy. J Bone Joint Surg Am 73(4):551, 1991.
28. Guthkelch AN: Occipital cranium bifdum. *Arch Dis Child* 45:104–109, 1972.
29. Hall WA, Albright AL, Brunberg JA: Diagnosis of tethered cords by magnetic resonance imaging. *Surg Neurol* 30(1):60, 1988.
30. Herman JM, McLone DG, Storrs BB, et al.: Analysis of 153 patients with

myelomeningocele or spinal lipoma reoperated upon for a tethered cord: Presentation, management and outcome. *Ped Neurosurg* 19(5):243, 1993.
31. Hoffman JJ, Raffel C: Craniofacial surgery, in, McLaurin RL, Venes JL, Schut L, Epstein F (ed). **Pediatric Neurosurgery. Surgery of the Developing Nervous System, 2.** Philadelphia: Saunders, 1989, p 120.
32. Hoffman HJ, Taecholarn C, Hendrick EB, et al.: Management of lipomyelomeningoceles: Experience at the Hospital for Sick Children, Toronto. J Neurosurg 62(1):1, 1985.
33. Hutchison JW, Stovring J, Turner PT: Occipital encephalocele with holoprosencephaly and aqueduct stenosis. *Surg Neurol* 12:331–335, 1979.
34. Ingraham FD, Swan H: Spina bifida and cranium bifidum. I. A survey of five hundred and forty-six cases. *N Engl J Med* 228:559–563, 1943.
35. Jimenez D, Barone CM: Evaluation and treatment of sincipital encephaloceles: Report of 38 consecutive cases. **Proceedings of the Pediatric Section of the AANS and CNS.** December 1–4, 1998, p 33.
36. Kaplan WE, McLone DG, Richards I: The urological manifestations of the tethered spinal cord. *J Urol* 5(140):1285, 1988.
37. Karch SB, Urich HL: Occipital encephalocele: A morphological study. *J Neurol Sci* 15:89–112, 1972.
38. La Marca F, Grant JA, Tomita T, et al.: Spinal lipomas in children: Outcome of 270 procedures. *Ped Neurosurg* 26(1):8, 1997.
39. Leblanc R, Tampieri D, Robataille Y et al.: Developmental anterobasal temporal encephalocele and temporal lobe epilepsy. *J Neurosurg* 74:933–939, 1991.
40. Leong AYS, Shaw CM: The pathology of occipital encephalocele and a discussion of the pathgenesis. *Pathology* 11:223–234, 1979.
41. Lichtenstein BW: Distant neuroanatomic complications of spina bifida (spinal dysraphism), hydrocephalus, Arnold-Chiari deformity, stenosis of the aqueduct of Sylvius, etc., pathogenesis and pathology. *Arch Neurol Psychiat* 47:195, 1942.
42. Locke MD, Sarwark JF: Orthopedic aspects of myelodysplasia in children. [Review]. *Cur Opin Pediatr* 8(1):65, 1996.
43. Lorber J: The prognosis of occipital encephalocele. *Dev Med Child Neurol* 13:75–86, 1967.
44. Luyendijk W: Intranasal encephaloceles: A survey of 8 neurosurgically treated cases. *Psychiat Neurol Neurochir* 72:77–87, 1969.
45. Macfarlane R, Rutka JT, Armstrong D et al.: Encephaloceles of the anterior cranial fossa. *Ped Neurosurg* 23:148–158, 1995.
46. Maiuri F, Corriero G, Gallicchio B, et al.: Late neurological dysfunction in adult lumbosacral lipoma. J Neurosurg Sci 31(1):7, 1987.
47. Matson DD: **Neurosurgery of Infancy and Childhood,** 2nd edition. Springfield: Thomas, 1969, pp 61–75.
48. McCarthy JG, La Trenta GS, Breitbart AS et al.: Hypertelorism correction in the young child. *Plast Reconstr Surg* 86:214–225, 1990.
49. McLaurin RL: Parietal cephaloceles. *Neurology* 14:764–772, 1964.
50. McLendon RE, Oakes WJ, Heinz ER, et al.: Adipose tissue in the filum terminale: A computed tomographic finding that may indicate tethering of the spinal cord. *Neurosurgery* 22(5):873, 1988.
51. McLone DG, Knepper PA: The cause of Chiari II malformation: A unified theory. *Ped Neurosurg* 15:1, 1989.
52. McLone DG, Dias MS, Goossens W et al.: Pathological changes in exposed neural tissue of fetal delayed splotch (Spd) mice. Childs Nerv Systm 13(1):1, 1997.
53. McLone DG, Raimondi AJ, Sommers MW: The results of early treatment of 100 con-

secutive newborns with myelomeningocele. Proceedings of the VII Cognress of European Society for Paediatric Neurosurgery. *Z Kinder Chir* 2:115, 1981.

54. Mealey J, Dzenitis AJ, Hockley AA: The prognosis of encephaloceles. *J. Neurosurg* 32:209–218, 1970.
55. Mulliken JB, Kaban LB, Evans CA et al.: Facial skeletal changes following hypertelorbitism correction. *Plast Reconstr Surg* 77:7–16, 1986.
56. Naidich TP, Fernbach SK, McLone DG, et al.: John Caffey Award. Sonography of the caudal spine and back: Congenital anomalies in children. *Am J Roentgenol* 142(6):1229, 1984.
57. Naidich TP, McLone DG: Spinal dysraphism, in, Newton TH, Potts DG (ed): **Modern Neuroradiology Volume 1. Computed Tomography of the Spine and Spinal Cord,** 1. San Francisco, New York: Clavadel Press, 1983, p 299.
58. Osaka K, Matsumoto S, Tanimura T: Myeloschisis in early human embryos. *Childs Brain* 4(6):347, 1978.
59. Padget DH: Neuroschisis and human embryonic maldevelopment: New evidence on anencephaly, spina bifida and diverse mammalian defects. *J Neuropathol Exp Neurol* 29:192–216, 1970.
60. Padget DH: Development of so-called dysraphism: With embryologic evidence of clinical Arnold-Chiari and Dandy-Walker malformations. *Johns Hopkins Medical Journal* 130:127, 1972.
61. Padget DH, Lindenberg R: Inverse cerebellum morphogenetically related to Dandy-Walker and Arnold-Chiari syndromes: Bizarre malformed brain with occipital encephalocele. *Johns Hopkins Medical Journal* 131:228, 1972.
62. Pierre-Kahn A, Lacombe J, Pichon J, et al.: Intraspinal lipomas with spina bifida: Prognosis and treatment in 73 cases. *J Neurosurg* 65(6):756, 1986.
63. Pierre-Kahn A, Zerah M, Renier D, et al.: Congenital lumbosacral lipomas. [Review] Childs Nerv Sys 13(6):298, 1997.
64. Pierre-Kahn A, Zerah M, Renier D: Lipomes malformatifs intra-rachidiens. Attitude therapeutique. *Neuro-Chirurgie* 41(suppl 1):114, 1995.
65. Raffel C, Litofsky S, McComb JG: Central nervous system malformations and the Vater association. *Ped Neurosurg* 16:170–173, 1990.
66. Rahman NY: Nasal encephalocele: Treatment by trans-cranial operation. *J Neurol Sci* 42:73–85, 1979.
67. Sarwark JF, Weber DT, Gabrieli AP, et al.: Tethered cord syndrome in low motor level children with myelomeningocele. *Ped Neurosurg* 25(6):295, 1996.
68. Sathi S, Madsen JR, Bauer S, et al.: Effect of surgical repair on the neurologic function in infants with lipomeningocele. *Ped Neurosurg* 19(5):256, 1993.
69. Sato K, Shimoji T, Sumie H, et al.: Surgically confirmed myelographic classification of congenital intraspinal lipoma in the lumbosacral region. *Childs Nerv Syst,* 1(1):3, 1985.
70. Schoenwolf G, Desmond ME: Neural tube occlusion precedes rapid brain enlargement. *J Exp Zool* 30:405, 1984.
71. Schut L, Bruce DA, Sutton LN: The management of the child with a lipomyelomeningocele. *Clin Neurosurg* 30:464, 1983.
72. Sedano HO, Cohen MM, Jirasek J, et al: Frontonasal dysplasia. *J Pediatr* 76:906–913, 1970.
73. Sever LE, Sanders M, Monsen R: An epidemiologic study of neural tube defects in Los Angeles count. I. Prevalence at birth based on multiple sources of case ascertainment. *Teratology* 25:315–321, 1982.
74. Simpson DA, David DJ, White J: Cephaloceles: Treatment outcome and antenatal diagnosis. *Neurosurgery* 15:14–21, 1984.

75. Smith MT, Huntington HW: Inverse cerebellum and occipital encephalocele: A dorsal fusion defect uniting the Arnold-Chiari and Dandy-Walker spectrum. *Neurology* 27:246–251, 1977.
76. Sternberg H: Zur formalen Genese der vorderen Hirnbrucke (Encephalomeningocele anterior). *Wien Med Wochenschr* 79:462–466, 1929.
77. Streeter GL: Factors involved in the formation of the filum terminale. *Am J Anat* 25:1, 1919.
78. Sutton LN: Lipomyelomeningocele. [Review] *Neurosurg Clin N Am* 6(2):325, 1995.
79. Suwanwela C: Craniomeningocele and encephalomeningocele, in, Sano K, Ishii S (ed): **Recent Progress in Neurological Surgery, Proceedings of the Symposia of the Fifth International Congress of Neurological Surgery.** Amsterdam, Excerpta Medica, 1974, p. 49.
80. Suwanwela C, Hongsaprabhas C: Fronto-ethmoidal encephalomeningocele. *J Neurosurg* 25:172–182, 1966.
81. Suwanwela C, Suwanwela N: A morphological classification of sincipital encephalomeningocele. *J Neurosurg* 36:201–211, 1972.
82. Walsh JW, Markesbery WR: Histological features of congenital lipomas of the lower spinal canal. *J Neurosurg* 52(4):564, 1980.
83. Warf BC, Scott RM, Barnes PD, et al.: Tethered spinal cord in patients with anorectal and urogenital malformations. *Ped Neurosurg* 19(1):25, 1993.
84. Whatmore WJ: Sincipital encephalomeningoceles. *Br J Surg* 60:261–270, 1973.
85. Wippold FJ, Citrin C, Barkovich AJ, et al.: Evaluation of MR in spinal dysraphism with lipoma: Comparison with metrizamide computed tomography. *Ped Radiol* 17(3):184, 1987.
86. Yokota A, Matsukado Y, Fuwa I et al.: Anterior basal encephalocele of the neonatal and infantile period. *Neurosurgery* 19:468–477, 1986.

CHAPTER

20

Moyamoya Syndrome: A Surgically Treatable Cause of Stroke in the Pediatric Patient

R. MICHAEL SCOTT, M.D.

Stroke in a child can be due to a myriad of etiologies, such as embolization from cardiac sources, disturbances of coagulation, metabolic disorders, and trauma (15). One of the treatable causes of stroke in this population that warrants neurosurgical assessment and treatment is Moyamoya syndrome.

Moyamoya syndrome is a progressive occlusive cerebrovascular disorder characterized by: 1) progressive stenosis of the supraclinoid carotid arteries and branches of the Circle of Willis, and 2) the nearly simultaneous development of profuse arterial collaterals at the base of the brain which pass through the basal ganglia supplying distal circulation to the brain.

Review of published series of pediatric stroke patients suggests that about 6% of pediatric strokes are caused by Moyamoya syndrome (9, 12), but that the rate may be as high as 12% in certain populations (9). The clinical presentation of most patients with Moyamoya syndrome is cerebral ischemia. In my own series of 100 patients under age 21, 66 presented with stroke and 18 with transient ischemic attacks (TIA). The syndrome passes through well-defined arteriographic changes, which were first described by Suzuki (8, 13). Initially, the apex of the suprasellar intracranial internal carotid artery becomes stenotic (Suzuki stages 1 and 2). As the stenosis progresses, the basal collateral vessels (the moyamoya circulation) begin to form and dilate, and become visible on angiography (Suzuki stages 3 and 4). It is during these stages that the vast majority of pediatric patients become symptomatic. During the final stages of the process, extracranial to intracranial collateral pathways—which are already developing through the anterior skull base, over the convexity, and around major dural venous sinuses—enlarge to become the major source of intracranial circulation while the carotids are occluding (Suzuki stages 5 and 6). In my experience with more than 130 children and adults with the syndrome, the course of this progression has been extraordinarily variable, with certain patients having a rapidly progressive syndrome that causes multiple strokes over the course of only a year or two, and others having an extremely slow progression, with symptom-free intervals of up to eight years in one case (11). In the course of following pediatric patients with Moyamoya syndrome for more than two decades, I have never seen a patient in whom the arteriographic process did not progress and in whom the clinical syndrome did not similarly evolve while the patient was untreated, although the rate of progression of the clinical syndrome and arteriographic process is unpredictable (15).

The prognosis of a pediatric patient with Moyamoya syndrome seems to be most directly related to the extent of disease and infarction at diagnosis rather than to age of onset. For example, all children in my series under five years of age with significant bilateral infarcts at presentation were developmentally delayed at long-term follow-up despite surgery that was successful in preventing additional stroke. Older children also tended to have developmental problems if they had suffered bilateral strokes at initial diagnosis. Although children have a remarkable capacity to recover from strokes that might incapacitate older patients, their recovery abilities should not be overstated, since many children with even small strokes will later in life be shown to have difficulties with schooling or job performance. Children with large bilateral strokes suffered at an early age will be severely delayed and may have chronic seizure disorders. A single large dominant hemisphere infarct also may lead to a poor long-term outcome at any age. However, multiple small infarcts, particularly frontal or large nondominant strokes, may not have such a poor prognosis; many of these children are educable and capable of leading independent and productive lives.

Predictions and prognosis in a given child is largely based on common sense interpretation of imaging studies and neurologic deficit. A presentation of TIAs only, even if accompanied by severe arteriographic disease, frequently carries an excellent prognosis if surgical revascularization is carried out before infarction occurs. It is not wise to wait for evidence of stroke before recommending surgery in this patient population, however, since in my series, a number of such patients went on to develop strokes while under observation. The long-term outlook for a successfully treated pediatric patient remains unknown, simply because of the relatively recent recognition of the syndrome and the short period of follow-up available in many of the published series; however, the patients in our surgical series who have been followed for more than ten years into adulthood have been symptom free. Three of our patients have become pregnant and gone through pregnancies and delivery (two

Cesarean sections and two vaginal deliveries) without incident. One of their children, however, has gone on to develop Moyamoya syndrome himself, and underwent surgery at 21 months of age after a hemisphere stroke was diagnosed. One mother, unaffected herself, has had three children with the syndrome, each by different fathers. One young female patient with the syndrome, however, has an unaffected identical twin, which indicates that there must be a multifactorial etiology to the syndrome.

Diagnosis of the syndrome is probably made most easily by magnetic resonance imaging (MRI) and magnetic resonance angiography (MRA) although cerebral angiography is the only certain way of making the diagnosis. MRI typically shows diminished flow voids in the internal carotid and middle cerebral arteries. Axial and sagittal T-1 images, as well as proton density and T2 weighted images, may demonstrate flow voids in the basal ganglia that result from the enlarged moyamoya collateral in these structures (3). MRI will detect small infarcts in the cortex and demonstrate the gyriform enhancement noted occasionally on computed tomography (CT) scans, which connotes either borderline perfusion, ischemia, or infarction. MRA can frequently detect the presence of Moyamoya syndrome (6, 16), but it may also misdiagnose the extent of arterial occlusion, most commonly by underestimating its degree or failing to detect the moyamoya vessels themselves. MRA combined with conventional MRI is said to have a sensitivity of approximately 92% (6). Some authorities have suggested that MR alone may obviate the need for standard angiography, at least in terms of making a nonquantitative diagnosis (3). Recent reports have suggested that gradient-echo and diffusion-weighted images may demonstrate ischemic areas of the brain earlier and more definitively than other techniques (2).

The role of quantitative cerebral blood flow studies in the evaluation of these patients has been emphasized by certain authors (5). Cerebral angiography remains the standard for diagnosis in this condition, and I believe that it is an essential part of the patient's diagnostic management. The study should include selective external as well as internal carotid injections. The purpose of these selective studies is to document preoperatively the extent of preexisting collateral from the external circulation so that proposed surgical procedure will not interfere with it, and to demonstrate by flow patterns and leptomeningeal collateral pathways where obvious watershed areas in the circulation are located.

Perhaps of greatest importance to the neurosurgeon is that the syndrome can develop in neurosurgical patients previously treated for brain tumors or other neurosurgical conditions in whom sequential scanning routinely carried out for the primary condition may reveal the development of Moyamoya syndrome. It is a condition that should be suspected when certain syndromic patients under chronic medical management suffer stroke or TIAs. My own series has included patients with neurofibromatosis, Down syndrome, prior cranial irradiation or intrathecal chemotherapy, hemoglobinopathies, etc. (Table 20.1).

When to operate in a given patient with Moyamoya syndrome is difficult to summarize in a presentation of this type, but in general, most patients with the syndrome are considered candidates for the procedure provided the diagnosis is clearly established by angiographic criteria. Since all patients with the syndrome appear to progress both neurologically and clinically over time, I usually recommend surgery when the process has been diagnosed before further symptoms develop. In the case of patients already affected by stroke and neurologic deficits, the decision to operate is based on whether there is additional brain tissue at risk for stroke and whether the patient's quality of life is such that further deficits would represent an intolerable burden to the family and patient. It is a highly individualized decision-making process, and at least two patients not operated on for a variety of reasons have gone on to die, one of renal failure and another of repetitive strokes.

In my opinion, the role of surgery in the treatment of this syndrome has been firmly established. To evaluate various treatment regimens critically, however, it is often necessary to utilize the patient's own past history as a measure of treatment success, and follow-up for at least

TABLE 20.1
Clinical Associations in a Surgical Series of 100 Consecutive Children with Moyamoya Syndrome

Asian ancestry	13
Neurofibromatosis	13
Prior cranial X-irradiation	10
Brain tumors	9
Down syndrome	9
Surgery for congenital cardiac anomalies	8
Hemoglobinopathies	4
Renal artery stenosis	3
Giant facial hemangiomas	3
Mother or sibling with Moyamoya syndrome	2
Intrathecal chemotherapy and low-dose cranial irradiation	2
Graves disease	1
[No known risk factors	46]

(Scott RM. Unpublished data. The numbers exceed 100 because of a combination of risk factors in certain patients, e.g., Down syndrome and congenital cardiac anomalies.)

five years and probably ten may be necessary in order to determine the efficacy of a treatment modality. The role of surgery in this syndrome is further complicated by the fact that ischemic symptoms have a dual etiology, with some symptoms certainly resulting from emboli from thrombus formation at proximal vessel stenoses. For this reason, all of our patients are kept on aspirin indefinitely. There is no evidence, however, that aspirin or any other medication reverses or stops the progression of the arterial stenoses that lead to the development of symptoms in so many patients. Anticoagulants, such as coumadin, are contraindicated because of the risk of spontaneous bleeding from the abnormal moyamoya vessels, and coumadin is particularly contraindicated in children, who are prone to unpredictable trauma as well.

The surgical procedures for Moyamoya syndrome all increase surface collateral flow to the brain by using the external carotid circulation in some form as a donor supply. These techniques are probably particularly effective in moyamoya patients since these patients have increased levels of growth factors in their cerebrospinal fluid (CSF) that attract the ingrowth of new blood vessels from any source (7). Virtually any pathway through the skull, dura, and arachnoid that a surgeon can create will allow the development of some type of collateralization to the brain's surface, and even burr holes where the dura and arachnoid are opened can provide pathways for collateral in a certain number of patients. In our pediatric and adult patients, we use a technique that fixes the intact superficial temporal artery to the pial surface after a wide opening of the dura and arachnoid ("pial synangiosis") (1). Simply described, this surgical procedure involves the dissection of the superficial temporal artery, the placement of a craniotomy directly beneath the intact vessel, a stellate dural opening and wide microsurgical opening of the arachnoid over the surgical field, and the affixing of the intact superficial temporal artery to the pial surface with multiple sutures of 10-0 nylon. The postoperative arteriograms in these patients demonstrate very dramatic collateralization to the brain over the hemisphere through the craniotomy, not only from the donor superficial temporal artery, but also from other meningeal and scalp arteries near the craniotomy site. The spectacular postoperative arteriographic results are mirrored by the stable long-term neurological status of most of these patients, whose transient ischemic attacks diminish in frequency and intensity following surgery and who do not develop additional strokes over the long term.

The exceptions to this postoperative pattern, in a pediatric series averaging more than a five-year mean follow-up, are three children who developed strokes or transient ischemic attacks in the distribution of the posterior cerebral artery. In each case, the follow-up arteriograms demonstrated progressive involvement of the posterior cerebral arteries and apex of the basilar artery in vascular territories not sufficiently collateralized by the anterior circulation surgical procedures. This late complication may be seen more frequently as patients are followed for prolonged periods, although many pediatric patients on postoperative arteriography appear to have excellent perfusion of the posterior cerebral circulation, either via native collateral or through the surgically-induced pathways.

The risks of surgery in patients with Moyamoya syndrome are similar to those of patients being considered for carotid endarterectomy and other surgical procedures for stroke, and are most directly related to neurologic instability at the time of surgery. Moyamoya patients are notoriously poor anesthetic risks for any surgical procedure, and several of the patients in my series developed their first symptoms or stroke following a general anesthetic for another purpose. Anesthesia in these patients requires meticulous management of fluid balance, blood pressure, and blood gases. We also employ intraoperative EEG monitoring with a full scalp electrode array to aid in anesthetic management. Because anesthetic risks are so significant, we try to operate on both hemispheres under the same anesthetic to reduce the number of inductions and wake-ups, and to minimize time off antiplatelet agents. Our anesthesia service has developed a protocol for the perioperative management of the pediatric moyamoya patient, (12) and all patients are admitted the night before surgery for intravenous hydration.

Some symptoms seen in the moyamoya population are probably not helped by surgery and require careful medical management. Headache, for example, has been a particularly troublesome symptom in certain patients. The headache often mimics typical migraine, and seems to respond to the usual medications, although a variety of antimigraine medications may need to be tried before consistent relief is obtained. TIAs may persist in certain patients as well, although they are never as severe or frequent as preoperatively. They almost always disappear within a year of the procedure.

Future areas for research and therapy may involve the use of growth factors, either applied topically or systemically, to induce the development of new blood vessels to the brain, along with attempts to block or alter the underlying process that leads to the formation of the arteriopathy. Many of the genetically determined conditions associated with the development of Moyamoya syndrome have in common an alteration of arterial wall anatomy or cardiac structure, and gene therapy targeted toward these conditions may provide therapeutic benefit in certain patients. Recent work in our laboratories has demonstrated that intracellular adhesion molecules are elevated in the cerebrospinal fluid and blood of patients with Moyamoya syndrome, which suggests that a chronic inflammatory process is taking place within the cerebral circulation of these children. The development of an effective blockade of this pathway may also provide an opportunity for novel therapy for the condition.

REFERENCES

1. Adelson PD, Scott RM. Pial synangiosis for moyamoya syndrome in children. **Ped Neurosurg** 23:26–33, 1995.
2. Chabbert V, Ranjeva J, Sevely A, Boetto S, Berru I, Manelfe C. Diffusion and magnetization transfer-weighted RI in childhood moyamoya. **Neuroradiology** 40:267–271, 1998.
3. Chang K, Yi J, Han M, Kim I. Imaging findings of moyamoya disease. **J Korean Med Sci** 5:85–90, 1990.
4. Giroud M, Lemesele G, Madinier G, Manceau E, Osseby G, Dumas R. Stroke in children under 16 years of age: Clinical and etiological difference with adults. **Acta Neurol Scand**, 96:401–406, 1997.
5. Golby AJ, Marks MP, Thompson RC, Steinberg GK. Direct and combined revascularization in pediatric moyamoya disease. **Neurosurgery** 45:50–60, 1999.
6. Katz D, Marks M, Napel S, Bracci P, Roberts S. Circle of Willis: Evaluation with spiral CT, angiography, MRA, and conventional angiography. **Radiol** 195:445–449, 1995.
7. Malek A, Connors S, Robertson R, Scott RM, Elevation of cerebrospinal fluid levels of basic fibroblast growth factor in moyamoya and central nervous system disorders. **Pediatr Neurosurg** 27:182–189, 1997.
8. Matsushima Y, Aoyagi M, Niimi Y, Masaoka H, Ohno K. Symptoms and their pattern of progression in childhood moyamoya disease. **Brain Dev** 12:784–789, 1990.
9. Nagaraya D, Verma A, Taly A, Kumar M, Jayakumar P. Cerebrovascular disease in children. **Acta Neurol Scand** 90:251–255, 1994.
10. Roach ES, Riela AR. **Pediatric Cerebrovascular Disorders,** 2nd Edition. New York: Futura, Cermont 1995, pp 4–5.
11. Scott RM. Surgical treatment of moyamoya syndrome in children, in **Concepts in Pediatric Neurosurgery,** P. Chapman, (ed) New York, S Karger: 1985, pp 192–212.
12. Soriano S, Sethna N, Scott RM. Anesthetic management of children with moyamoya syndrome. **Anesth Analg** 77:1066–1070, 1993.
13. Suzuki J, Takaku A, Cerebrovascular "moyamoya" disease: A disease showing abnormal net-like vessels in base of brain. **Arch Neurol** 20:288–299, 1969.
14. Takeshita M, Kagawa M, Izawa M, Kitamura K. Hemorrhagic stroke in infancy, childhood, and adolescence. **Surg Neurol** 26:496–500, 1986.
15. Takeuchi K, Shimizu K. Hypoplasia of the bilateral internal carotid arteries. **Brain Nerve** 9:37–43, 1957.
16. Yamada I, Suzuki S, Matsushima Y. Moyamoya disease: Comparison of assessment with MR angiography and MR imaging versus conventional angiography. **Radiol** 196:211–218, 1996.

CHAPTER

21

Indications and Outcomes for Lobectomy, Corpus Callosotomy, and Hemispherectomy in Pediatric Neurosurgical Patients

BENJAMIN S. CARSON, SR., M.D.

INTRODUCTION

More than 1% of the population of the United States suffers from some form of epilepsy. The vast majority of these cases start during childhood, with the peak incidence of seizure activity occurring during the first year of life. Many epileptic patients are, in fact, surgical candidates, but only a small fraction are ever considered for neurosurgical intervention for a variety of reasons. The results of seizure surgery are particularly gratifying, and it is important that these good results be disseminated throughout the medical community as well as throughout the population at-large to give the maximum number of epileptic patients an opportunity to live seizure-free and drug-free lives.

Seizure surgery candidate selection and workup is generally done by epileptologists, who most frequently are neurologists. The candidate selection and workup is as important as the surgery itself, since superb surgery on an inappropriate candidate will lead to a poor outcome just as inferior surgery on a superb candidate will lead to a poor outcome. Frequently, the parents of pediatric seizure patients who are being considered for surgical intervention are anxious to proceed with a definitive procedure, and it becomes important for the entire medical team to emphasize patience and a meticulous investigation prior to subjecting a patient to potentially irreversible surgical effects.

At least 10% and possibly as many as 25% of seizure patients have medically intractable seizures (10, 20). Clearly, any candidate being considered for seizure surgery must have seizures that cannot be readily controlled through medical management. Nevertheless, 10 to 25% of one percent of the total United States population constitutes a huge number of potential candidates for seizure surgery and highlights the magnitude of the problem.

Seizures in the pediatric population can be a more urgent problem than in the mature brain because there are several mechanisms through which the seizures can have a deleterious effect on the developing brain. It has been shown that induced electroconvulsive activity in rat pups done at frequent intervals can reduce brain protein and myelin and cause dissociation of ribosomes (14, 22, 35). Additionally, early status epilepticus can produce delays in neuronal maturation, and frequent seizures can induce cytotoxic damage (21). N-methyl-D-aspartate (NMDA) and glutumate, for example, are released by seizure-induced hypoxia, producing cytopathic changes that can lead to cell death (30). Anti-epileptic drugs (AED) may also potentially have deleterious effects on the developing nervous system, providing another rationale for early surgical management of intractable seizures, which potentially could accelerate the possibility of discontinuing such drugs.

We will limit the discussion in this chapter to cerebral hemispherectomy, lobectomy and cortical resections, and corpus callosotomy as surgical methods for treatment of intractable seizures. Certain prerequisites must be met when considering pediatric patients for seizure surgery (*Table 21.1*): 1) The seizures have to be debilitating in nature. Since children generally do not drive automobiles or operate dangerous machinery, the occasional annoying seizure certainly does not constitute a debilitating situation in this population as it might in the adult population. However, one has to consider not only the frequency of the seizures but the effect that the seizures are having on the individual's neurologic development and emotional stability when determining if, in fact, seizures are debilitating. 2) Intractability. It is generally unwise to consider a candidate for seizure surgery whose seizures can be controlled with anti-epileptic drugs. In some cases, modification of diets, including the use of the Ketogenic Diet with or without the use of anti-epileptic drugs, can effectively reduce or eliminate the seizure activity.

3) Good localization of seizure focus. Except in the case of corpus callosotomy and vagal nerve stimulation, surgical intervention for intractable seizures should be predicated on excellent localization of the

TABLE 21.1
Indications for Seizure Sugery (Resections)

- Debilitating seizure
- Intractability
- Good localization of focus
- Little risk of postoperative deficits
- Good understanding and strong desire (patient and/or family)

seizure focus. It is necessary for the epileptologist to go to whatever lengths are necessary to identify the seizure focus prior to recommending surgical intervention. In many cases, external electroencephalographic data alone, in conjunction with the clinical evaluation, will provide adequate localization for surgery, although this is less commonly the case now that we have the ability to be so precise as to eliminate most guesswork. 4) There must be little risk of postoperative neurologic deficits. Obviously the benefit-to-risk ratio of seizure surgery must be heavily shifted in the patient's favor in terms of safety and subsequent quality of life. 5) The patient and/or family must have an excellent understanding of the benefits and risks of surgery as well as a very strong desire to proceed with surgical intervention. It is wise not only for the epileptologist but for the surgeon to go over the benefits and risks as well as complete rationale on multiple occasions with the patient and family prior to embarking upon any of the procedures in question. Unless there is a very strong desire on behalf of the patient and/or family to proceed with surgical intervention, the small percentage of cases in which there are short-term or long-term complications can become particularly trying for the practitioners involved.

In addition to meeting the aforementioned criteria, it is important for the medical team to understand that certain childhood seizure disorders can remit spontaneously, and the epileptologist must exclude such conditions before embarking on the surgical pathway (5).

Most pediatric seizure surgery is directed at simple partial seizures and complex partial seizures, although all types of intractable seizures can be considered (13). Many mitigating factors determine the timing of the surgery once a positive workup has been completed. The patient must be in good medical condition with the ability to withstand a prolonged period of monitoring with external or internal electrodes and have the ability to withstand potential surgical complications. The social situation of the patient must be taken into consideration. A strong social support network is not only desirable but essential to the evaluation and therapeutic success. Also, the experience and capacity of the medical teams involved in seizure surgery play an important role in determining what therapies should be offered and when referral to another medical center is indicated.

IMAGING AIDES

The success of seizure surgery has been greatly enhanced by a host of neuroimaging techniques including standard MRI, three-dimensional MRI, fluid attenuation inversion recovery (FLAIR) (*Fig. 21.1*), MR spectroscopy, CT scanning, MR angiography, angiography (WADA), and functional scans including PET, SPECT, and MRI (6, 19, 24, 34).

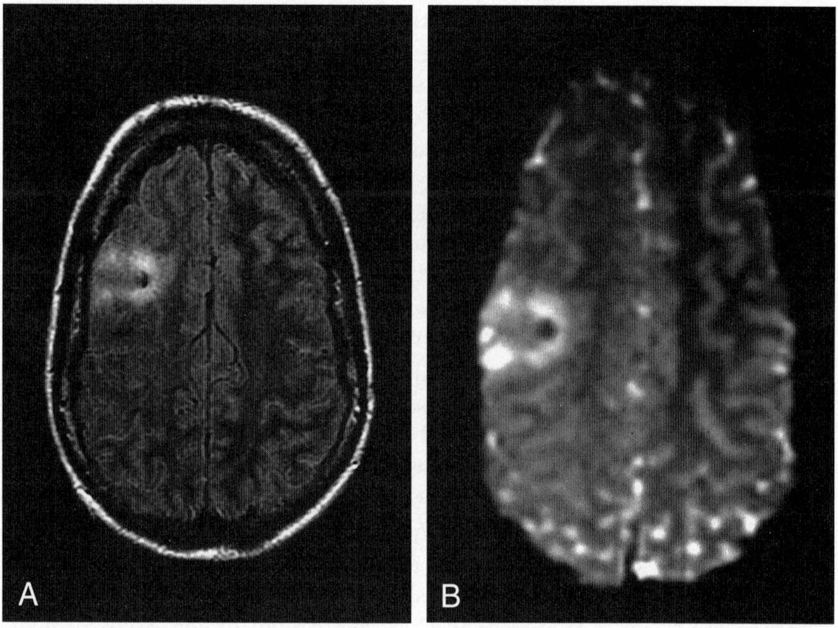

FIG. 21.1 Comparison of an epileptogenic lesional focus in a 15-year-old male with tuberous sclerosis using standard T2-weighted MR imaging (*A*) versus FLAIR (fluid attenuation inversion recovery) (*B*). Frontal lobectomy resulted in complete cessation of seizure activity.

These imaging techniques, when combined with careful history and physical exam and electrophysiologic data, provide a degree of accuracy that is astonishing compared to what was available just two decades ago. As these modalities continue to evolve, it is likely that surgical successes will become even more spectacular.

WHEN ARE GRID ELECTRODES NECESSARY?

Grid electrodes can be placed either epidurally or subdurally; however, the use of epidural grids is becoming less common because one can only retrieve data passively and does not have the ability to accurately stimulate the cortical surface. One should consider the use of subdural grids when results from external electrophysiologic monitoring are equivocal or inconsistent (1, 38). Sometimes, clinical and electrophysiologic or radiographic data do not all point to the same etiologic seizure focus, and in such cases, grid implants should be considered. Another indication would be when the resection area is in very close proximity to eloquent cerebral tissue, and extreme accuracy of resection is required to lessen the chances of negative neurologic sequelae. Questions involving the existence of a mirror or reflective seizure focus can frequently be answered by placing grids over the area of primary suspicion along with a few strip electrodes in appropriate locations on the opposite side (*Fig. 21.2*). It is easy to place a few strip electrodes on the opposite side or even inter-hemispherically when there is a significant index of suspicion for remote epileptic foci. It is much better to acquire all of the information during the first attempt, as reoperation for grid placement is not only difficult but quite unpleasant due to subdural scarring.

Depth electrodes can be very useful for mesial temporal seizure foci of unclear etiology with respect to side of origin in the adult population, but these are rarely useful in children. Fortunately, with the proper selection of grids and strips, mesial temporal monitoring can usually be accomplished without resorting to depth electrodes or sphenoidal electrodes.

CEREBRAL HEMISPHERECTOMY

Cerebral hemispherectomy refers to surgery in which all or large amounts of the cerebral tissue of one hemisphere are removed inclusive

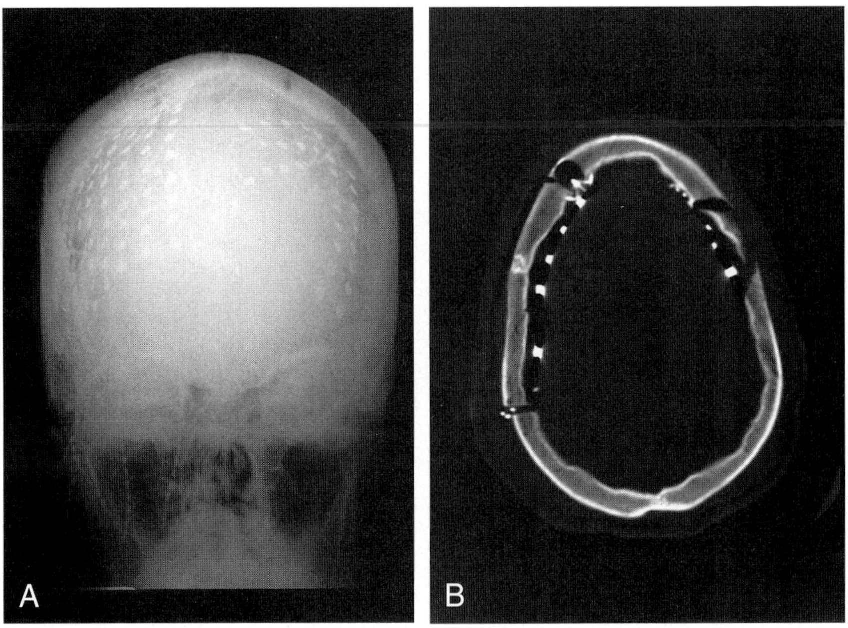

FIG. 21.2 (*A*) Plain skull x-ray demonstrating bilateral subdural grid electrode placement. (*B*) Bone window axial CT scan on the same patient.

TABLE 21.2
Posthemispherectomy Seizute Control

	Rasmussen's	Developmental
	%	
None/no drugs	55	25
None/drugs	18	10
Fewer	27	60
Same	0	5

of the motor and sensory cortex. It was first attempted by Walter Dandy in an effort to control a malignant glioma and has encountered varying degrees of enthusiasm and abhorrence in the neurosurgical community since that time (8). The term can include formal hemispherectomy, which includes resection of everything from the lateral ventricle outward, to hemi-decortication or hemi-corticectomy, in which the gray matter is removed and white matter is left over the ventricular surface as well as the basal ganglia and thalamic structures. Functional hemispherectomy can be done in a variety of ways, but essentially portions of the brain are left behind as a buttress, including frontal lobe and occipital lobe, which have been disconnected while the temporal lobe and central cortical core have been removed (23). Undoubtedly, further modifications will become popular in the near future as the number of centers performing various types of hemispherectomies continues to increase.

Between 1975 and 1994, 52 hemispherectomies were done at Johns Hopkins (7). The vast majority (greater than 90%) were done between 1985 and 1994. Thirty-one additional hemispherectomies have been done up until June, 1999. More than 90% of the patients who underwent hemispherectomy are seizure free or experienced a significant reduction in seizures (*Table 21.2*), whereas 44% of this group were in age-appropriate educational environments or able to work independently (*Table 21.3*). Eighteen patients were semi-independent and nine were dependent. The two most common groups of patients, undergoing cerebral hemispherectomy, were those with Rasmussen's encephalitis and

TABLE 21.3
Functional Outcome (H)

	Rasmussen's	Developmental
	%	
Dependent	9	30
Semi-dependent	23	50
Independent	68	20

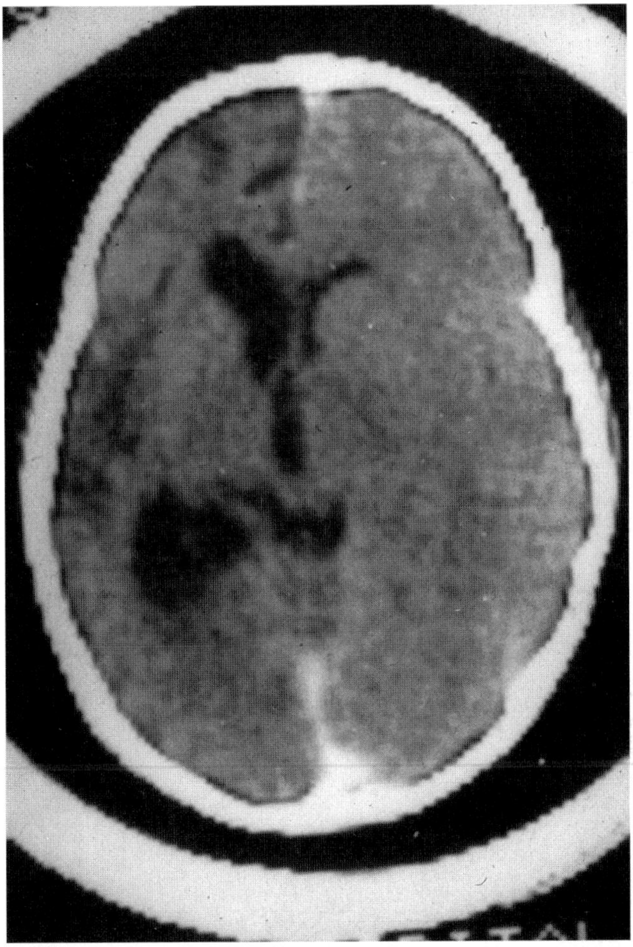

FIG. 21.3 Axial CT scan of a child with Rasmussen's encephalitis demonstrating hemicerebral atrophy, which is seen in advanced stages of the disease.

those with developmental disorders. Rasmussen's encephalitis is a nonspecific encephalitity characterized by progressively worsening seizures, hemiparesis, hemicerebral atrophy (*Fig. 21.3*), and a histologic picture consistent with viral encephalitis. Recent studies suggest that Rasmussen's encephalitis is actually a type of autoimmune phenomenon (4). Some potentially promising medical therapies take advantage of this newly found knowledge (3).

Developmental disorders of the brain in the hemispherectomy patients refer to conditions involving neuroglial disorganization and aberrant migration. One of the more common such conditions is hemimegalencephaly (*Fig. 21.4*).

In our original series of 52 hemispherectomy patients, 30 were right-sided and 22 were left-sided. The side of disease was not an important factor in determining which patients were good candidates for cerebral hemispherectomy. The patients with Rasmussen's encephalitis had an average age of 9.9 years at the time of surgery, whereas those with developmental disorders had an average age of 3.1 years at the time of

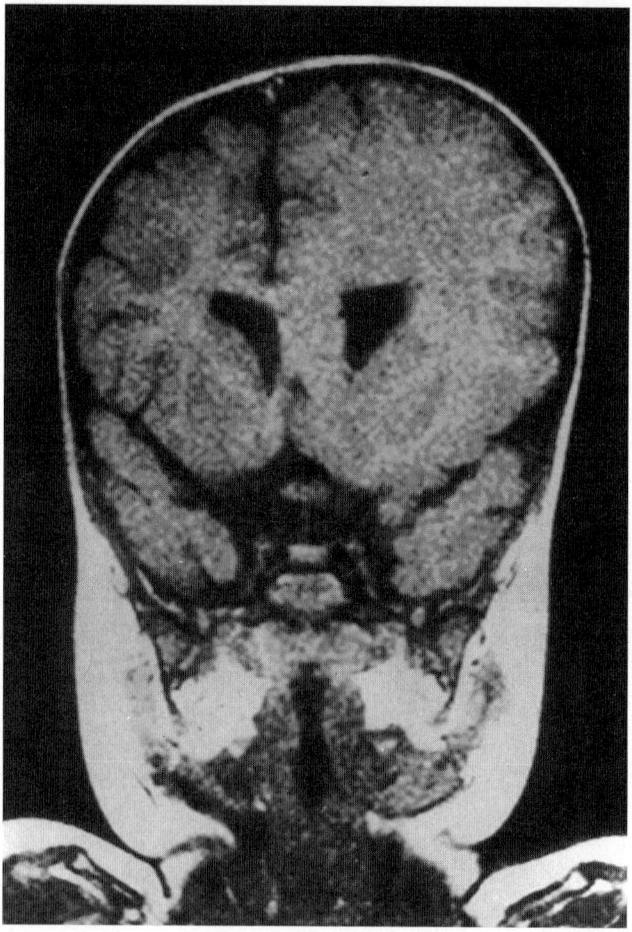

FIG. 21.4 Coronal MRI image of a child with hemimegalencephaly who subsequently successfully underwent cerebral hemispherectomy.

surgery. This is not surprising because we now feel that Rasmussen's encephalitis is an acquired disease process, whereas the developmental conditions are congenital in nature. Furthermore, it took less time (2.5 years) for the patients with developmental disorders to be brought to a surgical solution than it did for the patients with Rasmussen's encephalitis (3.9 years). A significant number of patients who underwent hemispherectomy had *had* previous focal resections exclusive of diagnostic biopsies. In some of those cases, the seizure activity declined transiently but almost always inexorably marched toward a state of intractability (7).

Initially, we preferred to do formal hemispherectomies, removing all four lobes of the brain en bloc. To do this, the brain had to be manipulated substantially, and it was later concluded that piecemeal dissections with a lobe by lobe approach would be more efficacious and less traumatic to the brainstem and remaining half of the brain. One appealing aspect of the en block resection was the relative paucity of blood loss since prior to significant dissection, the anterior, middle, and posterior cerebral arteries were clipped. After noting several cases in which the anterior cerebral arteries crossed each other on the corpus callosum, it was decided to abandon ligation of this artery to avoid the potential complication of compromising the other hemisphere. With the hemidecortication approach, we found that it was eminently possible to control most of the blood loss by creating a deep trough around the Silvian fissure and clipping or bipolaring and cutting all of the exiting branches of the middle cerebral artery. The sequence of lobe by lobe dissection is: temporal lobe, frontal lobe, parietal-temporal lobe, and occipital lobe. Once the parafalcine tissue is disconnected, it can be removed or left behind if the size and complexity of the draining parasaggital veins prove problematic (9).

Although we have experienced no deaths with hemispherectomy for several years, it should be noted that the early deaths that were experienced occurred at a time before we routinely used pediatric anesthe-

TABLE 21.4
Long-Term Posthemispherectomy Seizure Control

	Rasmussen's (12)	Developmental (10)
	%	
None/no drugs	58	40
None/drugs	8	30
Fewer	33	30
Same	0	0

TABLE 21.5
Long-Term Posthemispherectomy Functional Status

	Rasmussen's (12)	Developmental (10)
	%	
Dependent	8	20
Semi-dependent	33	50
Independent	58	30

siologists for all of our pediatric neurosurgery cases. The early deaths seem to be related to hypothermia and volume replacement issues.

Data for post-hemispherectomy seizure control and functional outcome indicate that hemispherectomy, in the appropriately selected patients, is dramatically successful both in the short-term and long-term (*Tables 21.4 and 21.5*). Although early hemispherectomy series reported high late complication rates (as high as 35 to 40%) (36, 37), we fortunately have not witnessed this. Perioperative complications have included infection, most of which were aseptic meningitis as well as hydrocephalus, most of which occurred early on before we adopted a practice of vigorous irrigation of all debris prior to closing. Other complications included bone loss, hemorrhage, and shifting of the midline (*Table 21.6*). Most patients are hospitalized for considerably less than 2 weeks before moving on to a rehabilitation setting, and in preadolescent hemispherectomy patients, the only functions that absolutely will not recover are vision (homonomous hemianopsia) and fine motor control.

We include a preliminary breakdown of the seizure status and functional status of 24 hemispherectomy patients that were done from 1995 to 1998 after our initially reported series. The findings are consistent with the previous data (*Table 21.7*).

LOBECTOMIES AND CORTICAL RESECTIONS

In the adult population, temporal lobectomy is the most common type of successful seizure surgery when the foci have been well localized. Ex-

TABLE 21.6
Perioperative Complications (H)

Infection	19% (aseptic meningitis included)
Hydroceopalus	33% (5% over last 5 years)
Bone loss	4%
Hemorrhage	20% (1 patient required surgery)
Shift	15%

TABLE 21.7
Hemispherectomy Review, 1995–1998: 24 Cases

		Seizure Status			Functional Status		
Age Group (years)	No.	*No Sz*	*No Sz/ Meds*	*Sz/Meds*	*Independ.*	*Semi-Depend.*	*Dependent*
0–2	3		3			2	1
3–5	8	7	1		6	2	
7–11	8	6	2		6	1	1
12–17	5	2	2	1	2	2	1

tratemporal epilepsy, however, is more common in infants and preadolescent children (12). Successful surgical outcomes with extratemporal resections in children are less frequent than with temporal lobectomy (18). Generally speaking, one can expect seizure remission (or near remission) rates of 60 to 80% after temporal lobectomy for temporal lobectomy epilepsy (TLE), whereas extratemporal resection remission rates run in the 60 to 70% range (11). The data acquired from the group of lobectomy patients from 1994 to 1998 at Johns Hopkins, in terms of seizure status and functional status, are presented in *Table 21.8.*

It should be noted that several recent reports of improved neuroimaging techniques have in many cases obviated the necessary for invasive neurophysiologic studies in TLE patients (28). It will be necessary to carefully analyze the data over the next several years regarding outcome of patients who have undergone temporal lobe resections based on clinical findings, EEG, and neuro-imaging versus patients who have undergone similar resections only after invasive monitoring. With or without invasive monitoring, in the hands of experienced clinicians and technically proficient surgeons, success rates, in terms of seizure freedom and excellent function, are high.

It is relatively rare to carry out parietal or occipital lobectomies in the pediatric population except as part of the cerebral hemispherectomy.

TABLE 21.8
Lobectomy Review, 1994–1998: 17 Cases

		Seizure Status			Functional Status		
Age Group (years)	No.	*No Sz*	*No Sz/ Meds*	*Sz/Meds*	*Independ.*	*Semi-Depend.*	*Dependent*
0–2	1	1			1		
3–5	1		1		1		
7–11	3	1	2		2	1	
12–22	12	1	11		9	3	

The vast majority of lobectomies carried out would be temporal lobectomies followed by frontal lobectomies. Cortical resections are frequently done rather than frontal lobectomies, but a simple cortical resection in the temporal lobe area is rare.

Before embarking upon temporal lobectomy, it is important to obtain a full history and physical examination of the patient and derive data from several standard electroencephalograms. In the pediatric population, video EEG monitoring has become very standard and provides necessary clinical and electrophysiologic correlation (27). In cases where seizure activity is rare but still enormously interfering and interictal data are not definitive, ambulatory EEG can be performed. This is similar to the Holter monitor used in cardiac patients. In addition to the aforementioned things, it is important to search for structural lesions that are not uncommon in the pediatric population with intractable seizures, and it is important to optimize medical therapy including looking at dietary options. Cognitive and psychiatric evaluations should be carried out, particularly given the large number of patients with temporal lobe epilepsy with aberrant neuropsychological manifestations (32). One should consider whether grids or depth electrodes are necessary, particularly in making the determination of medial primary seizure foci and hemispheric dominance.

CORPUS CALLOSOTOMY

Corpus Callosotomy (CC) is generally reserved for patients with life-altering generalized epilepsy of several kinds. Mental deficiencies are frequently noticed in this group of patients (16, 33). CC was developed as a pediatric procedure to treat lateralized seizures, and the most dramatic effects are seen in children with drop attacks (atonic seizures) (15, 29, 31). By interrupting the primary connection between the two hemispheres, the theory is that the electrical disturbance will remain in the hemisphere of initiation and not manifest itself in a generalized fashion, as it might if it were able to spread to the other side. *Table 21.9* depicts the type of seizure disorders that respond to corpus callosotomy.

Younger children who have undergone CC appear not to have as

TABLE 21.9
Seizure Types Responsive to Corpus Callostomy

- Myoclonic (atonic) [Lennox-Gastaut]
- Generalized tonic-clonic (secondary)
- Tonic
- Simple and complex partial seizures (less effective)

much of a problem with visual-tactile tasks as adolescents and adults (25). It is probable that plasticity plays a significant role in children who have undergone CC, accounting for this disparity (26).

The EEG in candidates for corpus callosotomy is frequently highly disorganized bilaterally, and the postoperative EEG data are not as impressive as that seen with other types of seizure surgery. However, it is not uncommon to see neuropsychological testing scores improve significantly after corpus callosotomy in children (2, 17). Although mental function has been included by some as a factor in determining which patients are good candidates for CC, it is not clear that mental function plays any significant predictive role when selecting patients for this procedure. We have performed three corpus callosotomies recently in patients with myoclonic seizures. In each case, seizures were reduced (more dramatically initially) but not eliminated. Although CC is a useful neurosurgical procedure in selected patients, medical advances and refinements in ablative techniques will hopefully one day eliminate its need as part of the neurosurgical armamentarium for intractable seizure disorders.

CONCLUSION

Intractable epilepsy in children is devastating both physically and emotionally for the patient and the family. The number of promising techniques for favorably altering or even eliminating the condition continues to be encouraging. The success rates for cerebral hemispherectomy and cortical resections and lobectomies are high in patients treated at epilepsy centers, and the complication rates are low. Given the successes of these techniques and the relatively small number of eligible candidates who benefit from these techniques, it is important to widely disseminate knowledge about the efficacy of epilepsy surgery in children while continuing to work to improve the lifestyles of this important group of patients.

REFERENCES

1. Adelson PD, Black PM, Madsen JR, et al: Use of subdural grids and strip electrodes to identify a seizure focus in children. **Pediatr Neurosurg** 22:174–180, 1995.
2. Amacher AL: Midline commissurotomy for the treatment of some cases of intractable epilepsy. **Childs Brain** 2:54–58, 1946.
3. Andrews PI, Dichter MA, Berkovic SF: Plasmapheresis in Rasmussen's encephalitis. **Neurology** 46:242–246, 1996.
4. Antozzi C, Graata T, Aurisano N, et al: Long-term selective IgG immuno-adsorption improves Rasmussen's encephalitis. **Neurology** 51:302–305, 1998.
5. Benbadis SR, Wyllie E: Evaluation of intractable seizures in children, in Albright L, Pollack I, Adelson D (eds): *Principles and Practice of Pediatric Neurosurgery,* 2nd Ed. New York, Thieme Medical Publishers, Inc., 1999.

6. Bergin PS, Fish DR, Shorvon SD, et al: Magnetic resonance imaging in partial epilepsy: Additional abnormalities shown with the fluid attenuated inversion recovery (FLAIR) pulse sequence. **J Neuro Neurosurg Psychiatry** 58:439–443, 1995.
7. Carson BS, Javedan SP, Freeman JM, Vining EPG, Zuckerberg AL, Lauer JA, Guarnieri M: Hemispherectomy: A hemidecortication approach and review of 52 cases from 1975–1994. **J Neurosurgery 84:903–911, 1996.**
8. Carson BS, Lauer JA, Guarnieri M: Hemispherectomy: A review. **Neurosurg Q** 6:155–175, 1996.
9. Carson BS, Zuckerberg AL: Hemispherectomy, in *Neurosurgical Operative Color Atlas.* Lebanon, American Association Neurological Surgeons, 1997.
10. Cowan LD, Bodensteiner JB, Leviton A, et al: Prevalence of the epilepsies in children and adolescents. **Epilepsia** 30:94–106, 1989.
11. Davidson S, Falconer MA: Outcome of surgery in 40 children with temporal-lobe epilepsy. **Lancet** 1:1260–1263, 1975.
12. Duchowny M: Epilepsy surgery in children. **Curr Opin Neurol** 8:112–116, 1995.
13. Duchowny MS: Pediatric epilepsy surgery: Special considerations, in Wyler AR, Hermann BP (eds): *The Surgical Management of Epilepsy.* Stoneham, Butterworth-Heinemann, 1994.
14. Dwyer BE, Wasterlain CG: Electroconvulsive seizures selectively impair myelin accumulation in the immature rat. **Exp Neurol** 78:616–628, 1982.
15. Fuiks KS, Wyler AR, Hermann BP, et al: Seizure outcome from anterior and complete corpus callosotomy. **J Neurosurg** 74:573–578, 1991.
16. Gates JR, Ritter FJ, Ragazzo PC, Reeves AG: Corpus callosum section in children: Seizure response, in Dychowny M, Resnick TJ, Alvarez LA (eds): *Pediatric Epilepsy Surgery.* New York, Demos, 1990.
17. Gates JR, Rosenfeld WE, Maxwell RE, Lyons RE: Response of multiple seizure types to corpus callosum section. **Epilepsia** 28:28–34, 1987.
18. Goldring S: Surgical management of epilepsy in children, in Engle J Jr (ed): *Surgical Treatment of the Epilepsies.* New York, Raven Press, 1987.
19. Graveline CJ, Mikulis DJ, Crawley AP, Hwang PA: Regionalized sensorimotor plasticity after hemispherectomy fMRI evaluation. **Pediatr Neurol** 19:337–342, 1998.
20. Hauser WA, Kurland LT: The epidemiology of epilepsy in Rochester, Minnesota. **Epilepsia** 16:1–66, 1975.
21. Holmes GL: Effect of serial seizures on subsequent kindling in the immature brain. **Dev Brain Res** 6:190–192, 1983.
22. Jorgensen OS, Dwyer BE, Wasterlain CG: Synaptic proteins after electroconvulsive seizures in immature rats. **J Neurochem** 35:123–137, 1980.
23. Kanev PM, Foley CM, Miles D: Ultrasound-tailored functional hemispherectomy for surgical control of seizures in children. **J Neurosurg** 86:762–767, 1997.
24. Kuzniecky R, Burgard S, Faught E, et al: Predictive value of MRI in temporal lobe epilepsy surgery. **Arch Neurol** 50:65–69, 1993.
25. Lassonde M, Sauerwein H, Geoffroy G, Decarie M: Effects of early and late transection of the corpus callosum in children: A study of tactile and tactuomotor transfer and integration. **Brain** 109:953–967, 1986.
26. Lassonde M, Sauerwein H, Geoffroy G, Decarie M: Long-term neuropsychological effects of corpus callosotomy in children, in Duchowny M, Resnick TJ, Alvarez LA (eds): *Pediatric Epilepsy Surgery.* New York, Demos, 1990.
27. Marks DA, Katz A, Scheyer R, et al: Clinical and electrographic effects of acute anticonvulsant withdrawal in epileptic patients. **Neurology** 41:508–512, 1991.
28. Meiners LC, Valk J, Jansen GH, van Veelen CW: MR contribution in surgery of epilepsy. **Eur Radiol** 9:493–507, 1999.

29. Oguni H, Olivier A, Andermann F, et al: Anterior callosotomy in the treatment of medically intractable epilepsies: A study of 43 patients with a mean follow-up of 39 months. **Ann Neurol** 30:357–364, 1991.
30. Olney JW, Collins RC, Sloviter RS: Excitotoxic mechanisms of epileptic brain damage, in Delgado-Escueta AV (ed): *Advances in Neurology,* Vol. 44. New York, Raven Press, 1986.
31. Reutons DC, Bye AM, Hopkins IJ, et al: Corpus callosotomy for intractable epilepsy: Seizure outcome and prognostic factors. **Epilepsia** 34:904–909, 1993.
32. Rutter M, Graham P, Yule W: A neuropsychiatric study in childhood, in: *Clinics in Developmental Medicine 35/36.* London, Spastics International Medical Publications, 1970.
33. Spencer DS, Spencer SS: Corpus callosotomy in the treatment of medically intractable secondarily generalized seizures of children. **Cleve Clin J Med** 56 (Suppl. Part 1):S69–S78, 1989.
34. Spencer S: The relative contributions of MRI, SPECT, PET imaging in epilepsy. **Epilepsia** 35 (Suppl. 6):S72–S89, 1994.
35. Wasterlain CF: Effect of epileptic seizures on brain ribosomes: Mechanisms and relationship to cerebral energy metabolism. **J Neurochem** 29:707–716, 1977.
36. White HH: Cerebral hemispherectomy in the treatment of infantile hemiplegia: Review of the literature and report of two cases. **Confin Neurol** 21:1–50, 1961.
37. Wilson PJE: Cerebral hemispherectomy for infantile hemiplegia: A report of 50 cases. **Brain** 93:147–180, 1970.
38. Wyllie E, Lüders H, Morris HH, et al: Subdural electrodes in the evaluation for epilepsy surgery in children and adults. **Neuropediatrics** 19:80–86, 1988.

CHAPTER

22

Epilepsy Surgery in Children

MOISE DANIELPOUR, M.D., WARWICK J. PEACOCK, M.D.

In 1886, Victor Horsley proved that epilepsy could be cured in some adults by resection of a seizure focus from the brain (52). In 1950, Krynauw reported success with treatment of childhood onset epilepsy. He performed cerebral hemispherectomy in 12 patients with infantile hemiplegic seizures (61). However, despite excellent results, treatment of childhood epilepsy continued to lag behind that of adults. Because of a fear of operating on the immature brain and the hope that the seizures might resolve spontaneously, epilepsy surgery was virtually restricted to temporal lobe epilepsy in adults. The fear of resective surgery in children with intractable epilepsy was further complicated by the fact that surgical protocols developed for treating adult epilepsy did not apply to children (105).

During the past two decades, there has been a renewed interest in surgical treatment of epilepsy in childhood (86). In younger patients, many seizure types appear to be suitable for resective surgery. Furthermore, a growing body of evidence suggests that seizures may have a deleterious effect on the developing brain and result in spectrum of developmental disorders that range from debilitating behavioral problems to mental retardation. Finally, the potential for functional recovery is greatest in the young child. It is wise to operate as soon as the seizures have proved refractory to appropriate anticonvulsant agents. Early curative surgery eliminates the adverse effects of seizures on the maturing brain and takes advantage of the plasticity of the immature brain (107).

To better understand the surgical treatment of epilepsy in children, it is helpful to summarize the basic concepts of brain development and plasticity, and to review the effects of intractable seizures on the child's brain. Taking into account both the knowledge of specific childhood seizure types and the advent of brain plasticity, we will review the protocols formulated for childhood epilepsy and appropriate choices of surgical procedures.

BRAIN DEVELOPMENT AND MATURATION

Central to the renaissance in the treatment of childhood epilepsy is the recognition that the dynamic development and plasticity of the young brain justified departure from the traditional dogmas and approaches to adult epilepsy surgery (85). Neuronal modification and neuroglial proliferation are the processes by which a child's brain undergoes maturation. The key to understanding the pathophysiology of brain plasticity is the time-dependent maturation of neuronal networks.

Dendrites undergo extensive branching and axonal growth cones migrate to their appropriate synaptic sites to create an intricate neuronal network during the first decade of life (89). This flurry of activity produces a peak in synaptic density in the brain at about eight years of age (89). There appears to be a period of synaptic and neuronal excess following which synaptic regression and selective cell death refines the nervous system. This reduction in synaptic density plateaus at about the age of 14 (8–10, 53, 90, 118). Neuronal plasticity is the capacity of the immature brain to modify existing pathways through axonal migration, dendritic proliferation, and cell death depending on surrounding electrical fields and other appropriate environmental stimuli (56).

The degree of plasticity seems to be age dependent. Experiments in hemispherectomized cats have demonstrated that the degree of functional recovery corresponds inversely with age at the time of operation. Villablanca et al. performed left-sided hemispherectomies on neonatal cats 5 to 15 days of age, and on adult cats. Late postoperative comparison revealed full recovery of motor and visual field deficits in the kittens but not the adult cats. Anatomical studies showed dramatic reorganization of cortical and subcortical projections in the kittens but not in their adult counterparts (118). Similar clinically recognized patterns of functional recovery probably occur in humans who have undergone hemispherectomy.

IMPACT OF SEIZURES ON THE DEVELOPING BRAIN

Substantial evidence suggests that frequent seizures interfere with the maturation of the brain. Collins et al. showed that seizures can induce secondary pathological changes in animals' brain. By exposing neurons to ictal activity, both locally and at a distance, they were able to demonstrate a combination of cortical axonal damage and subcortical dendritic changes. All of these changes resulted in extensive synaptic abnormalities (22).

Significant questions have been raised about the validity of extrapolation from animal epilepsy experiments to human disease. However, consistent with experimental data, histological examination of Golgi-Cox fixed brain blocks from autopsy or biopsy from patients with infantile spasm and dementia have shown decreases in dendritic length and reduced numbers of secondary and direct perikaryon branches (55).

These studies support the notion that seizure activity can adversely affect synaptogenesis and cerebral development in humans.

If repeated seizures do interfere with the establishment neuronal networks, the question arises as to the role of seizure type, duration, frequency, and interictal physiology in determining the extent of damage. For example, petit mal seizures can occur hundreds of times per day without evidence of developmental impairment, but comparable numbers of focal motor seizures can lead to focal abnormalities in the absence of underlying progressive disease (42, 60, 105).

Postictal depression and interictal spiking may also impair neuronal development. Release of endogenous opiods, coupled with possible depletion of neurotransmitters and neuronal exhaustion after an ictal episode, lead to a prolonged period of depressed activity (34, 35). Numerous depressions may, in turn, severely alter synaptogenesis and remodeling. Because of their considerable summated duration and presence of inhibitory postsynaptic potentials, frequent interictal epileptiform discharges can have a more deleterious effect on growth and development of neuronal networks than both ictal and postictal states combine (15, 23, 33, 45, 87–89, 98, 103, 104)

Shewmon and Erwin extended these findings to human patients. They demonstrated that a child shown visual stimuli at times corresponding to interictal spike wave discharges in the posterior temporal region failed to perceive more than 30% of the stimuli (104). Therefore, it is reasonable to infer that personality disorders associated with childhood temporal lobe epilepsy and the gradual decline of intellectual and psychosocial skills experienced by children with uncontrolled epilepsy might be accounted for by the frequent interictal discharges in the limbic system (13, 18, 50, 57, 58, 87, 88, 94, 96, 113–115). Resection of nociferous cortex often leads to resolution or partial elimination of behavioral disturbances.

Although the controversy continues over the impact of seizures on cerebral development, a large body of evidence suggest an adverse effect. It is, therefore, incumbent on the pediatric neurologist and neurosurgeon to evaluate medical intractability relatively quickly. By evaluating these children with intractable epilepsy as early as possible, one can minimize the potential damage during critical periods of brain development and maximize functional recovery that results from brain plasticity.

CHILDHOOD SEIZURE DISORDERS

According to the International Classification of Epileptic Seizures, seizures can be classified as either partial or generalized. The evaluation of children with partial onset seizures requires investigation of lateralization and localization of the area of seizure onset. It must then be determined whether resection of this area is possible without inflicting a new deficit or aggravating an old one. Some children with generalized seizures have also been helped by surgery (85). For instance, in patients with drop attacks caused by secondary bilateral synchrony, corpuscallostomy has been shown to interrupt the spread of epileptiform discharges from one hemisphere to the other. Furthermore, in selected patients with infantile spasms who are demonstrated to have a localized area of cortical abnormality, such as cortical dysplasia, resection of the area has been shown to eliminate seizures (12, 72, 82)

PARTIAL SEIZURES ASSOCIATED WITH HEMIPARESIS

Sturge-Weber Syndrome

Sturge-Weber syndrome is characterized by a small-vessel angiomatous malformation which involves the leptomeninges with or without a facial nevus. The disease process involves a single hemisphere and the ipsilateral face in the distribution of the first and second divisions of the trigeminal nerve. The underlying cerebral abnormalities include progressive cortical injury and calcification (111). Seizures usually develop within the first year of life. With the onset of uncontrollable seizures, patients may develop a progressive hemiparesis and hemianopsia, and become mentally retarded. If the seizures are medically intractable, surgery is recommended as early as possible to ensure minimal interference with development and maximal recovery (3, 4) Patients with a localized posterior lesion may require only a limited resection of the occipital and parietal lobes. Those with more diffuse hemispheric involvement accompanied by a hemiparesis are candidates for hemispherectomy.

Rasmussen's Encephalitis

In 1958, Rasmussen et al. initially described and performed a hemispherectomy for this syndrome (93). Patients typically present between four to nine years of age with the onset of infrequent partial seizures. Seizure frequency increases to the point of epilepsia partialis continua plus progressive hemiplegia and mental retardation (92). Magnetic resonance imaging (MRI) reveals increased signal intensity of the affected hemisphere, followed shortly thereafter by hemispheric atrophy. Pathological findings suggestive of encephalitis include perivascular lymphocytic cuffing. Since the inflammatory condition almost always spreads to the entire hemisphere, limited focal resection is not recommended. Instead, it is prudent to reserve resective surgery until there is a loss of digital dexterity in the affected hand.

Infantile Hemiplegic Epilepsy

This form of infantile hemiplegic epilepsy incorporates a number of disorders, all of which may lead to intractable partial seizures and hemiparesis. Most of the known underlying causes are congenital and include neuronal migrational defects, such as cortical dysplasia or hemimegalencephaly, and destructive lesions, such as congenital porencephaly or perinatal/postnatal cerebrovascular accidents (84). Seizures usually begin within the first few months of life, and the hemiparesis is noticed between the ages of three to six months. Many of these children will progress to intractable seizures and mental retardation. Imaging and examination of the surgical specimen often show infarction in the middle cerebral artery territory. Regardless of the cause, the neurosurgical treatment is hemispherectomy.

Complex Partial Epilepsy not Associated with Hemiparesis

Complex partial seizures of temporal lobe origin are the most common disorder in this category. They are not associated with hemiparesis and rarely result in severe mental retardation. However, the postulated adverse effects on development, accompanying psychosocial problems, and the effects of anticonvulsant medications can all be as equally debilitating. The best opportunity for surgical control of seizures and prevention of psychological and developmental handicaps is prior to puberty. Whereas in adults with poorly controlled epilepsy there is little urgency to operate, in young children with intractable seizures, surgery should be performed as early as possible to promote cerebral maturation and to take advantage of the available plasticity.

GENERALIZED OR SECONDARILY GENERALIZED SEIZURES

Infantile Spasms

Infantile spasm, also known as West's syndrome, is a characteristic triad of myoclonic seizures, a hypsarrhythmic pattern of electroencephalography (EEG), and, ultimately, profound mental retardation. The seizures are characterized by sudden flexion or extension of the extremities or trunk. They have been described clinically as salaam seizures, jackknife seizures, flexor or extensor spasms, and Blitskrampf–lightning attacks (38). Although seizure onset is usually between four to eight months of age, seizures can begin as late as 24 months. Some children respond to adrenocorticotropic hormone (ACTH) therapy. For others, the prognosis is extremely poor. In patients with poor medical control, workup should include a MRI, positron emission tomography (PET), and somatosensory evoked potentials (SSEP) to look for a zone of cortical abnormality. Surgical resection can be considered if an epileptogenic focus is localized.

Lennox-Gastaux Syndrome

Lennox-Gastaux Syndrome is a severe epileptic disorder of childhood identified by a range of intractable seizure types, mental retardation, and a slow spike and wave EEG pattern. In the past, children with Lennox-Gastaux and infantile spasms were not considered for surgical treatment because an isolated epileptogenic region could not be identified. Corpuscallosotomy had occasionally been performed as a palliative procedure. In some cases, PET has clearly demonstrated a localized area of interictal hypometabolism suggestive of a cortical abnormality, which has been supported by intraoperative electrocorticography (EcoG). Histopathological examination of surgical specimens have revealed the presence of structural abnormalities, such as cortical dysplasia or cystic gliosis.

SELECTION CRITERIA FOR PEDIATRIC EPILEPSY

The surgical approach to pediatric onset epilepsy was traditionally based on principles developed for treatment of adults. Despite most cases of epilepsy that begin in childhood, selection criteria for adult patients were applied unmodified to children. There has been a dramatic evolution in the treatment of epilepsy in children, with a departure from the treatment protocols of epilepsy in adults.

Since the maturing brain is adversely affected by frequent seizures and since it retains the capacity to recover from resective surgery, approaches for the surgical management of epilepsy in children are of necessity different from those used for adults. A number of principles used in evaluating adults with intractable epilepsy must be modified when evaluating children. Shewmon et al. defined the most significant ways in which the dynamic development and plasticity of the young brain justifies departure from the approaches to adult epilepsy surgery (105).

The traditional definition of medical intractability implies a minimum seizure frequency and a lengthy evaluation period needed to establish lack of responsiveness to all available drugs. In adults, it has been accepted that establishing medical intractability may take several years. In an adult having one to two seizures a month, it may take a significant time period, often several years, to establish medical intractability. In a child in whom seizures tend to occur more frequently, with 50 to 60 seizures per day a possibility, intractability can be rapidly established. In the young, it is not necessary to establish resistance to all classes of antiepileptic drugs. Therefore, medical intractability can often be determined in children within a few months or even weeks. The range of antiepileptic drugs available for children with epilepsy is much smaller than for their adult counterparts. Furthermore, certain pediatric conditions, such as Sturge-Weber, Rasmussen's encephalitis, or congenital brain malformations (50, 92, 93, 95), rarely respond to antiepileptic medications for an extended period of time. If a child does not respond to two or three appropriate antiepileptic drugs, it is extremely unlikely that he will respond to any medical regimen (105).

The toxic affects of anticonvulsants must also be considered when dealing with pediatric patients as candidates for operative intervention. Antiepileptic drugs have been shown to interfere with normal cerebral maturation. When administered to newborn rats, phenobarbital and valpric acid were associated with significantly smaller brain weights when compared to a control group (40, 62). Comparable affects have been observed in human babies who were exposed to anticonvulsant medications in utero (41). The literature concerning the neuronal toxicity of phenytoin is inconsistent, but a number of studies and case reports do implicate a deleterious affect on cerebellum (25, 28, 68, 69).

Adults who develop side effects from anticonvulsant medications will complain or simply modify their dosage. Children, on the other hand, tend not to or are unable to complain, and their parents frequently accept the induced apathy or hyperactivity in exchange for improved seizure control.

When considering resective surgery in the very young child, there is no minimum age for surgical candidacy. Although spontaneous remission of seizures is common for complex partial seizures without an associated structural lesion, partial epilepsies with known structural lesions and not controlled with first- and second-line drugs are unlikely to remit as the child grows (6, 26, 31, 48, 59, 95). In fact, the younger the surgical candidate, the more urgent the need to proceed with surgery. By offering surgical resection at the earliest appropriate time, adverse affects of antiepileptic medications and epileptiform discharges on brain development and behavior can be minimized, while at the same time, taking maximal advantage of brain plasticity in promoting functional recovery.

Severe developmental delay is not always a contraindication to surgical treatment of epilepsy. Intractable focal or unilateral seizures that arise from a localized area of cortical abnormality can adversely affect the functioning of the other hemisphere. This may lead to a child with a focal abnormality that is functionally severely disabled. The "nociferous cortex" has been shown to produce cytoarchitectural changes and synaptic disorganization at distant sites (11). Because of the widespread affects of a focal epileptogenic abnormality, a child who is having frequent seizures may appear severely delayed; however, once the "nociferous cortex" has been removed and the seizures brought under control, developmental progress may be dramatic (10, 16, 49, 64, 109, 110).

Secondarily generalized epilepsies, such as West and Lennox-Gastaux syndromes, are usually equated with diffuse cerebral abnormality (29, 30, 70). In some cases, these syndromes are due to focal or unilateral brain pathology (5, 24, 32, 39, 72) and respond favorably to surgical therapy (83, 106, 108). In eight cases of medically intractable infantile spasms, Shewmon et al. showed marked improvement with cortical resection (108). Angelini et al. reported on a patient who had disappearance of Lennox-Gastaux syndrome and whose seizures resolved following resection of temporal lobe glioma (7). Thus, there are some children with what appear to be generalized seizure disorder who may benefit from surgical intervention.

Unlike adults, the production of a new or the aggravation of an existing deficit may be acceptable in a child. In a child with frequent seizures and thus at high risk for severe developmental delay, a postresective hemiparesis or hemianopsia is probably an acceptable price to pay for seizure control and improvement in intellectual development. Also, the induced motor deficits will usually improve significantly with time. In patients with Rasmussen's encephalitis or Sturge-Weber syndrome, the underlying disease eventually leads to the same deficit, and earlier surgery promotes greater functional recovery and developmental progress. Furthermore, when focal motor seizures are frequent enough, the child may be more disabled from them then from a static hemiparesis following resective surgery. It is important to keep in mind that each case requires an individualized judgment. Therefore, many factors must be kept in mind when a child is considered as a potential candidate for seizure surgery.

PRESURGICAL EVALUATION

History and Physical Exam

A careful history and physical exam is paramount in evaluating a child's candidacy for epilepsy surgery. The family history may suggest the risk of a genetically transmitted condition, such as tuberous sclerosis. Obtaining an accurate developmental history is crucial for evaluating the impact of epilepsy, as well as setting realistic postoperative goals. Medical intractability can be evaluated with a precise history of the seizures as well as the previous and present anticonvulsant regimens. The presence of long-standing stable hemiparesis makes a child a candidate for hemispherectomy and therefore, the duration and permanence of any neurological deficits should be determined. The parents must be questioned about the handedness of the child and whether a change in handedness occurred since the onset of seizures. Of course, it is important to note whether speech has been altered in any way in relation to the seizures.

The physical exam may reveal cutaneous stigmata, such as hypomelanotic macules of tuberous sclerosis, the café au lait spots of neurofibromatosis, or facial angioma associated with Sturge-Weber syndrome.

Structural Imaging

MRI and computed tomography (CT) may reveal structural lesions in some children with intractable epilepsy. Abnormalities include cortical dysplasia, as seen in agyria-pachygyria, polymicrogyria, and an area of heterotopic gray matter that is sometimes seen as a thickened cortex with blurring of the gray-white matter junction (85). Areas for resection may be identified by comparing structural imaging data with functional abnormalities defined by EEG, PET and EcoG. Serial imaging is also instructive for detecting abnormalities since many changes are time-dependent (102).

Electroencephalography with Video Telemetry

All patients should undergo continuous EEG with video telemetry to localize the site and frequency of seizures. Whereas the ictal spike waves are paramount in localization of seizure onset in adults, in children, identifying nonepileptiform abnormalities is often as helpful in the localization of a zone of cortical abnormality. Focal burst suppression pattern, amplitude attenuation across all leads, attenuation of beta activity (fast frequency), and polymorphic delta activity can all help localize a zone of cortical abnormality (105). Sodium thiopentone injection may be used to highlight areas for resection as it differentiates the impaired beta activation with the enhanced beta activity of the surrounding normal cortex.

Localization of epileptic excitability is derived from ictal and interictal EEG recordings (80). In children with catastrophic epilepsy, the ictal onsets are often difficult to localize and sometimes anatomically labile (17). However, the presence of epileptiform discharges outside the suspected zone of abnormality does not necessarily indicate multifocal or diffuse epileptogenicity. In fact, the presence of bilaterally independent, multifocal interictal epileptiform discharges in a young child does not necessarily indicate widespread epileptogenicity and is not in itself a contraindication to resective surgery. If a resectable unilateral focus is strongly suggested by convergence of other types of evidence, patients may still be excellent candidates for resective surgery guided by intraoperative EcoG. In patients who have undergone hemispherectomy, contralateral epileptiform activity often resolves (19, 50, 122).

Functional Imaging

PET of the brain is a noninvasive means of measuring local rates of cerebral glucose utilization and has proven to be of great value in the selection of patients for epilepsy surgery (80). The disturbances of cerebral glucose utilization shown by FDG-PET correlate with areas of cortical dysfunction as demonstrated by EcoG (80). Interictal studies have reliably demonstrated a region of hypometabolism that will correspond with the zone of cortical abnormality established intraoperatively by EcoG. These findings usually correlate well with histopathological findings (20, 80). PET can be used without any significant complications to demonstrate a lesion in cases in which the only pathology is cytoarchitectural disturbances without corresponding abnormalities on CT and MRI (21). A potentially resectable epileptogenic zone may be missed on MRI but clearly seen as a focal area of interictal hypometabolism on PET and its boundaries confirmed on EcoG. Prior to the advent of PET, many children would not have been considered good candidates for resective surgical procedures because their seizure type appeared generalized or because of the absence of a lesion on MRI or CT. PET scanning is of great value in the localization of dysfunctional cortex in these children with uncontrollable epilepsy (20, 80).

In addition, PET is useful in confirming the normal functional status of areas outside of the proposed resection site (36). Since spike waves can propagate along corticocortical connections, spike waves that arise outside the primary focus may not necessarily indicate an independent epileptogenic zone (2, 112). When spiking is detected outside of the area localized by noninvasive testing and no other abnormalities, such as absent or attenuated fast activity, are present on EcoG, then the extent of resection is not extended solely to ablate spikes. Spiking outside the area of resection has typically abated postoperatively in the areas of normal functional status as assessed by preoperative PET study (80, 105).

Evoked Potentials

Median nerve somatosensory and visual evoked potentials are used to assess physiological disturbances in areas of cortical abnormality and to test the lateralization of cortical dysfunction. Determining the functional integrity of the opposite hemisphere is of utmost importance, especially in evaluating patients as candidates for hemispherectomy. Abnormalities in thalamocortical peak latency or amplitude of the hemisphere ipsilateral to the hemiplegia may be a contraindication to resective surgery. In uncooperative or very young patients, visual evoked potentials are sometimes of value in demonstrating a hemianopsia.

SURGICAL PROCEDURES

The surgical treatment of children with intractable epilepsy can be divided into three main groups. These are: 1) resections—hemispherectomy, multilobar, lobar, and focal resection, 2) disconnections—corpuscallasotomy and multiple subpial transection, and 3) stimulation—vagal nerve stimulation

Resections

HEMISPHERECTOMY

In 1928, Dandy performed a hemispherectomy on an adult patient with a glioma diffusely involving the right cerebral hemisphere. McKenzie was the first to perform a hemispherectomy for intractable seizures; the adult patient was relieved of her grand mal seizures and became more alert (65). In 1950, Krynauw reported on the use of hemispherectomy for treatment of intractable childhood epilepsy. He performed hemispherectomies on 12 children with infantile hemiplegia and intractable seizures, and noted functional recovery and good seizure control (61).

The use of hemispherectomy soon spread to medical centers worldwide but was virtually abandoned after long-term follow-up reports showed late hemorrhagic complications in some patients (43,81). A subdural hematoma in the hemicranial space was found in as many as 15 to 20% of cases, and comparable numbers of patients had superficial cerebral hemosiderosis.

Rasmussen observed that hemorrhagic problems did not occur in patients with large but subtotal hemispheric resection (91). This led him to devise a "functional" hemispherectomy that would retain the same benefits as the "anatomical" hemispherectomy but would reduce the incidence of postoperative complications. He described a technique that entailed the resection of the sensorimotor cortex and temporal lobe. The frontal and occipital lobes were left intact but he sectioned all the projection fibers to the brain stem and spinal cord, as well as all commissural fibers running through the corpus callosum.

Other modifications to hemispherectomy have been introduced, including hemidecortication, dural plication to reduce the size of the subdural space, and early postoperative shunting (119, 120, 123). A paper from the University of Minnesota reported a series of 17 patients who underwent classical anatomical hemispherectomy with a mean follow-up period of 28 years. The authors reported an excellent seizure control rate, with only one patient suffering a postoperative hemorrhage into the cerebrospinal fluid (CSF). The investigators concluded that "the incidence and severity of late hemorrhagic complications after hemispherectomy may have been overestimated and the classical operation, without modifications, is an effective and relatively safe one" (27).

With anatomical hemispherectomy, 81 to 85% of patients have been reported to be completely seizure-free or to have significant reduction in their seizure frequency (27, 92). Similar results were found in 34 patients in whom functional hemispherectomy was performed in Montreal after 1974 (119). Eighty-four percent of these patients have been seizure-free or have had a greater that 80% reduction in seizure frequency.

FOCAL, LOBAR, AND MULTILOBAR RESECTIONS

Focal, lobar, and multilobar resection can be used for resection of an epileptogenic focus in a nonhemiplegic child when the focus does not involve the sensorimotor or language cortex. In some patients, the occipital lobe must be removed, which may result in a subsequent visual field deficit. However, if the tissue is structurally abnormal, there may not be a significant change in the visual field.

TEMPORAL LOBECTOMY

Temporal lobectomies are the most common surgical procedure performed for epilepsy in adults (14, 37). Although they have also produced good rates of seizure control in children, temporal lobectomy is less frequently used before adolescence (71).

Advances in neuroimaging have greatly facilitated selection of patients for temporal lobectomy. PET studies may demonstrate lobar interictal hypometabolism that signifies dysfunction. MRI is now able to identify discrete mesial temporal lobe structures and thus identify hippocampal atrophy. Other detectable lesions, including hamartomas, gangliogliomas, astrocytomas, cavernomas, and cortical dysplasia, can also be identified.

At the University of California in Los Angeles, 33 children underwent temporal and extended temporal lobe resections for intractable seizures. Sixteen cases were diagnosed as having tumors. Other pathological diagnoses included cortical dysplasia and reactive changes. In 30 patients with follow-up ranging from eight months to five years, a total of 23 patients (77%) were seizure free. An additional three patients (10%) had a 50% reduction in seizure frequency. One patient had no change in seizure frequency. One child was seizure-free for one year postoperatively but experienced a breakthrough after his medication dosage was reduced.

Neurodevelopmental follow-up assessment showed improvement in all eight of the preschool-aged children after surgery. Improved school grades and performance were noted in eight children, but no change was observed in six children who also attended school. Behavior improvement was observed in six children (1, 85).

Disconnective Procedures

MULTIPLE SUBPIAL CORTICAL TRANSECTION

Frequently, patients will present with epileptogenic foci in eloquent areas. Using standard surgical resection techniques, the patient would be left with an unacceptable deficit. In order to address epileptogenic foci in an eloquent region, Morell et al. developed a technique called multiple subpial transection (MST) (76). The technique involves the selective disruption of short horizontal intracortical fibers at 5-mm intervals along gyri that exhibit epileptogenic activity. Critical to this technique is the sparing of vertically oriented incoming and outgoing neural elements, minimal trauma to the cortical blood supply, and preservation of an intact pial investment over the crown of the gyrus where it abuts the dura.

The rationale for this procedure rests on three different experimental findings. The first was the observation that there is a critical mass of side-to-side connectivity that is necessary for the generation of an epileptic spike, and that spread of the classic jacksonian march involved tangential intracortical fibers (73, 74, 114, 121). The second finding by Sperry et al. demonstrated that inserting mica chips into cortex from above did not interfere with learned behavior otherwise thought to depend on the treated cortex. The third set of findings were those of several different groups (8, 54, 78) that demonstrated a vertical columnar organization of axons entering and exiting the cerebral cortex. Morrell argued that by disrupting the tangential and horizontal fibers involved in the spread of epileptiform activity without disrupting the vertical columnar fibers, the capacity for the spread of epileptiform activity could be eliminated without disturbing the principal physiological action of that area of the cerebral cortex (73, 74, 76, 77).

In 45 patients treated by Morrell et al by transection and adjacent resection, 82% of patients showed at least a 90% reduction in their seizure frequency (75, 76). Of these patients, 25 patients (55%) are seizure free, 5 (11%) have rare seizures, 7 (16%) have a 90% reduction in seizure frequency, and 8 (18%) have not improved. Of the above group, 13 patients had only a transection and no resection of cortical tissue. In this subgroup of patients, seven patients (53%) are seizure free, one (7%) has rare seizures, two (15%) have a 90% reduction, and three (23%) are unimproved. In the two groups, one-third of the patients had a progressive disease (tumors, Rasmussen, subacute sclerosing panencephalitis) with anticipated long-term recurrence of disease. However, in none of the patients studied did the seizure foci recur in the transected cortical regions. Twenty-five of the 45 patients underwent transection in Brocas and Wernicke's area. None of these patients showed any decrease in verbal fluency as compared with preoperative testing. Only when comparing with age-matched controls was there a quantitative difference in verbal fluency. Four patients with the Landau-Kleffner syndrome who were mute for at least two years underwent transection of the entire perislyvian speech cortex. All 4 were able to talk and understand speech following surgery. In the 23 patients who underwent transection of precentral gyrus cortex, none experienced worsening in their ability to use the contralateral extremity for daily motor activities. Any motor deficits were unchanged from preoperative levels. In 19 patients, MST was performed in the postcentral gyrus without detectable loss of primary tactile modalities. Four patients demonstrated some degree of contralateral neglect. In two of these patients, the neglect completely resolved within six months. One patient exhibited contralateral neglect on careful examination at two-year follow-up. In one patient, the symptoms had persisted for four years. The remainder of patients showed no loss of two-point discrimination, baroagnosis, stereognosis, or tactile reading. In 6 of the 45 patients, the operation was complicated by a small, deep venous hemorrhage that resulted in transient loss of function. One patient experienced a small venous infarct, while another had a subcortical hemorrhage. In both these cases, the lesions occurred at a distance from the transection site (75, 76).

Evaluation of the functional outcome and the control of seizures following MST is very favorable. Therefore, MST permits an extension of surgical therapy to patients with epileptogenic foci in regions otherwise considered inoperable. Furthermore, the results of MST have shown that the procedure is not only curative in a large percentage of the patients who are candidates, but also can restore function to eloquent cortex, as demonstrated in patients with Landau-Kleffner syndrome.

CORPUSCALLOSOTOMY

Corpuscallosotomy is designed to prevent the propagation of seizures between hemispheres. Although by disconnecting the hemispheres one does not eliminate the primary seizure focus, one can prevent generalized tonic or atonic episodes that are manifested as drop attacks (79). Controlled drop attacks is crucial since children experiencing them often suffer from recurrent head and facial injuries. Corpuscallosotomy rarely produces a seizure-free state, but is successful if the child is no longer endangered by drop attacks.

Stimulation

VAGAL NERVE STIMULATION

The earliest reports of modulating seizure activity through afferent stimulation dates back to the teachings of Pelops, the master of Galen. Pelops described a technique that used ligatures applied to a limb as a means of aborting the progression of a focal seizure. Indeed, studies have shown the efficacy of cutaneous afferent stimulation in EEG synchronization. However, these methods are often associated with unacceptable levels of pain and unpleasant sensations (99). In animals, the vagus nerve has been known for many years to influence the EEG (128). In 1938, Bailey and Bremer reported alteration in the brain wave activity of cats after afferent vagal stimulation (9). In the subsequent 30 years, numerous researchers demonstrated additional changes in the EEG pattern of animals after vagal nerve stimulation (VNS). These findings led to the theory that appropriately timed stimulation of the vagus nerve may prevent or abort epileptiform activity (99, 101). Studies of generalized seizures induced by parenteral pentylenetetrazol (PTZ) or strychnine in anesthetized dogs revealed an inhibitory affect of VNS on ictal activity (126, 127). In primates, Lockard et al. showed an alteration in seizure frequency in two out of four monkeys undergoing VNS. They failed to demonstrate any changes in interictal spike activity, seizure severity, or seizure duration (63).

The vagus nerve innervates the pharynx, blood vessels, heart, lungs, and the gastrointestinal tract. However, most of the fibers within the nerve are afferent, transmitting impulses to parts of the brain, some of which are intimately involved with epilepsy, namely, the hippocampus, nucleus solitarius, and the hypothalamus. The exact mechanism by which VNS controls epileptiform activity is not fully understood. Much interest has centered on the effects of VNS at the level of the brainstem. Many authors have proposed that its antiepileptic actions relate to effects on the reticular activating system that projects to numerous basal forebrain structures (44, 120, 124, 125, 127, 128). Vagal afferents originate from peripheral receptors and project primarily to the nucleus of the solitary tract, which extends throughout the length of the brainstem. A small number of the vagal afferent fibers pass directly to the spinal trigeminal nucleus and the reticular formation. The nucleus of the solitary tract has widespread projections to the cerebral cortex, basal forebrain, thalamus, hypothalamus, amygdala, hippocampus, dorsal raphe, and cerebellum (67, 100).

At the molecular level, the action of VNS may depend on release of neurotransmitters that stabilize the cell membranes of hyperexcitable neurons. Although multiple neurotransmitters have been implicated in this role (46, 97, 99), most of the literature suggests that the antiepileptiform activity of VNS depends on widespread release of γ-aminobutyric acid (GABA) and glycine throughout the brain stem and cerebral cortex (118, 122, 123). This is supported by animal models (124, 125, 127).

Clinical Trials of VNS

Dr. Kiffen Penry implanted the first vagal nerve stimulator in 1990. Subsequently, two single-blinded pilot studies were carried out with 14 patients who had medication-resistent partial seizures (116, 117). Seizure frequency was reduced by greater than 50% in 36% of patients, and two patients became seizure free for greater than one year.

The largest multicenter trial of VNS (47) showed that 25% of patients with medically intractable seizures achieved a 50% reduction in seizure frequency. Another 10% achieved a 75% reduction, and less than 1% were seizure free with VNS.

The response of children with VNS is comparable to the results found in adults with partial epilepsy (51). Nineteen patients with medically and surgically intractable seizures underwent VNS from 2 to 30 months. Of the 19 patients, 6 (32%) had more than a 90% reduction in the number of seizures, and 10 (53%) had more than a 50% reduction in seizure frequency. Five patients required fewer antiepileptic medications, and one patient required an increase in medications.

Although the number of patients was small, the authors concluded that VNS in children has some advantages over medical management alone. They felt that the results with VNS in children were similar to the results of successful new anticonvulsant medications in a child with refractory epilepsy, with no relapses seen in responders. However, they advocated further studies in children to determine the specific role of VNS in the treatment of epilepsy in children.

REFERENCES

1. Adelson PD, Peacock, WJ, Chugani HT, et al. Temporal and extended temporal resections for the treatment of intractable seizures in early childhood. **Ped Neurosurg** 18:169–78, 1992.
2. Ajmone-Marsan C. Electrocorticography. **Handbook Electroencephalograp Clin Neurophysiol** 10C:1–46, 1973.
3. Alexander GL. Sturge-Weber Syndrome, in, Vinken PJ, Fruyn GW (ed). *Handbook of Clinical Neurology.* New York:Elsevier, 1977, pp 223–240.
4. Alexander GL, Norman, RN. *The Sturge-Weber Syndrome,* Bristol: John Wright & Sons, 1960.

5. Alvarez LA, Shinnar, S, Mosh, SL. Infantile spasms due to unilateral cerebral infarcts. **Pediatrics** 1024–1026, 1987.
6. Anderman F. Identification of candidates for surgical treatment of epilepsy, in, Engel J Jr (ed). *Surgical Treatment of the Epilepsies.* New York: Raven Press, 1987, pp 51–70.
7. Angelini L, Broggi, G, Riva, D, Lazzaro Solero C. A case of Lennox-Gastaut syndrome successfully treated by removal of a parietotemporal astrocytoma. **Epilepsia** 665–669, 1979.
8. Asanuma H, Sakata H. Functional organization of a cortical efferent system examined with focal depth stimulation in cats. **J Neurophysiol** 30:35–54, 1967.
9. Bailey P, Bremer F. A sensory cortical representation of the vagus nerve with a note on the effects of low blood pressure on the cortical electrogram. **J Neurophysiol** 1:405–412, 1938.
10. Basser LS. Hemiplegia of early onset and the faculty of speech with special reference to the effects of hemispherectomy. **Brain** 427–460, 1962.
11. Baumbach HD, Chow KL. Visuocortical epileptiform discharges in rabbits: Differential affects on neuronal development in the lateral geniculate nucleus and superior colliculus. **Brain Res** 209:61–76, 1981.
12. Branch CE, Dyken PR Choroid plexus papilloma and infantile spasms. **Ann Neurol** 302–304, 1979.
13. Brown SW, Reynolds EH Cognitive impairment in epileptic patients, in, Reynolds EH, Trimble MR (ed.) *Epilepsy and Psychiatry.* Edinburgh: Churchill Livingstone, 1981, pp 147–164.
14. Cahan DH, Sutherling W, McCullough AM, et al. Review of the 20 year UCLA experience with surgery for epilepsy. **Clev Clin Q** 313–318, 1984.
15. Caldecott-Hazard S, Engel J Jr. Limbic posticital events: Anatomical substrates and opiod receptor involvement. **Prog Neuropsychopharmacol Biol Psychiatry** 389–418, 1987.
16. Carlson J, Netley C., Hendrick EB, et al. A reexamination of intellectual disabilities in hemispherectomized patients. **Trans Am Neurol Assoc** 198–201, 1968.
17. Cavazzuti GB, Cappella L, Nalin A. Longitudinal study of epileptiform EEG patterns in normal children. **Epilepsia** 43–55, 1980.
18. Chaudry MR, Pond DA Mental deterioration in epileptic children. **J Neurol Neurosurg Psychiatry** 213–219, 1961.
19. Hendrick EB, Hoffman HJ, Hudson AR: Hemispherectomy in children. **Clin Neurosurg** 16:315–327, 1969.
20. Chugani HT, Phelps ME, Shields WD, Shewmon DA, et al. PET identifies cortical dysgenesis in cryptogenic cases for surgical treatment. **Ann Neurol** 27:487–497. 1990.
21. Chugani HT, Shewmon DA, Peacock WJ, Shields WD, Mazziotta JC, Phelps ME. Surgical treatment of intractable neonatal-onset seizures: The role of positron emission tomography. **Neurology** 38:1178–88, 1988.
22. Collins RC, Olney JW, Lothman EW. Metabolica and pathological consequences of focal seizures, in, Ward AA, Penry JK, Purpura DP (ed). *Epilepsy.* New York: Raven Press, 1983, pp 87–107.
23. Crowell RM. Distal effects of a focal epileptogenic process. **Brain Res** 137–154, 1970.
24. Cusmai R, Dulac O, Diebler C. Lesions focales dans les spasmes infantiles. **Neurophysiol Clin** 235–241, 1988.
25. Dam M. Chronic toxicity of antiepileptic drugs with respect to cerebellar and motor function, in, Oxley J, Janz D, Meinardi H, (ed). *Chronic Toxicity of Antiepileptic Drugs.* New York: Raven Press, 1983 pp 223–228.
26. Davidson S, Falconer MA Outcome of surgery in 40 children with temporal lobe epilepsy. **Lancet** 1260–1263, 1975.

27. Davies KG, Maxwell RE, French LA. Hemispherectomy for intractable seizures: Long-term results in 17 patients followed for up to 38 years. **J Neurosurg** 733–740, 1993.
28. De Bittencourt PRM. Cerebral and cerebellar atrophy in patients with severe epilepsy: A preliminary report, in, Oxley J, Janz D, Meinardi H, (ed). *Chronic Toxicity of Antiepileptic Drugs.* New York: Raven Press, 1983, pp 237–245.
29. Dreifuss FE. Goals of surgery for epilepsy, in, Engel J Jr, (ed). *Surgical Treatment of the Epilepsies.* New York: Raven Press, 1987, pp 31–49.
30. Dreifuss FE, Martine-Lange M, Roger J, Seino M, Wolf P, Dam M. **Epilepsia** 268–278, 1985.
31. Duchowny MS. The role of surgery in childhood epilepsy. **Int Pediatr** 205–211, 1987.
32. Dulac O, Chiron C, Jambaque I, Plouin P, Raynaud C. Infantile spasms. **Prog Clin Neurosci** 97–109, 1987.
33. Ebersole JS, Levine RA. Abnormal neuronal responses during evolution of a penicillin epileptic focus in cat visual cortex. **J Neurophysiol** 250–266, 1975.
34. Engel J Jr, Wilson CL. Evidence for enhanced synaptic inhibition in human epilepsy, in, Morselli PL, Nistico G, Engel J Jr (ed). *Neurotransmitters, Seizures and Epilepsy.* New York: Raven Press 1986, pp 1–10.
35. Engel J Jr, Ackermann RF, Caldecott-Hazard S, et al. Epileptic activation of antagonistic systems may explain paradoxical features of experimental and human epilepsy: A review and hypothesis, in, Wada JA (ed). *Kindling.* New York: Raven Press, 1981, pp 193–211.
36. Engel J Jr, Kuhl DE, Phelps ME, et al. Interictal cerebral glucose metabolism in partial epilepsy and its relation to EEG changes. **Ann Neurol** 150–217, 1982.
37. Falconer MA. Anterior temporal lobectomy for epilepsy, in, Logue V (ed). *Operative Surgery.* Philadelphia: J.B. Lippincott, 1971, pp 142.
38. Fuiks KS, Wyler AR, Hermann BP, et al. Seizure outcome from anterior and complete corpus callosotomy. **J Neurosurg** 573–578, 1991.
39. Gabriel YH. Unilateral hemispheric ganglioma with infantile spasms. **Ann Neurol** 287–288, 1980.
40. Glaser GH. Natural history of temporal lobe-limbic epilepsy, in, Engel J Jr (ed). *Surgical Treatment of Epilepsies.* New York: Raven Press 1987, pp 13–30.
41. Goldring S. Surgical management of epilepsy in children, in, Engel J Jr (ed). *Surgical Treatment of Epilepsies.* New York: Raven Press, 1987 pp 445–464.
42. Goulatia RA, Verma A, Mishra NK, et al. Disappearing CT lesions in epilepsy. **Epilepsia** 253–257, 1987.
43. Griffith HB. Cerebral hemispherectomy for infantile hemiplegia in the light of late results. **Ann R Coll Surg Engl** 183–201, 1967.
44. Group VNSS. A randomized controlled trial of chronic vagus nerve stimulation for treatment of medically intractable seizures. **Neurology** 45:224–230, 1995.
45. Gutnik MJ, Prince DA. Effects of projected cortical epileptiform discharges on neuronal activities in cat VPL: I. Interictal discharge. **J Neurophysiol** 1310–1327, 1974.
46. Hammond EJ, Uthman BM, Wilder BJ, et al. Neurochemical effects of vagus nerve stimulation in humans. **Brain Res** 583:300–303, 1992.
47. Handforth A, DeGiogio CM, Schachter SC, et al. Vagus nerve stimulation for partial-onset seizures: A randomized active-control trial. **Neurology** 51:48–55, 1998.
48. Harbord MG, Nanson JL. Temporal lobe epilepsy in childhood: A reappraisal of etiology and outcome. **Pediatr Neurol** 263–268, 1987.
49. Hillier WF, Jr. Total left cerebral hemispherectomy for malignant glioma. **Neurology** 718-721, 1954.

50. Hoffman HJ, Hendrick EB, Dennis M, Armstrong D. Hemispherectomy for Sturge-Weber syndrome. *Childs Brain.* 1979;5:233–248, 1979.
51. Horning GW, Murphy VJ, Schallert G, Tilton C. Left vagus nerve stimulation in children with refractory epilepsy: An update. **South Med J** 90:484–488, 1997.
52. Horsley SV. Brain-Surgery. **BMJ** 670–675, 1886.
53. Hovda DA, Villablanca JR. Differential brain stem nuclei degeneration after neonatal or adult cerebral hemispherectomy in cats. **Anat Rec** 56A, 1986.
54. Hubel DH, Wiesel TN. Receptive fields, binocular interaction and functional architecture in the cat's visual cortex. **J Physiol** 160:106–154, 1962.
55. Huttenlocher PP. Dendritic development in neocortex of children with mental defect and infantile spasms. **Neurology** 203–210, 1974.
56. Kellaway P. Afferent input: A critical factor in the ontogenesis of brain electrical activity, in, Burch N, Altshuber HL (ed). *Behavior and Brain Electrical Activity.* New York: Plenum Publishing, 1975, pp 391–420.
57. Kellaway P. The incidence, significance and natural history of spike foci in children, in, Henry CD (ed). *Current Clinical Neurophysiology: Update on EEG and Evoked Potentials.* Amsterdam: Elsevier North-Holland, 1980 pp 151–175.
58. Kennedy C, Ramirez LS. Brain damage as a cause of behavior disturbance in children, in, Birch HG (ed). *Brain Damage in Children: The Biological and Social Aspects.* Baltimore: Williams & Wilkins, 1964, pp 13–23.
59. Kotagal P, Rothner AD, Erenberg G, Cruse R., Wyllie E. Complex partial seizures of childhood onset: A five-year follow-up study. **Arch Neurol** 1177–1180, 1987.
60. Kramer RE, Luders H, Lesser RP, et al. Transient focal abnormalities of neuroimaging studies during focal status epilepticus. **Epilepsia** 628–632, 1987.
61. Krynauw R. Infantile hemiplegia treated by removing one cerebral hemisphere. **J Neurol Neurosurg Psychiatry** 243–267, 1950.
62. Lindsay J, Ounsted C, Richards P. Long-term outcome in children with temporal lobe seizures. V: Indications and contra-indications for neurosurgery. ***Dev Med Child Neurol*** 25–32, 1984.
63. Lockard JS, Congdon WC, DuCharme LL. Feasibility and safety of vagal stimulation in monkey model. **Epilepsia** 31(Suppl 2):S20–S26, 1990.
64. McFie J. The effects of hemispherectomy on intellectual functioning in cases of infantile hemiplegia. **J Neurol Neurosurg Psychiatry** 240–249, 1961.
65. McKenezie KG. The present status of a patient who had the right cerebra hemisphere removed. **JAMA** 1938:168, 1938.
66. McLachlan RS. Suppression of interictal spikes and seizures by stimulation of the vagus nerve. **Epilepsia** 34:918–923, 1933.
67. McLachlan RS. Vagus nerve stimulation for intractable epilepsy: A review. **J Clin Neurophysiol** 14:358–368, 1997.
68. McLain LW Jr, Martin JT, Allen JH. Cerebellar degeneration due to chronic phenytoin therapy. **Ann Neurol** 18–23, 1980.
69. Meistrup-Larsen KI, Hermann S, Permin, H. Chronic diphenylhydantoin encephalopathy in mentally retarded children and adolescent with severe epilepsy. **Acta Neurol Scand** 50–55, 1979.
70. Merlis JK. Proposal for an international classification of the epilepsies. **Epilepsia** 114–119, 1970.
71. Meyer FB, Marsh WR, Laws ER. Temporal lobectomy in children with epilepsy. **J Neurosurg** 695–696, 1983.

72. Mimaki T, Ono J, Yabuuchi H. Temporal lobe astrocytoma with infantile spasms. **Ann Neurol** 1983:695–696, 1983.
73. Morrell F. Callosal mechanisms in epileptogenesis: Identification of two distinct kinds of spread of epileptic activity, in, Reeves AG (ed). *Epilepsy and the Corpus Callosum.* New York: Plenum Press, 1985, pp 99–130.
74. Morrell F, Hanbery JW. A new surgical technique for the treatment of focal cortical epilepsy. **Electroencephalogr Clin Neurophysiol** 26:120, 1969.
75. Morrell F, Cooper M, Ali A, Smith MC, Pierre-Louis SJC, Whisler WW. Landau-Kleffner syndrome: Blood flow, metabolism and electrophysiologic studies. Epilepsia 31:672, 1990.
76. Morrell F, Whistler WW, Bleck TP. Multiple subpial transection: A new approach to the surgical treatment of focal epilepsy. **J Neurosurg** 70:231–239, 1989.
77. Morrell F, Whisler, WW, Smith MC. Multiple supial transection in Rasmussen's encephalitis, in, Andermann F (ed). *Chronic Encephalitis and Epilepsy: Rasmussen's Syndrome.* Boston: Butterworth-Heineman, 1991, pp 219–233.
78. Mountcastle VB. Modality and topographic properties of single neurons of cat's somatic sensory cortex. **J Neurophysiol** 20:408–434, 1957.
79. Oguni H, Olivier A, Andermenn F, et al. Anterior callosotomy in the treatment of medically intractable epilepsies: A study of 43 patients with a mean follow-up of 39 months. **Ann Neurol** 357–364, 1991.
80. Olson DM, Chugani HT, Shewmonb DA, et al. Electrocorticographic confirmation of focal positron emission tomographic abnormalities in children with intractable epilepsy. **Epilepsia** 31:731–739, 1990.
81. Oppenheimer DR, Griffith HB. Persistent intracranial bleeding as a complication of hemispherectomy. **J Neurol Neurosurg Psychiatry** 229–240, 1966.
82. Palm DG, Korinthenberg R. West syndrome and Lennox-Gastaux syndrome in children with porencephalic cysts: Long-term follow-up after neurosurgical treatment, in, Niedermeyer E, Degan R (ed). *The Lennox-Gastaux Syndrome.* New York: Alan R. Liss, 1988, pp 326–419.
83. Palm DG, Brandt M, Koringthenberg R. West and Lennox-Gastaut syndromes and other epilepsies with porencephalic cysts. **Clev Clin J Med** S286–S287, 1989.
84. Pavone L, Curatolo P, Rizzo R, et al. Epidermal nevus syndrome: A neurological variant with hemimegalencephaly, gyral formation, mental retardation, seizures, and facial hemihypertrophy. **Neurology** 266–271, 1991.
85. Peacock WJ. Neurosurgical aspects of epilepsy in children, in, Youmans JR (ed). *Neurological Surgery. Fourth Edition.* Philadelphia: W.B. Saunders Company, 1996, pp 3624–3642.
86. Peacock WJ. Personal communication. 1999.
87. Prince DA. Microelectrode studies of penicillin foci, in, Jasper HH, Ward AA Jr, Pope A (ed). *Basic Mechanisms of the Epilepsies.* Boston: Little, Brown & Co., 1969, pp 320–328.
88. Prince DA, Wildre BJ. Cortical mechanisms in epileptogenic foci: "Surround" inhibition. **Arch Neurol** 194–202, 1967.
89. Purpura DP. Dendritic differentiation in human cerebral cortex: Normal and aberrant developmental patterns. *Advances in Neurology.* 12:91–134, 1975.
90. Rabinowics T. The differential maturation of the human cerebral cortex, in, Falkner FT, JM (ed). *Human Growth.* New York: Plenum Publishing, 1979, pp 97–123.
91. Rasmussen T. Hemispherectomy for seizures revisited. **Can J Neurol Sci** 71–78, 1983.
92. Rasmussen T, Andermann F. Update on the syndrome of "chronic encephalitis" and epilepsy. **Cleve Clin J Med** S181–184, 1989.

93. Rasmussen T, Olszewski J, Lloyd-Smith D. Focal seizures due to chronic localized encephalitis. **Neurology** 433–455, 1958.
94. Rausch R, Crandall PH. Psychological status related to surgical control of temporal lobe seizures. **Epilepsia** 191–202, 1982.
95. Resnick TJ. Evaluation of children for epilepsy surgery. **Int Pediatr** 136–142, 1988.
96. Reynolds EH. Biological factors in psychological disorders associated with epilepsy, in, Reynolds EH, Trimble MR (ed). *Epilepsy and Psychiatry.* Edinburgh: Churchill Livingstone, 1981.
97. Ricardo JA, Koh ET. Anatomical evidence of direct projections from the nucleus of the solitry tract to the hypothalamus, amygdala, and other forebrain structures in the rat. **Brain Res** 153:1–26, 1978.
98. Rosen AD, Vastola EF, Hildenbrand ZJM. Visual radiation activity during a cortical penicilling discharge. **Exp Neurol** 1–11, 1973.
99. Rutecki P. Anatomical physiological and theoretical basis for the antiepileptic effect of vagus nerve stimulation. **Epilepsia** 31(Suppl 2):S1–S6, 1990.
100. Rutecki P. Anatomical, physiological and theoretical basis for the antiepileptic effect of vagus nerve stimulation. **Epilepsia** 299–304, 1993.
101. Salinski MC, Burchiel KJ. Vagus nerve stimulation has no effect on awake EEG rhythms in humans. **Epilepsia** 34:299–304, 1993.
102. Sankar R. Personal Communication. 1983.
103. Schwartzkroin PA, Van Duijn H, Prince DA. Effects of projected cortical epileptiform discharges on field potentials in the cat cuneate nucleus. **Exp. Neurol** 88–105, 1974.
104. Shewmon DA, Erwin RJ. The effect of focal interictal spikes on perception and reaction time: General considerations. **Electroencephalogr Clin Neurophysiol** 319–337, 1988.
105. Shewmon DA, Shields WD, Chugani HT, et al. Contrasts between pediatric and adult epilepsy surgery. Rationale and strategy for focal resection. **J Epilepsy** 3:141–155, 1990.
106. Shields WD, Chugani HT, Shewmon DA, Peacock WJ. Focal central nervous system lesions as a cause of infantile spasms. **Cleve Clin J Med** S291, 1989.
107. Shields WD, Peacock WP, Roper SN. Surgery for epilepsy: Special pediatric considerations. **Neurosurg Clin N Am** 4:301–310, 1993.
108. Shields WD, Shewmon DD, Chugani HT, Peacock WJ. The role of surgery in the treatment of infantile spasms. **J Epilepsy** 321–324, 1990.
109. Smith A. Dominant and nondominant hemispherectomy, in, Smith WL (ed). *Drugs, Development, and Cerebral Function.* Springfield: Charles C. Thomas, 1972, pp 37–68.
110. Smith A, Sugar O. Development of above normal language and intelligence 21 years after cerebral hemispherectomy. **Neurology** 813–818, 1975.
111. Sturge WA. A case of partial epilepsy, apparently due to a lesion on the vasomotor centers of the brain. **Trans Clin Soc Lond** 162–167, 1879.
112. Sutherling WW, Barth DS. Neocortical propagation of temporal lobe spike foci on magnetoencephalography and electroencephalography. **Ann Neurol** 25:373–381, 1989.
113. Taylor L. Psychological assessment of neurosurgical patients, in, Rasmussen TB (ed). *Functional Neurosurgery.* New York: Raven Press, 1979, pp 165–180.
114. Tharp BR. The penicillin focus: A study of field characteristics using cross-correlation analysis. **Electroencephalogr Clin Neurophysiol** 31:45–55, 1971.
115. Till K. Hemispherectomy for infantile hemiplegia. **Dev Med Child Neurol** 773–774, 1967.

116. Uthman BM, Wilder BJ, Hammond EJ, Reid SA. Efficacy and safety of vagus nerve stimulation in patients with complex partial seizures. **Epilepsia** S44–50, 1990.
117. Uthman BM, Wilder BJ, Penry JK, et al. Treatment of epilepsy by stimulation of the vagus nerve. **Neurology** 1338–1345, 1993.
118. Villablanca JR, Burgess JW, Olmstead CE. Recovery of function after neonatal or adult hemispherectomy in cats: Time course, movement, posture and sensorimotor tests. **Behav Brain Res** 19:205–226, 1986.
119. Villemure JG. Hemispherectomy techniques, in, Luners HO (ed). *Epilepsy Surgery.* New York: Raven Press, 199, pp 2569–578.
120. Villemure JG, Adams CBT, Hoffman JJ, et al. Hemispherectomy, in, Engel J Jr (ed). *Surgical Treatment of Epilepsies.* New York: Raven Press, 1993, pp 511–519.
121. Wilder BJ, Morrell F. Cellular behavior in secondary epileptic lesions. **Neurology** 17:1193–1204, 1967.
122. Wilson PJE. Cerebral hemispherectomy for infantile hemiplegia: A report of 50 cases. **Brain** 147–180, 1970.
123. Winston KR, Keasly W, Adler JR, et al. Cerebral hemicorticectomy for epilepsy. **J Neurosurg** 889–895, 1992.
124. Woodbury DM, Woodbury JW. Effects of vagal nerve stimulation on experimentally induced seizures in rats. **Epilepsia** 31(Suppl 2):S7–S19, 1990.
125. Woodbury JW, Woodbury DM. Vagal stimulation reduces the severity of maximal electroshock seizures in intact rats: Use of a cuff electrode for stimulating and recording. **Pacing Clin Electrophysiol** 14:94–107, 1991.
126. Zabara J. Peripheral control of hypersynchronous discharge in epilepsy (Abstract). **Electroencephalogr Clin Neurophysiol** 162, 1985.
127. Zabara J. Inhibition of experimental seizures in canines by repetitive vagal stimulation. **Epilepsia** 1005–1012, 1992.
128. Zanchetti A, Wang SC, Moruzzi G. The effect of vagal afferent stimulation on the EEG pattern of the cat. **Electroencephalogr Clin Neurophysiol** 4:357–361, 1952.

CHAPTER

23

Selective Dorsal Rhizotomy: An Excellent Therapeutic Option for Spastic Cerebral Palsy

T. S. PARK, M.D.

INTRODUCTION

Cerebral palsy (CP) is a persistent but not unchanging disorder of movement and posture, appearing early in life and caused by a nonprogressive disorder of the brain (5). The etiology of CP includes a group of divergent neurologic disorders. As a clinical syndrome, CP remains an important medical problem because of its continued high prevalence (59), the lifelong handicap, and the burdens it places on families and society (46, 48). In this nation alone, for example, approximately 500,000 children and adults suffer from CP, and approximately 8,600 new patients are diagnosed with it each year (26). The Advisory Council of the National Institute of Neurological Disorders and Stroke estimated recently that CP costs society $5 billion/year (38). Until a decade ago, neurosurgeons played a minimal role in care of the patients with CP, despite the fact that it is basically a neurologic disorder. Fortunately, this has changed with the utilization of selective dorsal rhizotomy (SDR) in treating spastic CP. This review examines evidence accumulated over the past decade regarding SDR and attempts to determine whether or not SDR is an acceptable option for patients with spastic CP.

CP is classified into several subtypes based on clinical features. *Table 23.1* illustrates the salient features of each subtype of CP. Spastic CP is the most common subtype, and more than 80% of patients are afflicted with spasticity of varying severity (47).

In 1962, Paine suggested the possibility of spontaneous improvement of CP (51). Likewise, in a multicenter study in the 1970s, 3 to 74% of children diagnosed with CP at 1 year of age became free of motor abnormality by age 7 years (47). Neither of the studies, however, examined specifically whether or not CP spasticity resolves spontaneously after age 2. Rather, the main message from the latter report is that CP cannot be diagnosed accurately during the first year of life, and diagnosis should be deferred until later years when delayed motor development is apparent.

TABLE 23.1
Subtypes of Cerebral Palsy

CP Subtypes	Main Clinical Features	Incidence (%)
Diplegia	Spastic weakness of lower extremities with no or minimal involvement of upper extremities	33
Quadriplegia	Spastic weakness of all extremities and trunk	29
Hemiplegia	Spastic weakness of unilateral upper and lower extremity	21
Dyskinetic/ataxic CP	Fluctuating muscle tone, athetosis, and motor weakness of all extremities	7
Mixed CP	Motor weakness with two or all of spasticity, dyskinesia, athetosis	10

In personal experience with over 1,000 children and adults with CP, the present author has not seen a single case, either mild or severe, in which CP spasticity that was detected after 2 years of age resolved spontaneously. Instead, a large number of adolescents and adults have been seen who were handicapped by lifelong CP spasticity and associated problems. The literature contains no report of a series of patients who showed spontaneous resolution of CP spasticity. Thus, it seems clear that CP spasticity, once developed, persists throughout a patient's life unless it is treated.

EFFECTS OF CP SPASTICITY

Harmful Effects

Abundant experimental data and clinical observations indicate that CP spasticity is harmful to patients at all ages and to pediatric patients in particular (*Table 23.2*). Normally, longitudinal muscle growth proceeds as new myofilaments and sarcomeres are added to the ends of the muscle fibers (76). The greatest increase in sarcomere numbers occurs at an early age; in general, the increase takes place much more actively during development than after maturation (76). Concurrent with the rapid addition of sarcomeres, longitudinal muscle growth also occurs most rapidly during development (78). The increase in the sarcomere number is not under direct neural control but is induced mainly by the amount of tension the muscle is subjected to, i.e., repeated muscle stretch (22, 32, 33). Thus when muscles are immobilized, there are rapid decreases in the numbers of already existing sarcomeres as well as in the number of new sarcomeres that should increase with normal development (22, 29, 34).

TABLE 23.2
Harmful Effects of Spasticity in Children With Spastic Cerebral Palsy

Reduction of protein synthesis in myocytes
Loss of sarcomeres
Reduction of muscle extensibility
Inhibition of longitudinal muscle growth
Shortening of muscle
Inhibition of voluntary movements
Development of muscle contractures
Development of bone and joint deformities

This information raises the possibility that spasticity inhibits longitudinal muscle growth. Ziv et al., who studied longitudinal muscle and bone growth in hereditary spastic mice, found that the muscle growth was 45% less than in control animals and was accompanied by substantially reduced bone growth (78). The observed spasticity-induced inhibition of muscle growth is in part related to spasticity-induced limitation of muscle stretch, because muscle fibers, when immobilized in a shortened position, suffer a rapid and substantial loss of sarcomeres (22, 29). The loss of sarcomeres accompanies reduced elasticity in the muscles (69) and makes muscles resistant to passive stretch (70). Additionally, muscles of children with spastic CP undergo atrophy of type I and II muscle fibers, concurrent with type II hypertrophy in some cases (11). These pathologic abnormalities result in abnormally shortened muscles and abnormally long tendons (70). Consequently, the muscles develop "muscle contracture," i.e., increased resistance of the muscle to passive stretch in the absence of muscle contraction. The muscle contractures typically worsen as a child grows (31) and produce various bone and joint deformities in the extremities (6).

Another important harmful effect of spasticity in CP is that it inhibits motor activities. The most compelling evidence for this is the fact that motor functions of patients improve following SDR (65). Some authors have contended that spasticity does not affect motor functioning in children with CP (39). That notion, however, was in part based on a study that examined the effect of spasticity on motor function of the upper extremities in adult patients with stroke, trauma, or multiple sclerosis (61), and significant differences have been shown between CP spasticity and spasticity of adulthood onset. For example, patients with CP lack normal reciprocal relaxation of the antagonist muscles during voluntary leg movements and instead exhibit co-contraction of agonist and antagonist muscles. In contrast, adult patients with spasticity of late onset do not exhibit such co-contraction of muscles during voluntary movements, and reciprocal relaxation of antagonist muscles is preserved (24). The spasticity-induced inhibition of motor activities in CP results in decreased muscle stretch in daily activities, which in turn contributes to muscle contractures and orthopedic deformities.

Beneficial Effects

Spasticity in CP, unlike spasticity following spinal cord injury, has no beneficial effects. Some clinicians feel that spasticity in a child with motor weakness helps the child execute movements. That idea, however, is at variance with the fact that reduction of spasticity after dorsal rhizotomy improves motor functions. For example, children with spastic CP who walk independently or with crutches and walkers invariably walk better after dorsal rhizotomy, and other gross motor functions improve as well.

For several decades, numerous varieties of orthopedic surgeries (6), physical therapy, braces, and assistive devices (36, 68) as well as oral antispasticity medications have been used for treatment of CP spasticity and associated deformities. Recent additions are intramuscular injection of botulinum-A toxin (Botox) (37) and intrathecal infusion of baclofen (3). The continuing effort to treat CP spasticity, with its associated problems, is testimony to the recognition of its major harmful effects. The national United Cerebral Palsy and Research Foundation, also recognizing the significant adverse effects of spasticity on patients

TABLE 23.3
Current Treatments for Cerebral Palsy Spasticity and Associated Deformities

Treatment	Comments
Antispasticity oral medication baclofen, benzodiazepine, clonidine	Unproven efficacy and potential side effects on developing brain
Intramuscular injection of botulinum-A toxin (Botox)	Temporary and limited reduction of spasticity; repeat injections required; long-term benefits unknown
Intrathecal baclofen infusion	Temporary reduction of spasticity; long-term outcome in CP spasticity unknown; potentially high expenses
Muscle and tendon releases	Morbidity includes permanent muscle weakness that produces deformities, abnormal posture, and gait pattern; no effect on spasticity itself
Selective dorsal rhizotomy	Morbidity includes spinal deformities, urinary incontinence, and sensory loss; permanent reduction of spasticity is possible
Physical therapy and braces	Improve muscle contractures but not spasticity itself

with CP, regards elimination of CP spasticity as one of its main priorities (see *www.ucpa.org*). Of all currently employed treatment modalities (*Table 23.3*), dorsal rhizotomy, as detailed below, is the only treatment that can permanently reduce CP spasticity.

SELECTIVE DORSAL RHIZOTOMY

Background

The use of dorsal rhizotomy in humans dates back to the early 1900s. Foerster reported on 88 children who underwent sectioning of the entire L2, -3, -5, and S1-2 dorsal spinal roots (L4 dorsal root spared) for "congenital spastic paraplegia" (20). He provided a clear description of improvements in the children's sitting and walking abilities. In the 1960s and 1970s, Gros in France and Fasano in Italy used electromyographic responses to electrical stimulation during dorsal rhizotomy in patients with spastic CP (18, 27). Fasano et al. subsequently modified the intraoperative electrical stimulation and coined the term "functional posterior rhizotomy" (19). In the late 1980s, Peacock presented his experience with what he called "selective posterior rhizotomy" (55, 56). Since 1986, a number of medical centers have used dorsal rhizotomy for spastic CP. At the same time, there has been close scrutiny of the procedure by neurosurgeons, orthopedists, therapists, pediatricians, neurologists, and biomedical engineers (17, 41, 44, 50, 62, 65, 73, 77). It is now clear that SDR can offer sustained reduction of CP spasticity, with minimal associated morbidity.

When dorsal rhizotomy was reintroduced, the main questions were 1) Does intraoperative electrophysiologic monitoring allow differentiation of the "abnormal" dorsal root fibers? 2) Does dorsal rhizotomy reduce spasticity and improve motor functions? 3) Who are candidates for the operation? and 4) What is the morbidity associated with the operation?

Intraoperative Electrophysiologic Monitoring

Fasano's intraoperative electrophysiologic monitoring technique for functional dorsal rhizotomy was apparently based on experimental studies by Decandia et al. (16) and Lloyd (40). In studies on cats, repeated high-frequency electrical stimulation of the afferent fibers elicited depression of motor neurons and monosynaptic reflex discharge. Fasano, having tried similar electrical stimulation on patients with spastic CP, interpreted the presence of the reflex discharge depression as "normal response" and the lack of the depression as "abnormal response" (18). His interpretation of electromyographic responses was, however, not based on additional studies of a control group to determine whether the "normal response" is unique to normal humans. Despite this limited background work, the intraoperative monitoring technique was accepted by neurosurgeons as standard practice. Compounding the lack of clarity surrounding the usefulness of the technique were various modifications made without a thorough evaluation of their validity (41, 64). At this time, it appears possible that intraoperative monitoring may be indeed invalid, as some speculated previously (14). However, the claim against its validity is based on anecdotal data, and only randomized human studies would resolve the issue. It should be noted that intraoperative electrophysiologic monitoring is only a small aspect of SDR, and persistent skepticism about it should not negate demonstrated benefits of the surgical procedure as a whole.

OUTCOME

Certainly, a critical issue is the surgical outcome. Because of the complex nature of CP, outcome studies of dorsal rhizotomy must address changes in spasticity, quantity and quality of motor functions, rate of orthopedic surgery, quality of life, as well as postoperative complications. Assessment of one or two of the items should not lead to a sweeping conclusion as has happened (44). A brief review of the reported outcome and personal experience with SDR for treatment of spastic CP is described below.

Spasticity

The consensus is that dorsal rhizotomy substantially changes muscle tone and reduces spasticity in CP (44, 55, 63). No other current treatment changes the severity of spasticity in CP as rapidly and profoundly as does dorsal rhizotomy. Spastic diplegic patients show consistent reduction of spasticity after dorsal rhizotomy, and often spasticity is eliminated completely. The likelihood of eliminating spasticity is highest in ambulatory children with mild spastic diplegia. More important, dorsal rhizotomy produces sustained reduction of spasticity. In a follow-up study of our spastic diplegic patients for 5 to 12 years after dorsal rhizotomy, recurrent spasticity was rare.

In contrast, spastic quadriplegic patients carry a substantial risk of recurrent spasticity following dorsal rhizotomy. It seems that the risk is closely related to the severity of CP, and the risk is highest among children with severe spastic quadriplegia. For example, the majority of spastic quadriplegic children, who cannot sit alone prior to rhizotomy, develop recurrent spasticity postoperatively. This should be taken into consideration in patient selection. The studies were well intended and conducted carefully, but all three provide inconclusive data. In particular, the study by McLaughlin et al. is limited in scope and has major shortcomings.

Hence, the results of the study do not justify their sweeping conclusion that "selective dorsal rhizotomy may not be an efficacious treatment for children with mild spastic diplegia." 1) The number of patients in the study was too small, with 21 patients in the dorsal rhizotomy group and 17 patients in the physical therapy group, and the study used GMFM to assess motor functions (60). In a power analysis to estimate sample size for GMFM assessment, we found that a minimum of 40 patients in each group is required to obtain 85% power. Thus, the small number of patients could affect statistical analysis of the data. 2) The follow-up period was only 24 months, so the study has not examined long-term effects of persistent spasticity. 3) GMFM assesses only the quantity and not the quality of motor functions. Additionally, GMFM cannot accurately assess changes in motor function in individuals with high motor function prior to treatment, as was the case with these patients, nor does it assess changes in the quality of life. 4) For quantitative measure of spasticity, the study used a device that oscillates the ankle joint in an arc at different rates to elicit reflex increases in the gastrocnemius-soleus muscles. The oscillation of the ankles in an arc would produce ankle clonus of varying intensity. Prior heel cord release would certainly affect the intensity of elicited spasticity, but the authors fail to clarify how many of their patients underwent heel cord release. Also, the device examines spasticity of only the ankle joint, leaving out most of the major muscles in the lower extremities. No other group has used or validated that particular technique for studying of CP spasticity. 5) In these patients, only 26% of all rootlets tested were sectioned. Not surprisingly, ankle clonus, which is an unequivocal sign of spasticity, persisted in 21% of patients in a follow-up. In our patients with spastic diplegia, 50 to 70% of rootlets are sectioned, and persistent ankle clonus in diplegic patients is exceedingly rare. The difference in surgical techniques is another variable that most likely impacted their results.

Gait

Gait is a part of gross motor function, but gait outcome is worthy of a separate review because it is a primary concern to many parents of children with CP. Gait outcome is assessed by detailed gait analysis and ambulation status. The gait analysis quantifies cadence (steps/min), velocity (m/s), stride length (m), pelvic tilt, hip extension and abduction, knee range, and ankle range. Several groups have conducted gait analysis before and after SDR (7, 8, 67, 71, 73). In general, the gait parameters improved following dorsal rhizotomy. Hip range, knee range, stride length, and velocity improved postoperatively, and the improvements in gait were sustained up to 10 years after the procedure (67).

Cadence and coronal plane motion of pelvis and hip remained unchanged (7, 73), and the only negative change was increased anterior pelvic tilt in the independent ambulators (7).

Studies conducted before the dorsal rhizotomy era showed that the outcome of gait is closely related with the subtypes of CP and milestones of motor development. All hemiplegics walk independently, and 87 to 91% of diplegics walk with or without an assistive device (9, 45). Among quadriplegics, 27 to 72% walk with assistive devices, and many are nonambulatory (9, 45, 75). Regarding the relation of motor development to gait outcome, it was shown that all children who could sit before 24 months of age walked independently or with assistive devices; 54% of children who could sit at 24 to 36 months of age could walk with or without support; and only 29% of children who could sit after 36 months attained ambulation (9).

Thus, the age of sitting is considered a predictor of independent or assisted ambulation, but it is not a predictor of independent ambulation in particular. We found that a child's ability to perform foot dorsiflexion is a useful predictor of independent ambulation after dorsal rhizotomy (13). In our experience, virtually all children who can dorsiflex the feet bilaterally without associated simultaneous movements of other joints either before or after dorsal rhizotomy become independent walkers. If the dorsiflexion is unilateral and without associated movements of other joints, there is a high chance for the child to become an independent walker, but the gait will be significantly abnormal because of the more affected extremity. If the dorsiflexion of the feet is bilateral but associated with other joint movements, there is a good chance for household independent walking. If voluntary dorsiflexion is lacking bilaterally, independent walking after dorsal rhizotomy is impossible, and the patient will need a walker or crutches. The predictive value of foot dorsiflexion stems from the fact that loss of voluntary toe and foot movements follows mild injury to the leg motor area, and impaired knee and hip movements follow more severe injury (21).

Orthopedic Surgery

Because spasticity is a major cause of muscle contractures and deformities, reduction of spasticity following dorsal rhizotomy may reduce the rate of orthopedic surgery in spastic CP. We reported that dorsal rhizotomy performed on patients 2 to 4 years of age indeed reduces the rate of orthopedic surgery for heel cord, hamstring, and adductor releases (12). In our experience, diplegic children who underwent dorsal rhizotomy between 2 and 4 years of age and walk independently rarely require orthopedic surgery later. In contrast, many of the children who walk with assistive devices or cannot walk after dorsal rhizotomy need orthopedic surgery for muscle contractures and deformities that increase with time. The reason for this is that even in the absence of spasticity, limitations on muscle stretching in daily activities is bound to produce muscle contractures. Additionally, dorsal rhizotomy performed after 6 years of age does not improve many of the fixed deformities, and muscle and tendon releases would be required. Thus, the relatively high incidence of orthopedic surgeries after dorsal rhizotomy reported by the three groups is not surprising (4, 10, 43). Many patients undergoing dorsal rhizotomy should have orthopedic follow-up.

Hip Deformities

Hip subluxation is a common problem in children with spastic CP, occurring in 3 to 59% of patients (42, 62). Hip subluxation tends to progress in children younger than 5 years who undergo remodeling of the hips (28, 74). The etiology of the hip deformities is multifactorial, but predominant spasticity in hip adductor and iliopsoas muscles combined with lack of normal weight-bearing play contributes to development of the hip deformities. By decreasing spasticity, dorsal rhizotomy may decrease the incidence of hip subluxation in children with CP. We examined changes in lateral hip migration in spastic diplegic and quadriplegic children undergoing SDR. First, 67 diplegics who were 2 to 11 years old at the time of surgery were followed for 6 to 46 months. Of all hips examined radiographically, 75% remained unchanged, 17% improved, and 7% worsened (53). Next, 45 quadriplegics were examined in a similar manner. In this group of children, 80% of hips remained unchanged, 9% improved, and 11% worsened (30). The results compare favorably to those of orthopedic surgeries (35) and indicate that SDR can stabilize the hips in spastic diplegic and quadriplegic children. It should be emphasized that some children show progressive hip subluxation after dorsal rhizotomy (25).

Long-Term Outcome

Long-term outcome of SDR was reported by a group in Cape Town, South Africa (4, 67). Fifty-one children with spastic CP who underwent dorsal rhizotomy 3 to 7 years before were studied. Ages at the time of dorsal rhizotomy ranged from 20 months to 14 years. They found that spasticity remained reduced in all patients, motor function continued to improve in 80%, sensory disturbances were insignificant, and 47% required orthopedic surgeries to improve further their functions (4). Others have also reported on long-term results (49). Repeat gait analysis 10 years after dorsal rhizotomy in children with spastic diplegia demonstrated sustained improvements of hip and knee ranges of motion, step length, and velocity (67).

MORBIDITY

The risk of SDR is low, and postoperative morbidity is within acceptable range. It is clear that the benefit of dorsal rhizotomy greatly outweighs the risks. Intraoperative untoward events are mild hyperthermia, cardiac arrhythmia, and bronchospasm; these are uncommon and inconsequential (72). Virtually all patients experience severe dysesthetic pain for 2 to 3 days and paresthesia in the lower extremities for a week. Potential early postoperative complications include severe motor weakness, neurogenic bladder, CSF leak, meningitis, ileus, bronchospasm, pneumonia, and urinary tract infection. Late complications include sensory loss, hyperesthesia, back pain, and postlaminectomy spinal deformities (1, 66). Progressive hip subluxation and heterotopic ossification near the osteotomized femur have been attributed to dorsal rhizotomy, although a causal relation remains to be established (25, 54).

The early neurologic complications are rare. In our series of 690 patients, we have not encountered motor weakness, CSF leak, meningitis, or neurogenic bladder, but a small number of patients developed bronchospasm, pneumonia, or urinary tract infection. Only two patients were hospitalized slightly longer than the usual 6 to 7 days because of pneumonia. Others have reported similar results (72).

The late morbidities, i.e., motor weakness, sensory loss, urinary incontinence, and spinal problems, are of primary concern. Late motor weakness directly related to dorsal rhizotomy has not occurred among our patients. Deterioration of motor functions years after dorsal rhizotomy does occur, but it always results from preexistent motor impairments and associated muscle contractures and deformities. Persistent sensory diminution of no clinical significance was seen in 3.8% of patients (66). Typically, the sensory abnormality is confined to a small area, and patients are often unaware of it. Loss of proprioception attributed to dorsal rhizotomy never occurred in our patients.

Persistent neurogenic bladder requiring intermittent catheterization that was attributed to dorsal rhizotomy occurred in 14.4% (2). Others have noted this complication in 1.3% (66). None of our patients required intermittent catheterization for more than 3 days after the procedure. Our experience is in agreement with that of others (72).

Spinal deformities, i.e., spondylosis, spondylolisthesis (58), lumbar spinal stenosis (23), and lumbar hyperlordosis (15), have been attributed to dorsal rhizotomy performed through a lumbosacral laminectomy or laminotomy. In a series of 99 patients, 20% developed isthmic spondylolysis or grade I spondylolisthesis following five-level lumbosacral laminectomies (58). The isthmic defects in 19 children involved L3–4, L4–5, or L5–S1 levels. Six children had spondylolisthesis. The majority of patients were ambulatory and active.

Spinal stenosis was seen in 1.5% of patients undergoing dorsal rhizotomy through a multilevel laminectomy or laminotomy (23). The spinal deformity became symptomatic 2 to 4 years after the operation and required decompressive procedures to relieve symptoms. Severe lumbar hyperlordosis was reported to occur in two adults with spastic quadriplegia who underwent multilevel laminectomies for dorsal rhizotomy (15). We have performed dorsal rhizotomies through an L1 or L1–2 laminectomy on 542 patients since 1991. Thus far, none of our patients has developed any spinal problem; our experience suggests that the risk of postrhizotomy spinal deformities is very low in patients undergoing dorsal rhizotomy through a limited laminectomy, as detailed previously (52).

INDICATIONS

Indications for SDR vary with centers. Our current indications for SDR are illustrated in *Table 23.4.* The primary indication for SDR is spastic diplegia and quadriplegia secondary to premature birth (*Table 23.5*). In spastic hemiplegic CP, spasticity is not a major cause of motor impairment, and reduction of spasticity does not significantly improve motor function.

Spasticity should be evident clinically and inhibit motor activities, especially walking. Ideally, patients should have sufficient motor strength and potential to make significant gains in motor functions postoperatively (*Table 23.6*). In some patients with spastic quadriplegia, dorsal rhizotomy is performed to improve sitting posture and upper extremity movements. In patients who are deemed likely to have no postoperative functional gains due to severe motor impairment, we do not recommend dorsal rhizotomy.

The optimal age for dorsal rhizotomy is 2 to 5 years (*Table 23.7*). SDR is not recommended for children under the age of 2 years because the di-

TABLE 23.4
Indications for Selective Dorsal Rhizotomy

Diagnosis—spastic diplegia or quadriplegia
Age—2 to 45 years
History of premature birth or neonatal asphyxia
Bilateral schizencephaly underlying spastic diplegia
Emerging locomotive functions
Potential for significant postoperative functional gains

TABLE 23.5
Subtypes of Spastic CP in 690 Patients Who Underwent Selective Dorsal Rhizotomy: SLCH Series 1987–1999

CP Subtypes	No. of Patients	%
Diplegia	527	76
Quadriplegia	154	22
Triplegia	7	<1
Hemiplegia	2	<1
Total	690	100

agnosis of CP is often erroneous at early ages (47). Early dorsal rhizotomy would minimize deleterious effects of spasticity on developing muscles and hence alleviate orthopedic deformities of the lower extremities. Adolescents and adults can also benefit from dorsal rhizotomy (57). The oldest patient in our series was 38 years old.

Some neurosurgeons consider high motivation and intelligence to be criteria for selection of patients. We do not include them in the selection criteria but regard them as factors favoring a good outcome. Walking ability in children is often dissociated from the intelligence level. Thus, many children with CP and mental retardation can walk independently whether or not they undergo dorsal rhizotomy. If a child appears to be motivated to execute motor activities, e.g., walking, it reflects preservation of the motor system rather than high motivation alone.

Prior orthopedic operations and orthopedic deformities must be taken into account in selecting patients. In patients with prior orthopedic operations, the released muscle is always weak to some degree, and full muscle strength cannot be restored in most cases. The muscle weakness will prevent certain kinds of functional gains that would otherwise follow dorsal rhizotomy. This possibility should be ascertained

TABLE 23.6
Prerhizotomy Ambulatory Functions in 690 Patients Who Underwent Selective Dorsal Rhizotomy for Spastic Cerebral Palsy: SLCH Series 1987–1999

Walking Ability	No. of Patients	%
Walking with walker	251	36
Walking with crutches or cane	38	6
Independent walking	199	29
Some locomotion	102	15
Crawling	81	12
No independent mobility	19	<3
Total	966	100

TABLE 23.7
Age At Time of Selective Dorsal Rhizotomy for Spastic Cerebral Palsy: SLCH Series 1987–1999

Age (Years)	No. of Patients	%
2–6	537	78
7–10	96	14
11–18	43	6
19–38	14	2
Total	690	100

during the preoperative evaluation. In general, however, dorsal rhizotomy improves mobility and gross motor functions even in patients with prior orthopedic surgeries.

Spinal deformities associated with CP include lumbar lordosis, spondylolysis, spondylolisthesis, and scoliosis. The spinal deformities are not a contraindication for dorsal rhizotomy performed through a single-level laminectomy. However, spinal deformities would preclude dorsal rhizotomy performed through a multilevel laminectomy or laminotomy.

In selection of adult patients over 18 years of age for rhizotomy, we take additional factors into consideration. Patients should ambulate independently or with crutches, have only mild fixed orthopedic deformities, experience no back pain, be committed to postoperative strengthening exercises, and be free of other major medical problems, including psychiatric disorders.

CONTRAINDICATIONS

If congenital hydrocephalus, neonatal bacterial meningitis, intrauterine encephalitis such as toxoplasmosis and cytomegalovirus infection, severe head trauma, and brain injury following drowning underlie the diagnosis of CP, SDR is not recommended (*Table 23.8*) because these disorders are likely associated with dystonia and rigidity as well as spasticity. The presence of extensive neuronal migration disorder is another contraindication. It should be noted, however, that schizencephaly involving the motor area is a rare cause of spastic diplegia, and these patients can show reduction of spasticity and functional improvements after dorsal rhizotomy. Severe basal ganglia damage following perinatal difficulties is a contraindication in young children under the age of 5 years. Dystonia manifests during the first 5 years of age. After age 5, however, dorsal rhizotomy can be considered even in the presence of demonstrable basal ganglia damage if spasticity is an overwhelming problem.

Predominant athetosis, ataxia, and dystonia are also contraindications. However, if spasticity concomitant with athetosis and dystonia

TABLE 23.8
Contraindications for Selective Dorsal Rhizotomy

CP associated with intrauterine encephalitis
Mixed CP with predominant dystonia, rigidity, athetosis, or ataxia
Spastic hemiplegia
CP due to widespread neuronal migration disorder
Severe head injury and hypoxic encephalopathy, e.g., after drowning, as a cause of CP
Familial spastic paraplegia and other progressive neurologic disorders
Severe basal ganglia damage in children younger than 5 years
Severe thoracolumbar scoliosis
Severe lumbar lordosis
Multiple prior muscle and tendon releases
Profound motor impairment with no head control
Psychiatric disorder in adults
Lack of commitment to carry out postoperative therapy

inhibits motor activities, dorsal rhizotomy can be offered. Dorsal rhizotomy in such children reduces spasticity, but their athetosis and dystonia remain unchanged postoperatively.

The presence of scoliosis, lumbar lordosis, and spondylolisthesis precludes dorsal rhizotomy performed through a multilevel lumbosacral laminectomy. However, these spinal deformities do not contraindicate dorsal rhizotomy performed through a single-level laminectomy.

In adults, severe depression and other psychiatric disorders are considered contraindications.

CONCLUSIONS

Information accumulated in the past decade strongly favors SDR as an excellent treatment option for many patients with spastic CP. The value of intraoperative electrophysiologic monitoring is still unproven. It is clear that SDR can produce a sustained reduction of spasticity, and long-term morbidity of the procedure is minimal. At this time, SDR is the only treatment available that can permanently reduce CP spasticity. Accumulated data on the surgical outcome is overwhelmingly in favor of SDR. In light of the available information, physicians caring for patients with CP have an obligation to inform them of SDR when discussing treatment options. Future investigations should further refine criteria for selection of appropriate candidates for SDR, examine long-term benefits of SDR, and explore the utilization of SDR for adult patients.

REFERENCES

1. Abbott R: Complications with selective posterior rhizotomy. **Pediatr Neurosurg** 18:43–47, 1992.

2. Abbott R, Johann-Murphy M, Shiminski-Maher T, Quartermain D, Forem SL, Gold JT, Epstein FJ: Selective dorsal rhizotomy: Outcome and complications in treating spastic cerebral palsy. **Neurosurgery** 33:851–857, 1993.
3. Albright AL, Cervi A, Singletary J: Intrathecal baclofen for spasticity in cerebral palsy. **JAMA** 265:1418–1422, 1991.
4. Arens LJ, Peacock WJ, Peter J: Selective posterior rhizotomy: A long-term follow-up study. **Childs Nerv Syst** 5:148–152, 1989.
5. Bax MC: Terminology and classification of cerebral palsy. **Dev Med Child Neurol** 6:295–307, 1964.
6. Bleck EE: *Orthopaedic Management in Cerebral Palsy.* London, MacKeith Press, 1987, pp 1–497.
7. Boscarino LF, Ounpuu S, Davis RB, Gage JR, DeLuca PA: Effects of selective dorsal rhizotomy on gait in children with cerebral palsy. **J Pediatr Orthop** 13:174–179, 1993.
8. Cahan L, Adams J, Perry J, Beeler L: Instrumented gait analysis after selective dorsal rhizotomy. **Dev Med Child Neurol** 32:1037–1043, 1990.
9. Campos da Paz A, Burnett SM, Braga LW: Walking prognosis in cerebral palsy: A 22-year retrospective analysis. **Dev Med Child Neurol** 36:130–134, 1994.
10. Carroll KL, Moore KR, Stevens PM: Orthopedic procedures after rhizotomy. **J Pediatr Orthop** 18:69–74, 1998.
11. Castle ME, Reyman TA, Schneider M: Pathology of spastic muscle in cerebral palsy. **Clin Orthop** 142:223–233, 1979.
12. Chicoine MR, Park TS, Kaufman BA: Selective dorsal rhizotomy and rates of orthopedic surgery in children with spastic cerebral palsy. **J Neurosurg** 86:34–39, 1997.
13. Chicoine MR, Park TS, Vogler GP, Kaufman BA: Predictors of ability to walk after selective dorsal rhizotomy in children with cerebral palsy. **Neurosurgery** 38:711–714, 1996.
14. Cohen AR, Webster HC: How selective is selective posterior rhizotomy? **Surg Neurol** 35:267–272, 1991.
15. Crawford K, Karol LA, Herring JA: Severe lumbar lordosis after dorsal rhizotomy. **J Pediatr Orthopaedics** 16:336–339, 1996.
16. Decandia M, Provini L, Taborikova H: Mechanisms of the reflex discharge depression in the spinal motoneurone during repetitive orthodromic stimulation. **Brain Res** 4:284–291, 1967.
17. Engsberg JR, Olree KS, Ross SA, Park TS: Spasticity and strength changes as a function of selective dorsal rhizotomy. **J Neurosurg** 88:1020–1026, 1998.
18. Fasano VA, Barolat-Romana G, Zeme S, Sguazzi A: Electrophysiological assessment of spinal circuits in spasticity by direct dorsal root stimulation. **Neurosurg** 4:146–151, 1979.
19. Fasano V, Urciuoli R, Broggi G, Barolat-Romana G, Benech F, Ivaldi A, Sguazzi A: New aspects in the surgical treatment of cerebral palsy. **Acta Neurochir Suppl** 24:53–57, 1977.
20. Foerster O: On the indications and results of the excision of posterior spinal nerve roots in men. **Surg Gynecol Obstet** 16:463–474, 1913.
21. Foerster O: The motor cortex in man in the light of Hughlings Jackson's doctrines. **Brain** 59:135–159, 1936.
22. Goldspink G, Tabary C, Tabary JC, Tardieu C, Tardieu G: Effect of denervation on the adaptation of sarcomere number and muscle extensibility to the functional length of the muscle. **J Physiol** 236:733–742, 1974.

23. Gooch JL, Walker ML: Spinal stenosis after total lumbar laminectomy for selective dorsal rhizotomy. **Pediatr Neurosurg** 25:28–30, 1996.
24. Gottlieb GL, Myklebust BM, Penn RD, Agarwal GC: Reciprocal excitation of muscle antagonists by the primary afferent pathway. **Exp Brain Res** 46:454–456, 1982.
25. Greene WB, Dietz FR, Goldberg MJ, Gross RH, Miller F, Sussman MD: Rapid progression of hip subluxation in cerebral palsy after selective posterior rhizotomy. **J Pediatr Orthop** 11:494–497, 1991.
26. Grether JK, Cummins SK, Nelson KB: The California cerebral palsy project. **Paediatr Perinat Epidemiol** 6:339–351, 1992.
27. Gros C: Spasticity-clinical classification and surgical treatment. **Acta Neurol Scand Suppl** 42:55–97, 1966.
28. Harris NH, Lloyd-Roberts GC, Gallien R: Acetabular development in congenital dislocation of the hip. **J Bone Joint Surg** 57B:46–52, 1975.
29. Hayat A, Tardieu C, Tabary JC, Tabary C: Effects of denervation on the reduction of sarcomere number in cat soleus muscle immobilized in shortened position during seven days. **J Physiol (Lond)** 74:563–567, 1978.
30. Heim RC, Park TS, Vogler GP, Kaufman BA, Noetzel MJ, Ortman MR: Changes in hip migration after selective dorsal rhizotomy for spastic quadriplegia in cerebral palsy. **J Neurosurg** 82:567–571, 1995.
31. Hoffer MM, Knoebel RT, Roberts R: Contractures in cerebral palsy. **Clin Orthop** 219:70–77, 1987.
32. Holly RG, Barnett JG, Ashmore CR, Taylor RG, Mole PA: Stretch-induced growth in chicken wing muscles: A new model of stretch hypertrophy. **Am J Physiol** 238:C62–C71, 1980.
33. Huet de la Tour E, Tabary JC, Tabary C, Tardieu C: The respective roles of muscle length and muscle tension in sarcomere number adaptation of guinea-pig soleus muscle. **J Physiol (Lond)** 75:589–592, 1979.
34. Jackson ST, Hoffer MM, Parrish N: Brachial-plexus palsy in the newborn. **J Bone Joint Surg** 70A:1217–1220, 1988.
35. Kalen V, Bleck E: Prevention of spastic paralytic dislocation of the hip. **Dev Med Child Neurol** 27:17–24, 1985.
36. Knutson LM, Clark DE: Orthotic devices for ambulation in children with cerebral palsy and myelomeningocele. **Phys Ther** 71:947–960, 1991.
37. Koman LA, Mooney JF, Smith BP, Goodman A, Mulvaney T: Management of spasticity in cerebral palsy with botulinum-A toxin: Report of a preliminary randomized, double-blind trial. **J Pediatr Orthop** 14:299–303, 1994.
38. Kuban KC, Leviton A: Cerebral palsy. **N Engl J Med** 330:188–195, 1994.
39. Landau W, Hunt C: Dorsal rhizotomy: A treatment of unproven efficacy. **J Child Neurol** 5:174–178, 1990.
40. Lloyd DP: Monosynaptic reflex response of individual motoneurons as a function of frequency. **J Gen Physiol** 40:435–450, 1957.
41. Logigian EL, Shefner JM, Goumnerova L, Scott RM, Soriano SG, Madsen J: The critical importance of stimulus intensity in intraoperative monitoring for partial dorsal rhizotomy. **Muscle Nerve** 19:415–422, 1996.
42. Lonstein JE, Beck K: Hip dislocation and subluxation in cerebral palsy. **J Pediatr Orthop** 6:521–526, 1986.
43. Marty GR, Dias LS, Gaebler-Spira D: Selective posterior rhizotomy and soft-tissue procedures for the treatment of cerebral diplegia. **J Bone Joint Surg** 77:713–718, 1995.
44. McLaughlin JF, Bjornson KF, Astley SJ, Graubert C, Hays RM, Roberts TS, Price R,

Temkin N: Selective dorsal rhizotomy: Efficacy and safety in an investigator-masked randomized clinical trial. **Dev Med Child Neurol** 40:220–232, 1998.
45. Molnar GE, Gordon SU: Cerebral palsy: Predictive value of selected clinical signs for early prognostication of motor function. **Arch Phys Med Rehabil** 57:153–158, 1976.
46. Murphy KP, Molnar GE, Lankasky K: Medical and functional status of adults with cerebral palsy. **Dev Med Child Neurol** 37:1075–1084, 1995.
47. Nelson KB, Ellenberg JH: Children who "outgrew" cerebral palsy. **Pediatrics** 69:529–536, 1982.
48. Newacheck PW, Taylor WR: Childhood chronic illness: Prevalence, severity, and impact. **Am J Public Health** 82:364–371, 1992.
49. Nishida T, Thatcher SW, Marty GR: Selective posterior rhizotomy for children with cerebral palsy: A 7-year experience. **Childs Nerv Syst** 11:374–380, 1995.
50. Oppenheim WL: Selective posterior rhizotomy for spastic cerebral palsy: A review. **Clin Orthop** 253:20–29, 1990.
51. Paine RS: On the treatment of cerebral palsy: The outcome of 177 patients, 74 totally untreated. **Pediatrics** 605–616, 1962.
52. Park TS: Selective dorsal rhizotomy for the spasticity of cerebral palsy. **Neurosurg Oper Atlas** 4:183–190, 1995.
53. Park TS, Vogler GP, Phillips LH II, Kaufman BA, Ortman MR, McClure SM, Gaffney PE: Effects of selective dorsal rhizotomy for spastic diplegia on hip migration in cerebral palsy. **Pediatr Neurosurg** 20:43–49, 1994.
54. Payne LZ, DeLuca PA: Heterotopic ossification after rhizotomy and femoral osteotomy. **J Pediatr Orthop** 13:733–738, 1993.
55. Peacock W, Staudt L: Functional outcomes following selective posterior rhizotomy in children with cerebral palsy. **J Neurosurg** 74:380–385, 1991.
56. Peacock WJ, Arens LJ: Selective posterior rhizotomy for the relief of spasticity in cerebral palsy. **S Afr Med J** 62:119–124, 1982.
57. Peter JC, Arens LJ: Selective posterior lumbosacral rhizotomy in teenagers and young adults with spastic cerebral palsy. **Br J Neurosurg** 8:135–139, 1994.
58. Peter JC, Hoffman EB, Arens LJ: Spondylolysis and spondylolisthesis after five-level lumbosacral laminectomy for selective posterior rhizotomy in cerebral palsy. **Childs Nerv Syst** 9:285–288, 1993.
59. Rosen MG, Dickinson JC: The incidence of cerebral palsy. **Am J Obstet Gynecol** 167:417–423, 1992.
60. Russell DJ, Rosenbaum PL, Cadman DT, Gowland C, Hardy S, Jarvis S: The gross motor function measure: A means to evaluate the effects of physical therapy. **Dev Med Child Neurol** 31:341–352, 1989.
61. Sahrmann SA, Norton BJ: The relationship of voluntary movement to spasticity in the upper motor neuron syndrome. **Ann Neurol** 2:460–465, 1977.
62. Samilson RL, Tsou P, Aamoth G, Green WM: Dislocation and subluxation of the hip in cerebral palsy. **J Bone Joint Surg** 54A:863–873, 1972.
63. Steinbok P, Gustavsson B, Kestle JR, Reiner A, Cochrane DD: Relationship of intraoperative electrophysiological criteria to outcome after selective functional posterior rhizotomy. **J Neurosurg** 83:18–26, 1995.
64. Steinbok P, Kestle JR: Variation between centers in electrophysiologic techniques used in lumbosacral selective dorsal rhizotomy for spastic cerebral palsy. **Pediatr Neurosurg** 25:233–239, 1996.
65. Steinbok P, Reiner AM, Beauchamp R, Armstrong RW, Cochrane DD: A randomized clinical trial to compare selective posterior rhizotomy plus physiotherapy with

physiotherapy alone in children with spastic diplegic cerebral palsy. **Dev Med Child Neurol** 39:178–184, 1997.

66. Steinbok P, Schrag C: Complications after selective posterior rhizotomy for spasticity in children with cerebral palsy. **Pediatr Neurosurg** 28:300–313, 1998.
67. Subramanian N, Vaughan CL, Peter JC, Arens LJ: Gait before and 10 years after rhizotomy in children with cerebral palsy spasticity. **J Neurosurg** 88:1014–1019, 1998.
68. Syer-Acevedo J: Physical therapy for the child with cerebral palsy. **Pediatr Phys Ther** 89–134, 1994.
69. Tabary JC, Tardieu C: Experimental rapid sarcomere loss with concomitant hypoextensibility. **Muscle Nerve** 4:198–203, 1981.
70. Tardieu C, Huet de la Tour E, Bret MD, Tardieu G: Muscle hypoextensibility in children with cerebral palsy: I. Clinical and experimental observations. **Arch Phys Med Rehabil** 63:97–102, 1982.
71. Thomas SS, Aiona MD, Pierce R, Piatt JH: Gait changes in children with spastic diplegia after selective dorsal rhizotomy. **J Pediatr Orthop** 16:747–752, 1996.
72. Van De Wiele BM, Staudt L, Rubinstien EH, Nuwer M, Peacock WJ: Perioperative complications in children undergoing selective posterior rhizotomy: A review of 105 cases. **Paediatr Anaesth** 6:479–486, 1996.
73. Vaughan C, Berman B, Peacock W: Cerebral palsy rhizotomy: A 3-year follow-up evaluation with gaits analysis. **J Neurosurg** 74:178–184, 1991.
74. Vidal J, Deguillaume P, Vidal M: The anatomy of the dysplastic hip in cerebral palsy related to prognosis and treatment. **Int Orthop** 9:105–110, 1985.
75. Watt JM, Robertson CM, Grace MG: Early prognosis for ambulation of neonatal intensive care survivors with cerebral palsy. **Dev Med Child Neurol** 31:766–773, 1989.
76. Williams PE, Goldspink G: Longitudinal growth of striated muscle fibres. **J Cell Sci** 9:751–767, 1971.
77. Wright FV, Sheil EM, Drake JM, Wedge JH, Naumann S: Evaluation of selective dorsal rhizotomy for the reduction of spasticity in cerebral palsy: A randomized controlled trial. **Dev Med Child Neurol** 40:239–247, 1998 (comment).
78. Ziv I, Blackburn N, Rang M, Koreska J: Muscle growth in normal and spastic mice. **Dev Med Child Neurol** 26:94–99, 1984.

CHAPTER

24

Baclofen Infusion for Spastic Cerebral Palsy

PAUL STEINBOK, M.B.B.S., B.SC, F.R.C.S.C.,
MAUREEN O'DONNELL, M.D., M.SC., F.R.C.P.C.

Intrathecal baclofen, which was first introduced by Penn and Kroin (42) in 1984, is well established as an effective treatment of spasticity of both spinal and cerebral origin. In the adult population, the treatment is used predominantly for spasticity of spinal origin. This review focuses on the use of intrathecal baclofen for treatment of spasticity in children. In the pediatric population, spasticity is almost always of cerebral origin, and occurs most commonly in the context of a diagnosis of cerebral palsy.

NATURE OF MOTOR DISORDER IN SPASTIC CEREBRAL PALSY

The motor disorder in children with spastic cerebral palsy is complex, and results from a combination of spasticity, weakness, incoordination, excessive reflex irradiation, muscle and joint contractures, and impaired sensory perception. The spasticity is but one element of an upper motor neuron syndrome. Invariably there is associated weakness and usually some incoordination of the affected limbs. Increased tone is usually not the result of spasticity alone, and there is typically some dystonia or athetosis in addition to the spasticity. In children with spastic quadriplegia, the hypertonia may be more the result of rigidity than spasticity, and because of the therapeutic implications, it is important to determine how much of the hypertonia is attributed to spasticity. Spasticity implies a velocity-dependent increase in muscle tone, typically demonstrated as a clasp-knife response, and is associated with exaggerated deep tendon reflexes. In addition to the spasticity and weakness, children with spastic cerebral palsy demonstrate reflex irradiation to other muscle groups, which results in difficulty isolating movements in the affected limbs. They have cocontraction of agonists and antagonists, rather than the normal pattern in which antagonists of contracting muscles relax. They also demonstrate mirror movements, such that, for example, when they try to extend the knee on one side, the other knee extends at the same time. As the child gets older, contractures and deformities of the spine and extremities often develop, with hip dislocations, knee flexion contractures, rocker bottom feet, and scoliosis commonly adding to the motor disability.

BACLOFEN

Baclofen (β-[4-chlorophenyl]-GABA) is a synthetic gamma-aminobutyric acid (GABA) agonist that acts selectively on both pre- and postsynaptic $GABA_B$ receptors to reduce excitatory synaptic transmission. Activation of presynaptic $GABA_B$ receptors by baclofen results in a decreased release of excitatory neurotransmitters, such as glutamate and aspartate, but the mechanism for this effect is not clear (22). Most studies have suggested that the presynaptic effect of baclofen is related to a restriction of calcium influx into the presynaptic terminals. Activation of postsynaptic $GABA_B$ receptors by baclofen causes increased potassium conductance at postsynaptic terminals, which results in prolonged hyperpolarization of the neuronal membrane and decreased neuronal activity (22).

$GABA_B$ receptors are located throughout the central nervous system but are particularly concentrated in the thalamus and in layers II and III of the dorsal gray matter of the spinal cord (45). Baclofen relieves spasticity by its action on the spinal cord receptors, whereas the major side effects of sedation and respiratory depression reflect the supraspinal effects of the drug.

ORAL BACLOFEN

Baclofen has been used orally since the early 1970s as an antispastic agent. The drug is absorbed well after oral administration but has low lipid solubility and does not cross the blood–brain barrier readily (1). The usual starting dose in children is 5 to 10 mg daily in three divided doses, working up to doses as high as 160 mg daily, with the usual therapeutic doses in the range of 40 to 60 mg/d (1). Oral baclofen has been shown in a number of randomized controlled studies involving children and adults to improve spasticity associated with spinal cord lesions (39). Oral baclofen has not been as effective in reducing spasticity of cerebral origin, and specifically in children with cerebral palsy (39). The value of oral baclofen has been limited by the common occurrence of sedation at the dose levels needed for relief of spasticity. Other less frequent side effects have included behavioral changes, confusion, ataxia, urinary frequency, and insomnia (1, 39). These limiting adverse effects are probably related to the effects of baclofen on intracranial $GABA_B$ receptors.

INTRATHECAL BACLOFEN

Because the target site of action for relief of spasticity by baclofen is the $GABA_B$ receptors in the superficial layers of the spinal cord, and baclofen does not cross the blood–brain barrier readily, it was rationalized that direct instillation of the drug into the spinal subarachnoid fluid might relieve spasticity, while minimizing the centrally mediated side effects. Lumbar cerebrospinal fluid (CSF) levels of baclofen with oral administration of doses as high as 100 mg/d were never more than 12 ng/ml (24, 36). With continuous intrathecal infusions of baclofen of 50 to 1200 μg/d in patients, lumbar CSF baclofen levels ranged from 130 to 950 ng/ml (36). Intraspinal subarachnoid baclofen does diffuse in a cephalad direction in the CSF by bulk flow, as does any hydrophilic compound. With a continuous infusion into the subarachnoid space at the L1 level, the concentration in the cisterna magna is one-quarter of that in the lumbar subarachnoid space (28), which explains why the effect is more marked in the lower than the upper limbs. Because the concentrations of baclofen typically achieved with continuous intrathecal infusions are 10 to 80 times that present after oral administration, and the CSF levels at the level of the cisterna magna are only one-quarter of those in the lumbar CSF, other factors have to be hypothesized to explain why sedation is seen relatively infrequently with intrathecal baclofen. It may be that the intracranial $GABA_B$ receptors are not as close to the surface as the spinal $GABA_B$ receptors, and because the baclofen diffuses poorly into neural tissue, the baclofen tissue concentration at the intracranial receptor sites is relatively less than at the spinal receptor sites (38).

A bolus injection of intrathecal baclofen at the T12 level typically reduces lower limb spasticity in approximately 60 minutes, affects upper extremities by approximately 2 hours, has its maximal effect at approximately 4 hours, and the effect wears off by 8 to 10 hours (7, 35). There is wide individual variation in the pharmacokinetics of intrathecal baclofen, with the elimination half-life ranging from 0.9 to 5 hours (43, 48). To achieve a clinically useful, prolonged effect, intrathecal baclofen must be administered by continuous infusion via an implanted pump.

PUMP TECHNOLOGY

Two basic types of implantable pumps are available: programmable and nonprogrammable. In children with spasticity of cerebral origin, the severity of spasticity tends to fluctuate and the ability to program the rate of infusion of intrathecal baclofen is often helpful. The only programmable pump available, the Synchromed pump (Medtronic, Inc., Minneapolis, MN; (*Fig. 24.1*), is a battery-powered pump. It is adjusted

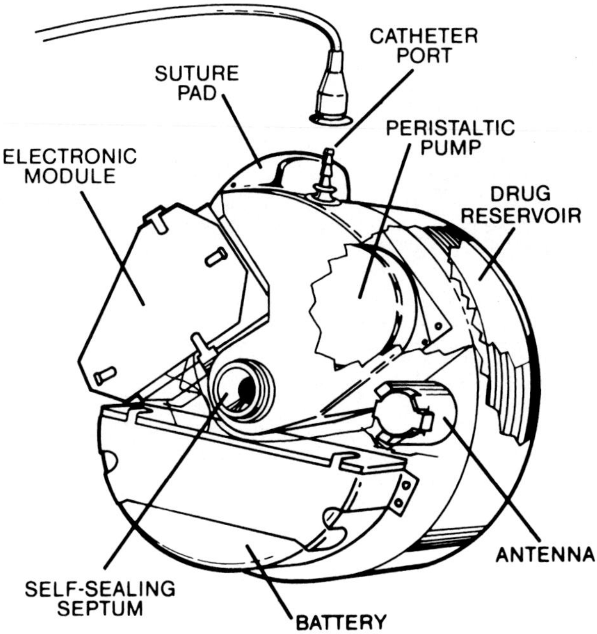

FIG. 24.1 Line drawing showing the essential features of the Synchromed programmable pump. Courtesy, Medtronic, Inc., Minneapolis, MN.

using a radiofrequency-controlled external wand and programming computer (*Fig. 24.2*) to deliver variable flow rates, either continuous and/or bolus infusions, or a set total dose. The pump is powered by a lithium thionyl–chloride battery, which lasts for 5 to 7 years, at which time the pump must be replaced. The pump contains a drug reservoir and is covered by a titanium casing with a central aperture that can be punctured for filling of the chamber. The standard pump, with an 18-ml reservoir, has a diameter of 7.5 cm and a thickness of 2.8 cm, approximately the size of an ice hockey puck. The pediatric version has the same diameter, but is 2.3 cm in thickness and the reservoir has a capacity of 10 ml.

The nonprogrammable implantable pumps, such as the Arrow (Arrow International, Inc., Reading, PA), Isomed (Medtronic, Inc., Minneapolis, MN), and Anschutz (Tricumed GmbH, Kiel, Germany) pumps (*Fig. 24.3*) deliver a fixed flow rate, and work by expressing fluid by expansion of a propellant gas, which is compressed by refilling the pump. In the nonprogrammable pumps, the rate of infusion is set by the manufacturer and the inability to change the rate is a major disadvantage. These pumps do have the advantage that, in theory, they have an in-

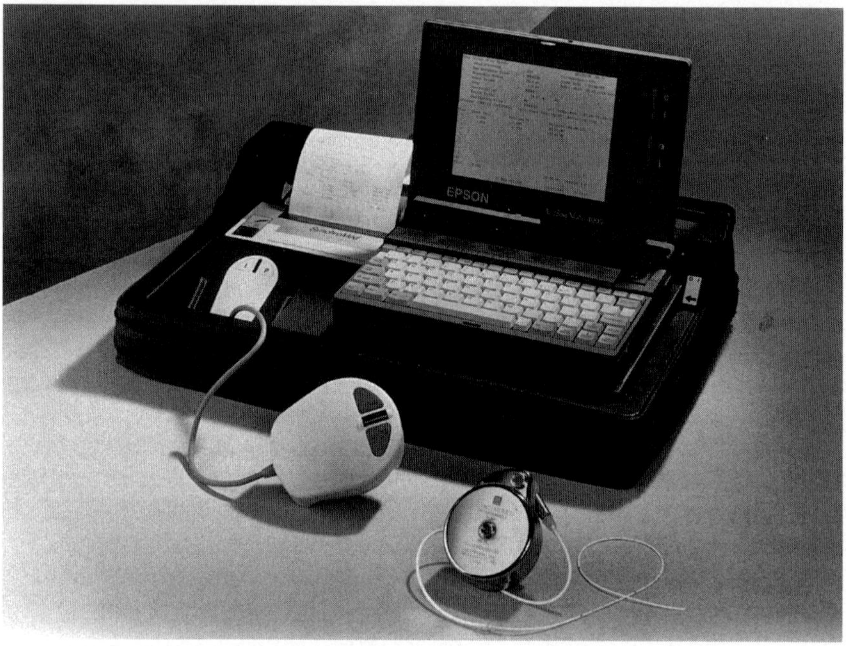

FIG. 24.2 The programming device and computer for the Synchromed pump, with a Synchromed pump and attached catheter in the foreground. Courtesy, Medtronic, Inc., Minneapolis, MN.

definite life span, but in practice, the pumps usually have to be replaced because of some malfunction within 10 years. The nonprogrammable pumps are more tapered than the Synchromed pump, and may be easier to implant in a small child. The delivery systems cost between US $5000 and US $10,000 at the time of writing, with the programmable Synchromed pump costing slightly more than the nonprogrammable pumps.

In most centers a screening trial of injections of baclofen into the spinal subarachnoid space is performed to determine which patients are likely to benefit from continuous intrathecal baclofen. Responders to this preliminary trial have a pump implanted for long-term continuous infusion. In children with spasticity, the screening trial involves boluses of intrathecal baclofen, which may be administered using repeated lumbar punctures to inject the drug, or by repeated injections into a lumbar subarachnoid catheter coming externally or into an implanted reservoir attached to a lumbar subarachnoid catheter. The tone in the limbs is assessed by a physiotherapist, before and at multiple

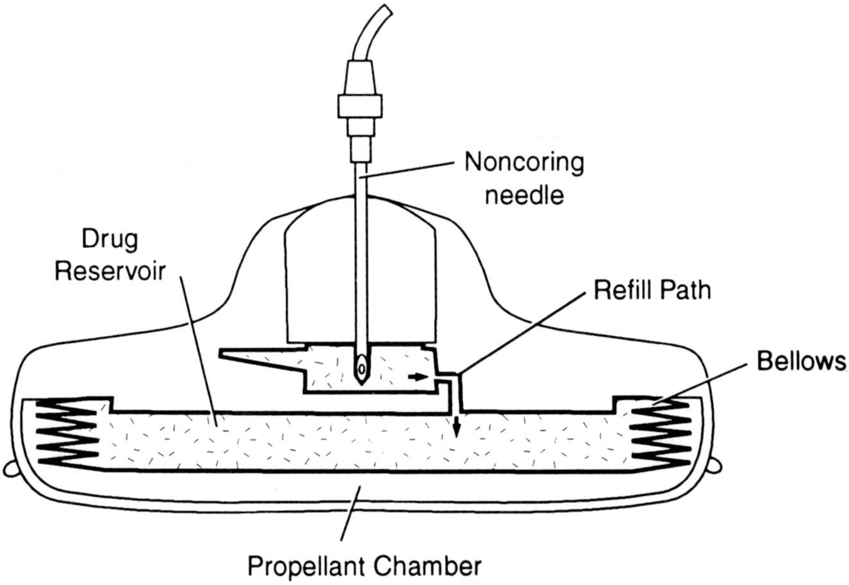

FIG. 24.3 Line drawing showing the essential features of the Arrow nonprogrammable pump. Other nonprogrammable pumps use a similar mechanism.

time periods during the first 8 hours after each bolus injection, using a quantitative scale such as the Ashworth scale (*Table 24.1*). During this trial it is important to avoid being misled by a placebo effect, and often placebo and baclofen are injected in a blinded fashion. This is particularly important in patients whose tone fluctuates from time to time. In most patients in whom there is a response to the intrathecal bolus of baclofen, the spasticity is reduced so dramatically that a placebo trial may appear superfluous, and some workers no longer use a placebo control (2). The initial dose of baclofen is usually 25 μg, and it can be doubled each day to a maximum of 100 μg until a response is achieved or it is determined that the patient is a nonresponder. In children with cerebral palsy, muscle tone in the lower extremities decreased by 1 point or more on the Ashworth scale, which was considered to be clinically significant, in 68% of patients after a 25-μg dose, and in an additional 17% of patients after a 50- or 100-μg dose of baclofen (1). The response to intrathecal boluses of baclofen is useful in determining whether the patient is likely to respond to a continuous intrathecal infusion, but the response does not predict the functional outcome with continuous intrathecal baclofen (2).

TABLE 24.1
Ashworth Scale for Grading Spasticity

Score	Definition
0	Hypotonic: less than normal muscle tone, floppy
1	Normal: no increase in muscle tone
2	Mild: slight increase in tone, "catch" in limb movement or minimal resistance to movement through less than half the range
3	Moderate: more marked increase in tone through most of the range of motion but affected part is easily moved
4	Severe: considerable increase in tone, passive movement difficult
5	Extreme: affected part rigid in flexion or extension

The risks associated with these screening trials are small. Meningitis is a possibility, especially if a lumbar subarachnoid catheter or implanted reservoir is used for multiple injections (10). Sedation has been the most common adverse neurological effect of bolus doses of baclofen, and has been noted with doses as low as 10 μg (2, 10).

PUMP IMPLANTATION AND FOLLOW-UP

In patients with a successful response to screening doses of intrathecal baclofen, a pump is implanted into a subcutaneous pocket in the anterior abdominal wall. A catheter is inserted into the lumbar subarachnoid space at the L3–L4 or L4–L5 level, and is threaded superiorly to place the tip at the T11–T12 level in patients with disabling lower limb spasticity. If the intent is to reduce upper limb spasticity as well, the catheter may be threaded higher into the midthoracic region. This can be performed most precisely under fluoroscopic control, but can also be achieved by measuring the length of catheter to be inserted and directing it superiorly. The catheter is inserted via a Tuohy needle. The technique that we use, in an attempt to avoid displacement of the catheter or CSF leak, is to insert a Tuohy needle into the subarachnoid space. With the needle still in position, a small incision is made incorporating the needle, and a figure-of-eight suture is placed into the lumbar fascia around the needle. The catheter is threaded into the subarachnoid space, the Tuohy needle is removed, and the figure-of-eight suture is tied snugly around the catheter. The catheter is then pulled through a subcutaneous tunnel into the anterior abdominal wall, where it is connected to the pump. The pump is filled with intrathecal baclofen and, if programmable, the pump is programmed in the operating room. Our practice has been to perform the procedures as day surgery in an acute care hospital, but the children return to a rehabilitation facility for observation for at least 24 hours after surgery.

Thereafter, the pump is refilled every 2 to 3 months, and is reprogrammed as necessary. The refilling is often delegated to the family physician or a clinic nurse, but the reprogramming is performed under the direction of the team involved in the intrathecal baclofen program. The daily dose of baclofen varies from 25 to 1000 μg/d, and each patient has to be titrated initially to determine the best dose and schedule. The daily doses of intrathecal baclofen usually have to be increased during the first year to control spasticity, and this then tends to stabilize.

OUTCOMES

We review the efficacy or "outcome" of intrathecal baclofen in children with cerebral palsy while considering the quality of the evidence supporting the treatment's use and the "dimensions" or "domains" in which that treatment has been demonstrated to have an effect. The National Center for Medical Rehabilitation Research has proposed that outcomes be considered in one of five dimensions (*Table 24.2*). These comprise pathophysiology, impairment, functional limitation, disability, and societal limitation.

TABLE 24.2
National Center for Medical Rehabilitation Research Model of Dimensions of the Disabling Process

Dimension	Definition
Pathophysiology	Defines the cellular and molecular processes of injury or disease pertinent to a particular condition.
Impairment	Involves dysfunction of the organ system level resulting from a disease process or injury. Examples of impairment level outcomes include tone, spasms, or strength.
Functional limitation	Defines limitations to the set of skills required to perform specific activities, either of the whole body or body segments. Examples include limitations in gait, sitting, or manipulating objects.
Disability	Defines difficulties in carrying out the role or function expected for an individual such as attending school, returning to work, partaking in age-appropriate recreation, or performing activities of daily living.
Societal limitation	Represents the barriers placed by society that limit full participation by people with disabilities. These barriers may be physical, economic, or attitudinal. Examples include wheelchair-unfriendly architecture or the inability to afford a power wheelchair.

The majority of work studying the efficacy of intrathecal baclofen has come from study of adults with spinal cord injury in whom there is strong evidence of efficacy of intrathecal baclofen. This evidence comes from both double-blind, placebo-controlled trials (14), as well as a number of open trials (21, 31, 33). These studies demonstrate statistically significant effects on outcomes in the impairment dimension, including decreases in lower extremity tone (using the Ashworth scale) and decreased spasms. The improved spasticity and spasms is said to be associated with less discomfort and easier care. However, in this adult spinal cord group there is little scientifically documented evidence of positive outcomes in the dimensions of functional limitation, disability, or societal limitation, such as activities of daily living, motor performance, self-care, or participation in school or work.

Much less is known about the efficacy of intrathecal baclofen in treatment of spasticity of cerebral origin, particularly as it relates to children. Most of the studies of intrathecal baclofen for children are case reports or case series (3, 5, 10, 17–19, 27, 29, 41, 50). Although these case series can be helpful and can provide direction for additional systematic study, their results must be approached with caution. Almeida et al. (8) and Armstrong et al. (10) reported N-of-1 randomized clinical trials, which provide stronger evidence of the treatment's efficacy. In the study by Armstrong et al. (10), the randomized trial involved only bolus doses of intrathecal baclofen, and this part of the study was undertaken to determine whether the patients improved enough to justify implantation of the continuous infusion pump. The strongest study design (and therefore the strongest evidence) is presented by Albright et al. (7) in the only double-blind, placebo-controlled study reported to date. Their study involved 19 children and 4 adults with spasticity resulting from cerebral palsy or of other cerebral origin who participated in a randomized, multiple crossover study of bolus doses (not continuous infusion) of intrathecal baclofen.

These studies have provided evidence of efficacy of intrathecal baclofen at the "impairment" level (e.g., tone, clonus, spasms, strength, and range of motion). In the randomized study of Albright et al. (7), lower extremity muscle tone, as measured by the Ashworth scale, was significantly reduced, but a significant change in upper extremity muscle tone could not be demonstrated. In a later retrospective case series there was a mild reduction in spasticity in the upper limbs, which was similar to that noted in patients treated by selective dorsal rhizotomy (4). Almeida et al. (8) and Latash and Penn (29) reported significant improvements in ankle clonus, exaggerated reflexes, and spasms. In their case series of children receiving continuous infusion of intrathecal baclofen, Armstrong et al. (10) identified a significant decrease in hip adductor tone, as measured on the Ashworth scale, with a lesser improvement in elbow flexor spasticity. The N-of-1 study by Almeida et al. (8) also demonstrated a desirable short-term improvement in range of movement, but this did not persist over time. Although a number of the case series studies have examined the effect of intrathecal baclofen on range of motion and the need for subsequent orthopedic procedures, at this time there is only weak evidence of efficacy in this regard (18). An effect on motor control, relating particularly to the upper limb has been sought but is not yet strongly supported (3, 4, 7, 8, 29).

Outcomes within the dimension of "functional limitation," such as activities of daily living, have been examined less frequently. In the N-of-1 study by Almeida et al. (8), self-reported improvement in dressing, transferring, and toileting was documented in the one patient studied, but there was no improvement in the gross motor function measure (GMFM) during the randomized trial. Albright et al. (3) also determined that children previously able to perform self-care rated their own self-care as improved. For both these studies, one must be cautious about the self-reported outcome measure used. In the case series reported by Gerszten et al. (17), the effect of intrathecal baclofen on ambulation was assessed in 24 children who were ambulatory to some extent with or without assistive devices before the intervention. Gait was felt to be improved in 20 of the 24 children, as reported by the patients or their families. The level of ambulation, as graded retrospectively using a four-level functional scale, improved in 9 patients, remained the same in 12, and was worse in 3 patients. Thus, there is only weak evidence of improved gross motor function after intrathecal baclofen administration in children with spastic cerebral palsy.

Regarding the "disability" and "societal limitation" dimensions, no significant evidence of the efficacy of intrathecal baclofen has been demonstrated. This means that at this time there is no evidence that intrathecal baclofen increases a child's ability to attend school, to participate in developmentally appropriate activities, or to have an improved quality of life. Thus, although there is a demonstrated effectiveness of intrathecal baclofen on the treatment of spasticity, spasms, and exaggerated reflex responses for children with spasticity of cerebral origin, further study is required to delineate its effect on gross and fine motor function, activities of daily living, and quality of life.

COMPLICATIONS

Complications associated with intrathecal baclofen are common, and may be related to the drug, or to local problems with the surgical procedure or the hardware. The most common drug-related problem from intrathecal baclofen is mild sedation, which requires a decrease in the dose of the drug. Less commonly there may be dizziness, blurred vision, and slurred speech (1, 40). An increased frequency or precipitation of seizures has also been reported (14, 26, 47). Life-threatening overdoses, characterized by severe respiratory depression, coma, hypotension, and bradycardia, also occur. In most cases, the overdose was associated with the use of bolus doses of intrathecal baclofen, especially when the bolus was administered in addition to a continuous infusion or when intrathecal baclofen was used concurrently with oral baclofen, but programming errors or pump malfunction have also been responsible (10, 30, 38). In patients with suspected drug overdose, the diagnosis is supported by the findings of weakness, flaccidity, and areflexia in both lower and upper limbs. These patients should be admitted to an intensive care unit, where ventilatory support should be provided if needed. Intrathecal infusion should be discontinued and/or the pump reservoir emptied of baclofen. Intravenous physostigmine has been used with variable success in the treatment of overdoses (15, 37, 49), and because of the potential side effects is not recommended. Removal of baclofen from the lumbar subarachnoid space via lumbar puncture may be helpful (1, 15). With appropriate supportive care, the outcome after overdose has been good uniformly, with no lasting sequelae. A complication that is related to the expected reduction in lower limb tone with intrathecal baclofen is deep venous thrombosis in the lower limbs and pulmonary embolus. This was noted in the adult population but not in children (9, 13).

Sudden withdrawal of intrathecal baclofen after long-term use, as might occur with a blockage to the system or pump failure, may result in hallucinations, seizures, confusion, psychotic behavior, rebound severe spasticity, and hyperthermia (25, 32, 46). If the diagnosis is made, reinfusion of baclofen into the subarachnoid space via the pump as a bolus or by lumbar puncture may reverse the symptoms, and in patients with hyperthermia, dantrolene has been useful (23, 46). If it is decided to discontinue continuous intrathecal baclofen, this should be done gradually, and the patient should be placed on oral baclofen.

Failure of the pump occurs in 5 to 10% of patients, and requires replacement (14, 40). Other local problems related to the infusion system are common, and include seromas around the pump, erosion of the skin over the pump, disconnection at a connector site, a break in the catheter, kinking of the catheter, displacement of the intrathecal catheter, and leak of CSF at the catheter insertion site (1, 10, 16). Some of these complication have been reduced as surgeons have gained experience with inserting the pumps and with improved catheter systems, particularly with the development of thicker walled catheters (44). However, even in recent series, reoperations for catheter-related problems are performed in more than 20% of patients (1, 38). In children, the local problems tend to be aggravated. The pumps are large and protrude markedly in the anterior abdominal wall, especially in young or very thin children (*Fig. 24.4*). In spastic quadriplegic children, who are often restrained in a wheelchair and who tend to be thin, the protruding pump may be irritated repeatedly by the restraints that are used, leading to a higher incidence of local complications. Another potential complication of the administration of intrathecal baclofen is spinal arachnoiditis, associated with the drug or the catheter, but there is no definite case report of such a complication (11).

As in any surgery involving implants, infection is a major concern. Local infection of the wound or subcutaneous pump pocket has been reported in as many as 20% of patients (16, 34). Pump erosion through the skin with subsequent contamination of the pump is not unusual, especially in children. Local infection can sometimes be eradicated with the use of systemic antibiotics, but more often the pump has to be removed. Meningitis has been documented, both during the trial of repeated intrathecal injections before insertion of the pump and after pump implantation (10, 34, 30). Treatment of meningitis using systemic antibiotics in addition to intrathecal antibiotics administered through the pump reservoir or side port of the pump may be successful, and avoids removal of the pump (34).

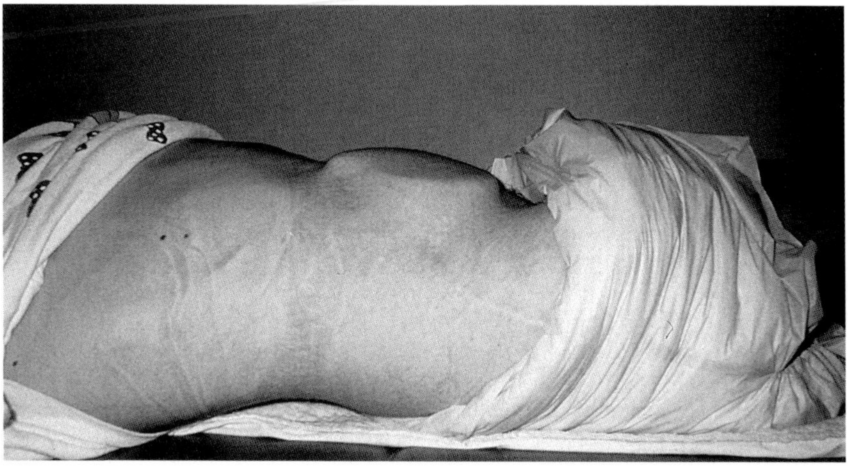

FIG. 24.4 A photograph of a 9-year-old child with an implanted Synchromed pump demonstrating the marked protrusion of the pump in the anterior abdominal wall.

An additional consideration is that continuous intrathecal baclofen requires chronic medical attention to refill the pump, to adjust the dose to obtain the desired effect, to replace the pump when the battery fails, and to address the various complications mentioned previously. Should spasticity recur in a patient receiving continuous intrathecal baclofen, one needs to determine whether tolerance to the drug has occurred or whether there is a problem with the delivery of the drug intrathecally. Hence, pump failure or some mechanical problem with the system has to be ruled out. Plain anteroposterior and lateral radiographs of the infusion system may demonstrate an obvious break or disconnection, or may show that the catheter has migrated out of the subarachnoid space. If the system appears intact and is positioned appropriately, a number of techniques may be helpful in determining the cause of the problem (1). If a programmable pump has been used, the pump can be programmed to deliver a bolus of baclofen to determine whether this relieves spasticity. Radioactive isotope or water-soluble contrast material can be injected into the reservoir, and after a few hours to allow the material to reach the end of the catheter, a scan or radiograph can be acquired. The infusion rate can be increased or a bolus can be administered to speed up the investigation, but if this is done, the baclofen should be removed from the reservoir first. Even then there is a risk of creating an overdose because the baclofen in the catheter is infused rapidly into the subarachnoid space. If there is a side port associated with the pump, the contrast material or radionuclide can be injected into the side port to outline the catheter system immediately. Assay of CSF obtained by lumbar puncture for the concentration of baclofen may also be helpful.

MANAGEMENT

The goals of management of the child with spasticity of cerebral origin are improved motor function, increased mobility, increased independence, decreased painful spasms, and, for severely affected quadriplegics, increased ease of care. It is critical for all parties involved, including the caregivers, to appreciate that the goals of treatment are not simply relief of spasticity or improved range of movement.

SELECTION OF PATIENTS FOR NEUROSURGICAL TREATMENT

To make the most appropriate recommendations, the treating physicians must be familiar with and must be prepared to discuss the pros and cons of the various options available. These include physiotherapy; occupational therapy; oral spasmolytics; orthopedic procedures, such as tendon lengthening; botulinum toxin injections; therapeutic electrical stimulation; and selective dorsal rhizotomies.

In children in whom the functionally important spasticity is predominantly in one muscle group (e.g., the ankle plantar flexors or hamstrings), consideration is given to simpler orthopedic tendon lengthening or botulinum toxin. We recognize that even when the functionally important spasticity affects one muscle group there is usually spasticity throughout the lower limbs, and one can argue for performing a dorsal rhizotomy or using intrathecal baclofen to decrease the lower limb spasticity more diffusely in this patient population. However, we opt for a simpler procedure if the functional results might reasonably be expected to be similar.

If the child might benefit functionally from relieving spasticity diffusely in the lower limbs, one considers options such as intrathecal baclofen or dorsal rhizotomy. The ambulatory potential must be assessed, and an attempt is made to determine whether reduction in lower limb spasticity might be detrimental to the child's ambulatory function, because the child is using the spasticity to support weight in the upright position. This is one of the most difficult issues. Children who are walking independently without a walker or crutches, and younger children who crawl on their knees and arms, in our experience, have enough underlying strength in the lower limbs and are not a concern. For the other patients, the child's ability to rise in a slow, graded fashion from the squatting position is assessed. If the child is able to do this with the examiner supporting the arms or upper body minimally, the probability is high that there is adequate underlying quadriceps strength to support the child's weight if the spasticity is reduced. One clearly needs to be concerned about this issue in children with ambulatory potential, but even in spastic quadriplegics, in whom ambulation is not a realistic goal, one also needs to be concerned. Many of these children, who get around in a wheelchair, use their spasticity to assist in standing transfers. They may be worse functionally if that spasticity is reduced and they are no longer able to support their weight. This may not appear to be a major issue in the young child, who is easily lifted, but it attains increasing importance as the child gets older, heavier, and more difficult to lift.

If it is determined that treatment of the spasticity is indicated, one then needs to decide which intervention would be most appropriate. Intrathecal baclofen is the intervention of choice in spastic, dystonic, and children who are quadriplegic from near drowning (10). In patients in whom dystonia, rather than spasticity, is the inhibiting function, preliminary studies suggest that intrathecal baclofen may be indicated (6). Children with spastic, quadriplegic cerebral palsy affecting the upper limbs more than lower limbs, or with severe opisthotonic posturing, may be considered for intrathecal baclofen because it may be possible to increase the dose of baclofen or direct the subarachnoid catheter higher in the spinal canal such that upper limb spasticity is reduced (20).

Intrathecal baclofen is often proposed in preference to rhizotomy in children with spastic diplegic cerebral palsy, when there is concern that spasticity is needed for standing or walking support (2). The argument is that the dose of baclofen can be titrated, and in the worse-case scenario, if the result is unsatisfactory, the treatment is reversible. This concern about the possible loss of ability to stand or walk may be more theoretical than real. Our experience has been that these patients, about whom we have agonized, have done well after selective dorsal rhizotomy, with no child losing the ability to walk or to stand after that procedure. Hence, our preference has been to recommend a selective dorsal rhizotomy in this situation as opposed to intrathecal baclofen.

Other indications for intrathecal baclofen include older patients with diplegia, particularly those older than 16 years, and children with spastic quadriplegia in whom lower limb spasticity is disabling or making care difficult (2). These children may also meet the criteria to be considered for selective dorsal rhizotomy, and there are no studies that compare these two treatment modalities in these populations. In these situations, when either intrathecal baclofen or selective dorsal rhizotomy can be considered to be equally effective and indicated options, our practice has been to recommend a rhizotomy. Our rationale is that, compared with intrathecal baclofen, selective dorsal rhizotomy requires little long-term management, does not require reoperation, has fewer complications, has been better documented to be effective in improving function, and is less costly overall to the health care system (50).

CONCLUSIONS

The management of motor impairment in the child with spastic cerebral palsy should be multidisciplinary, and usually involves a physiotherapist, occupational therapist, developmental pediatrician, orthopedic surgeon, and orthotist, in addition to the neurosurgeon. The neurosurgeon is usually asked for an opinion regarding the management of the spasticity. It is important that he/she appreciates the various neurosurgical and non-neurosurgical interventions available for the relief of spasticity, but also recognizes that the goal of treatment is not the relief of spasticity per se, but the improvement of motor function. The neurosurgeon should work as part of a team to identify the best management option to optimize the functional outcome. Furthermore, if a neurosurgical intervention directed at the relief of spasticity is felt to be indicated, the best outcome is achieved with input from physiotherapists, occupational therapists, orthotists, and orthopedic surgeons during the postoperative period.

REFERENCES

1. Albright AL: Baclofen in the treatment of cerebral palsy. **J Child Neurol** 11:77–83, 1996.
2. Albright AL: Intrathecal baclofen in cerebral palsy movement disorders. **J Child Neurol** 11:S29–S35, 1996.
3. Albright AL, Barron WB, Fasick MP, Polinko P, Janosky J: Continuous intrathecal baclofen infusion for spasticity of cerebral origin. **JAMA** 270:2475–2477, 1993.
4. Albright AL, Barry MJ, Fasick MP, Janosky J: Effects of continuous intrathecal baclofen infusion and selective posterior rhizotomy on upper extremity spasticity. **Pediatr Neurosurg** 23:82–85, 1995.
5. Albright AL, Barry MJ, Hoffmann P: Intrathecal L-baclofen for cerebral spasticity: Case report. **Neurology** 45:2110–2111, 1995.
6. Albright AL, Barry MJ, Painter MJ, Shultz B: Infusion of intrathecal baclofen for generalized dystonia in cerebral palsy. **J Neurosurg** 88:73–76, 1998.
7. Albright AL, Cervi A, Singletary J: Intrathecal baclofen for spasticity in cerebral palsy. **J Am Med Assoc** 265:1418–1422, 1991.
8. Almeida GL, Campbell SK, Girolami GL, Penn RD, Corcos DM: Multidimensional assessment of motor function in a child with cerebral palsy following intrathecal administration of baclofen. **Phys Ther** 77:751–764, 1997.
9. Armstrong RW: Intrathecal baclofen and spasticity: What do we know and what do we need to know? **Dev Med Child Neurol** 34:739–745, 1992.
10. Armstrong RW, Steinbok P, Cochrane DD, Kube SD, Fife SE, Farrell K: Intrathecally administered baclofen for treatment of children with spasticity of cerebral origin. **J Neurosurg** 87:409–414, 1997.
11. Armstrong RW, Steinbok P, Farrell K, Cochrane D, Norman MG, Kube S: Continuous intrathecal baclofen treatment of severe spasms in two children with spinal-cord injury. **Dev Med Child Neurol** 34:731–738, 1992.
12. Bohannon RW, Smith MB: Interrater reliability of a modified Ashworth scale. **Phys Ther** 67:206–207, 1987.
13. Broseta J, Morales F, Garcia–March G, et al: Use of intrathecal baclofen administered by programmable infusion pumps in resistent spasticity. **Acta Neurochir Suppl** 46:39–45, 1989.
14. Coffey RJ, Cahill D, Steers W, et al: Intrathecal baclofen for intractable spasticity of spinal origin: Results of a long-term multicenter study. **J Neurosurg** 78:226–232, 1993.
15. Delhaas EM, Brouwers JR: Intrathecal baclofen overdose: Report of 7 events in 5 patients and review of the literature. **Int J Clin Pharmacol Ther Toxicol** 29:274–280, 1991.
16. Gardner B, Jamous A, Teddy P, et al: Intrathecal baclofen—a multicentre clinical comparison of the Medtronics Programmable, Cordis Secor and Constant Infusion Infusaid drug delivery systems. **Paraplegia** 33:551–554, 1995.
17. Gerszten PC, Albright AL, Barry MJ: Effect on ambulation of continuous intrathecal baclofen infusion. **Pediatr Neurosurg** 27:40–44, 1997.
18. Gerszten PC, Albright AL, Johnstone GF: Intrathecal baclofen infusion and subsequent orthopedic surgery in patients with spastic cerebral palsy. **J Neurosurg** 88:1009–1013, 1998.

19. Gilmartin R, Rawlins P: Seizures in epileptic cerebral palsy patients receiving intrathecal baclofen infusion. **Epilepsia** 36:12, 1995.
20. Hugenholtz H, Nelson RF, Dehoux E: Intrathecal baclofen—the importance of catheter position. **Can J Neurol Sci** 20:165–167, 1993.
21. Hugenholtz H, Nelson RF, Dehoux E, Bickerton R: Intrathecal baclofen for intractable spinal spasticity—a double-blind cross-over comparison with placebo in 6 patients. **Can J Neurol Sci** 19:188–195, 1992.
22. Kerr DIB, Ong J: $GABA_B$ receptors. **Pharmacol Ther** 67:187–246, 1995.
23. Khorasani A, Peruzzi WT: Dantrolene treatment for abrupt intrathecal baclofen withdrawal. **Anesth Analg** 80:1054–1056, 1995.
24. Knuttson E, Lindblom U, Beissinger RL, Martenson A: Plasma and cerebrospinal fluid levels of baclofen (Lioresal) at optimal therapeutic responses in spastic paraparesis. **J Neurol Sci** 23:473–484, 1974.
25. Kofler M, Arturo LA: Prolonged seizure activity after baclofen withdrawal. **Neurology** 42:697–698, 1992.
26. Kofler M, Kronenberg MF, Rifici C, Saltuari L, Bauer G: Epileptic seizures associated with intrathecal baclofen application. **Neurology** 44:25–27, 1994.
27. Krach L, Gilmartin R, Bruce D, Storrs B, Abbott R, Ward J: Functional changes noted following treatments of individuals with cerebral palsy with intrathecal baclofen. **Dev Med Child Neurol** 39; suppl 75:12–13, 1997.
28. Kroin JS, Ali A, York M, Penn RD: The distribution of medication along the spinal canal after chronic intrathecal administration. **Neurosurgery** 33:226–230, 1993.
29. Latash ML, Penn RD: Changes in voluntary motor control induced by intrathecal baclofen in patients with spasticity of different etiology. **Physiother Res Int** 1:229–246, 1996.
30. Lazorthes Y, Sallerin–Caute B, Verdie JC, Bastide R, Carillo JP: Chronic intrathecal baclofen administration for control of severe spasticity. **J Neurosurg** 72:393–402, 1990.
31. Loubser PG, Narayan RK, Sandin KJ, Donovan WH, Russell KD: Continuous infusion of intrathecal baclofen: Long-term effects on spasticity in spinal cord injury. **Paraplegia** 29:48–64, 1991.
32. Mandac BR, Hurvitz EA, Nelson VS: Hyperthermia associated with baclofen withdrawal and increased spasticity. **Arch Phys Med Rehabil** 74:96–97, 1993.
33. Meythaler JM, Steers WD, Tuel SM, Cross LL, Haworth CS: Continuous intrathecal baclofen in spinal cord spasticity. A prospective study. **Am J Phys Med Rehabil** 71:321–327, 1992.
34. Müller H: Treatment of severe spasticity: Results of a multicenter trial conducted in Germany involving the intrathecal infusion of baclofen by an implantable drug delivery system, in Lakke JPWF, Delhaas EM, Rutgers AWF (eds.): *Parenteral Drug Therapy in Spasticity and Parkinsons Disease.* Lancaster, Parthenon, 1992, pp 103–113.
35. Muller H, Zierski J, Dralle D, Hoffmann O, Michaelis G: Intrathecal baclofen in spasticity, in Muller H, Zierski J, Penn RD (eds.): *Local Spinal Therapy of Spasticity.* Berlin, Springer-Verlag, 1988, pp 155–214.
36. Muller H, Zierski J, Dralle D, Kraus D, Mutschler E: Pharmacokinetics of intrathecal baclofen, in Muller H, Zierski J, Penn RD (eds.): *Local Spinal Therapy of Spasticity.* Berlin, Springer-Verlag, 1988, pp 223–226.
37. Muller–Schwefe G, Penn RD: Physostigmine in the treatment of intrathecal baclofen overdose. Report of three cases. **J Neurosurg** 71:273–275, 1989.
38. Ochs GA: Intrathecal baclofen. **Baillieres Clin Neurol** 2:73–86, 1993.

39. O'Donnell M, Armstrong R: Pharmacologic interventions for management of spasticity in cerebral palsy. **Ment Retard Dev Disabil Res Rev** 3:204–211, 1997.
40. Penn RD: Intrathecal baclofen for spasticity of spinal origin: Seven years of experience. **J Neurosurg** 77:236–240, 1992.
41. Penn RD, Gianino JM, York MM: Intrathecal baclofen for motor disorders. **Move Disord** 10:675–677, 1995.
42. Penn RD, Kroin JS: Intrathecal baclofen alleviates spinal cord spasticity. **Lancet** 1:1078, 1984.
43. Penn RD, Kroin JS: Long-term intrathecal baclofen infusion for treatment of spasticity. **J Neurosurg** 66:181–185, 1987.
44. Penn RD, York MM, Paice JA: Catheter systems for intrathecal drug delivery. **J Neurosurg** 83:215–217, 1995.
45. Price GW, Wilkin GP, Turnbull MJ, Bowery MG: Are baclofen-sensitive $GABA_b$ receptors present on primary afferent terminals of the spinal core? **Nature** 307:71–74, 1984.
46. Reeves RK, Stolp–Smith KA, Christopherson MW: Hyperthermia, rhabdomyolysis, and disseminated intravascular coagulation associated with baclofen pump catheter failure. **Arch Phys Med Rehabil** 79:353–356, 1998.
47. Rifici C, Kofler M, Kronenberg M, Kofler A, Bramanti P, Saltuari L: Intrathecal baclofen application in patients with supraspinal spasticity secondary to severe traumatic brain injury. **Funct Neurol** 9:29–34, 1994.
48. Sallerin–Caute B, Lazorthes Y, Monsarrat B, Cros J, Bastide R: CSF baclofen levels after intrathecal administration in severe spasticity. **Eur J Clin Pharmacol** 40:363–365, 1991.
49. Saltuari L, Baumgartner H, Kofler M, et al: Failure of physostigmine in treatment of acute severe intrathecal baclofen intoxication. **N Engl J Med** 322:1533–1534, 1990.
50. Steinbok P, Daneshvar H, Evans D, Kestle JR: Cost analysis of continuous intrathecal baclofen versus selective functional posterior rhizotomy in the treatment of spastic quadriplegia associated with cerebral palsy. **Pediatr Neurosurg** 22:255–264, 1995.

IV

General Scientific Session IV
Lumbar Interbody Fusions

CHAPTER

25

The Biomechanics of Lumbar Interbody Fusion and Sagittal Plane Balance

GREGORY J. PRZYBYLSKI, M.D.

Since the application of threaded fusion cages in the treatment of intervertebral disc disorders (25, 33) there has been a growing interest in the use of anterior and posterior surgical approaches for placement of interbody devices to achieve a lumbar fusion. The search for alternative fusion methods has been prompted in part by the dissatisfaction with significant perioperative pain and reduced fusion rates associated with posterolateral graft placement. The more limited spinal exposure needed for placement of interbody devices as well as the intervertebral placement of graft material allowing for graft compression may overcome the limitations observed with interbody devices. Moreover, improvements in surgical instrumentation and development of a variety of intervertebral devices have allowed greater ease of placement through both anterior and posterior surgical approaches.

However, the biomechanical effects of these devices have not been examined with the same scrutiny that has been applied to posterolateral fixation and fusion methods. Yet the growing popularity of these interbody constructs has fostered interest in studying the biomechanical differences between devices to determine whether a particular implant is ideally suited for achieving successful internal fixation and arthrodesis of the lumbar spine. The biomechanical effects of various constructs should be examined to facilitate an understanding of the predicted consequences of these devices on spinal motion. This review considers the concept of an ideal curvature of the lumbar spine in terms of sagittal plane balance. Moreover, the structural mechanics of intervertebral arthrodesis and instrumentation techniques are evaluated in comparison with posterolateral techniques to serve as a basis for choosing a method that best supports the goal of spinal stabilization.

The configuration of the spine can become altered with degenerative disease and may contribute to painful conditions of mechanical instability. Progressive loss of water turgor in the intervertebral disc with aging results in interspace collapse and loss of the wedge-shaped contour, thereby reducing segmental lordosis. Different instrumentation techniques can have a variety of effects on spinal alignment. The concept of sagittal plane balance considers the relationship of the lumbosacral junction and pelvis relative to the center of gravity of the torso to estimate an ideal lumbar curvature. To understand this concept better, the definition of sagittal plane balance, sacral inclination, sacropelvic angle, and lumbar lordosis are examined. Normative values are reviewed and compared with values in symptomatic patients to determine whether certain patterns can be associated with painful conditions. Lastly, the concepts are applied to the lumbar spine to suggest the lumbar curve that may be ideal to achieve with internal fixation.

Determination of sagittal plane balance is made from a lateral 36 inch standing radiograph of the entire spinal column that includes the pelvis and the acetabulae (18). A vertical plumb line is drawn from the center of the inferior end plate of the 7th cervical vertebra toward the pelvis. The location of a sacral point relative to the plumb line contributes to spinal balance. Sacral reference points that have been used include the anterosuperior and posterosuperior corners of the 1st sacral vertebra. Additional, related measures include the sacral inclination and lumbar lordosis. The angle formed by the intersection of a line tangential to the posterior margin of S1 with a vertical line through the posterosuperior corner of S1 defines the sacral inclination. The pelvic hip axis is identified as the midpoint of a line joining the centers of the femoral heads. A line projected from this point to the posterosuperior corner of S1 represents the pelvic radius. This allows calculation of the sacropelvic angle between this line and a vertical line passing through the pelvic hip axis. Sacropelvic translation is then measured as the distance between vertical lines drawn through the hip axis and the posterosuperior corner of S1. Lastly, overall lumbar lordosis can be measured as the Cobb angle from the superior end plates of the first lumbar and sacral segments, whereas individual segmental measures can be made from the superior end plates of adjacent vertebrae (18).

Normative values have been measured from standing radiographs in several studies examining 150 normal volunteers (9, 18). The plumb line typically intersects the superior end plate of the sacrum near the posterior corner and gradually moves anteriorly with age. This is accompanied by a loss of distal lordosis without a corresponding increase in thoracic kyphosis. The mean sacral inclination of 50 $\pm$ 7.7 degrees becomes slightly reduced to 46 $\pm$ 9 degrees with age. Most of the lumbar lordosis occurs at the two lowest intervertebral joints. Although the overall mean lordosis in younger patients of -61 ± 12 degrees is similar to the mean lumbar lordosis of -64 ± 10 degrees in older patients, segmental values were reduced at the lumbosacral junction (*Fig. 25.1*).

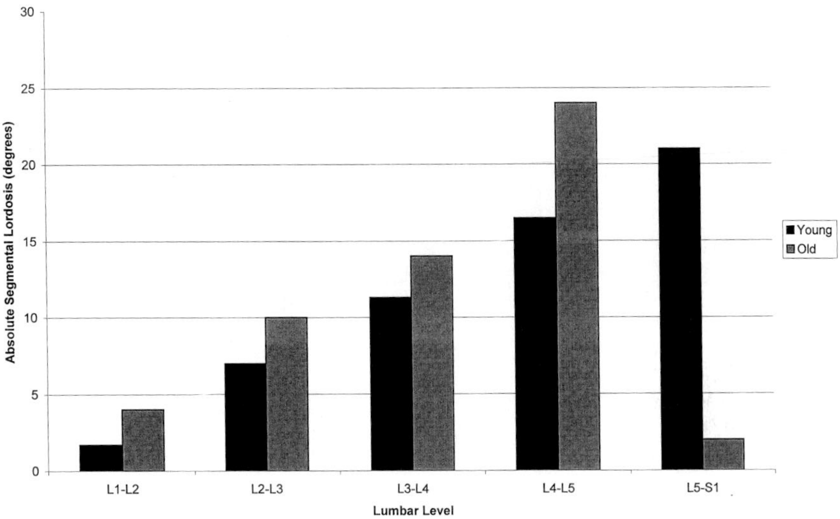

FIG. 25.1 Histogram comparing the segmental lordosis in young and old asymptomatic volunteers.

Comparisons have been made between asymptomatic volunteers and patients with a variety of low back problems including degenerative disc disease, low-grade degenerative spondylolisthesis, and scoliosis. The location of the plumb line dropped from C7 relative to the sacrum was similar in all symptomatic conditions studied when compared with the volunteers. However, their balance was achieved through a variety of mechanisms in each of the conditions examined (*Fig. 25.2*). For example, sacral inclination increased in patients with lumbar disc disease, whereas the sacropelvic angle increased with spondylolisthesis (19). The total lordosis was reduced with both degenerative lumbar disc disease and scoliosis, but increased with spondylolisthesis accompanied by an increased sacropelvic angle. The L5–S1 Cobb angle was smaller in degenerative disc disease, whereas the L4–L5 Cobb angle increased in spondylolisthesis. Lastly, the L1–L2 Cobb angle was reduced in scoliosis. A close correlation was observed between lumbar lordosis and sagittal balance through pelvic rotation and translation. For example, loss of lordosis resulting in a more anterior location of the C7 plumb line relative to the sacrum was associated with posterior sacropelvic translation.

Ideally, the torso is balanced when the center of gravity is centered over the hips (18), thereby necessitating proximity of the C7 plumb line to the posterior corner of the 1st sacral segment. Reduction in distal lumbar lordosis was associated with posterior pelvic rotation. However, this increases the distance between the hip and S1. Although it is un-

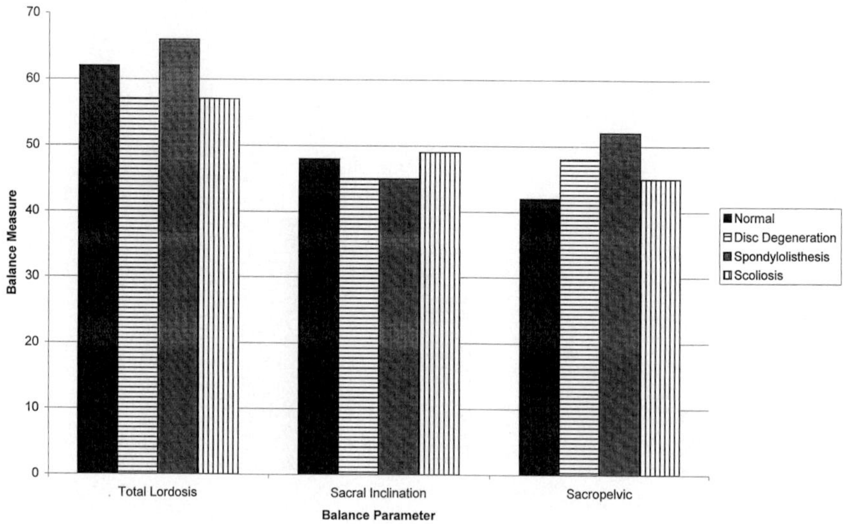

FIG. 25.2 Histogram comparing parameters of sagittal balance among normal volunteers and patients with degenerative disc disease, spondylolisthesis, and scoliosis.

certain whether the position of the lumbar vertebrae alters symptoms, it has been suggested that maintenance of a lower lumbar lordosis achieves the ideal alignment to maintain the sacrum in line with the hip joints (19).

However, if a goal of operative stabilization of lumbar spinal disorders is to maintain distal lumbar lordosis, then one may be concerned about placement of interbody devices that may reduce the difference between the anterior and the posterior intervertebral heights, resulting in more parallel end plates. Because one must also consider the structural mechanics of the intervertebral prostheses, it would be helpful to evaluate the biomechanical differences observed among a variety of interbody arthrodesis and instrumentation techniques to determine their effect when compared with common posterolateral methods.

Traditional posterolateral fusion begins to develop stiffness at 4 weeks in a sheep model (22). Subsequently, reduced forces are measured in the pedicle fixation devices at 8 weeks. Greater stiffness of the bone mass was observed in instrumented segments when compared with noninstrumented levels. Histologically, more woven bone was observed at the instrumented levels. However, solid arthrodesis was achieved by 16 weeks, regardless of the use of internal fixation. Placement of the fusion mass closer to the instantaneous axis of rotation of the lumbar intervertebral joint increases the moment of inertia, thereby achieving a better stabilizing fusion (42). However, even with a solid posterolateral fusion mass, some bending occurs within the fused bone, just as bending occurs in normal bone. Under axial compression, axial displacement and flexion rotation are predicted. However, a concurrent facet fusion can reduce this posterior movement, permitting a stiffer posterolateral fusion (37).

Because the instantaneous axis of rotation is located within the posterior portion of the interspace, one might expect improved stiffness with an interbody arthrodesis (44). Finite element modeling predicted a more rigid fusion with interbody techniques (37). However, the stiffness is least in extension. A cadaveric study (4) predicted increased intradiscal pressure as well as greater intervertebral motion adjacent to the level of an anterior lumbar interbody fusion (ALIF). This effect may be more prominent with interbody techniques compared with posterolateral fusion (7).

When comparing interbody fusion methods, stiffness of anterior techniques is greater in torsion and bending when compared with posterior approaches (40). Moreover, open ALIF has resulted in greater stiffness than with laparoscopic techniques. Greater removal of the annular ligament with additional room for anterior grafts may facilitate the onset of fusion (34). Given the greater removal of the facet joints with posterior lumbar interbody fusion (PLIF), one might predict reduced stiffness in extension, axial rotation, and lateral bending (26, 36).

Posterolateral arthrodesis is often supplemented with pedicle fixation. These devices predominantly impart greater flexion stiffness (23). Bending moments increase within the pedicle screw with as little as a 7-degree cephalad angulation relative to the rod (28, 43). Similarly, short screw lengths $<$40mm and incomplete insertion also increase bending moments in the pedicle screw (28). However, cancellous bone density had a limited effect on screw bending failure (29). In addition, cross-linking can stiffen the construct in axial rotation (26). The addition of a sublaminar hook adjacent to the screw significantly improves stiffness as well (3, 14, 16). Stiffer fixation can be achieved with translaminar facet screw fixation in flexion, whereas pedicle screw fixation was stiffer in extension (5, 15). Pedicle fixation contributes more to flexion stiffness than to lateral bending stiffness (23).

Given the rigidity of most spinal implants, one might anticipate an effect of implants on bone healing. Kanayama et al. (21) showed earlier bone healing with the use of implants. Although the fusion becomes stiffer, concurrent osteopenia in the vertebra can be seen (27, 30). However, stress shielding was not observed in a goat model (20). Moreover, bone density itself may not alter the force required to achieve bending failure of the screw (29). Feighan et al. (8) showed more successful union with increasing instrumentation rigidity in a rabbit model.

Increased rotation and facet motion are observed at adjacent levels to a spinal segment instrumented with pedicle fixation (6, 12, 13, 31). Although the goal of establishing a lumbar lordosis may encourage in situ bending, this maneuver increases bone–screw interface failure with less than 10 degrees of bending without significantly increasing the lordosis (41). The stronger anterior longitudinal ligament resists tensile forces induced during bending, resulting in failure at the weaker bone–screw interface. Lastly, simple compression reduces the axial compressive force (24).

A variety of interbody devices have been used for facilitating intervertebral arthrodesis. The pullout strength and failure force in axial compression of bone was less than that of cages (1). However, the femoral ring was stiffer in flexion than threaded cages and stiffer than corticocancellous bone in both flexion and axial compression, whereas threaded cages were stiffer in axial rotation (10, 11). The range of motion and the breadth of the neutral zone were similar when comparing tricortical bone graft and titanium fiber mesh devices in a PLIF model (17). However, stiffness was least when comparing bone graft with a threaded titanium interbody device in a calf model, particularly in torsion (2). Interspace height loss was greater for the bone dowel than a cage in a sheep model (35). In fact, only the cage maintained any distraction at 6 months, yet the dowel was stiffer in lateral bending than the cage (35, 36). The orientation of the cage did not appear to affect motion when facets are intact, thereby supporting either anterior or lateral cage placement (36).

When comparing interbody devices with pedicle fixation, stiffness, particularly in extension, is greater with pedicle fixation (11). Translaminar facet screws can reverse the reduction in extension stiffness seen with ALIF devices (39). When comparing various cage designs, anterior placement of the threaded intervertebral fusion device (Danek, Memphis, TN) was stiffer in extension than the Bagby and Kuslich (BAK) device (Spine-Tech, Minneapolis, MN), whereas the BAK cage was stiffer in axial compression (32). Greater adjacent-level motion is seen with ALIF alone when compared with a posterolateral fusion alone. Moreover, ALIF causes similar adjacent-level effects as a circumferential fusion (7).

Limitations of applying the various balance parameters examined include a highly variable vertical spinal axis among people. Often, there is a compensatory rotation or translation of the pelvis for changes in the lumbar lordosis. Moreover, alterations in hip, knee, and ankle position can affect the pelvic position in the setting of spinal rigidity (38). There remains uncertainty regarding the ideal balance position and its clinical significance. Lastly, the degree of reduction in segmental and overall lordosis from cylindrical cages is unknown.

Similarly, interpretation of differences among the biomechanical parameters examined is limited. The relationship of biomechanical properties to clinical outcomes is unknown. In addition, most in vivo biomechanical studies were performed in quadrupeds. Results may not be applicable in biped models. Lastly, most in vitro instrumentation studies are performed in aged cadavers, in which significant changes in material properties have occurred.

In conclusion, sagittal plane balance can be evaluated in several ways, including measures of the location of the sacrum relative to the C7 plumb line as well as the degree of sacropelvic translation. Loss of distal lordosis may be associated with altered balance. Consequently, fixation devices may be better if the lordosis can be preserved. The removal of the lumbar facets in PLIF approaches causes reduced stiffness. Although interbody devices are stiffer than pedicle fixation in compression, these are least stiff in extension. Posterolateral fusions are associated with some bending, which can be reduced with concurrent facet fusion, which will add stiffness. Lastly, interbody fusions alone increase adjacent-level motion more than posterolateral fusions. An understanding of the biomechanical effects of spinal instrumentation can help the spinal surgeon better choose the technique for achieving spinal stabilization.

REFERENCES

1. Brantigan JW, Stefee AD, Geiger JM: A carbon fiber implant to aid interbody lumbar fusion. Mechanical testing. **Spine** 16:S277–S282, 1991.
2. Brodke DS, Dick JC, Kunz DN, McCabe R, Zdeblick TA: Posterior lumbar interbody fusion. A biomechanical comparison, including a new threaded cage. **Spine** 22:26–31, 1997.
3. Chiba M, McClain RF, Yerby SA, Moseley TA, Smith TS, Benson DR: Short segment pedicle instrumentation. Biomechanical analysis of supplemental hook fixation. **Spine** 21:288–294, 1996.
4. Chow DH, Luk KD, Evans JH, Leong JC: Effects of short anterior lumbar interbody fusion on biomechanics of neighboring unfused segments. **Spine** 21:549–555, 1996.
5. Deguchi M, Cheng BC, Sato K, Matsuyama Y, Zdeblick TA: Biomechanical evaluation of translaminar facet joint fixation. A comparative study of poly-l-lactide pins, screws, and pedicle fixation. **Spine** 23:1307–1312, 1998.
6. Dekutowski MB, Schendel MJ, Ogilvie JW, Olsewski JM, Wallace LJ, Lewis JL: Comparison of in vivo and in vitro adjacent segment motion after lumbar fusion. **Spine** 19:1745–1751, 1994.
7. Esses SI, Doherty BJ, Crawford MJ, Dreyzin V: Kinematic evaluation of lumbar fusion techniques. **Spine** 21:676–684, 1996.
8. Feighan JE, Stevenson S, Emery SE: Biologic and biomechanic evaluation of posterior lumbar fusion in the rabbit. The effect of fixation rigidity. **Spine** 20:1561–1567, 1995.

9. Gelb DE, Lenke LG, Bridwell KH, Blanke K, McEnery KW: An analysis of sagittal spinal alignment in 100 asymptomatic middle and older aged volunteers. **Spine** 20:1351–1358, 1995.
10. Glazer PA, Colliou O, Klisch SM, Bradford DS, Bueff HU, Lotz JC: Biomechanical analysis of multilevel fixation methods in the lumbar spine. **Spine** 22:171–182, 1997.
11. Glazer PA, Colliou O, Lotz JC, Bradford DS: Biomechanical analysis of lumbosacral fixation. **Spine** 21:1211–1222, 1996.
12. Gunzburg R, Hutton WC: Effects of posterior instrumentation on axial rotation of the lumbar spine: An in vitro biomechanical study. **J Spinal Disord** 8:103–110, 1995.
13. Ha KY, Schendel MJ, Lewis JL, Ogilvie JW: Effect of immobilization and configuration on lumbar adjacent-segment biomechanics. **J Spinal Disord** 6:99–105, 1993.
14. Hasegawa K, Takahashi HE, Uchiyama S, et al.: An experimental study of a combination method using a pedicle screw and laminar hook for the osteoporotic spine. **Spine** 22:958–962, 1997.
15. Heggeness MH, Esses SI: Translaminar facet joint screw fixation for lumbar and lumbosacral fusion. A clinical and biomechanical study. **Spine** 16:S266–S269, 1991.
16. Hilibrand AS, Moore DC, Graziano GP: The role of pedicolaminar fixation in compromised pedicle bone. **Spine** 21:445–451, 1996.
17. Hoshijima K, Nightingale RW, Yu JR, et al.: Strength and stability of posterior lumbar interbody fusion. Comparison of titanium fiber mesh implant and tricortical bone graft. **Spine** 22:1181–1188, 1997.
18. Jackson RP, McManus AC: Radiographic analysis of sagittal plane alignment and balance in standing volunteers and patients with low back pain matched for age, sex, and size. A prospective controlled clinical study. **Spine** 19:1611–1618, 1994.
19. Jackson RP, Peterson MD, McManus AC, Hales C: Compensatory spinopelvic balance over the hip axis and better reliability in measuring lordosis to the pelvic radius on standing lateral radiographs of adult volunteers and patients. **Spine** 23:1750–1767, 1998.
20. Johnston CE, Welch RD, Baker KJ, Ashman RB: Effect of spinal construct stiffness on short segment fusion mass incorporation. **Spine** 20:2400–2407, 1995.
21. Kanayama M, Cunningham BW, Sefter JC, et al.: Does spinal instrumentation influence the healing process of posterolateral spinal fusion? An in vivo animal model. **Spine** 24:1058–1065, 1999.
22. Kanayama M, Cunningham BW, Weis JC, Parker LM, Kaneda K, McAfee PC: Maturation of the posterolateral spinal fusion and its effect on load-sharing of spinal instrumentation. An in vivo sheep model. **J Bone Joint Surg Am** 79A:1710–1720, 1997.
23. Kotani Y, Cunningham BW, Cappucino A, Kaneda K, McAfee PC: The role of spinal instrumentation in augmenting lumbar posterolateral fusion. **Spine** 21:278–287, 1996.
24. Krodel A. Mechanical principles of compressive interbody fusion. **Spine** 21:821–826, 1996.
25. Kuslich SD, Ulstrom CL, Grifith SL, Ahern JW, Dowdle JD: The Bagby and Kuslich method of lumbar interbody fusion. History, techniques, and 2-year follow-up results of a United States prospective, multicenter study. **Spine** 23:1267–1279, 1998.
26. Lund T, Oxland TR, Jost B, et al.: Interbody cage stabilization in the lumbar spine: Biomechanical evaluation of cage design, posterior instrumentation and bone density. **J Bone Joint Surg Br** 80B:351–359, 1998.

27. McAfee PC, Farey ID, Sutterlin CE, Gurr KR, Warden KE, Cunningham BW: The effect of spinal implant rigidity on vertebral bone density. A canine model. **Spine** 16:S190–S197, 1991.
28. McKinley TO, McLain RF, Yerby SA, Sharkey NA, Sarigul–Klijn N, Smith TS: Characteristics of pedicle screw loading. Effect of surgical technique on intravertebral and intrapedicular bending moments. **Spine** 24:18–24, 1999.
29. McLain RF, McKinley TO, Yerby SA, Smith TS, Sarigul–Klijn N: The effect of bone quality on pedicle screw loading in axial instability. A synthetic model. **Spine** 22:1454–1460, 1997.
30. Myers MA, Casciani T, Whitebeck MG, Puzas JE: Vertebral body osteopenia associated with posterolateral spine fusion in humans. **Spine** 21:2368–2371, 1996.
31. Nagata H, Schendel MJ, Transfeldt EE, Lewis JL: The effects of immobilization of long segments of the spine on the adjacent and distal facet force and lumbosacral motion. **Spine** 18:2471–2479, 1993.
32. Rapoff AJ, Ghanayem AJ, Zdeblick TA: Biomechanical comparison of posterior lumbar interbody fusion cages. **Spine** 22:2375–2379, 1997.
33. Ray CD. Threaded titanium cages for lumbar interbody fusions. **Spine** 22:667–669, 1997.
34. Riley LH, Eck JC, Yoshida H, et al.: Laparoscopic assisted fusion of the lumbar spine. A biomechanical and histologic analysis of the open versus laparoscopic technique in an animal model. **Spine** 22:1407–1412, 1997.
35. Sandhu HS, Turner S, Kabo JM, et al.: Distractive properties of a threaded interbody fusion device. An in vivo model. **Spine** 21:1201–1210, 1996.
36. Tencer AF, Hampton D, Eddy S. Biomechanical properties of threaded inserts for lumbar interbody spinal fusion. **Spine** 20:2408–2414, 1995.
37. Totoribe K, Tajima N, Chosa E: A biomechanical study of posterolateral fusion using a three-dimensional nonlinear finite element method. **J Orthop Sci** 4:115–126, 1999.
38. Van Royen BJ, Toussaint HM, Kingma, et al.: Accuracy of the sagittal vertical axis in a standing lateral radiograph as a measurement of balance in spinal deformities. **Eur Spine J** 7:408–412, 1998.
39. Volkman T, Horton WC, Hutton WC: Transfacet screws with lumbar interbody reconstruction: Biomechanical study of motion segment stiffness. **J Spinal Disord** 9:425–432, 1996.
40. Voor MJ, Mehta S, Wang M, Mahan J, Johnson JR: Biomechanical evaluation of posterior and anterior lumbar interbody fusion techniques. **J Spinal Disord** 11:328–334, 1998.
41. Voor MJ, Roberts CS, Rose SM, Glassman SD: Biomechanics of in situ rod contouring of short segment pedicle screw instrumentation in the thoracolumbar spine. **J Spinal Disord** 10:106–116, 1997.
42. White AA, Panjabi MM: Clinical biomechanics of the spine. 2nd ed. Philadelphia, JB Lippincott, 1990, p 563.
43. Youssef JA, McKinley TO, Yerby SA, McLain RF: Characteristics of pedicle screw loading. Effect of sagittal insertion angle on intrapedicular bending moments. **Spine** 24:1077–1081, 1999.
44. Zdeblick TA, Smith GR, Warden KE, Eng MB, McAfee PC: Two-point fixation of the lumbar spine. Differential stability in rotation. **Spine** 16:S298–S301, 1991.

CHAPTER

26

Posterior Lumbar Interbody Fusion (PLIF): Past, Present, and Future

PAUL M. LIN, M.D.

This chapter discusses the work of Dr. Ralph Cloward, a pioneer in posterior lumbar interbody fusion (PLIF) surgery, and subsequently modified by the author. As described by Dr. Vince Traynellis, the Scientific Program Chairman of the 1999 CNS annual meeting, "The works of Dr. Cloward and Dr. Lin represent the standard by which all new techniques must be measured." I am grateful to Dr. Traynellis for the opportunity here to review PLIF of the past, comment on the state-of-the-art PLIF of the present, and express my hope for the future.

THE PAST: BACKGROUND HISTORY AND EVOLUTION OF THE PROCEDURE

Dr. Ralph Cloward performed the first PLIF in 1940 (5), earning the title "Father of PLIF." His work on PLIF was first published in the *Journal of Neurosurgery* (6) and his seminal work was presented in 1953, at what was then called the Cushing Society (7).

Dr. Cloward was an exceptionally skillful and technically innovative neurosurgeon. He always loved to use very fine and sharp osteotomes for the bony dissection. Rightfully, he has been called the "Michelangelo of Neurosurgery." Because of this extraordinary technical superiority, none of his contemporary orthopedic colleagues was able even to come close to replicating his excellent results. Anecdotal experiences were reflective of a low fusion rate and high incidence of complications. Neurosurgeons in that era were not interested in performing spinal fusions, and PLIF was eschewed for almost 40 years. Except for one other paper by Cloward that appeared in 1963 in *Clinical Orthopedics* (8), there was a long hiatus from presentations or publications on PLIF in the neurosurgical or orthopedic communities.

A breakthrough came in 1977 with the publication *Neurosurgery* of an article by Lin entitled "A Technical Modification of Cloward's Posterior Lumbar Interbody Fusion" (16). This paper was also presented at the Congress of Neurological Surgeon's Meeting in 1976, albeit at the postconvention symposium. Twenty-three years had elapsed since Cloward's original paper at the Cushing Society's meeting. In 1981 a live telecast of a PLIF procedure was broadcast in Philadelphia (22), and demonstrated that this technically demanding neurosurgical procedure could be done successfully by any careful and trained neurosurgeon. This telecast was repeated again in 1983 (23) in front of 200 physicians during the First International Symposium on PLIF sponsored by Temple University School of Medicine. The enthusiasm for PLIF had been planted and began to grow.

Lin's modification of Cloward's PLIF stressed the importance of adhering to four sound biomechanical principles to enhance a high rate of osteosynthesis (16, 18, 19).

1. Preservation of the posterior portion of the motion segment. Emphasis is placed on preserving the locking mechanism of the facet by performing a mesial facetectomy only. This improves the stability of the PLIF construct. (Fig. 26.1) The current reliance of an internal fixator, the screw-plate pedicle system, grew out of this concern. The preservation of the supraspinous and the interspinous ligaments is

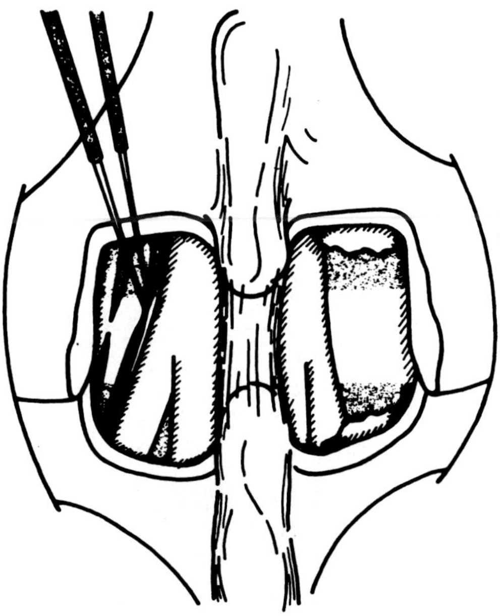

FIG. 26.1 After mesial facectectomy, the spinous process, supraspinous ligaments, and facet are preserved. Control of epidural hemorrhage by bi-polar or insulated coagulation forceps is used on the left side. On the right side, the epidural hemorrhage is controlled by surgical tampons. Impacted surgical tampons also push the nerve root medially and expose the disc space without requiring use of nerve root retractor. Source: *Clinical Orthopaedics and Related Research,* 1983, 180:154–168 Fig. 3.

very important for the muscle to assert its stabilizing influence through proper reattachment.

2. Total Discectomy. About 80% of the disc space should be excavated. A larger area of bony contact between the grafts with the vertebral bodies heightens the chances of successful interbody fusion.
3. Partial decortication of the endplates, as with anterior cervical interbody fusion, total decortication down to the bleeding marrow is not needed nor desirable. Removal of the endplate increases the probability of subsidence of graft or implants. The subchondral endplate is not a cortical bone and, in fact, it serves as nutrient membrane to the intervertebral disc.
4. Unigraft concept. Four to six unicortical peg grafts are used, with the cortical bone of the peg grafts parallel to the longitudinal axis of the body. Every effort is then made to fill all of the remaining empty spaces with cancellous bone strips and packing of the autogenous cancellous bone strips in between the unicortical peg grafts, the high density cancellous graft. The construct, therefore, acts functionally and mechanically as a one piece "unigraft," similar to the anterior interbody cervical fusion (Fig. 26.2).

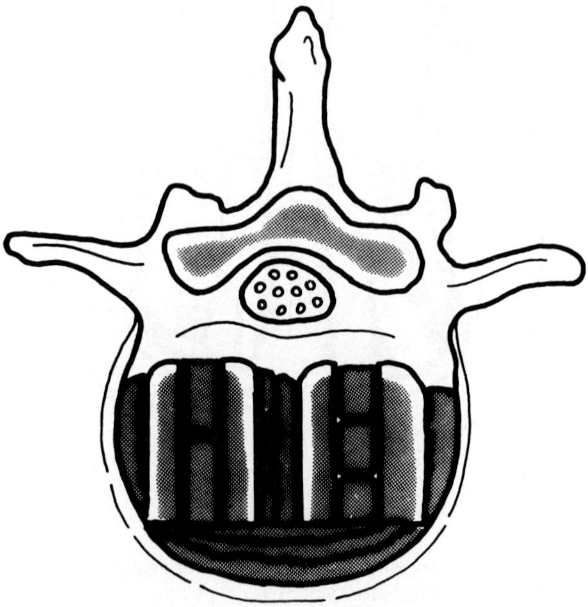

FIG. 26.2 Compact sandwiched cortical peg grafts interfacing tightly with impacted cancellous strips. Source: *Clinical Orthopaedics and Related Research,* 1983, 180:154–168 Fig 10 ABC.

Clinical results of PLIF are superior when there is osteosynthesis or solid fusion. The three determinants for an osteosynthesis are:

1) stable construct of the PLIF, 2) large amounts of bone grafts, and 3) adequate osteogenicity of the graft construct (17–19, 27, 28).

The radiologic indication of computed tomographic osteosynthesis is evidence of remodeling of the interbody graft (27). As seen on the computed tomographic (CT) scan, the interbody graft should give the appearance of a remodeled vertebral body—a cortical ring and cancellous marrow or centrum, the "Ring" sign (17) (Fig. 26.3). Other secondary radiologic evidence includes:

1. Absorption of anterior intervertebral spurs (19) (Fig. 26.4);
2. Anterior progression of the graft (19) (Fig. 26.5);
3. Formation of continuous posterior or anterior intervertebral cortex (19) (Fig. 26.6);
4. Spontaneous facet fusion (19, 21) (Fig. 26.7);
5. Increased bone density at the interpedicular line in A-P radiograph, the line of stress (Wolffe's Law) (18, 21) (Fig. 26.8);
6. Trabeculation pattern of the graft, the presence of haversian canals on lateral radiograph (18, 21) (Fig. 26.9); and,
7. Loss of osteoblastic activity and graft-host interfaces on radiograph (17, 21).

Currently, PLIF is undergoing a renaissance of sorts, as evidenced by the enthusiasm generated on this topic at this convention. Let me take this opportunity to introduce the contributions of a group of PLIF surgeons whom I call the "PLIF Millenium Club." The club has 12 members, each of whom has performed over 1000 PLIFs. Many have made significant modifications and contributions to the original PLIF described by Cloward. Listed below in alphabetical order are the members and their contributions to PLIF:

1. Horst Blume—Unilateral chip-dowel autograft (1, 2).
2. J.W. Simmons—Autogenous chip grafts from neural arch (34).
3. John Collis—Clowardian technique, xenograft, disc replacement concept (9).
4. William Duffy—High density autogenous cancellous graft.
5. Charles Hunter—Trapezoid shape autograft to prevent retropulsion (14).
6. John Jackson—Midas Rex for discectomy and posterior interspinous wiring (dorsal tension band) (15).
7. Paul M. Lin—Preservation of posterior segment and autograft (16, 18, 19, 20, 21).
8. Gabriel Ma—Mortising chisel instrumentation, allograft (24).

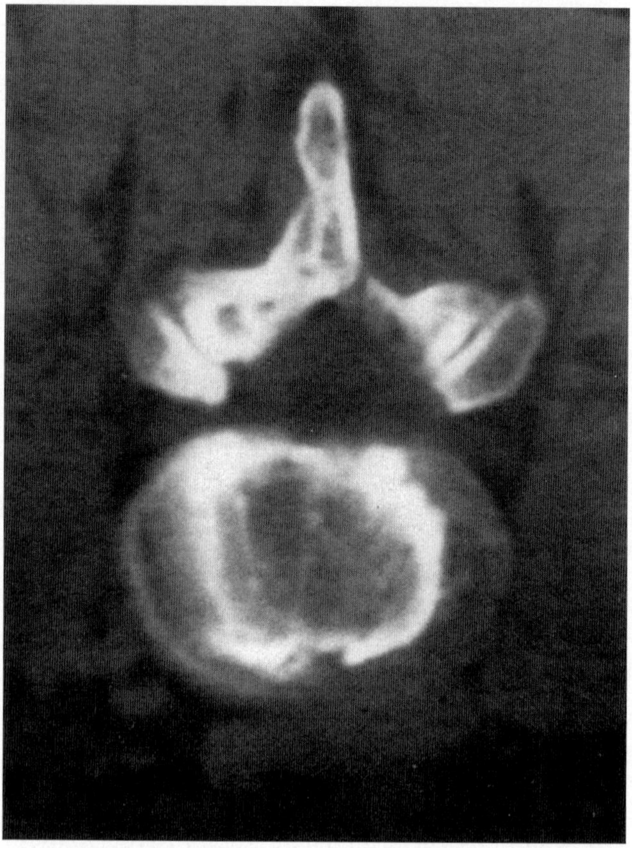

FIG. 26.3 Full maturation of an L4-5 autograft, only 9 months after a PLIF. Note that the remodeling has given the graft the osseous characteristics of a vertebral body (i.e., a cortical ring and a cancellous centrum). Source: *Clinical Orthopaedics and Related Research,* 1989, 242:158–163, Fig. 5

9. P.S. Ramani—Mixed allograft and autograft (29).
10. Alastair Robson—Clowardian technique.
11. Miyuki Takeda—Bicortical autograft (37).
12. Tomio Yamamoto—Clowardian technique.

Other significant PLIF surgeons reside in Germany, France, and New Zealand. Needless to say, to become a "PLIF Millenium Club member," a PLIF surgeon must have good results and the support of the referring medical community.

Arthur Steffee's introduction of the pedicular screw, plate assembly, and various other interbody prostheses, cages, or screws codified the be-

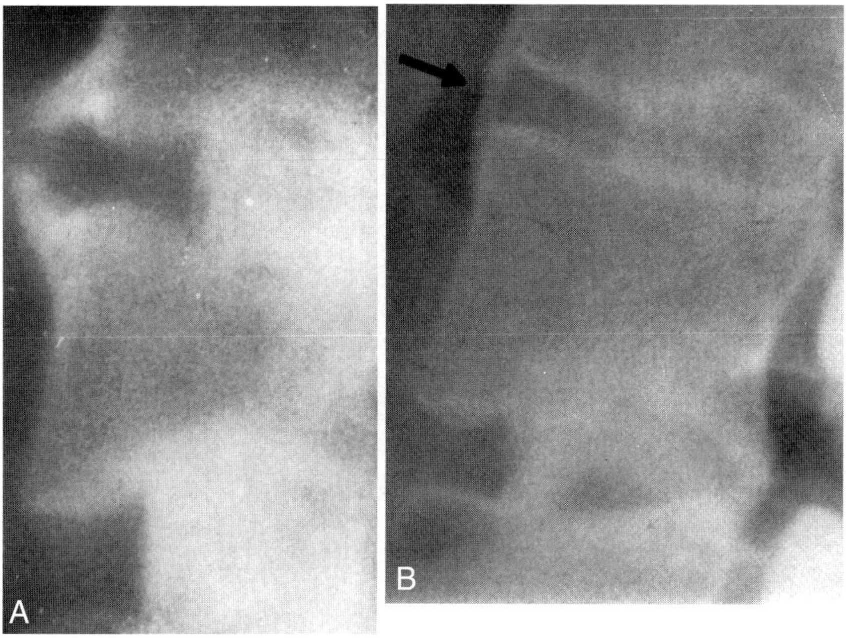

FIG. 26.4 AB (A) Film taken 4 months after PLIF at L 3-4. Note the reactive changes of the anterior limiting membrane between the spurs. (B) Film taken 1 year after the surgery. Note the disappearance of the anterior spur and the calcification of the anterior limiting membrane. Source: *Clinical Orthopaedics and Related Research,* 1985, 193:90–102, Fig. 4AB.

ginning of the modern PLIF era (35, 36). The advantage of an internal fixator is clear—it increases the stability of the PLIF construct, and by derivation, a better fusion rate. However, an internal fixator takes away the natural compressive movements that are highly desirable for rapid physiological osteosynthesis of an interbody fusion. The introduction of various types of hardware in PLIF has actually delayed the recognizable radiological evidence of PLIF from 6 to 12 months. Currently, the overdependence on mechanical devices has become so pervasive that there are young spine surgeons who attempt to learn how to insert lumbar interbody cages, screw, and plates without ever performing or witnessing a "traditional" PLIF. Instead of emphasizing the need of osteosynthesis in a physiological setting, we are now totally dependent on mechanical devices to hold the two vertebral bodies together—a mechanical "fusion" but not necessarily a physiologic osteosynthesis. Lack of motion on dynamic films does not equate to the presence of osteosynthesis.

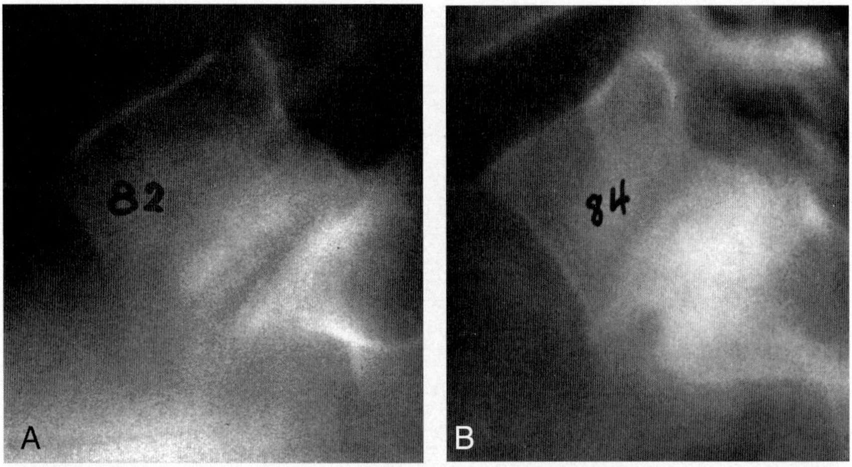

FIG. 26.5 Lateral tomogram obtained after L5-S1 PLIF, showing an anterior progression of the graft that suggests maturation and remodeling. (A) 4 months after surgery. (B) 2 years after surgery. Note rounding off of the posterior graft with adjoing cortices. Source: *Clinical Orthopaedics and Related Research,* 1985, 193:90–102, Fig. 3 AB.

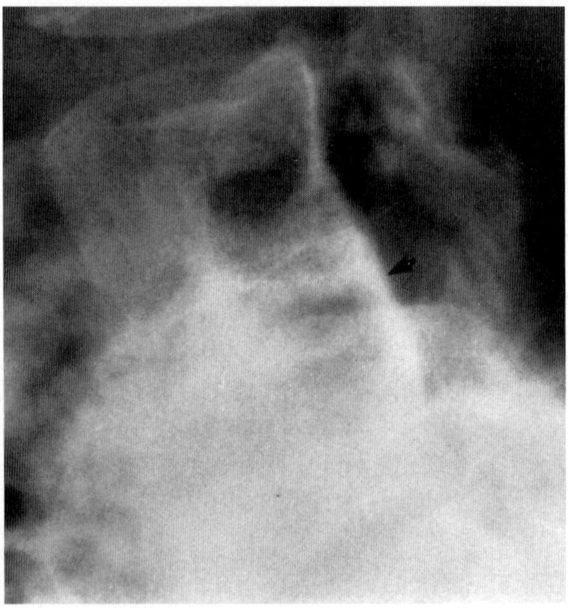

FIG. 26.6 Lateral radiograph obtained 1 year after PLIF. Note posteriorly the continuing cortical line between the adjoining vertebral body and the posterior graft of the disc space.

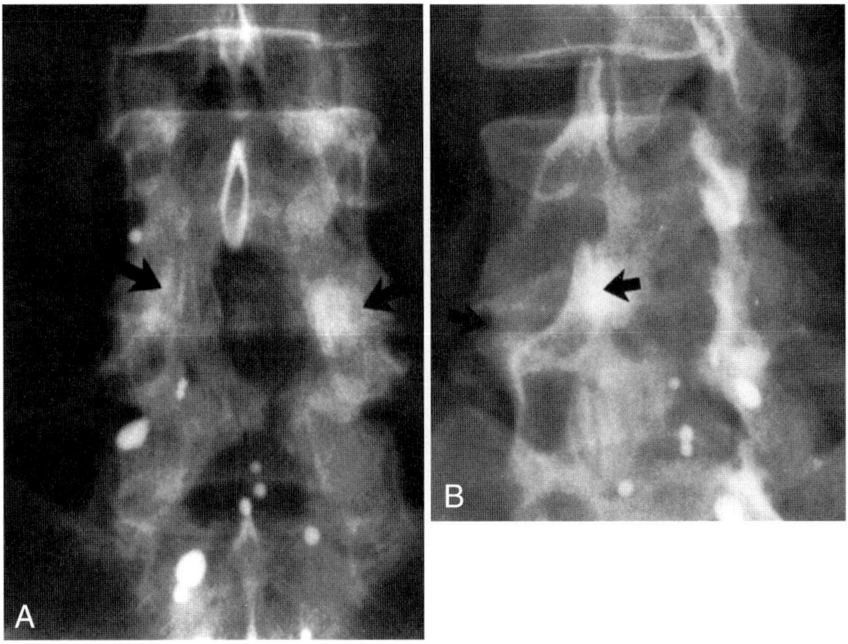

FIG. 26.7 Spontaneous facet fusion as seen 8 years after PLIF. (A) Anteroposterior radiograph. (B) Right oblique radiograph. Arrow indicates spontaneous facet fusion.

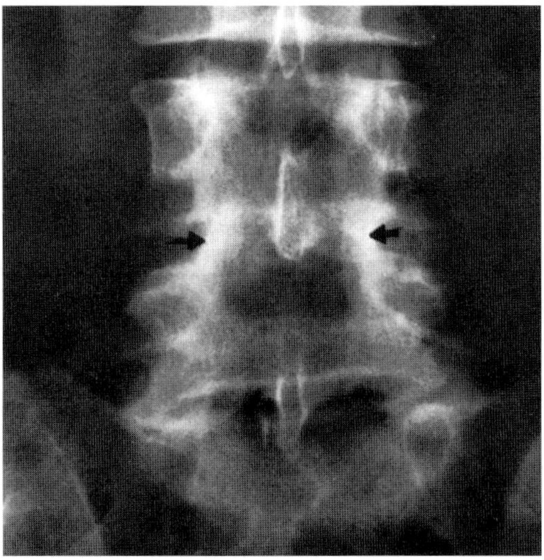

FIG. 26.8 Increased interpedicular bone density in a mature PLIF, as seen on an anteroposterior radiograph. This represents bone reaction to the external stress (Wolffe's Law). Source: *Clinical Orthopaedics and Related Research,* 1983, 180:154–168, Fig. 13B.

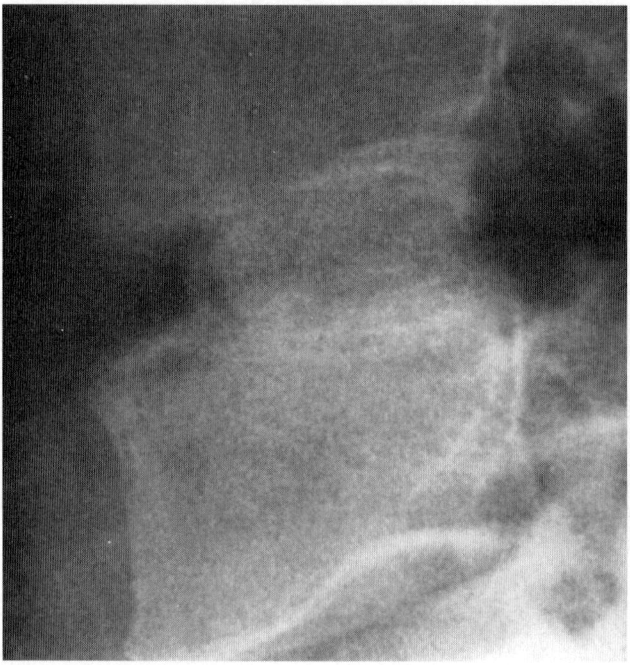

FIG. 26.9 Lateral radiograph showing trabeculation of the graft. This is an anatomic fusion, or an arthrodesis. Source: *Clinical Orthopaedic & Related Resources,* 1989, 242:158–163, Fig. 2.

My presentation will focus now on a critical review of the result of PLIF performed in the earlier noninstrumented era as compared to the present, where PLIF is being performed almost totally dependant on mechanical stabilizing devices. The fusion rate reported by Cloward in 1953 was 96% in 162 cases (6), perhaps an unrealistically high standard for ordinary mortal spine surgeons (like most of us). Despite the use of destabilizing total facetectomy, Cloward's success depended on compressive forces from the large brick-like symmetrical graft construct induced by maximal distraction of the interspace. In 1983, I reported an 88% fusion rate among 465 cases (18, 26). This was very similar to Ray's review of 13 PLIF surgeons (30, 31) who reported an average fusion rate of 89% among 2,580 uninstrumented PLIF cases.

These figures are not as high as the fusion rates in the modern instrumented series of 98.9% reported by Brantigan among 178 cases (4), in which a carbon fiber cage was used. Likewise, in 1997, Ray reported fusion in 96% of 236 cases (30, 32) using a threaded cage. I believe that PLIF performed with current technology with heavy reliance on various types of implants or internal fixators has a 10% advantage of fusion rate as compared to the conventional PLIF performed in my generation. In this current litigious environment, this 10% difference in fusion rate could be critical.

However, there are some legitimate criticisms of the current instrumented PLIF procedure.

1. High cost. The cost of modern hardware for PLIF is between $2,500 to $5,000 for each level. The final hospital charge to the patient is usually twice that amount. Factoring the extra cost for operating room charges and surgeon's reimbursement for the extra procedures, the total extra cost of a PLIF procedure is about $25,000. When you consider that 70,000 lumbar spinal fusions are performed each year in the U.S., the total added cost to society would be 1.75 billion dollars (3, 11, 31).
2. Clinical result of uninstrumented PLIF is not directly related to a successful fusion. Unlike PLIF done with instrumentation, failure of the traditional PLIF does not necessarily result in clinical failure. As long as the posterior segment is intact, a 10% rate of pseudoarthrosis does not mean a 10% clinical failure rate (20). This implies that the additional cost of the instruments may not be justified.
3. An unsuccessful traditional PLIF can be redone with instrumentation. A failed instrumented PLIF is more difficult to correct and refuse. In my personal series of 1989, 20% of my PLIFs were instrumented, with a fusion rate of 97.5% (39/40) (20, 21). I believe instrumentation has its role, but it is not automatic nor universal. Perhaps only half of the cases require the benefit of an internal fixator, such as those with various destabilizing pathology or those that were destabilized intraoperatively, those PLIF should have the benefit of an internal fixator.

THE FUTURE: THE IMPACT OF TECHNOLOGY

I believe the future will bring even better PLIF results based on the following:

1. Improved magnification and lighting analogous to the improvement in microsurgical or endoscopic surgery (12);
2. Improved discectomy technique using a power tool such as Midas Rex or Power Wisk with intraoperative fluroscopic control;
3. Improved technique to generate maximal impaction using power injected BMP-enriched Grafton gel (13, 25), or the autogenous cancellous bone mush inserted in and around the prosthesis;
4. If done without instrumentation, routine use of dorsal tension band with cable (Songer);

5. Improved autograft harvesting technique, such as using an endoscope or other percutaneous methodology;
6. Consideration of the use of biocompatible and degradable miniosteosynthetic material for fixation devices such as resorbable polyevolactide (PLLA). As reported this year in the *Journal of Neurosurgery* (May 1999), osteosynthesis has been shown to be enhanced using the PLLA screw and plate (26);
7. Additional research on the methods to attain physiological osteosynthesis and less dependence on hardware. The use of recombinant human bone Morphogenic Protein 2 (rhBMP2) has shown great promise in an experimental setting (10, 25, 33). Without fusion and osteosynthesis, eventually subsidence of the implants within the vertebral body would occur, as the implant materials are much harder than the surrounding cancellous bone marrow of the vertebral body of the host. This complication would become more evident as the patient population ages; and
8. Interbody fusion is undoubtedly the fusion site of choice in the lumbar area. The posterior approach (as in PLIF) has the distinct advantage of being able to achieve satisfactory neural decompression, but the PLIF surgeon of the future should also be equally familiar with the indications and proper techniques in performing an anterior lumbar interbody fusion (ALIF).

I have spent the last 15 years of my neurosurgical career, prior to my retirement from surgical practice in 1988, seeking to further the cause of PLIF. Today, I speak for Dr. Cloward and myself to remind you that PLIF is very much alive and well.

REFERENCES

1. Blume HG. Unilateral lumbar interbody fusion (posterior approach) utilizing dowel grafts, in Lin, PM (ed). *Posterior Lumbar Interbody Fusion,* Springfield, IL: Charles C. Thomas, 1982, p. 252–275.
2. Blume HG. Unilateral posterior interbody fusion. Simplified dowel technique. **Clin Orthop** 193:75–84, 1985.
3. Branch CL. Instrumentation after anterior cervical fusion. **Clin Neurosurg** 45:22–24, 1998.
4. Brantigan JW. Lumbar interbody fusion using the Brantigan I/F Cage for PLIF and the VSP pedicle screw system: Two year results of a Food and Drug Administration IDE clinical trial. March 12, 1999, page 14.
5. Cloward RB. New treatment for ruptured intervertebral disc. Annual Meeting of Hawaii Territorial Medical Association, May 1945.
6. Cloward RB. The treatment of ruptured intervertebral discs by vertebral body fusion. Indications, operative technique, after care. **J Neurosurg** 10:154, 1953.
7. Cloward RB. History of PLIF—Forty years of personal experience, in, Lin, PM (ed). Lumbar Interbody Fusion. Springfield: Charles C. Thomas, 1982, pp 58–71.

8. Cloward RB. Lesions of the intervertebral discs and their treatment by interbody fusion methods: The painful disk. **Clin Orthop** 27:51, 1963.
9. Collis JS. Total disc replacement: A modified posterior lumbar interbody fusion: Report of 750 cases. **Clin Orthop** 193:64–67, 1985.
10. Cook SD, Dalton JE, Tan EH et al: In vivo evaluation of recombinant human osteogenic protein (rh OP-1) implants as a bone graft substitute for spinal fusion. **Spine** 19:1655–1663, 1994.
11. Geer CP, Papadopoulos SM: Instrumentation after anterior cervical fusion. **Clin Neurosurg** 45:25–29, 1998.
12. Haid RW. Neurosurgery of the spine in the year 2001: A four year review. **Clin Neurosurg** 45:153–159, 1998.
13. Helm GA, Sheehan JM, Sheehan JP, et al. Utilization of type I collagen gel, demineralized bone matrix, and bone morphogenetic protein-2 to enhance autologous bone lumbar spinal fusion. **J Neurosurg** 86:93–100, 1997.
14. Hutter CG. Spinal stenosis and posterior lumbar interbody fusion. **Clin Orthop** 193:103–114, 1985.
15. Jackson JD. Posterior lumbar interbody fusion utilizing power instrumentation and posterior wire stabilization, in, Lin & Gill (ed). *Lumbar Interbody Fusion.* Rockville, MD: Aspen Publications, 1989, pp. 233–241.
16. Lin PM. A technical modification of Cloward's posterior lumbar interbody fusion. **Neurosurg** 1:118–124, 1977.
17. Lin PM. Radiographic evidence of posterior lumbar interbody fusion with an emphasis on Computerized Tomographic Scanning. **Clin Orthop** 242:158–163, 1989.
18. Lin PM, Cautilli RA, Joyce MF. Posterior lumbar interbody fusion. **Clin Orthop** 180:154–168, 1983.
19. Lin PM. Posterior lumbar interbody fusion technique: Complications and pitfalls. **Clin Orthop** 193:90–102, 1985.
20. Lin PM. Techniques and complications of Posterior Lumbar Interbody Fusion, Chapter 15, in Lin & Gill (ed.) *Lumbar Interbody Fusion.* Rockville, MD: Aspen Publications, 1989, pp. 171–198.
21. Lin PM. Radiologic evidence of PLIF, Chapter 5, in Lin & Gill (ed.) *Lumbar Interbody Fusion.* Rockville, MD: Aspen Publications, 1989, pp. 55–69.
22. Lin PM. Posterior lumbar interbody fusion: A live video surgical clinic. PLIF Workshop Temple University School of Medicine, April 21–25, 1981, Philadelphia, PA.
23. Lin PM. Posterior Lumbar Interbody Fusion: A live telecast. First International Symposium on PLIF, April 20–23, 1983, Philadelphia, PA.
24. Ma GW. Posterior lumbar interbody fusion with specialized instruments. **Clin Orthop** 193:57–63, 1985.
25. Muschler GF, Hypodo A, Manning T, et al: Evaluation of human bone morphogenic protein 2 in a canine spinal fusion model. **Clin Orthop** 308:229–240, 1994.
26. Peltoniemi HH, Tulamo RM, Toivonen T, et al: Biodegradable semirigid plate and miniscrew fixation compared with rigid titanium fixation in experimental calvarial osteotomy. **J Neurosurg** 90:910–917, 1999.
27. Prolo DJ, Oklund SA, Buthcher M. Toward uniformity in evaluating results of lumbar spine operations: A paradigm applied to PLIF. **Spine** 11:601–606, 1986.
28. Prolo DJ. Osteosynthesis in lumbar interbody fusion, in, Lin & Gill (ed). *Lumbar Interbody Fusion.* Rockville, MD: Aspen Publications, 1989, pp 71–78.
29. Ramani PS (ed). *Posterior Lumbar Interbody Fusion.* Bombay, India: Associated Personnel Services Publication, 1989, p 121.
30. Ray CD. Threaded titanium cages for lumbar interbody fusions. **Spine** 22:667–680, 1997.

31. Ray CD. Threaded fusion cages for lumbar interbody fusions: An economic comparison with 360 fusions. **Spine** 22:681–685, 1997.
32. Ray CD. Spinal interbody fusions: A review, featuring new generation techniques. **Neurosurg Q** 7:135–156, 1997.
33. Schimandle JH, Boden SD, Hutton WC. Experimental spinal fusion with recombinant human bone morphogenic protein-2. **Spine** 20:1326–1337, 1995.
34. Simmons JW. Posterior lumbar interbody fusion with posterior elements as chip grafts. **Clin Orthop** 193:85–89, 1985.
35. Steffee AD. The variable screw placement system with posterior lumbar interbody fusion, in, Lin & Gill (ed). *Lumbar Interbody Fusion*. Rockville, MD: Aspen Publications, 1989, pp 81–93.
36. Steffee AD, Biscuip R, Sitkowski D. Segmental spine plates with pedicle screw fixation. **Clin Orthop** 203:45–53, 1986.
37. Takeda M. Experience in posterior lumbar interbody fusion: Unicortical versus bicortical autologous grafts. **Clin Orthop** 193:120–126, 1985.

CHAPTER

27

Posterolateral Fusion of the Lumbar Spine: Rationale, Indications, Techniques, and Results

MARK N. HADLEY, M.D.

Instability of the lumbar spine is a common and important clinical entity in the practice of neurological surgery and orthopedic spinal surgery. Lumbar instability is a cause of severe back pain and disability, and contributes to sciatica and/or neurogenic claudication in affected patients. Stabilization and fusion of unstable or "hypermobile" lumbar spinal segments often provides clinical benefit in terms of pain relief and improved patient function. A variety of methods have been used in an effort to provide stabilization and fusion of the lumbar spine in humans. This review provides a brief overview of the time-tested technique of noninstrumented posterolateral lumbar spine fusion in the treatment of lumbar spinal instability.

HISTORICAL PERSPECTIVE AND RATIONALE

Fusion of the lumbosacral spine developed as an adaptation of techniques described by Hadra (15), Lange (25), Abbe (1), Hibbs (21), and others (3) for the surgical correction and stabilization of the thoracic spine in the treatment of patients with Pott's disease. These reports, dating from the turn of the century, describe attempted fixation of thoracic spinal deformities using various types of segmented and nonsegmented instrumentation, often, but not necessarily, using additional bone as the fusion substrate (15, 25). Abbe (1) and Hibbs (21) documented the first successful posterior lumbar spinal fusion procedures, independently, both in 1911. Hibbs' (21) technique of autologous harvest of adjacent spinal laminae as a dorsal onlay graft became the most popular and the most frequently used (*Fig. 27.1*).

Posterior and posterolateral fusion techniques were adopted in the treatment of patients with traumatic fracture injuries, infections, scoliosis, and as secondary procedures for patients with pseudarthrosis or other failed spinal procedures. Despite variations and modifications of surgical techniques, including the use of autologous iliac crest graft as

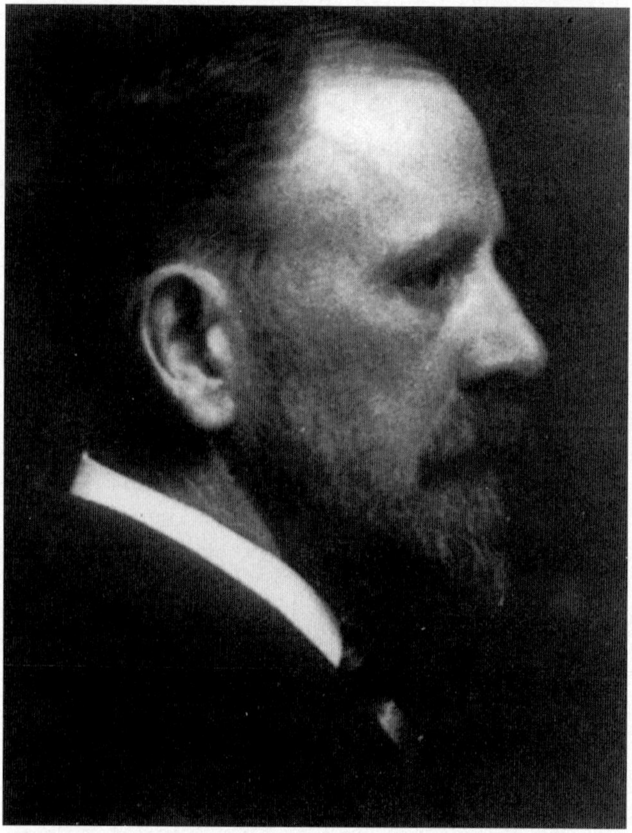

FIG. 27.1 Russel Hibbs first reported the use of autologous bone graft as only fusion substrate (*from,* Albertsone GD, Benzel EC. In: E Benzel (ed) Spine Surgery (Vol 1) Techniques, Complication Avoidance, and Management. Chapter 1, History. Churchill Livingstone, Philadelphia, PA, 1999, p. 11).

the fusion substrate, early experience with attempted dorsolateral arthrodesis was poor (3, 6, 10).

Despite high failure rates (pseudarthrosis), the concept of and rationale for posterior spinal fusion appeared sound. The surgical exposure would become common and straightforward. Posterolateral fusion could be used in conjunction with posterior discectomy or decompression procedures, and could be combined with posterior fixation instrumentation, be it wires, rods, or other devices. By itself, however, posterolateral fusion could not correct deformity, nor was it particularly successful in the treatment of spinal instability with deformity, either acute fracture–dislocation injury or progressive scoliosis (3, 10, 30).

With the advent of the science of spinal biomechanics and a better appreciation of the advantages and limitations of spinal instrumentation, more appropriate and discriminate use of fusion and internal fixation procedures occurred. In 1963, Holdsworth (23) introduced his classification scheme for characterization and treatment of subaxial spinal fractures. His contributions and those of others helped clinicians better appreciate, identify, and treat mechanical instability of the spine. Paul Harrington (18, 19), the "Father of Modern Spinal Instrumentation," made his keen observations known in the 1960s and 1970s (*Fig. 27.2*). His conclusions that because spinal instruments fail over time they should be applied as

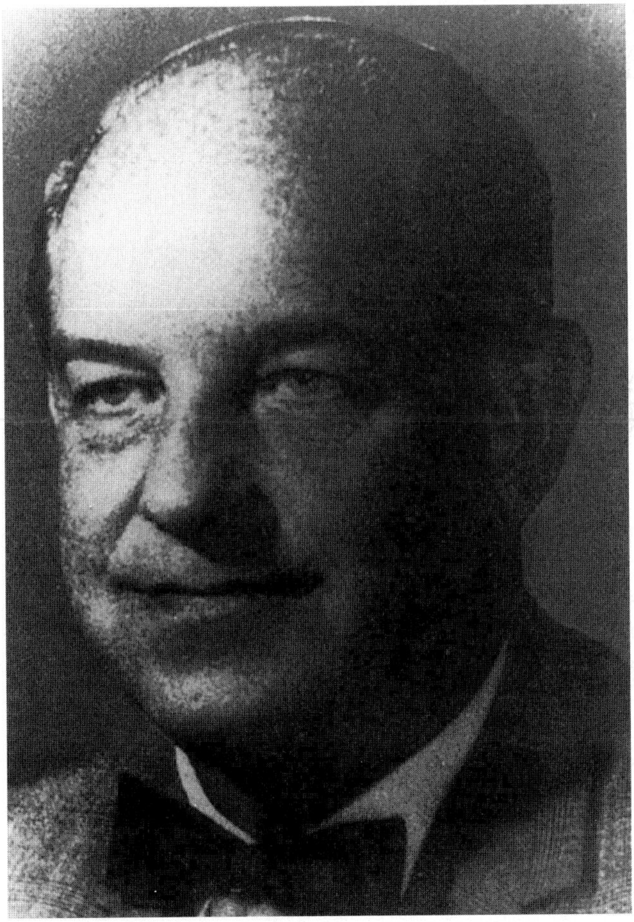

FIG. 27.2 Paul Harrington, pioneer of spinal instrumentation as adjunct to fusion (*from,* Albertsone GD, Benzel EC. In: E Benzel (ed) Spine Surgery (Vol 1) Techniques, Complication Avoidance, and Management. Chapter 1, History. Churchill Livingstone, Philadelphia, PA, 1999, p. 14).

temporary adjuncts to attempted fusion, and that after implant failure, successful fusion will maintain correction and stability, helped to reshape spinal surgery and became the foundation of modern spinal correction and surgical stabilization. As surgeons became familiar with the principles of clinical mechanics, the use of spinal instrumentation, and the biology of bone healing and fusion, success with spinal fusion procedures, with or without instrumentation, became common.

INDICATIONS

Posterolateral fusion procedures have been advocated in the treatment of patients with pain and dysfunction from lumbar or lumbosacral spinal instability, either primary or secondary (2, 12–14, 17, 24, 30). Primary instability of the spine is described as what occurs de novo, and includes patients with acute spinal instability as a result of trauma, infection, or neoplasm, and those with chronic progressive instability resulting from scoliotic deformity, degenerative disc disease with facet osteoarthritis, degenerative scoliosis with spinal stenosis, and isthmic spondylolisthesis.

Secondary spinal instability is what occurs after surgical procedural intervention. Examples include instability after decompression for stenosis and instability because of a failed attempt at fusion (pseudarthrosis). Fusion procedures, therefore, have been suggested as adjunctive treatment for patients who have the potential to develop instability as a result of surgical treatment of lumbar spine pathology. A patient with multilevel stenosis and degenerative spondylolisthesis who requires extensive decompression represents a common clinical scenario for which fusion is used.

A number of investigators have attempted to characterize patient clinical and radiographic criteria, which help to define the need for lumbar spinal fusion. We prefer the scheme described by Sonntag and Marciano (30), reported in 1995. Their extensive literature review resulted in the characterization of three different "grades" or "classes" of pathology that warrant spinal fusion as an adjunct to the treatment of patients with lumbar spine disorders.

Pathology for which fusion is recommended

Two- or three-column injury/instability, such as trauma, tumor, or infection
Iatrogenic instability
Isthmic spondylolisthesis

Pathology for which fusion may be beneficial, and relative indications for surgery

Degenerative spondylolisthesis
Abnormal movement on dynamic films with appropriate pain or neurological deficit
"Mechanical" back pain

Pathology that rarely requires lumbar spinal fusion as an adjunct to direct treatment, or decompression

Routine discectomy
Abnormal radiograph without appropriate findings
Stable spinal stenosis

A host of factors must be assessed when determining whether any patient, irrespective of the pathology involved, is a candidate for lumbar spinal fusion. In addition to defining correctly the patient's pathology and the degree of or potential for lumbar instability, the patient's medical health, mental health, life expectancy, and potential for realization of the clinical benefit from surgery must be considered.

TECHNIQUES

There are two basic techniques of posterolateral spinal fusion exclusive of posterior lumbar interbody fusion: the intertransverse fusion method (*Fig. 27.3*) and the interlaminar fusion method (2, 24, 31) (*Fig. 27.4*). They differ in the amount of dorsolateral exposure obtained and the amount of bone surface area involved in the attempted arthrodesis. Unilateral procedures and lateral-only procedures have been described (16). Most surgeons use the bilateral intertransverse method, particularly after lumbar decompression, to maximize the area of bone surface–graft interface, without fusion mass compromise medially at the site of decompression.

Several investigators have defined the relevant anatomy and vascular supply of the dorsolateral lumbar spine (27, 28, 31). Meticulous exposure and decortication of the transverse processes, lateral aspects of the pars, the involved facet complex, and the remaining laminae, without devascularization of these structures or the adjacent musculature, has been cited as essential to successful intertransverse posterolateral fusion. Avoidance of compromise of the uninvolved superior facet complex is another critical component of long-term success. Abundant autologous fusion substrate placed in contact with the exposed, decorticated dorsolateral surfaces of the spinal segments being treated completes the procedure. Denuding, decortication, and packing of the involved facet joints with fusion substrate have been described as components of both the intertransverse and interlaminar fusion methods (10, 24, 27, 28, 31).

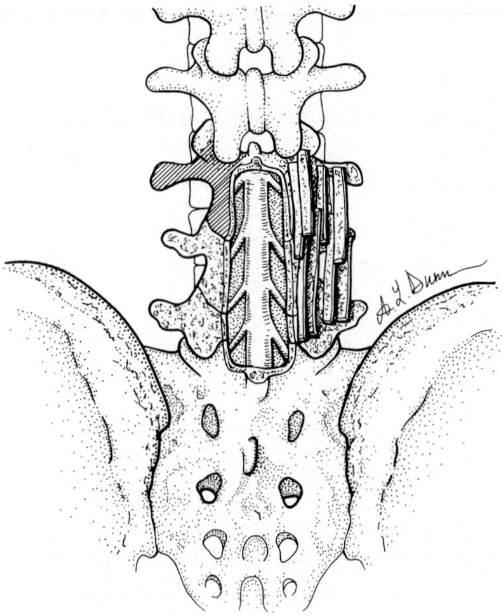

FIG. 27.3 Dorsolateral lumbar intertransverse fusion (*from,* Kaptain GJ, Shaffrey CL, Halliday AL, Schneier IM, Jane JA. In: E Benzel (ed) Spine Surgery (Vol 1) Techniques, Complication Avoidance, and Management. Chapter 25, Dorsal and Lateral Thoracic and lumbar Fusion. Churhill Livingstone, Philadelphia, PA, 1999, p. 352).

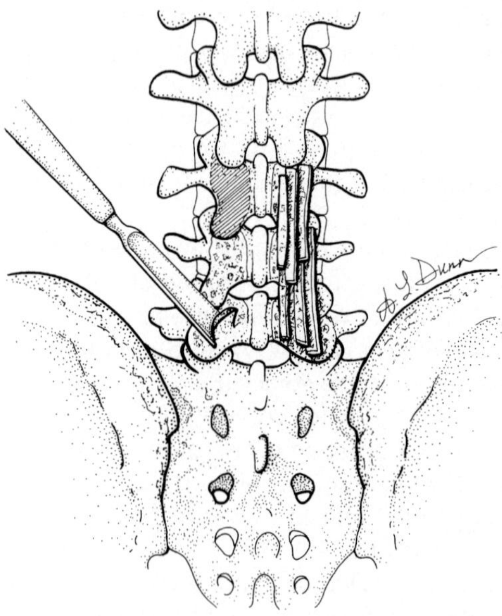

FIG. 27.4 Dorsolateral lumbar interlaminar fusion (*from,* Kaptain GJ, Shaffrey CL, Halliday AL, Schneier IM, Jane JA. In: E Benzel (ed) Spine Surgery (Vol 1) Techniques, Complication Avoidance, and Management. Chapter 25, Dorsal and Lateral Thoracic and lumbar Fusion. Churhill Livingstone, Philadelphia, PA, 1999, p. 352).

RESULTS

The success of posterolateral fusion for lumbar spine instability depends on the pathological process being treated, the number of levels involved, and the observer's definition of success. Reported fusion rates for posterolateral fusion procedures for lumbosacral spinal instability range from 60 to 95% (3–5, 9–11, 16, 20, 24, 26–33).

In comparison with other noninstrumented lumbar fusion methods, posterolateral fusion resulted in arthrodesis more consistently than other techniques. McNab and Dall (28) compared the incidence of pseudarthrosis after posterolateral fusion, posterior fusion, and anterior lumbar interbody fusion (ALIF). Arthrodesis was accomplished in 93% of patients who underwent posterolateral intertransverse fusion procedures. Patients who had posterior interlaminar fusion procedures had an 80% fusion success rate. Only 70% of patients who underwent attempted ALIF procedures achieved arthrodesis (28). Several authors have cited a difference between clinical outcome and radiographic evidence of fusion (4, 11, 31, 32). In general, clinical "success," a good or excellent clinical result, correlates with segmental arthrodesis confirmed on posttreatment radiographs. Stauffer and Coventry (31) noted that 72% of Mayo Clinic patients treated with posterolateral fusion, who had confirmed arthrodesis, reported a good clinical result. Interestingly, 18% of their patients with postoperative pseudarthrosis also indicated good clinical outcome.

In the 1970s, 1980s, and early 1990s, bilateral posterolateral fusion of the lumbar spine became the gold standard with which other fusion techniques were compared (2, 4, 5, 9–11, 20, 24, 26, 30–33). Noninstrumented posterolateral lumbar fusion in the treatment of lumbar or lumbosacral spinal instability was relatively easy to perform, had good clinical and radiographic success rates, and was associated with

TABLE 27.1
Decomposition with Posterolateral Fusion Without Instrumentation

Author	Number of Patients	Number Fused	Percentage
Feffer*	8	8	100%
Herkowitz*	25	16	64%
Lombardi*	21	19	90%
Zdeblick*	10	6	60%
Bernhardt	27	20	74%
France	28	19	64%
Stauffer	143	115	80%
Thomsen	66	56	85%
Axelsson	70	54	77%

*spondylolisthesis only

relatively few complications. This was particularly true when used in the treatment of moderate lumbar spinal instability without deformity. Failure rates of posterolateral fusion were highest in patients with prior fusion failure (pseudarthrosis), marked instability (fractures, progressive deformity, or dynamic spondylolisthesis), or multilevel disease with instability. For these disorders, internal fixation devices were offered as adjuncts to posterolateral fusion. Fusion success rates of instrumented procedures for patients with these conditions were reportedly superior to those without instrumentation (5, 7, 8, 22, 29, 33). The use of internal fixation as an adjunct to fusion in the treatment of lumbar instability of all types is now commonplace.

It has been difficult to assess accurately and to compare outcome results of noninstrumented posterolateral fusion procedures with those of instrumented lumbar fusion procedures. There are a variety of reasons for this, the most important of which has been the lack of good-quality comparative studies assessing randomized patients with similar disorders prospectively, treated with and without instrumentation. A number of retrospective reviews suggest better radiographic and clinical success with the use of internal fixation as an adjunct to fusion (5, 7, 8, 22, 29). Several retrospective studies noted better, earlier correction of deformity in the lumbosacral spine and increased "stiffness" or rigidity of the segments under treatment with the added use of internal fixation compared with noninstrumented posterolateral fusion methods (5, 9). Posterolateral bone fusion mass as determined by postoperative radiographs is less robust after instrumented fusion procedures, presumably the result of less surface area to place fusion substrate in contact with the dorsolateral surfaces of the segments to be fused. Despite 2-year fusion rates that are similar statistically to noninstrumented methods, and an increase in complications associated with instrumentation, proponents of internal fixation as an adjunct to lumbar fusion argue that multisegment instability, marked acute fracture disruption, spinal deformity, neoplastic spinal instability, and dynamic spondylolisthetic instability are treated more successfully with instrumentation and fusion rather than dorsolateral fusion alone (5, 7, 8, 22, 29, 33).

Two recent studies of patients with degenerative lumbar spinal instability shed some light on this issue (11, 32). Both are prospective, randomized assessments of posterolateral lumbar fusion procedures performed with or without transpedicular internal fixation. With minor caveats, both have good clinical and radiographic follow-up 2 years after surgery.

Thomsen et al. (32) received the 1997 Volvo Award for their clinical assessment of posterolateral fusion with and without Cotrel–Dubous-

TABLE 27.2
Prospective Comparison of Lumbar Fusion with and without Instrumentation

	France	Thomsen
Fusion*		
No Instrumentation	64%	85%
Yes Instrumentation	76%	68%
Satisfaction*		
No Instrumentation	56%	80%
Yes Instrumentation	57%	82%
Complication		
No Instrumentation	NA	1%
Yes Instrumentation	N/A	5%
Reoperation		
No Instrumentation	11%	6%
Yes Instrumentation	17%	19%

*two year follow-up

set pedical screw fixation. Their group noted no statistically significant difference in fusion success rates and found equally high global patient satisfaction between instrumented (82%) and noninstrumented (74%) fusion patients. In a study by France et al. (11), published in 1999, single-level posterolateral lumbar fusion procedures with instrumentation had a higher rate of fusion (86%) than noninstrumented fusion procedures (71%). Oddly, the reverse was true for multilevel procedures. The overall fusion success rate for instrumented procedures was 74% compared with 64% for posterolateral fusion without internal fixation. Clinical outcomes were similar for the two groups. Both studies cited increased operative time, instrumentation-related complications, and a higher rate of reoperation in the instrumentation-with-fusion groups. Neither study provided data to support the use of added instrumentation in attempted elective lumbar posterolateral fusion procedures.

The conclusions from these studies raise the question of the efficacy of the routine use of instrumentation as an adjunct to fusion in the treatment of lumbar spinal instability. Although segmental pedicle screw rod/plate fixation appears to provide benefit to selected patients who require fusion for lumbar spinal instability, instrumentation is not required to achieve arthrodesis or clinical success in all patients who require lumbar stabilization and arthrodesis. Posterolateral lumbar and lumbosacral spinal fusion methods without instrumentation remain important, even contemporary, techniques in the armamentarium of the spinal surgeon who treats patients with lumbar spinal instability (*Fig. 27.5*). Careful patient selection, good judgment, and meticulous surgical technique can improve the clinical and radi-

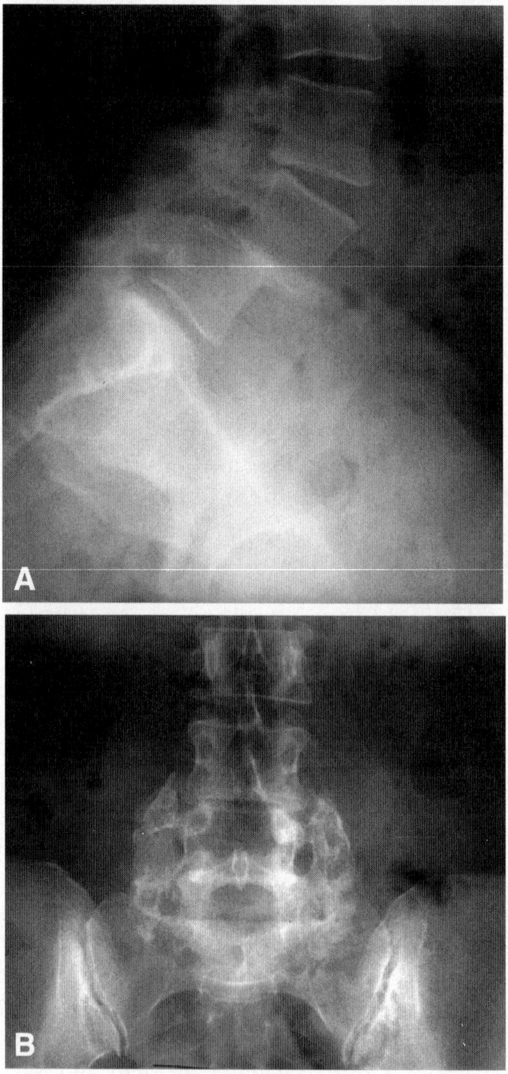

FIG. 27.5 (*A*) Patient with grade II spondylolisthesis and instability treated with decompression and dorsolateral intertransverse fusion 4 years ago. (*B*) Note robust fusion bilateral fusion mass.

ographic success rates of these procedures, irrespective of whether added instrumentation is used or not.

REFERENCES

1. Abbe R: Spinal surgery: A report of eight cases. **Med Rec** 38:85–92, 1890.
2. Abraham DJ, Herkowitz HN, Katz JN: Indications for thoracic and lumbar spine fusion and trends in use. **Orthop Clin North Am** 29:803–811, 1998.
3. Albertstone CD, Benzel EC: History, in Benzel EC (ed.): *Spine Surgery Volume 1.* New York, Churchill Livingstone, 1999, pp 1–21.
4. Axelsson P, Johnsson R, Stromqvist B, Arvidsson M, Herrlin K: Posterolateral lumbar fusion. Outcome of 71 consecutive operations after 4 (2–7) years. **Acta Orthop Scand** 65:309–314, 1994.
5. Bernhardt M, Swartz DE, Clothiaux PL, Crowell RR, White AA III: Posterolateral lumbar and lumbosacral fusion with and without pedicle screw internal fixation. **Clin Orthop Rel Res** 284:109–115, 1992.
6. Boucher HH: A method of spinal fusion. **J Bone Joint Surg Br** 41B:248–259, 1959.
7. Bridwell KW, et al.: Role of fusion and instrumentation in the treatment of degenerative spondylolisthesis. **J Spinal Disord** 6:461–472, 1993.
8. Chang K, McAfee P: Degenerative spondylolisthesis and degenerative scoliosis treated with a combination segmental rod–plate and transpedicular screw instrumentation system: A preliminary report. **J Spinal Disord** 1:247–256, 1989.
9. Feffer HL, Weisel S, et al.: Degenerative spondylolisthesis: To fuse or not to fuse. **Spine** 10:286–289, 1985.
10. Fessler RG, Locantro J: Indications and techniques for stabilization in degenerative disease of the lumbar spine, in Tindall GT, Cooper PR, Barrow DL (eds.): *The Practice of Neurosurgery. Volume III.* Baltimore, Williams & Wilkins, 1996, pp 2521–2539.
11. France JC, Yaszemski MJ, Lauerman WC, et al.: A randomized prospective study of posterolateral lumbar fusion. **Spine** 24:553–560, 1999.
12. Frymoyer JW: Low back pain. The role of spine fusion. **Neurosurg Clin North Am** 2:933–954, 1991.
13. Frymoyer JW: Segmental instability, in Frymoyer JW (ed.): *The Adult Spine: Principles and Practice.* New York, Raven Press, 1991, pp 1873–1891.
14. Frymoyer JW, Selby DK: Segmental instability: Rationale for treatment. **Spine** 10:280–286, 1985.
15. Hadra BE: Wiring the spinous processes in Pott's disease. **Trans Am Orthop Assoc** 4:206–210, 1891.
16. Hambly MF, Wiltse LL, Peek RD, DiMartino PP, Darakjian HE: Unilateral lumbar fusion. **Spine** 16:S295–S297, 1991.
17. Hanley EN Jr.: The indications for lumbar spinal fusion with and without instrumentation. **Spine** 20:143S–153S, 1995.
18. Harrington PR: Treatment of scoliosis. **J Bone Joint Surg Am** 44A:591–610, 1962.
19. Harrington PR: The history and development of Harrington instrumentation. **Clin Orthop Rel Res** 93:110–112, 1973.
20. Herkowitz H, Kurz L: Degenerative lumbar spondylolisthesis with spinal stenosis. **J Bone Joint Surg Am** 3A:802–808, 1991.
21. Hibbs RA: An operation for progressive spinal deformities. **N Y Med J** 93:1013–1016, 1911.

22. Hirabayashi S, Kiyoshi K, Kwoki T: Cotrel Dubousset pedicle screw system for various spinal disorders. **Spine** 16:1298–1304, 1991.
23. Holdsworth FW: Fractures, dislocations, and fracture–dislocation of the spine. **J Bone Joint Surg Br** 45B:6–20, 1963.
24. Kaptain GJ, Shaffrey CI, Halliday AL, Schneier IM, Jane JA: Dorsal and lateral thoracic and lumbar fusion, in Benzel EC (ed.): *Spine Surgery Volume 1.* New York, Churchill Livingstone, 1999, pp 347–358.
25. Lange F: Support of the spondylitic spine by means of buried steel bars attached to the vertebrae. **Am J Orthop Surg** 8:334–336, 1910.
26. Lombardi J, Wiltse L, et al.: Treatment of degenerative spondylolisthesis. **Spine** 10:821–827, 1985.
27. MacNab I: The blood supply of the lumbar spine and its application to the technique of intertransverse lumbar fusion. **J Bone Joint Surg Br** 53B:628–638, 1971.
28. MacNab I, Dall D: The blood supply of the lumbar spine and its application to the technique of intertransverse lumbar fusion. **J Bone Joint Surg Br** 54:1195, 1972.
29. Mardjetko SM, Connolly PJ, Shott S: Degenerative lumbar spondylolisthesis: A meta-analysis of literature 1970–1993. **Spine** 19:2256S–2265S, 1994.
30. Sonntag VKH, Marciano FF: Is fusion indicated for lumbar spinal disorders? **Spine** 20:138S–142S, 1995.
31. Stauffer RN, Coventry MB: Posterolateral lumbar-spine fusion. **J Bone Joint Surg Am** 54A:1195–1204, 1972.
32. Thomsen KT, Christensen FB, Eiskjaer SP, Hansen ES, Fruensgaard S, Bunger CE: 1997 Volvo award winner in clinical studies. The effect of pedicle screw instrumentation on functional outcome and fusion rates in posterolateral lumbar spine fusion: A prospective, randomized clinical study. **Spine** 22:2813–2822, 1997.
33. Zdeblick T: A prospective, randomized study of lumbar fusion: Preliminary results. **Spine** 18:983–991, 1993.

CHAPTER

28

The Role of Pedicle Screw Fixation for Lumbar Spinal Stabilization and Fusion

CURTIS A. DICKMAN, M.D., PAUL W. DETWILER, M.S., M.D., RANDALL W. PORTER, M.D.

Various techniques for posterior fixation and fusion of the spine have been developed (13, 15). Pedicle screws have been employed clinically with widespread use for more than 20 years and have become the gold standard for posterolateral fixation and fusion of the lumbar spine and sacrum (2, 24). Essentially, pedicle screws provide the most rigid mechanical fixation available for the lumbosacral spine. Cases of overt spinal instability require instrumentation with pedicle screw fixation. The goal of placing pedicle screw instrumentation is to immobilize and to stabilize spinal motion segments as an adjunct to posterolateral spinal fusion or interbody fusion. This technique offers a number of significant clinical and biomechanical benefits compared with other methods of fusing and fixating the lumbosacral spine. Primarily, pedicle screws exploit the unique cylindrical anatomy of lumbar pedicles to provide a strong and rigid bone anchor within the vertebrae, which avoids contact of the hardware with the dura (17).

HISTORY

Pedicle screw instrumentation was first used for lumbosacral fixation in the 1970s by Roy–Camille, et al. (21) and Steffee et al. (23). In the 1980s and 1990s, pedicle screws gained widespread popularity clinically for fixating the lumbosacral spine. Other techniques include noninstrumented fusions, which are used when degenerative conditions exist without overt hypermobility or instability of the spine. Noninstrumented lumbosacral fusion can be performed with facet grafting; intertransverse posterolateral bone grafting; posterior lumbar interbody fusion (PLIF) using cages, dowels, or grafts; or anterior lumbar interbody fusion (ALIF) using cages, dowels, or grafts. Other lumbosacral fixation techniques include posterior hook–rods, wires and rods, translaminar facet screws, and anterior screw plates and screw rods.

Pedicle screws have superior biomechanical characteristics to other lumbar spinal fixation devices. They provide significantly more rigid immobilization of the spine and fixate fewer motion segments compared with hook–rods, and wires and rods. Pedicle screws can be used after a laminectomy has been performed, unlike hooks or wires attached to posterior rods. Anterolateral spinal screw plates and rods cannot be used to fixate L5 or the sacrum. In comparison, pedicle screws have greater versatility and can be inserted into the thoracic or lumbar pedicles, into the sacral pedicles, or into the sacral alae. Pedicle screws remain the most common method of fixating the lumbar spine while an arthrodesis is forming because of their versatility, ease of use, mechanical superiority, and ability to minimize the number of segments that are fused.

Interbody cages, bone dowels, and bone grafts *do not* provide fixation of the spine. They do not immobilize unstable motion segments. However, they can be used to supply bone graft for arthrodesis with the graft material placed under compression, which facilitates graft incorporation. Interbody dowels and grafts can be used to distract and to hold open stenotic, degenerated neural foramen and can provide tension to lax spinal ligaments to add partial stability to a degenerated motion segment. However, these devices serve only as *mechanical spacers* between the vertebral bodies and do *not* rigidly fixate the vertebrae. Therefore, they should not be used as stand-alone devices when the spine is grossly unstable, which occurs with cases of spondylolisthesis, kyphotic deformities, spinal fractures, ligament disruption, or angular instability of the spine. In these instances, pedicle screws or anterior screw plates are required to provide stability.

REGULATORY STATUS OF PEDICLE SCREWS

The regulatory status of pedicle screws had been based upon the Medical Devices Act of 1976, which gave the Food and Drug Administration (FDA) the authority to regulate labeling of medical implants and classified medical devices into previously available implants (preamendment devices) and new devices. Dr. Paul Harrington had devised and used pedicle screws attached to rods to treat grade III and IV spondylolisthesis before 1976. Therefore, pedicle screws were found to be acceptable by the FDA for labeling for this indication *only*. All other clinical uses were considered “off-label” use.

To address the regulatory mismatch between the limited labeling and the widespread clinical use of pedicle screws for spinal fixation, in 1992 the FDA approached the American Association of Orthopedic Surgeons (AAOS), Scoliosis Research Society (SRS), the North American Spine Society (NASS), the American Association of Neurological Surgeons (AANS), the Congress of Neurological Surgeons (CNS), and spinal implant manufacturers to create a scientific study to assess pedicle screw safety and efficacy. This collaborative initiative by the FDA was a novel landmark approach in which the FDA participated in creating the design of a scientific study to assess the safety and efficacy of a medical device. The conduct of the study, collection of data, and publication of the results was performed by the scientific committee without any FDA involvement in these later phases.

The Historical Cohort Study of Pedicle Screw Fixation and Thoracic, Lumbar, and Sacral Fusions (28) was conducted in 1993 by Drs. Hansen Yuan (representing NASS), Steven Garfin (representing AAOS), Stephen Martjetko (representing SRS), and Curtis Dickman (representing AANS and CNS). This study assessed retrospectively more than 3000 patients with spinal fusion. The two diagnoses that were studied included degenerative spondylolisthesis and lumbar spinal fractures. In both groups, patients treated with pedicle screws were compared with control patients who were treated with noninstrumented fusions (for degenerative spondylolisthesis) and other spinal fixation devices (for spinal fractures). More than 300 spinal surgeons contributed patients to this study.

The patient population consisted of 2684 patients with degenerative spondylolisthesis (2177 were in the pedicle screw fixation group) and 814 patients with spinal fractures (586 of whom received pedicle screw instrumentation). The fusion rate of patients treated for degenerative spondylolisthesis with pedicle screw fixation was 89%, which was significantly higher than the 70% fusion rate without spinal instrumentation. For the patients with spinal fractures, the fusion rate was 89% for those receiving pedicle screw fixation and 81% for those with other types of spinal fixation devices.

The concurrent control group was a strength of the Cohort Study (28). Furthermore, selection bias was minimized by requiring participating surgeons to submit data on all eligible patients with degenerative spondylolisthesis or fractures (inclusion criteria were based on the specific diagnoses of degenerative spondylolisthesis and spinal fracture). Outcome variables included pain, fusion, function, and neurological status. The study demonstrated excellent safety and efficacy data that substantiated the use of pedicle screws. As a result of this study and the assessment of all other available information from the medical literature (6, 10, 26–29), on July 22, 1994, the FDA advisory panel unanimously recommended that the Orthopedic and Rehabilitation Devices Advisory Panel of the FDA reclassify pedicle screws from class III to class II devices (10). Four years later, on August 26, 1998, the FDA finally adopted the recommendations, and the final reclassification of pedicle screws became effective.

INDICATIONS FOR PEDICLE SCREWS

As a result of the FDA reclassification, pedicle screws are class II devices and are labeled for use for degenerative and isthmic spondylolisthesis, fractures and dislocations, spinal deformities (kyphosis, scoliosis), spinal tumors, and treatment of failed prior fusion (pseudarthrosis). The use is restricted to the thoracic and lumbar spine and sacrum. Use of these implants in the cervical spine or for other indications (e.g., infections, congenital malformations, and so on) are considered off-label uses of these devices.

Relative contraindications to the use of pedicle screws include morbid obesity, active infection, osteopenia, osteoporosis, and medical illnesses that preclude surgery (4, 6–8, 22, 25–27, 29).

BIOMECHANICS OF PEDICLE SCREW FIXATION

There is a large volume of literature that demonstrates the significant biomechanical advantages of pedicle screw fixation for rigidly stabilizing the lumbosacral spine (3, 5, 11–13, 26). Pedicle screws are attached bilaterally to the vertebrae, and adjacent vertebrae are connected with rods or plates. The attachments are often reinforced with cross-linking devices for additional rigidity of the construct. Pedicle screws resist shear loads (translational spinal motion) and torsional loads (bending and rotational motion). These fixation devices can be used to apply compressive or distractive forces, or bending moments to individual vertebral segments, thereby facilitating correction of spinal deformities. The three-column rigid spinal fixation provided by pedicle screws is markedly stiffer and controls spinal motion significantly more effectively than hook–rods and wires with rods that are not rigidly attached to the vertebrae.

The strength of fixation provided by pedicle screws is dependent on the patient's bone density and the diameter of the screws that are used. Screw pullout is dependent on bone density. Soft osteopenic bones will not hold screws well. Screw breakage is dependent on the third power of the screw diameter. Therefore, using the widest diameter screw possible (i.e., 60 to 70% of the diameter of the pedicle) reduces the risk of screw failure. Pedicle screws are also susceptible to bending loads that can cause screws to fracture. Therefore, if anterior column defects are present (i.e., vertebral body destruction or large gaps in the surfaces of the vertebral bodies or end plates), an anterior reconstructive graft should be placed to "load share" and to minimize mechanical stress that could cause the screws to break.

PEDICLE SCREWS, CAGES, AND SPINAL INSTABILITY

To examine the relative merits and pitfalls of pedicle screws compared with interbody cages and bone dowels in the unstable lumbar spine, we conducted a recent biomechanical study in our laboratory at the Barrow Neurological Institute (Cagli et al., unpublished). A grade I spondylolisthesis was created in human cadaveric lumbar spines by resecting the facets, removing the disc material, and elevating the spinal ligaments. The biomechanical effects were compared using pedicle screws alone, threaded interbody cages or bone dowels alone, and pedicle screws plus cages or dowels. The devices were loaded using physiological range nondestructive bending moments and shear loads.

Our study demonstrated significant superiority of pedicle screw fixation in this model of spinal instability. Pedicle screws controlled 80 to 90% of the motion of the destabilized motion segment, compared with the 30 to 40% stabilizing effect provided by threaded interbody cages or bone dowels. Furthermore, cages and dowels were susceptible to significant loosening and displacement when fatigued with cyclic loads. Adding cages or dowels to pedicle screws increased the stability of the fixation by an additional 5 to 10% (Figs. 28.1 and 28.2). The results of this study clearly demonstrate that *when the spine is grossly unstable* (i.e., spondylolisthesis or angular deformity) *or when spinal ligaments are disrupted, interbody cages should* not *be used alone.* They should be supplemented with pedicle screws.

SURGICAL TECHNIQUE

Typically, preoperative evaluation includes plain radiography, magnetic resonance imaging (MRI) or myelography, and computed tomography (CT) myelography. These studies provide vital information regarding the extent of instability, the decompression needed, and the appropriate levels of fixation. The diameter of a pedicle screw should be no more than two-thirds the width of the pedicle, and the screws should be inserted through no more than 80% of the length of the vertebral body.

The patient is placed in a prone position, and a dorsal midline incision is made. The paraspinal muscles are dissected medially to laterally, exposing subperiosteally the spinous processes, laminae, facets, and transverse processes. The transverse processes are not exposed above or below the fusion site to avoid unintentional fusion of adjacent levels.

The predetermined levels are decompressed by removing the lamina, and the nerve roots and foramina are decompressed. Herniated disc fragments are removed when necessary. Once the decompression is complete, the pedicle screws are placed. The key to the safe and effective placement of pedicle screws is to identify specific pedicle landmarks (16, 20, 21). The pedicle is located at the intersection of a line through the middle of the transverse process (axial plane) and the

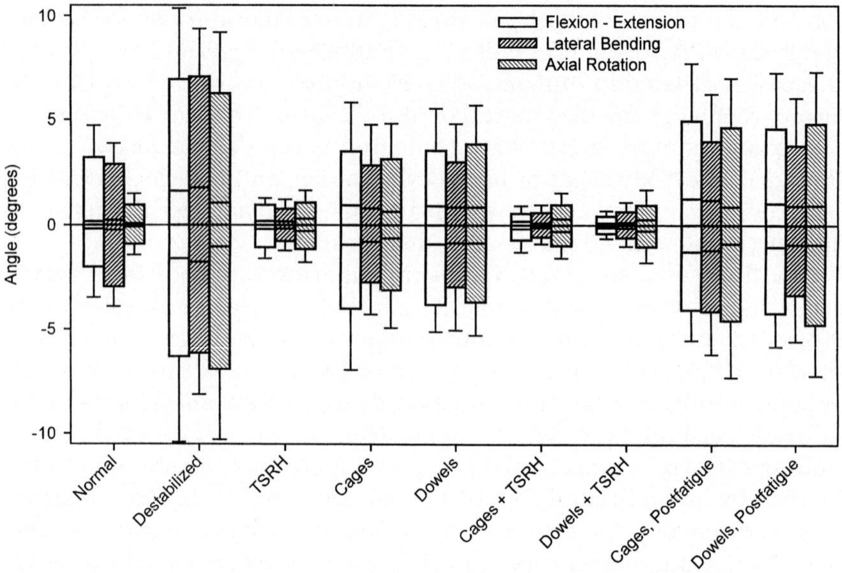

FIG. 28.1. Comparison of the biomechanical performance of pedicle screws and interbody cages, rotational motion TSRH = Texas Scottish Rite Hospital.

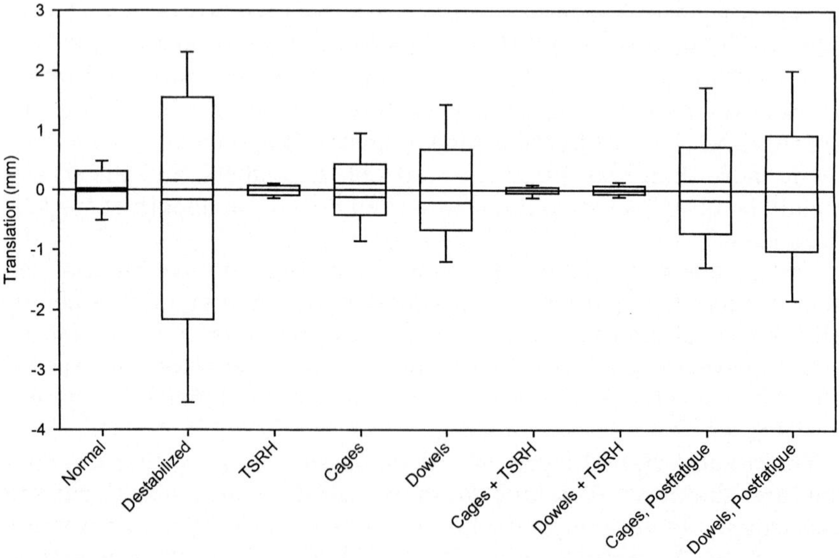

FIG. 28.2. Comparison of the biomechanical performance of pedicle screws and interbody cages, translational motion. TSRH = Texas Scottish Rite Hospital.

sagittal plane line through the lateral superior facet. The superior, medial, and inferior surfaces of the pedicle within the spinal canal can be defined by palpation and often can be visualized directly after decompression. The intended trajectory is then verified using the fluoroscopic C-arm in the anteroposterior and lateral positions. In the sacrum, the point overlying the pedicle is usually near the inferolateral portion of the S1 facet.

At all levels to be instrumented, bone over the entry point is decorticated with a high-speed drill or rongeur, and a T-handle probe is advanced through the center of the pedicle into the vertebral body. Anteroposterior fluoroscopic views can be used to confirm the proper position within the center of the pedicle. Typically, the pedicle is oriented 0 degrees (perpendicular to the vertebral body) at L1, 5 degrees medially at L2, 10 degrees medially at L3, 15 degrees medially at L4, 20 degrees medially at L5, and 25 degrees medially at S1. After the pedicle has been tapped, a pedicle probe is used to verify that the tap did not penetrate the cortical bone. The length of the pedicle screw needed is determined by measuring the vertebral body diameter using preoperative radiographic studies in the axial plane (CT and MRI).

The screw is advanced under lateral fluoroscopic guidance. Next, a rod is fashioned to fit between the most superior and the most inferior pedicle screws on both sides. A malleable endotracheal tube stylette can serve as a template for the rod, which is then cut and bent to match the template. The pedicle screw is attached to the rod with eyebolt connectors. Spondylolisthesis or spinal deformities can be reduced using in situ bending irons, distractors, compressors, and the corkscrew device. If rotational instability is present or more than one level is to be instrumented, cross-linking is indicated.

The articular facet surfaces and the posterior cortical surfaces of the transverse processes at the levels to be fused are decorticated with a Leksell rongeur or a drill. Dissection ventral to the transverse process can injure the nerve root or ganglia and should be avoided. Autogenous bone obtained either from the decompression site or the iliac crest is packed over the decorticated transverse processes. To augment the fusion further, the facet joint capsule is interrupted and the articular surfaces are decorticated. The joint is then packed with cancellous bone graft.

Postoperative management involves early mobilization in a thoracolumbosacral orthosis. Anteroposterior and lateral radiographs are obtained in the recovery room and at follow-up examinations to evaluate the integrity of the instrumentation and the status of the arthrodesis. Lateral dynamic flexion–extension radiographs are obtained 3 months after surgery.

CLINICAL DATA REGARDING PEDICLE SCREWS

Extensive data exist that substantiate the superb clinical performance of pedicle screws for lumbosacral spinal fixation and fusion. The most informative sources arise from a meta-analysis of the peer-reviewed medical literature; the results of the Cohort Study prospective, randomized clinical studies; and additional literature review (1, 2, 4–7, 9, 14, 15, 18, 19, 21, 22, 24–29).

The most useful clinical reports have based their analyses on the performance of pedicle screws compared with other treatments (i.e., noninstrumented fusions or fusions with other types of spinal instrumentation) for *specific* pathological categories. The two pathologies that have received the majority of attention in the literature are degenerative lumbar spondylolisthesis and lumbar fractures. These two discrete pathologies are both well studied.

The literature that addresses pedicle screw fixation for other pathologies (e.g., as a spinal deformity, scoliosis, isthmic spondylolisthesis, spinal tumors or infections, repair of pseudarthrosis, and so on) is less extensive and not as rich as the literature for fractures and degenerative spondylolisthesis. Furthermore, many literature reports lump together the assessment of pedicle screws for a wide variety of pathologies, which yields limited useful information.

It is extremely important that clinical studies regarding pedicle screws assess the role of factors that inhibit spinal fusion such as cigarette smoking; prior failed fusion (pseudarthrosis); use of steroidal and nonsteroidal anti-inflammatory medications; osteoporosis; and metabolic, hormonal, or nutritional deficiencies (diabetes, obesity, etc.). In addition, the studies must carefully measure outcomes (pain, neurological function, overall functional capacity) and complications.

DEGENERATIVE SPONDYLOLISTHESIS

Patients with degenerative lumbar spondylolisthesis have a significantly better clinical outcome if a decompression and a fusion are performed, compared with a decompression without fusion (7, 18). A literature meta-analysis demonstrated that only 69% of patients had satisfactory clinical outcomes with decompression alone, compared with 86 to 90% of patients treated with decompression and spinal fusion (7, 18). The results of posterolateral spinal fusion with bone graft alone without instrumentation have been extremely variable, ranging from 46 to almost 100% for degenerative spinal conditions (29).

Comparisons of fusion rates and clinical outcomes for patients with degenerative spondylolisthesis demonstrate significantly better results with pedicle screw fixation compared with noninstrumented fusions

(27–29). Furthermore, using rigid spinal fixation with screws and rods results in a significantly greater fusion rate than nonrigid pedicle screw–plate systems (29). Zdeblick (29) performed a prospective, randomized study of 124 patients with degenerative lumbar pathology using noninstrumented fusion, semirigid screw plates, and rigid screw rods. He found that the fusion rate and clinical outcome were both significantly enhanced by adding increasingly rigid spinal fixation (Table 28.1) (29).

In the Cohort Study (28), the fusion rates, functional outcome, and pain outcome for degenerative spondylolisthesis were all significantly better in the patients treated with pedicle screws compared with the 513 noninstrumented control patients (Table 28.2).

LUMBAR SPINAL FRACTURES

A meta-analysis of the medical literature for unstable fractures of the thoracic and lumbar spine (6) demonstrated significantly greater fusion rates with pedicle screw fixation (99.4%, n = 543) compared with anterior spinal instrumentation (94.8%, n = 223) and with hook–rod instrumentation (96.9%, n = 48). There were no significant differences between the different types of instrumentation for treating spinal fractures with regard to pain outcome, neurological outcome, or functional outcome.

The Cohort Study (28) demonstrated an 89% fusion rate for patients receiving pedicle screws compared with 81% for patients with other types of spinal fixation devices. The clinical outcome, as measured by

TABLE 28.1
Outcome of Degenerative Pathology

Technique	Fusion Rate	Good or Excellent Clinical Results
No instrumentation	65%[a]	71%
Semirigid pedicle screw plates	77%	89%
Rigid pedicle screw–rods	95%[a]	95%

[a]Statistically significant.

TABLE 28.2
Cohort Study: Results for Degenerative Spondylolisthesis

Characteristic	Pedicle Screws	Noninstrumented Controls
n	2177	513
Fusion rate	89%	70%
Good or excellent functional outcome	90%	87%
Good or excellent pain outcome	92%	84%

functional status, neurological function, pain outcome, and complication rate, did not differ significantly between patients treated with pedicle screws (n = 514) and those treated with other types of spinal instrumentation (n = 228).

The Cohort Study (28) demonstrated equivalent performance of pedicle screws for lumbar fractures compared with other types of spinal fixation. Furthermore, there were several clear-cut advantages of pedicle screws compared with other spinal fixation devices (hook–rod instrumentation and Luque rods with wires) that included fusion of fewer spinal motion segments and preservation of more normal spinal motion.

COMPLICATIONS

Complications of pedicle screws can be minimized using basic tenets including meticulous hemostasis, microsurgical dissection, fluoroscopic guidance, frameless stereotaxis, definition of pertinent bony anatomy, aseptic technique, perioperative antibiotics, multilayer closure, and drains when indicated (5, 16, 17, 19–21, 28).

In the Cohort Study (28), the infection rate was 3% in both the pedicle screw and the control groups. Rates of infection reported elsewhere in the literature range from 2 to 15% for noninstrumented and instrumented spinal fusions (5, 17, 19). In the Cohort Study (28) hardware failure, including screw fracture, pullout, or loosening was rare, occurring in approximately 7% of the cases, and was comparable with the hardware failure rates that occurred with other types of spinal instrumentation. The rate of cerebrospinal fluid (CSF) leaks was low (0.5% in the pedicle screw fixation group and 0.7% in the noninstrumented group treated for degenerative spondylolisthesis) (28). CSF leaks have a 0.5 to 5% incidence in the literature for all types of spinal fusion procedures, regardless of whether instrumentation is used. Pedicle screws do not appear to be associated with a higher incidence of CSF leakage and dural tears. The rate of new perioperative spinal cord injury was extremely low, 0.2% in all groups in the Cohort Study (28) and in the literature. Permanent, new radicular pain occurred in 1.5% and 1.8% of the control groups in the Cohort Study (28). In the literature, new radiculopathy has been reported to occur in 0.5% to 8% of patients with pedicle screws.

CASE EXAMPLES

Failure of Interbody Implants Alone for Grade II Spondylolisthesis

A 33-year-old woman with severe left L5 radicular pain and foot drop was treated conservatively for 12 months with chiropractic manipulation, epidural steroid blocks, physical therapy, exercise, and nonsteroidal anti-inflammatory agents. Radiographic imaging revealed grade II spondylolisthesis at L5–S1 with significant foraminal stenosis at the same level. Laparoscopic placement of interbody cages at L5–S1 reduced the spondylolisthesis by 70% (Fig. 28.3A). Immediately after surgery her back and leg pain was relieved, but it recurred transiently 1 month later. Lateral lumbar spine radiographs (Fig. 28.3B) demonstrated a 5-mm increase in the anterior subluxation of L5 on S1. The threaded interbody cages and L5 had resubluxed simultaneously 5 mm anteriorly. CT demonstrated no prominence of the cages beyond the borders of L5 and no vascular compression. The patient wore a corset and reported complete resolution of her back and radicular pain at her 1-year follow-up examination (Fig. 28.3C). The subluxation at L5–S1 had not increased on lateral radiographs. This is an example of loss of reduction of a grade II spondylolisthesis with threaded interbody cages alone. Fortunately, the patient fused in a partially subluxed position without vascular impingement or neurological sequelae. This demonstrates the pitfalls of using cages as stand-alone devices for mobile spondylolistheses or spondylolistheses that are greater than grade I. If cages are used in this instance, they should be supplemented with pedicle screws. Alternatively, pedicle screws can be used alone as the sole treatment without interbody grafting.

PLIF Combined with Pedicle Screw Instrumentation and Posterolateral Fusion

A 38-year-old man presented with a 2-year history of left L4 radicular pain that worsened with walking and standing, and was relieved by lying down. He had been treated conservatively by a number of physicians but his symptoms failed to improve. His neurological examination was significant for leg weakness (4/5) in the left quadriceps and extensor hallucis longus.

Radiographic evaluation of the lumbar spine, including MRI, demonstrated grade I spondylolisthesis at L4–L5 with foraminal stenosis attributable to a far-lateral herniated disc. The herniated disc was resected and his radicular pain was relieved completely.

The patient's symptoms recurred 5 months after surgery. He developed back and radicular pain, and neurological deficits that were disabling and protracted. Dynamic radiographic studies, including flexion–extension films of the lumbar spine, revealed 9 mm of subluxation in the neutral position that increased to 14 mm during flexion. The patient underwent a posterior approach with bone graft PLIF and pedicle screw fixation at L4–L5 (Fig. 28.4). At his 18-month follow-up examination, he was neurologically intact and had no back pain or radicular

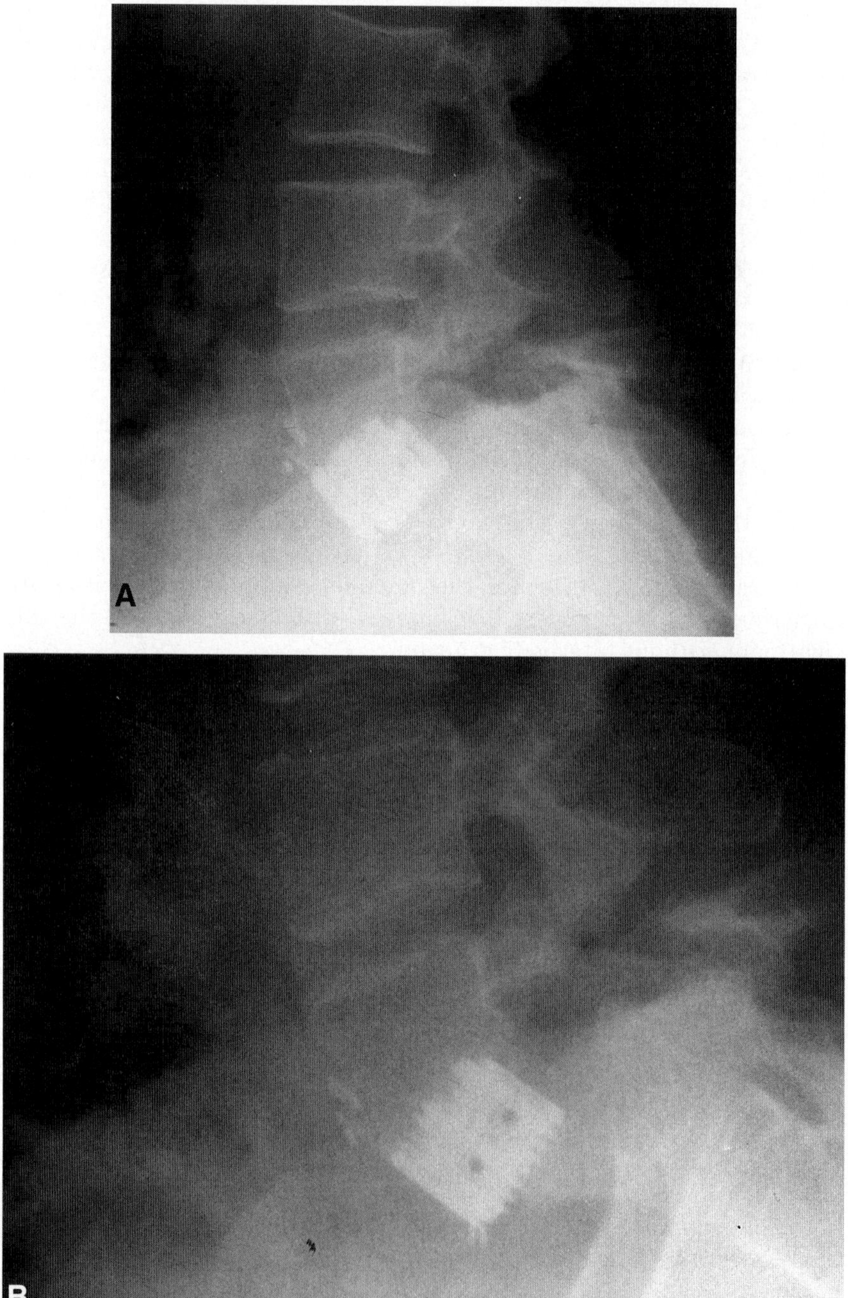
A
B

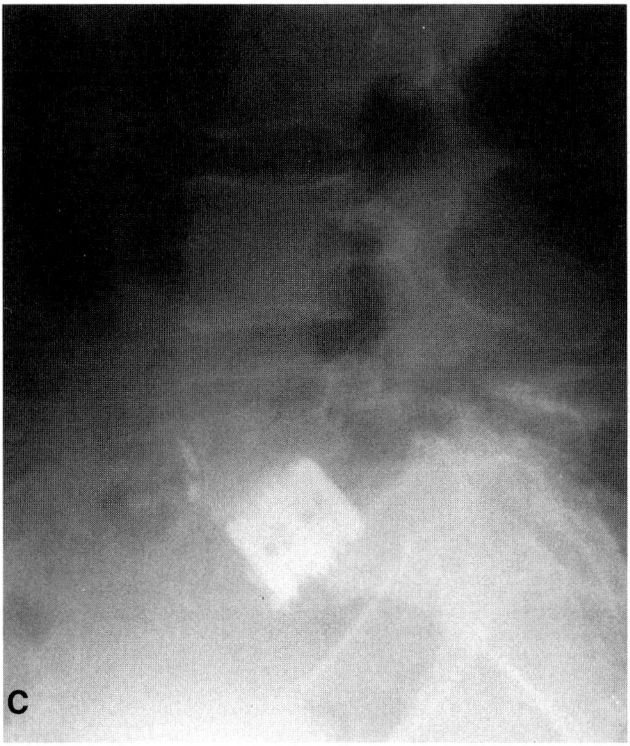

FIG. 28.3. (*A*) Lateral lumbar radiograph of a 33-year-old woman who underwent laparoscopic placement of threaded interbody fusion cages at L5–S1. She had debilitating pain in the back and left L5 distribution and weakness attributable to grade II spondylolisthesis. The spondylolisthesis was reduced completely by the placement of threaded interbody titanium cages, and the patient's pain was relieved. (*B*) Lateral lumbar radiograph 1 month after surgery showing a 5-mm increase in the subluxation at L5–S1. The patient's back and left lower extremity pain recurred transiently after activity and then resolved. She was treated nonsurgically with a corset. (*C*) A 12-month follow-up radiograph showing no increased slippage. The patient now has very mild, occasional lower back pain but no radicular symptoms or neurological deficits. She is significantly improved clinically with resolution of her neurological deficits, symptoms, and radicular and back pain.

pain. Plain radiographs of the lumbar spine, including static and dynamic radiographs, demonstrated stable spinal alignment and a well-formed interbody fusion.

ALIF Combined with Pedicle Screw Fixation

A 59-year-old woman presented with a 6-month history of progressive, sharp stabbing pain that radiated from her buttock into her left

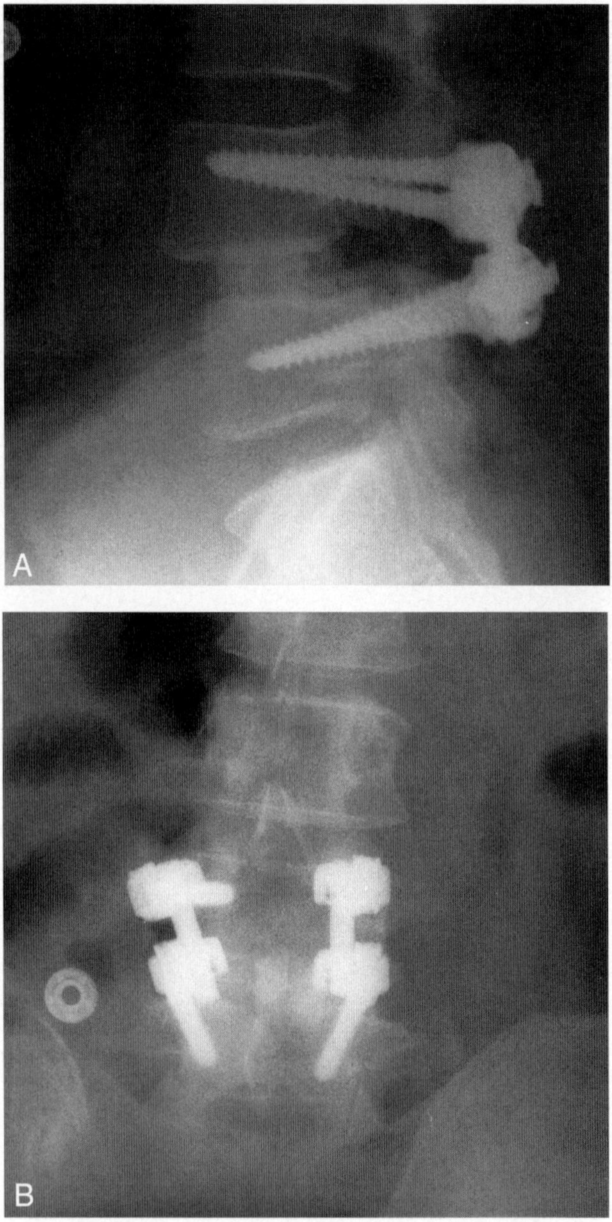

FIG. 28.4. Lateral (*A*) and anteroposterior (*B*) lumbar radiographs of a 38-year-old man who underwent posterior lumbar interbody fusion and pedicle screw placement for a hypermobile grade I spondylolisthesis at L4–L5 after a far-lateral herniated disc was resected.

leg, and severe mechanical back pain. She had undergone three previous lumbar surgeries. At age 55, she had undergone a multi-level lumbar discectomy and fusion using pedicle screws that had relieved her radicular pain. Two years later, her hardware failed and she developed a recurrent disc herniation. The recurrent herniated disc was resected, and her spinal instrumentation was removed except for a retained portion of a fractured pedicle screw. Approximately 1 year later, a new herniated disc was resected. She did well for approximately 4 months, when severe, agonizing back pain and left-side lumbar radicular pain developed suddenly. The pain radiated across the buttock into the anterolateral portion of the left thigh. Before this recurrence, she had been walking 5 miles a day and was swimming regularly. After the sciatica and mechanical back pain recurred, she was unable to engage in activities of daily living.

Imaging studies, including dynamic myelography and CT myelography, demonstrated grade I spondylolisthesis at L3–L4 and L4–L5 (Fig. 28.5A and B), and lumbar stenosis at L3–L4 with foraminal stenosis on the left (Fig. 28.5C). At L5, a fractured pedicle screw was retained within the vertebral body and pedicle on the left. At L4–S1, there was severe bilateral neural foraminal stenosis. There was no evidence of a posterolateral fusion mass at any spinal level. An interbody arthrodesis had formed in the L4–L5 segment. ALIF was performed at L3–L4 and at L5–S1 to reduce the spondylolisthesis and to treat the foraminal stenosis (Fig. 28.5D). This was followed by pedicle screw instrumentation and posterolateral intertransverse process fusion from L3–S1 (Fig. 28.5E and F). At her 8-month follow-up examination, the patient had a very mild residual lumbar aching pain. She has had complete relief of her radicular pain, mechanical back pain, and neurological deficits.

CONCLUSION

Pedicle screws are rigid, structural fixators that are reliable, effective, stand-alone devices that have withstood the test of time. Fusion rates with pedicle screws range from 85 to 95%, and 90 to 95% of the motion of the destabilized segment is controlled with pedicle screw fixation (4, 5, 17, 19, 22, 24, 25, 29). Interbody fusion with cages and dowels alone, specifically for mobile spondylolisthesis, relies on ligamentous integrity and hence provides inadequate stability. Threaded cages or bone dowels should *not* be used alone to treat spondylolistheses that are mobile or greater than grade I. The efficacy of pedicle screws depends on the integrity of the bone, and they clearly outperform cages and dowels when spinal instability exists. Pedicle screws provide rigid segmental spinal fixation whereas cages provide only an interposition strut that does not fixate the spine.

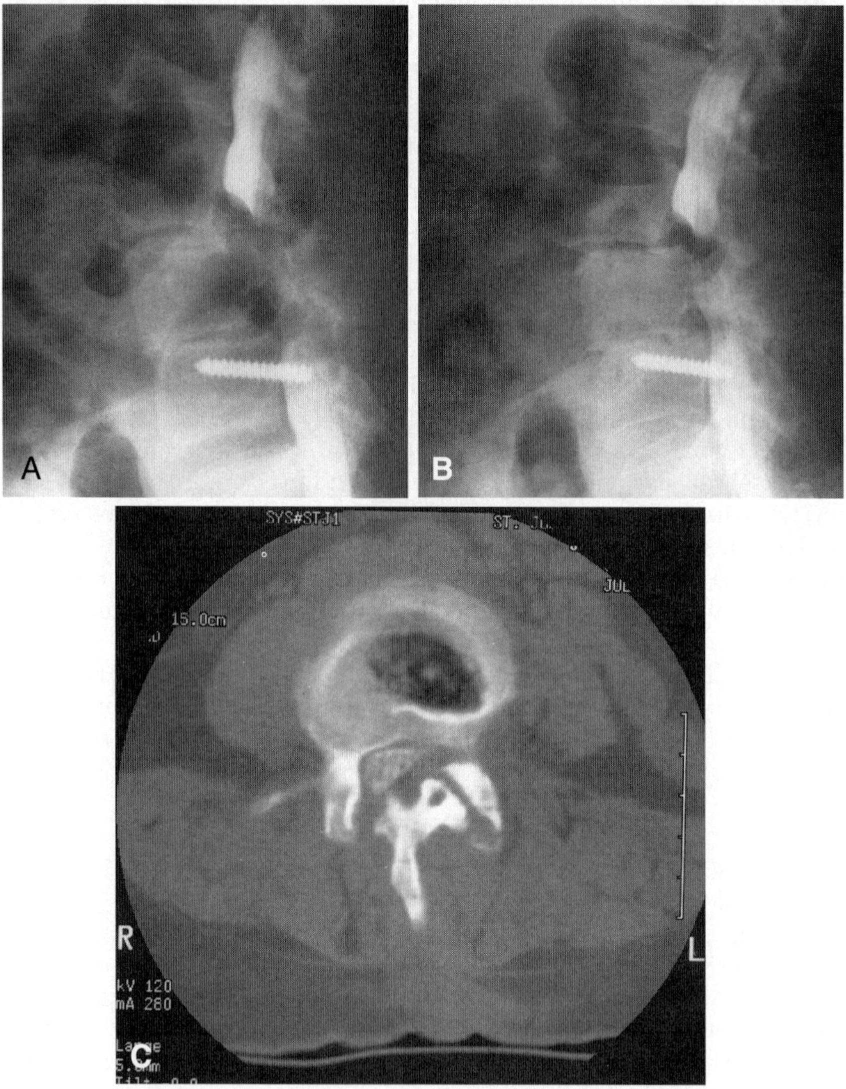

Fig. 28.5. Lateral lumbar myelograms in flexion (A) and extension (B) demonstrating hypermobility at L3–L4 and a fixed nonmobile listhesis at L4–L5. (C) Computed tomographic myelogram demonstrating spinal stenosis at L3–L4. The stenosis is most pronounced on the left side of L3–L4.

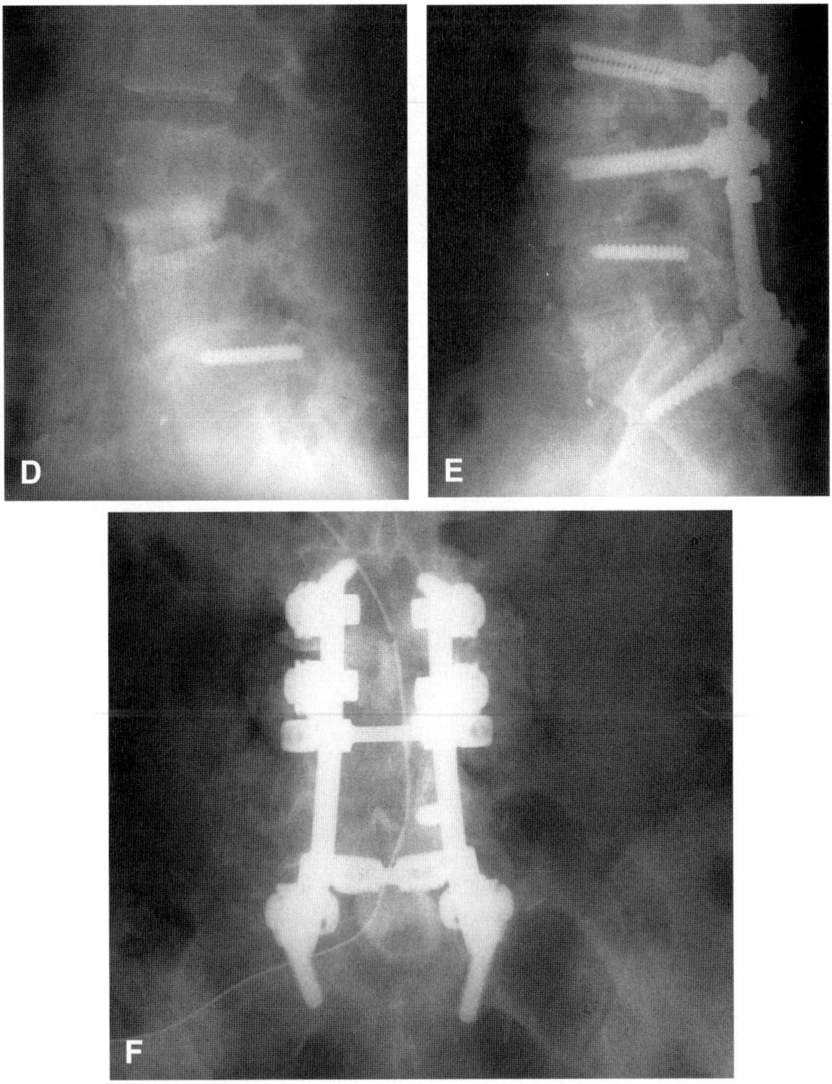

FIG. 28.5 (D) Lateral radiograph obtained after the L3–L4 spondylolisthesis was reduced and the foraminal stenosis at L3–L4 and L5–S1 was treated with anterior lumbar interbody fusion using threaded allograft bone dowels packed with autograft. Lateral (E) and anteroposterior (F) radiographs showing the posterolateral intertransverse process fusion and anterior interbody bone grafts augmented with pedicle screw instrumentation from L3 to S1.

REFERENCES

1. Brantigan JW, Steffee AD: A carbon fiber implant to aid interbody lumbar fusion. Two-year clinical results in the first 26 patients. **Spine** 18:2106–2117, 1993.
2. Bridwell KH, Sedgewick TA, O'Brien MF, et al. The role of fusion and instrumentation in the treatment of degenerative spondylolisthesis with spinal stenosis. **J Spinal Disord** 6:461–472, 1992.
3. Brodke DS, Dick JC, Kunz DN, et al. Posterior lumbar interbody fusion. A biomechanical comparison, including a new threaded cage. **Spine** 22:26–31, 1997.
4. Buttermann GR, Garvey TA, Hunt AF, et al. Lumbar fusion results related to diagnosis. **Spine** 23:116–127, 1998.
5. Dickman CA, Fessler RG, MacMillan M, et al. Transpedicular screw–rod fixation of the lumbar spine: Operative technique and outcomes in 104 cases. **J Neurosurg** 77:860–870, 1992.
6. Dickman CA, Yahiro MA, Lu HTC, et al. Surgical treatment alternatives for fixation of unstable fractures of the thoracic and lumbar spine. A meta-analysis. **Spine** 19:2266S–2273S, 1994.
7. Fischgrund JS, Mackay M, Herkowitz HN, et al. Degenerative lumbar spondylolisthesis with spinal stenosis: A prospective, randomized study comparing decompressive laminectomy and arthrodesis with and without spinal instrumentation. **Spine** 22:2807–2812, 1997.
8. Franklin GM, Haug J, Heyer NJ, et al. Outcome of lumbar fusion in Washington State Workers Compensation. **Spine** 19:1897–1903, 1994.
9. Fredrickson BE, Baker D, McHolick WJ, et al. The natural history of spondylolysis and spondylolisthesis. **J Bone Joint Surg Am** 66A:699–707, 1984.
10. Garfin SR. Editorial. **Spine** 19:2254S–2255S, 1994.
11. Glazer PA, Colliou O, Klisch SM, et al. Biomechanical analysis of multilevel fixation methods in the lumbar spine. **Spine** 22:171–182, 1997.
12. Glazer PA, Colliou O, Lotz JC, et al. Biomechanical analysis of lumbosacral fixation. **Spine** 21:1211–1222, 1996.
13. Goel VK, Pope MH. Biomechanics of fusion and stabilization. **Spine** 20:85S–99S, 1995.
14. Hanley EN Jr. Decompression and distraction–derotation arthrodesis for degenerative spondylolisthesis. **Spine** 11:269–276, 1986.
15. Herkowitz HN, Kurz LT. Degenerative lumbar spondylolisthesis with spinal stenosis. A prospective study comparing decompression with decompression and intertransverse process arthrodesis. **J Bone Joint Surg Am** 73A:802–808, 1991.
16. Laine T, Schlenzka D, Makitalo K, et al. Improved accuracy of pedicle screw insertion with computer-assisted surgery. A prospective clinical trial of 30 patients. **Spine** 22:1254–1258, 1997.
17. Lin PM. Posterior lumbar interbody fusion technique: Complications and pitfalls. **Clin Orthop** 193:90–102, 1985.
18. Mardjetko SM, Connolly PJ, Shott S. Degenerative lumbar spondylolisthesis. A meta-analysis of literature 1970–1993. **Spine** 19:2256S–2265S, 1994.
19. Masferrer R, Gomez CH, Karahalios DG, et al. Efficacy of pedicle screw fixation in the treatment of spinal instability and failed back surgery: A 5-year review. **J Neurosurg** 89:371–377, 1998.
20. Robertson PA, Novotny JE, Grobler LJ, et al. Reliability of axial landmarks for pedicle screw placement in the lower lumbar spine. **Spine** 23:60–66, 1998.
21. Roy–Camille R, Saillant G, Mazel C. Internal fixation of the lumbar spine with pedicle screw plating. **Clin Orthop** 203:7–17, 1986.

22. Schnee CL, Freese A, Ansell LV: Outcome analysis for adults with spondylolisthesis treated with posterolateral fusion and transpedicular screw fixation. **J Neurosurg** 86:56–63, 1997.
23. Steffee AD, Biscup RS, Sitkowski DJ. Segmental spine plates with pedicle screw fixation. A new internal fixation device for disorders of the lumbar and thoracolumbar spine. **Clin Orthop** 203:45–53, 1986.
24. Suk S-I, Lee C-K, Kim W-J, et al. Adding posterior lumbar interbody fusion to pedicle screw fixation and posterolateral fusion after decompression in spondylolytic spondylolisthesis. **Spine** 22:210–220, 1997.
25. Thomsen K, Christensen FB, Eiskjaer SP, et al. The effect of pedicle screw instrumentation on functional outcome and fusion rates in posterolateral lumbar spinal fusion: A prospective, randomized clinical study. **Spine** 22:2813–2822, 1997.
26. Yahiro MA. Comprehensive literature review. Pedicle screw fixation devices. **Spine** 19:2274S–2278S, 1994.
27. Yahiro MA. Review of the Historical Cohort Study of Pedicle Screw Fixation in Thoracic, Lumbar, and Sacral Spinal Fusions report. **Spine** 19:2297S–2299S, 1994.
28. Yuan HA, Garfin SR, Dickman CA, et al. A historical cohort study of pedicle screw fixation in thoracic, lumbar, and sacral spinal fusions. **Spine** 19:2279S–2296S, 1994.
29. Zdeblick TA. A prospective, randomized study of lumbar fusion. Preliminary results. **Spine** 18:983–991, 1993.

CHAPTER

29

Posterior Lumbar Interbody Fusion: Indications, Techniques, and Results

MARK R. MCLAUGHLIN, M.D., REGIS W. HAID, JR., M.D., GERALD E. RODTS, JR., M.D., BRIAN R. SUBACH, M.D.

"Those who do not remember the past are condemned to repeat it."

—George Santayana

HISTORY

Hibbs and Albee (7) were the first to introduce stabilization of the spine in 1911. They reported the use of an interlaminar fusion technique for the treatment of the unstable spine secondary to Pott's disease. This technique became a popular treatment for lumbar instability secondary to infectious diseases of the spine, but ultimately was extended to other pathological lesions and regions of the spine. In 1936, Mercer (11) theorized that the ideal operation for stabilization of the spine was an interbody fusion. He lamented that the procedure was impossible to perform at that time given the existing equipment and sophistication of spinal surgery. The first posterior lumbar interbody fusion (PLIF) was reported by Jaslow (9) in 1946, when he utilized a bone peg that was placed within the lumbar interspace after discectomy. He augmented this with autogenous bone chips placed posteriorly that were harvested from the posterior elements. Variations of this procedure were reported sporadically throughout the years, including the anterior lumbar interbody approach introduced by Hodgson and Stock (8) in 1956.

The visionary report of Cloward brought PLIF into mainstream spinal surgery. Cloward (4), in his landmark presentation at the American Association of Neurological Surgeons Meeting and subsequent publication, reported his results in treating 100 lumbar intervertebral disc herniations with PLIF. It was his belief that interbody fusion should be used as a first-line strategy in treating ruptured lumbar disc disease. Although it is now known that simple lumbar disc herniations refractory to conservative therapy have excellent long-term outcomes with limited discectomy alone, the treatment for recurrent disc herniations is still less clear.

INDICATIONS

The indications for PLIF in recent years have ranged in spectrum from gross spinal instability to severe degenerative disc disease. We are all familiar with the passionate arguments for and against the surgical treatment of low back pain secondary to segmental instability. Our indications for this procedure are based on an understanding of the pathophysiology of the degenerative cascade and the magnitude of disability and dysfunction that the patient experiences. This is coupled with the correlation of objective diagnostic (and potentially therapeutic) management interventions, and an overall philosophy that has developed by our experience and others in treating patients with lumbar degenerative disease. (5, 6, 12, 15, 16).

Candidates for PLIF include patients with degenerative disc disease characterized by segmental disc degeneration with Modic changes with or without foraminal stenosis demonstrated with magnetic resonance imaging (MRI) or computed tomography (CT) myelography. These patients must have a clinical history consistent with mechanical low back pain with or without leg pain. Other candidates include patients with degenerative lumbar instability, recurrent lumbar disc herniations, spondylolisthesis (less than grade III), postsurgical spinal instability, and pseudoarthrosis after attempted posterior fusions.

Plain films should demonstrate disc space collapse, and parasagittal CT or MRI reconstructions usually show impingement of the neural foramen by the superior facet of the inferior vertebrae. Provocative discography is used occasionally in patients with multi-level degenerative changes to identify the possible pain generator. Although discography traditionally focused on disc morphology, its current application is based on the reproduction of a patient's particular pain (i.e., concordant pain). Specifically, needles are placed into the disc of interest as well as into adjacent discs. Sterile saline solution, anesthetic, or contrast material is injected. A positive discogram recreates the patient's pain at the appropriate level of interest. Injection at adjacent levels should produce no pain or "discordant" pain (dissimilar from the patient's described pain in terms of location and intensity). Patients considered to be poor candidates for interbody fusion have inappropriate responses to discography. The usefulness of discography is controversial and patient selection can be complicated.

FRONT, BACK, OR NEITHER?

We would consider absolute contraindications to interbody fusion (either anterior or posterior) to be patients with multilevel disc disease with a nondiagnostic discogram, single-level disease, with radicular pain only (little or no mechanical back pain), and patients with severe osteoporosis. Relative contraindications for interbody fusion include patients who are actively smoking, patients with multilevel disease with more than one level positive on discogram, and patients with significant co-morbid illnesses.

When attempting to determine the best approach for an interbody fusion (i.e., anterior versus posterior), it is important to consider evidence of posterior pathology such as a disc fragment in the canal, facet hypertrophy, lateral recess, or central spinal stenosis. These findings would clearly cause us to favor a posterior approach. Contraindications specific to anterior approaches may include multiple prior abdominal procedures (which have led to adhesions). Also, severe atherosclerosis may preclude mobilization of the aorta and iliac vessels in fusions at or above the L5–S1 level. Relative contraindications to posterior procedures include patients with multiple prior posterior surgeries and significant scar formation. With advances in technology it is anticipated that some posterior pathology such as free fragments may eventually be addressed from an anterior approach similar to anterior cervical discectomy.

MODERN AGE PLIF

During the last 10 years it has been fascinating to see the development of modern age PLIF. There are few spinal procedures that have undergone such revolution in technology and frequency. The introduction of pedicle screw fixation by Roy–Camille for posterior stabilization stimulated a resurgence of posterolateral fusions. This was followed by the development of better instrumentation systems for the delivery and stability of the intervertebral disc space. Placement of threaded, cylindrical titanium cages grew in popularity because of the theoretical advantages of interbody fusion and axial load resistance compared with pedicle screw fixation (10, 13, 14). The improved instrumentation systems stimulated an explosion of interbody procedures because the original procedure was refined to the point that interbody fusions were easier to perform with less risk. The improved technology also allowed for more reliable placement of interbody prostheses. After the initial reports of good success with threaded, cylindrical titanium cages, various modifications of the implant device have been created.

Our group has experienced an evolution of philosophy regarding instrumentation for patients undergoing PLIF. Several years ago we began using "stand-alone" threaded titanium cages packed with morselized autograft as our first-line PLIF procedure. Using this technique, we began to find similar stability rates and clinical outcomes compared with our previous standard posterolateral fusion techniques.

Although the early stability rates for our stand-alone PLIFs were the same (approximately 91% in our series) (2) compared with previous posterolateral fusion procedures, we were concerned about the extensive disruption of the posterior tension band required to place these devices. Because of this and to increase our stability percentage, we began to supplement the stand-alone PLIF procedure with pedicle screw fixation. This made more sense to us from a theoretical and biomechanical standpoint because we were restoring the posterior tension band. With the addition of pedicle screw fixation, we were able to achieve a 100% stability rate. Despite this, we still struggled with the difficulty of determining radiologically whether fusion occurred in these patients because of metallic artifact. We also wondered what the long-term implications were of implanting a device with such a different modulus of elasticity compared with native bone.

Because of this we switched to threaded cortical bone dowels that were packed with morselized autograft, hoping to find a better way to determine fusion and to provide patients with a more physiological implant. We found that it was much easier to determine fusion status when using allograft implants. Long-term follow-up demonstrated osseous integration of the cortical bone with identical stability rates to our metallic implants with tension band constructs.

Unfortunately, during the period of using cylindrical cages (both metallic and allograft bone), we also experienced our highest number of nerve root injuries and cerebrospinal fluid leaks. The problem with cylindrical devices is that they are as wide as they are tall. To achieve optimal distraction and to increase joint stiffness, a prerequisite for successful fusion, large cylinders had to be placed. This required extensive dural and nerve root retraction, and caused our subsequent morbidities.

The introduction of rectangular cages added a significant advantage to PLIF (1, 3). Rectangular implants are considerably easier to navigate through the window of the superior and inferior nerve roots because of the more slender width in the sagittal plane. Although width is decreased, height is not sacrificed. Therefore the same distractive force achieved with large cylindrical devices is replicated with rectangular cages without the additional nerve root retraction. We were finally able to achieve the desired disc space distraction without the associated morbidity.

The most commonly used rectangular devices include carbon fiber, titanium, and allograft bone. The vast majority of metallic rectangular devices are used in Europe. We prefer using allograft bone implants because they offer structural stability under compression with a similar modulus of elasticity to the vertebral bodies. They also do not cause ar-

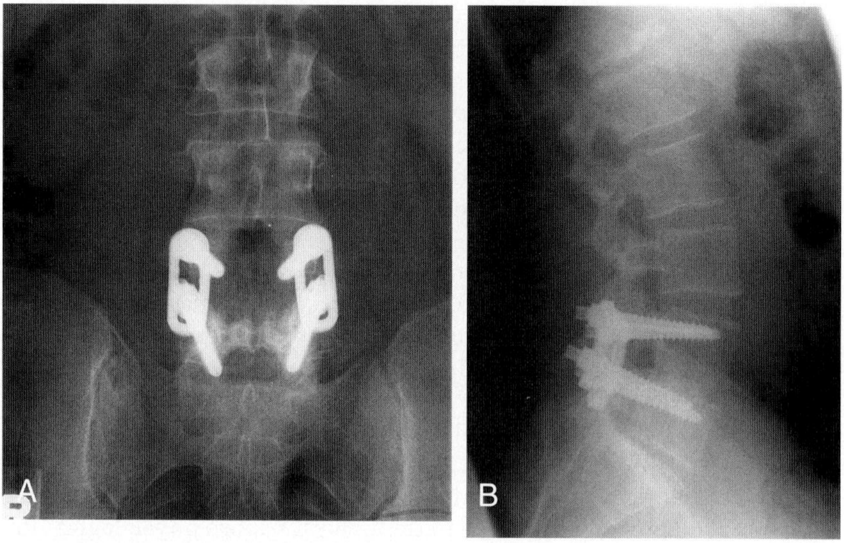

FIG. 29.1 (*A*) Anteroposterior plain radiograph of a patient 18 months after L4–L5 posterior lumbar interbody fusion with pedicle screw fixation. (*B*) Lateral plain radiograph of the same patient. Notice that the bone wedge appears to be well integrated within the subchondral end plates, indicating fusion.

tifact, allowing for better assessment of fusion, and they can undergo osseous integration (*Fig. 29.1*). Moreover, the allograft implants are shaped lordotically in the axial plane, allowing the surgeon to restore lumbar lordosis at the diseased segment. In addition to the placement of the allograft implant we always supplement this construct with morselized autologous iliac crest graft within the interspace between the implants and pedicle screw fixation (*Fig. 29.2*).

TECHNIQUE

Despite the technology and instrumentation that has made this procedure considerably easier to perform than years ago, PLIF is still a difficult and technically demanding procedure. Only expeditious completion of each step of the procedure coupled with meticulous hemostasis will result in technical success with minimal morbidity. We have come to order the sequence of this operation in such a way that formalizes the teaching of the procedure and allows for a logical, streamlined approach to completing the task at hand with minimized blood loss. Rarely do we deviate from this sequence.

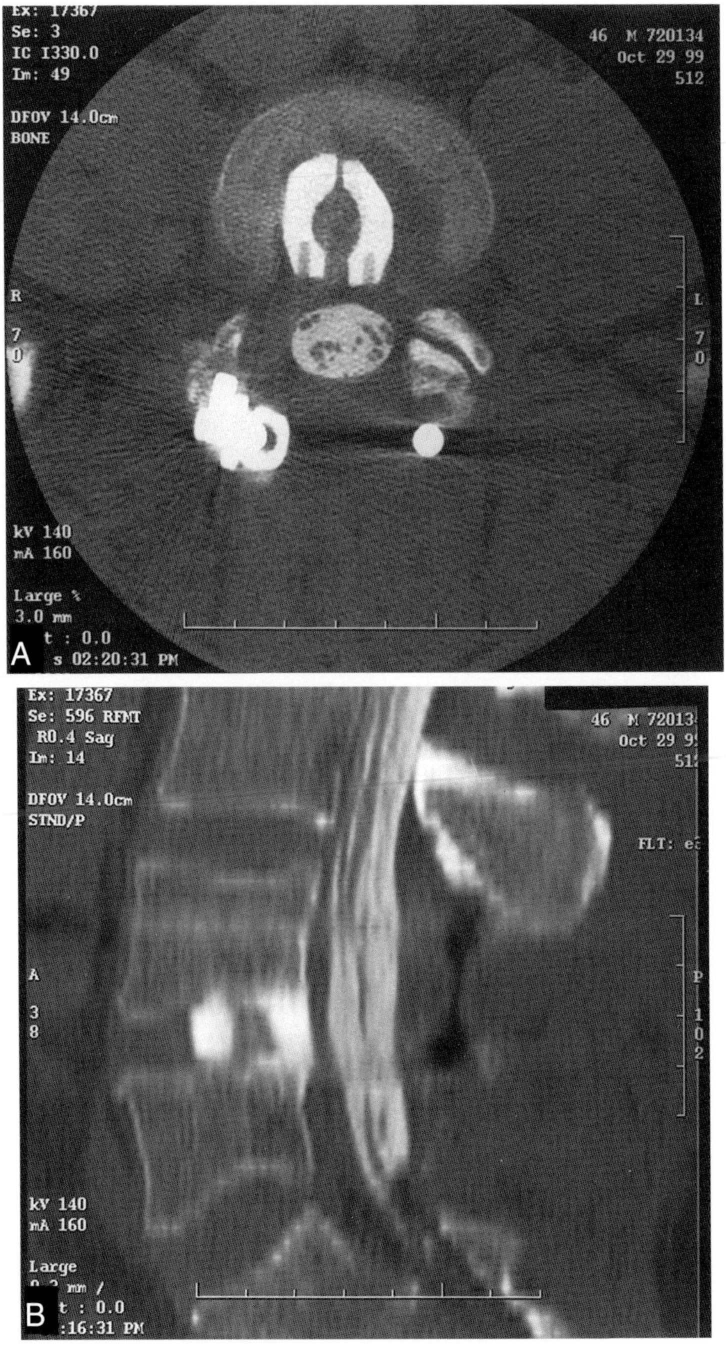
Ex: 17367
Se: 3
IC I330.0
Im: 49
DFOV 14.0cm
BONE
46 M 720134
Oct 29 99
512
R
L
kV 140
mA 160
Large
3.0 mm
t : 0.0
s 02:20:31 PM
A
Ex: 17367
Se: 596 RFMT
R0.4 Sag
Im: 14
DFOV 14.0cm
STND/P
A
P
kV 140
mA 160
Large
t : 0.0
:16:31 PM
B

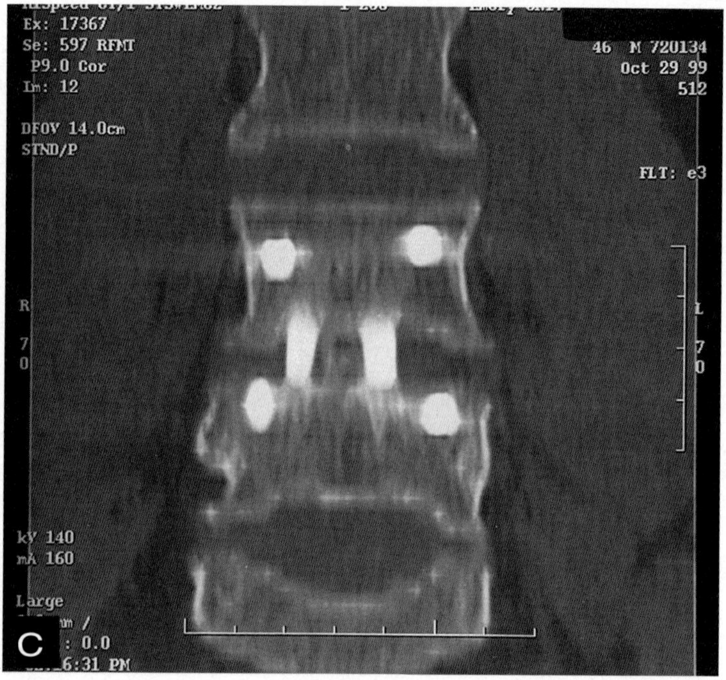

FIG. 29.2 (*A*) Axial computed tomographic (CT) scan of a patient 14 months after posterior lumbar interbody fusion with pedicle screw fixation. The bone wedges have a concavity that allows placement of morselized autograft within the central portion of the interspace. (*B*) Reformatted sagittal CT reconstruction of the same patient demonstrating osseous integration of the bone wedge. (*C*) Reformatted coronal CT reconstruction of the same patient demonstrating the incorporation of the bone graft allowing for easy assessment of fusion with allograft cortical bone wedges.

THE PROCEDURE: OVERALL PRINCIPLES

It has our belief that a wide exposure with a generous skin incision and deep muscle-relaxing incisions offers the best visualization for the surgeon and least postoperative pain for the patient. We routinely use "one-twitch" paralysis to improve muscle relaxation. Adequate muscle relaxation coupled with wide exposure decreases the paraspinous muscular injury incurred with vigorous retraction. Before making the skin incision, the proper size of the implant is determined by templating an adjacent normal level to determine optimal distraction. Pedicle screw length is also determined by measuring the length of the pedicles on axial CT. This information is conveyed to the scrub nurse before beginning to minimize intraoperative delays.

Step 1: Harvest Autologous Bone

At the beginning of the procedure, after the midline incision is made, we dissect a suprafascial plane through the same lumbar incision to identify the posterior superior iliac spine (PSIS). The fascia is then opened over the PSIS and the area is dissected in a subperiosteal fashion to expose the entire roof of the PSIS. The gluteus musculature is not dissected off the ileum when exposing the PSIS, because this results in significantly increased post-operative graft site pain. Using an osteotome, the cortical bone of the PSIS is chipped off to expose the cancellous undersurface. A large bone gouge is used to harvest the cancellous bone from the ileum. Using the gouge in a rotating fashion, the cancellous bone can be removed without violating the cortex, and the bone can be undermined within the intact pelvic wing. Usually, in an adult, approximately 20 to 30 cc of autologous graft can be harvested from this region. The bone is then morselized and stored for use later during the procedure. We have found that this technique, first described by Cloward as a PUCA-style graft, yields high-quality bone graft with less graft site pain compared with other grafting procedures.

The graft site is then irrigated with antibiotic and packed with gel foam. The fascial opening is then closed in a watertight fashion, and the dead space created by the suprafascial approach is also closed. Although the graft can be taken at any time during the procedure, we have found that harvesting graft first, before any epidural dissection, minimizes blood loss later in the procedure.

Step 2: Obtain Wide Bony Exposure

After the bone graft has been harvested, the midline incision is deepened and the spinous processes are identified. In a subperiosteal fashion, the muscle is dissected laterally to the base of the transverse processes. The pars intra-articularis must be identified and clearly dissected from the soft tissues. The intersection of the pars intra-articularis and the base of the transverse process marks the pedicle entry site. The pars intra-articularis also marks the region of the exiting nerve root. Because we supplement all PLIFs with pedicle screw tension band constructs, we prefer to mark our preliminary pedicle entry sites before the bony decompression. These preliminary sites will be reconfirmed later using fluoroscopy and by direct palpation of the pedicle from within the canal.

Before proceeding to the next step, the base of the transverse process and the pars intra-articularis of the superior and inferior vertebrae to be fused should be well visualized. The surgeon should have a "mind's-eye" view of where the exiting and traversing nerve roots are under the bone, before the decompression.

Step 3: Perform the Decompression

At this point, the spinous processes and lamina are removed to decompress the spinal canal and to give the surgeon an intra-canal view of the pedicles. Although many stylized sketches of a minimal laminectomy defect have been propagated by commercial advertisements, we have found that a complete laminectomy of the superior and inferior vertebrae is the best way to ensure adequate visualization of the nerve roots. We prefer to use a high-speed drill to thin the posterior elements and the lateral bony overhang. This tends to minimize blood loss during this portion of the procedure, and eases the bony removal with the Kerrison rongeur. After the laminae have been removed, we use a bone chisel to remove the medial portion of the facet joint. We have found chisels to be especially effective at removing the medial portion of the superior facet of the inferior vertebrae. Another approach we have used is to create an iatrogenic pars defect through the superior vertebrae, which disarticulates the inferior facet, which can then be removed, completely exposing the superior facet of the inferior vertebrae. During the removal of the lateral bony wall we try to cut only bone and to leave the ligamentum flavum in the lateral recess for a later point during the dissection. This removal of bone without the ligament again minimizes blood loss from the epidural plexus during this step of the procedure.

Step 4: Follow the Nerve Roots

After a wide decompression and facetectomy is performed, the pedicles of the superior and inferior vertebrae can be visualized and palpated. Using a Woodson or dental dissector, the course of the nerve is followed laterally into the foramen. A generous foraminotomy is then performed to approximately 1 cm lateral to the origin of the nerve root at the superior and inferior level. This bony removal allows for adequate exposure of the true axilla of the superior nerve root to be performed in the next step. Moreover, this generous foraminotomy ensures adequate decompression of any symptomatic nerve roots.

Step 5: Find the True Axilla of the Superior Nerve Root

After completing the foraminotomy it is important to remove the lateral bony overhang comprised by the inferior facet of the superior vertebrae that sometimes interferes with placement of interbody devices. After this is removed, the epidural veins within the lateral gutter are coagulated and cut, and the remaining ligamentum flavum is removed. The coagulation of epidural veins and removal of ligamentum flavum should only be performed after both the superior and inferior nerve roots are well visualized. Using meticulous bipolar electrocautery to the veins located in the axilla of the superior nerve root, the surgeon can then divide the tethering venous plexus to expose the true axilla of the nerve root. This dissection affords the surgeon a slightly larger portal of entry for the interbody prosthesis, gives more laxity to the superior nerve root during dural retraction, and minimizes the chances for dural tears or nerve root injury.

Step 6: Place the Pedicle Screws

At this point during the operation the surgeon can easily construct a three-dimensional mind's-eye view of the size, diameter, and trajectory of the pedicles. The preliminary pedicle entry sites are checked and verified with C-arm fluoroscopy. At this point, necessary adjustments can be made and the pedicles are then probed, tapped, and screwed under fluoroscopic guidance. We prefer to use the TSRH instrumentation system (Medtronic Sofamor Danek, Memphis, TN). When tapping the pedicle, it is important to remember that if the entry site has been chosen correctly, then the tap almost guides itself down the pedicle. No downward pressure needs to be applied to the tap for it to enter the pedicle. After tapping, the screw is placed and should easily follow the tapped channel. The pedicle screw depth can be estimated by lateral fluoroscopy and should incorporate approximately 80% of the vertebral body. It has been our preference to place the pedicle screws before performing the PLIF. The reason for this is that if a dural tear is encountered during the PLIF portion of the procedure, the epidural bleeding can be difficult to control because of the loss of the tamponade of the thecal sac turgor. This epidural bleeding can be significant enough to prohibit placement of the interbody device. If the dural tear is encountered before placement of pedicle screws, then the epidural bleeding continues during the 15 minutes of pedicle screw placement.

Step 7: Perform a Generous Discectomy

After placement of the pedicle screws and generous debulking and coagulation of the lateral recess epidural plexus and ligamentum flavum, a generous discectomy is performed on both sides of the thecal sac. We generally perform the discectomy using standard annulotomy, curettage, and pituitary rongeur removal of the nucleus pulposus. Although the PLIF instruments perform a significant discectomy with the reamers and scrapers, we have found that the effectiveness of these instruments is enhanced if the disc has been debulked. A standard discectomy does not add significant time to the procedure, and it augments the surface area for fusion. Moreover, particularly with the newer systems, inadequate discectomy can occasionally lead to the distracter plugs kicking out after initial placement.

Step 8: Perform the PLIF

At this point we proceed with the PLIF. It is our preference to use the Tangent instrumentation system (Medtronic Sofamor Danek) and to place rectangular, lordotically shaped cortical allograft bone wedges. It has been our experience that this system offers the best distraction and structural support with the least amount of nerve root retraction. There are numerous other instrumentation systems available, and the details of their implementation can be obtained from the manufacturer's literature. We address only the Tangent system method.

After a generous standard discectomy is performed, distractors are hammered into place under direct fluoroscopic guidance. These distracters are then sequentially dialed up to larger sizes until the desired distraction is achieved. After the desired distraction is obtained, one distracter is left in place on one side of the thecal sac. On the contralateral side of the thecal sac, a rotating cutter is then hammered into position under fluoroscopic guidance. The guide is typically hammered to a depth of 30 to 40 mm, depending on the size of the vertebral body. Because the rotator cutter is flanged in the middle, it is important to rotate the instrument several times as it is hammered down. This prevents the rotator cutter from being too difficult to rotate at its peak depth. Next, the remaining loose disc material is removed from the interspace. An end plate scraper is then placed within the disc space and the end plates are denuded of their cartilage. We use short stroking movements with the end plate scraper to minimize pullout of the instrument.

After the end plate has been prepared, a channel cutter is then placed at the dorsal aspect of the interspace. Using fluoroscopy, the ideal entry and trajectory of the channel cutter is approximated to cut a channel of bone approximately 1 to 2 mm into the end plate of both the superior and inferior vertebral bodies. The trajectory of this instrument is checked several times as it is hammered into the interspace. If the trajectory veers off the ideal pathway, the channel cutter is backed out and a new trajectory is taken. This is important because if a channel is not cut in the ideal position, the graft can be placed partially into the vertebral body. This is undesirable because the distractive force of the graft will be lost and it will not be aligned with the contralateral graft. After the channel has been cut, a pituitary rongeur is again used to remove any loose debris within the interspace. At this point the prechosen allograft implant is then tamped into place. Usually we countersink the graft approximately 2 mm.

Once the first graft is placed, attention is then turned to the contralateral side, the distracter is removed and the rotator cutter, end plate scrapper, channel cutter sequence is repeated. After the channel is cut and the remaining interspace debris is removed, we then pack the disc space with approximately 10 cc of morselized autologous bone graft that was harvested earlier during the operation. Using the distracters and a bone spatula, this bone is packed within the interspace and medially toward the contralateral allograft implant. Then the second allograft implant is tamped and countersunk into position.

The wound is then irrigated thoroughly and the remaining bone surfaces are decorticated. The rod connector construct is then placed onto the pedicle screws and is tightened under mild compression. Because these grafts are only countersunk 1 to 2 mm, the implants sit within the joint's instantaneous axis of rotation. We feel that gentle compression of the graft increases the chances for osseous union because the graft is placed under stress, a necessary component for bone growth (Wolff's Law). Also, because a posterior tension band construct is created with the "lock-down" of the posterior elements, we have found our patients to have less postoperative pain than patients undergoing this operation with stand-alone devices. Because the interbody fusion is performed in conjunction with pedicle screw fixation, we do not perform a traditional posterolateral fusion with muscle dissection out to the tips of the transverse processes. Any remaining bone is placed over the remaining decorticated bone surfaces. Before closure, it is important to check all exposed nerve roots to verify adequate decompression and to make sure that loose autograft has not accidentally fallen into the neural foramen. After this step, a large drain is placed and the wound is closed in three layers with a watertight fascial closure.

RESULTS

Review of our stand-alone PLIF series with titanium cages demonstrated a 91% stability rate defined as absence of movement on flexion–extension radiographs (2). We did not calculate a fusion rate for this series because it is our belief that true fusion is difficult or impossible to determine because of metallic artifact, even with CT reformatted images. We were able to obtain a 100% stability rate when we supplemented the metallic cages with pedicle screw fixation, but again were unable to determine fusion rate. Combining our stand-alone series and the metallic-cage-with-pedicle-screw-fixation series , we found our incidence of transient nerve root injury to be as high as 10%. Permanent nerve root injury with titanium cages was 5% in the combined series. The intraoperative cerebrospinal fluid leak in this series was 9% (2). Although these complication rates were consistent with other published reports, we felt they were unacceptably high.

The overall satisfactory results defined as excellent or good Prolo outcomes was 70% in our series of PLIF patients using threaded cortical bone dowels packed with morselized autograft bone and pedicle screw supplementation (2). We achieved a 95% fusion rate at the 1-year follow-up examination, defined as an increase in subchondral end plate sclerosis, the presence of bridging bone incorporating the bone graft, and an absence of lucency around the threaded cortical bone dowel. We found a similar incidence of complications using cylindrical bone dowels, including a 5% incidence of permanent nerve root injury (2).

During the last 18 months, we have switched almost exclusively to using rectangular bone wedges (Tangent, Medtronic Sofamor Danek). We have performed this procedure in approximately 70 patients. Preliminary follow-up of this patient series has demonstrated a similar fusion and stability rate compared with cylinders with pedicle screw fixation without nerve root injury in all cases. We believe the introduction of rectangular devices that decrease nerve root retraction will significantly reduce the morbidity of this operation yet still produce excellent fusion rates.

CONCLUSION

The treatment of degenerative lumbar disease has undergone a revolution in the last 20 years. Newer techniques and better instrumentation systems have allowed spine surgeons to do today what was previously impossible. PLIF is an excellent example in the medical literature of an idea that came before its time. Some of the earliest descriptions of PLIF, once abandoned by surgeons as a dangerous, high-morbidity operation, are now well-accepted techniques that are strikingly similar to their original descriptions. It would behoove us to think more about the ideas of our predecessors.

REFERENCES

1. Agazzi S, Reverdin A, May D: Posterior lumbar interbody fusion with cages: An independent review of 71 cases. **J Neurosurg** 91:186–192, 1999.
2. Barnes B, McLaughlin MR, Birch B, Rodts GE, Haid RW: Threaded cortical bone dowels for lumbar interbody fusion: Technique and short term results. **Neurosurg Focus** 7:1–4, 1999.
3. Brantigan JW, Steffee AD: A carbon fiber implant to aid interbody lumbar fusion: Two-year clinical results in the first 26 patients. **Spine** 18:2106–2116, 1993.
4. Cloward RB: The treatment of ruptured lumbar intervertebral discs by vertebral body fusion. **J Neurosurg** 10:154–168, 1953.
5. Dickman CA: Internal fixation and fusion of the lumbar spine using threaded interbody cages. **BNI Quarterly** 3:4–25, 1997.
6. Dunsker SB: Lumbar spine stabilization: Indications, in (Black PM, ed.): *Clinical Neurosurgery. Vol. 36.* Baltimore, Williams and Wilkins, 1988, pp 147–158.

7. Hibbs RA, Albee FH: An operation for progressive spinal deformities. **N Y State J Med** 93:1013, 1911.
8. Hodgson AR, Stock FE: Anterior spinal fusion: A preliminary communication on the radical treatment of Pott's disease and Pott's paraplegia. **Br J Surg** 44:266–275, 1956.
9. Jaslow IA: Intercorporal bone graft in spinal fusion after disc removal. **Surg Gynecol Obstet** 82:215–218, 1946.
10. Kuslich SD, Ulstrom CL, Griffith SL, Ahern JW, Dowdle JD: Lumbar interbody fusion: History, techniques, and 2-year follow-up results of a United States prospective, multicenter trial. **Spine** 23:1267–1279,1998.
11. Mercer W: Spondylolisthesis with a description of a new method of operative treatment and notes of 10 cases. **Edinburgh Med J** 43:545–572, 1936.
12. O'Brien JP: The role of fusion for chronic low back pain. **Orthop Clin North Am** 44:639–645, 1989.
13. Onesti ST, Ashkenazi E: Instrumentation, technique and technology. **Neurosurgery** 42:200–205, 1998.
14. Ray CD: Threaded titanium cages for lumbar interbody fusions. **Spine** 22:667–680, 1997.
15. Simmons JW: Posterior lumbar interbody fusion, in Frymoyer JW (ed.): *The Adult Spine.* New York, Raven Press, 1991, pp 1961–1987.
16. Truumees E, Sidhu K, Fischgrund JS: Indications for fusion in lumbar disc disease. **Semin Spine Surg** 11:147–162, 1999.

CHAPTER

30

The Role of Anterior Lumbar Interbody Allograft Bone Dowel Fusion as an Adjunct to Posterior Segmental Lumbar Fixation

HARSIMRAN S. BRARA, M.D., RICHARD G. FESSLER, M.D., PH.D.

Anterior lumbar interbody fusion (ALIF) was first described in 1932 by Capener (2) for the treatment of spondylolisthesis. Since then it has been used for a variety of pathologies, including spinal instability (4, 5, 15, 16), tumors, infection, and disabling low back pain resulting from failed low back surgery (1, 6, 7, 9, 10, 13, 16). Recently, laparoscopic and "mini open" laparotomy techniques have been described that achieve the same end through much less destructive procedures (11, 12, 14).

Symptomatic lumbar pseudoarthrosis resulting in intractable back pain with or without leg symptoms is a complex but increasingly common clinical problem. Various authors have suggested posterior instrumentation (3), ALIF (12), or combined anterior fusion and posterior instrumentation to treat these patients (7). Although there is limited literature examining circumferential lumbar fusions, the most appropriate setting in which to employ this approach may be the patient with the failed prior fusion. Primary short-segment posterolateral fusions with pedicle screw instrumentation systems can achieve a solid osseous union in more than 90% of patients (3). However, revision posterolateral fusion is less successful in achieving segmental arthrodesis. Anterior flexion, which creates stress on the posterior rod construct, may contribute to the failure of the primary fusion. Circumferential fusion, however, enables anterior column reconstruction along with segment stabilization. Therefore, lumbar lordosis may be restored by the placement of an anterior bone dowel or metallic cage, in a system that load shares with the posterior pedicle screw and rod instrumentation.

We present the results of a series of patients undergoing either ALIF alone or in combination with posterior instrumentation (Fig. 30.1). Results are analyzed both in terms of fusion rates and in terms of clinical outcome assessed by the Prolo Scale.

CLINICAL MATERIALS AND METHODS

Patient Population

Between July 1992 and July 1998, 27 patients with symptomatic lumbar pseudoarthrosis, or demonstrated, significant symptomatic lumbar instability in association with spondylolisthesis or advanced degenerative scoliosis were treated surgically with primary or revision fusion surgery. All patients underwent an ALIF procedure and 21 patients underwent circumferential fusion.

There were 11 men and 16 women that met the inclusion criteria. Their mean age was 51.9 years. Twenty-two of the patients had previously undergone an instrumented posterolateral fusion. Six patients underwent an anterior interbody fusion alone, whereas the remainder underwent circumferential fusion with the revision of their posterolateral fusion.

The mean preoperative duration of symptoms was 8.3 years and the mean follow-up period was 10.7 months (range, 4–72 months). Charts were reviewed to determine the operative blood loss, operative time, and perioperative or long-term complications. All patients were available for follow-up study by reviewing their outpatient chart or by speaking with them in a telephone interview. Telephone interviews were used to extend follow-up study in patients for whom there was limited outpatient follow-up data. Prolo Scale functional outcome scores were assigned to serve as the outcome measure at the point of most recent follow-up.

Radiographic evidence of fusion was assessed at each clinic visit with plain lumbar spine radiographs. Computed tomographic (CT) scans were obtained in patients with equivocal plain radiographs and continued symptomatology.

Management Protocol

Preoperatively, all patients underwent magnetic resonance imaging (MRI) examination, and CT scans as well plain lumbar radiographs with flexion–extension views to document their instability or their pseudoarthrosis from prior fusion attempts were acquired. Myelography with postmyelogram CT was obtained in all patients with preexisting metallic implants.

Patients had to fail an extensive course of nonoperative therapies before being considered for a lumbar fusion, regardless of whether it was primary or revision surgery. Conservative measures included wearing a TLSO brace, epidural corticosteroid injections, physical therapy, and structured narcotic analgesic programs.

Intraoperatively, cell saver was used to minimize the need for blood transfusions. Preoperative antibiotics were administered and the patients were maintained on postoperative antibiotics for at least 1 day.

Surgical Technique

ALIF was performed using allograft threaded cortical bone dowels filled with autograft bone. The retroperitoneal approaches via a minimally invasive open approach through a 4-cm flank incision or an endoscopic retroperitoneal approach were used to accomplish the anterior fusion.

The patient was then repositioned on a radiolucent operating table, and fluoroscopy with a C-arm image intensifier was used in all patients for the placement of the pedicle screws. Copious amounts of autograft iliac crest bone graft was harvested and used for the posterolateral onlay fusion. Meticulous attention was devoted to establishing a healthy, well-decorticated surgical bed for the onlay autograft.

RESULTS

Follow-up data for all 27 patients were available. The 11 men and 16 women (mean age, 51.9 years) undergoing lumbar interbody fusion with or without a posterior fusion between 1992 and 1998 at the University of Florida had preoperative symptoms for an average of 8.3 years. Twenty-two of the 28 patients had undergone a prior posterolateral fusion.

The mean follow-up interval was 10.7 months (range, 4–72 months). The average hospital stay was 4.8 days, and the average operative blood loss was 316 ml. Fusion was accomplished in 2 of 6 patients (33%) with anterior fusion alone and in 18 of 21 patients (85.6%) with circumferential fusions. The average Prolo Scale outcome scores assigned at the time of the most recent follow-up study was 8.8 points; the average preoperative Prolo Scale score was 6.3 points.

Significant complications arose in three patients. Two patients developed incisional hernias requiring operative repair and one patient fractured the allograft bone dowel, necessitating revision surgery. Delayed and less significant complications occurred in two patients. One patient had signs and symptoms of left S1 nerve root irritation without radiographic evidence of screw malpositioning. The patient improved after removal of the posterior instrumentation. A second patient developed a superficial wound infection that was treated successfully with a course of oral antibiotics. There were no significant general medical complications.

DISCUSSION

ALIF has the advantage of anterior column reconstruction in a load-sharing environment but also has the disadvantage of allowing unrestricted distractive forces in extension. Circumferential fusion retains the advantage of anterior column reconstruction while adding the advantage of segmental stabilization. The results of the current study clearly demonstrate that circumferential stabilization achieves a superior fusion rate

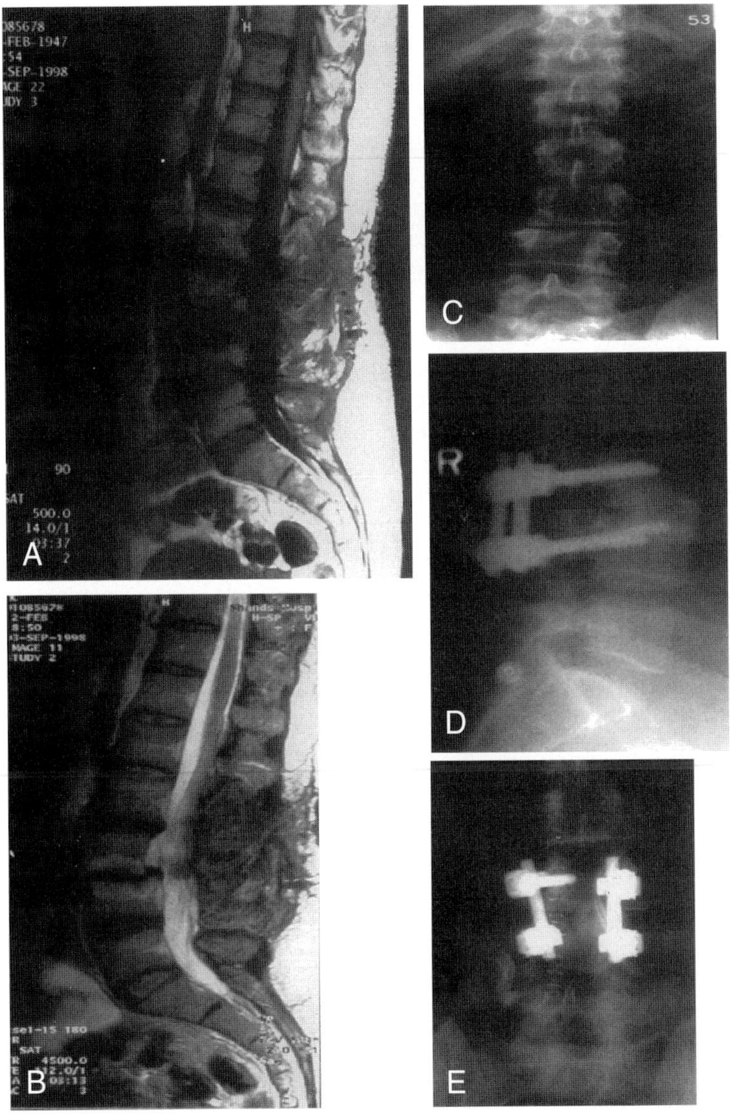

FIG. 30.1 Our illustrative case is a 51-year-old white woman with a 6-year history of progressive low back pain and left thigh pain after a decompressive laminectomy performed 7 years earlier. (*A, B*) Sagittal T1 and T2 magnetic resonance images illustrating the L3–L4 disc space collapse and vertebral end plate changes. (*C*) Anteroposterior films demonstrating the lateral listhesis. (*D, E*) At L3–L4 it was only possible to place one lumbar interbody allograft dowel before performing the posterior pedicle screw fusion. The reduction in both the sagittal and coronal planes is evident. The patient experienced marked improvement in her pain and was rendered far more functional as a result of the surgery.

to anterior interbody fusion alone. This result is consistent with other reports of both anterior and circumferential stabilization. Although Kuslich (8) reported a 90% fusion rate with BAK fusion alone, few others have achieved this result. Vamvanij et al. (17) reported a 60% fusion rate for anterior fusion alone compared with an 88% fusion rate for circumferential fusion. Wang et al. (18) reported a 95% fusion rate in patients with an anterior interbody fusion with posterior pedicle screw instrumentation.

The results of the current study also suggest improved functional outcome as assessed by the Prolo functional outcomes scale. Prolo Scale scores increased approximately 25% above presurgical levels.

Complications observed in the current series were primarily unrelated to the spinal allograft itself. One allograft fracture was observed that did result in revision surgery. This fracture was observed in the ALIF-alone group. No graft-related complications were observed in the ALIF-plus-posterior instrumentation group. Two incisional hernias were observed and two minor complications were also noted.

CONCLUSIONS

ALIF via a minimally invasive open or endoscopic technique is a useful adjunct to enhance the chance for achieving a solid arthrodesis in patients who are otherwise at a high risk for failure of fusion.

ALIF alone may not be a sufficient stand-alone method to achieve lumbar fusion in patients with significant instability or prior failed posterolateral lumbar fusion.

REFERENCES

1. Böhm H, Harms J, Donk R, Zielke K: Correction and stabilization of angular kyphosis. **Clin Orthop** 258:56–61, 1990.
2. Capener N: Spondylolisthesis. **Br J Surg** 19:374–386, 1932.
3. Dickman C, Fessler RG, MacMillan M, Haid RW: Transpedicular screw rod fixation of the lumbar spine: Operative technique and outcome in 104 cases. **J Neurosurg** 77:525–530, 1992.
4. Gertzbein SD, Court–Brown CM, Jacobs RR, et al.: Decompression and circumferential stabilization of unstable spinal fractures. **Spine** 13:392–395, 1988.
5. Grob D, Scheier HJG, Dvorak J, Siegrist H, Rubeli M, Joller R: Circumferential fusion of the lumbar and lumbosacral spine. **Arch Orthop Trauma Surg** 111:20–25, 1991.
6. Kozak JA, Heilman AE, O'Brien JP: Anterior lumbar fusion options. **Clin Orthop** 300:45–51, 1994.
7. Kozak JA, O'Brien JP: Simultaneous combined anterior and posterior fusion: An independent analysis of a treatment for the disabled low-back pain patient. **Spine** 15:322–328, 1990.
8. Kuslich SD, Ulstrom CL, Griffith SL, Ahern AW, Dowdle JD: The Boghy and Kuslich method of lumbar interbody fusion. **Spine** 23:1267–1279, 1998.

9. Linson MA, Williams H: Anterior and combined anteroposterior fusion for the lumbar disc pain: A preliminary study. **Spine** 16:143–145, 1991.
10. Louw JA: Spinal tuberculosis with neurological deficit. **J Bone Joint Surg Br** 72B:686–693, 1990.
11. Mayer M: A new microsurgical technique for minimally invasive anterior lumbar interbody fusion. **Spine** 22:691–700, 1997.
12. McAfee PC, Regan JJ, Geis P, Fedder IL: Minimally invasive anterior retroperitoneal approach to the lumbar spine. **Spine** 23:1476–1484, 1998.
13. O'Brien JP, Dawson MHO, Heard CW, Momberger G, Weatherley CR: Simultaneous combined anterior and posterior fusion: A surgical solution for failed spinal surgery with a brief review of the first 150 patients. **Clin Orthop** 203:191–195, 1986.
14. Regan JJ, Aronoff RS, Ohnmeiss DD, Sengupta DK: Laparoscopic approach to L4–L5 for interbody fusion using BAK cages: Experience in 58 cages. **Spine** 24:2171–2174, 1999.
15. Smith MD, Bohlman HH: Spondylolisthesis treated by a single-stage operation combining decompression with in-situ posterolateral and anterior fusion. **J Bone Joint Surg Am** 72A:415–421, 1990.
16. Spencer DL, DeWald RL: Simultaneous anterior and posterior surgical approach to the thoracic and lumbar spine. **Spine** 4:29–36, 1979.
17. Vamvanij V, Frederickson BE, Thorpe JM, Stadnick ME, Yuan HA: Surgical treatment of internal disc disruption: An outcome study of four fusion techniques. **J Spinal Disord** 11:375–382, 1998.
18. Wang J, Kim DJ, Yun YH: Posterior pedicle screw instrumentation and anterior interbody fusion in adult lumbar spondylosis or grade I spondylolisthesis with segmental instability. **J Spinal Disord** 9:83–88, 1996.

CHAPTER

31

Open Anterior Lumbar Interbody Fusion

CHARLES J. RIEDEL, M.D.

Anterior lumbar interbody fusion (ALIF) was described originally in the early 1930s for the treatment of spondylolisthesis (1). The popularity of the procedure has waxed and waned considerably during the decades since then, as the result of an evolving understanding of the degenerative process, pain generation, the biomechanics and consequences of different types of lumbar fusion, and changing technology, especially instrumentation.

INDICATIONS

Spondylolisthesis remains one of the most frequent indications for ALIF. ALIF is also a very useful option in revision surgery when a pseudoarthrosis exists after posterior or posterolateral fusion. When antibiotic therapy alone fails to eradicate an infectious discitis, ALIF allows aggressive debridement and eliminates the extremely painful motion segment. The most common use of anterior fusion surgery currently, however, and also the most controversial, is almost certainly in the treatment of internal disc disruption, other forms of degenerative disc conditions, and the so-called *failed back syndrome.*

FUSION OPTIONS

No approach for lumbar fusion is regarded universally as optimal. A variety of options are available to the spinal surgeon, each with unique advantages and disadvantages. These include posterior fusion, posterolateral intertransverse fusion, posterior lumbar interbody fusion (PLIF), and ALIF, which may be carried out with an open exposure or laparoscopically. Each of these may be supplemented with instrumentation. Few prospective, controlled studies compare clinical outcomes directly among different types of fusions, and therefore the type of fusion selected is tailored to the specific clinical situation and the surgeon's preference.

There are inherent disadvantages in posterior approaches. PLIF carries with it a high incidence of dysesthesias because of root retraction.

Several cases of cauda equina syndrome have been reported. Often, a considerable portion of the facets must be resected to gain adequate exposure for graft and device placement, which can lead to loss of construct strength, particularly in torsion. Because of the restrictions imposed by the thecal sac and nerve roots, it is often difficult to distract the interspace and place as large a cage or graft as can be accomplished anteriorly. Epidural fibrosis can be particularly intense. Even with more advanced devices, posterior dislodgment can occur.

Posterolateral fusion has its own limitations. Stripping of the paraspinous muscles by necessity results in partial devascularization and denervation. This can result in weakness and atrophy of these muscles, which are crucial to improved back function. This is sometimes referred to as *fusion disease.* These fusions are also less stiff mechanically and are only an indirect approach to treating what is a main source of pain[em]namely, the intervertebral disc. Lastly, interbody fusions have the advantage of being under compression.

BIOMECHANICAL ADVANTAGES OF ALIF

A number of studies suggest biomechanical advantages to ALIFs. Zdeblick et al. (21) used a simple model of two-point fixation with Steinmann pins in human cadaveric spines to demonstrate that fixation of the vertebral bodies eliminated intervertebral motion more effectively than fixation of the transverse processes, the pedicles, or the lamina. This was particularly true after disruption of the annulus fibrosis. In a cadaveric spine model that used polymethyl methacrylate to simulate posterior, posterolateral, or anterior fusion, anterior fusion increased stiffness 80%, whereas posterolateral fusion resulted in an increase of only 40% and posterior fusion a mere 10% (12). Also, posterior fusion allowed anterior motion with bending.

There is an important clinical correlate to these biomechanical observations. Goldner et al. (8) reported 100 patients with interbody fusions. Included in this group were patients who had solid posterior fusions but whose persistent back pain was relieved by anterior fusion. More recently Weatherley et al. (20) reported five patients with solid posterolateral or posterior fusions who had persistent low back pain without radicular pain. Discography suggested that the fused segment was the source of the pain. Four of the five patients underwent ALIF with complete relief of their pain.

In another biomechanical study, Chen et al. (3) demonstrated that anterior interbody distraction can significantly increase the height of the posterior disc, the cross sectional area, and the volume of the neuroforamina in the degenerative lumbar spine. This represents a potentially obvious advantage of the anterior approach over posterior approaches to help relieve nerve root compression.

As is often the case, however, biomechanical findings do not necessarily transfer to clinical findings. In a clinical study by Dennis et al. (5), disc height could be increased 89% or 9.5 mm initially with anterior fusions using autologous, cadaveric, or mixed iliac crest grafts. With long-term follow-up, however, all disc space heights diminished and nearly half the disc spaces were narrower than preoperatively. Femoral ring allograft, which has more structural strength, did better at sustaining the disc height, but still 41% of disc spaces were narrower at the follow-up than before surgery (11). This loss of disc height is multifactorial, including graft subsidence and remodeling.

There may be a price to pay for the increased stiffness of anterior fusion. Many, although not all, surgeons believe that accelerated degeneration may occur next to a lumbar fusion. Several biomechanical studies have shown that in cadaveric spine models with simulated anterior interbody fusions, the adjacent segments have increased motion (4, 12). Esses et al. (6) have shown that, in fact, ALIF increases adjacent segment motion more than posterolateral fusion. Interestingly, circumferential fusion does not have any more deleterious effects on adjacent segment motion than anterior fusion alone.

Once again, however, the biomechanical data are not necessarily reflected in the clinical situation. Penta et al. (16) looked at magnetic resonance images in patients with anterior lumbar fusions and 10 years of follow-up. They were unable to detect accelerated degeneration at adjacent segments. Their study was not well controlled.

Luk et al. (13) used flexion–extension radiographs to determine adjacent segment motion in patients who had previously undergone anterior fusions and were pain free. They compared this group with a group of age-matched asymptomatic control subjects and discovered that motion at segments adjacent to the fused level in the operated group was reduced compared with the control group, as was overall spinal motion. They suggest that hypermobility cannot explain accelerated degeneration.

SURGICAL TECHNIQUES

Anterior exposure can be obtained either transperitoneally or via a retroperitoneal approach. Recent advances in less invasive approaches have significantly reduced perioperative discomfort and hospital stays. Key to this has been smaller incisions with muscle sparing rather than muscle-cutting exposure of the retroperitoneal space. Microsurgical techniques have been applied by some surgeons. The relevant anatomy is primarily vascular. The L5–S1 level can be exposed readily between the iliac vessels because it usually lies below the bifurcation of the aorta and vena cava. L4–L5 is most commonly exposed by mobilizing the vessels from left to right. This may require dividing the segmental artery and vein as well as the ascending lumbar vein. This can be accomplished laparoscopically, but it is considerably more difficult and carries more risk than when the exposure is performed open.

A large array of new techniques is available to the surgeon for performing the actual fusion. The availability and ease of use of threaded titanium cages has certainly been one of the reasons for the recent resurgence of anterior interbody fusions. These were originally designed to be placed in an anteroposterior orientation. In biomechanical testing, however, the cages provide equal stiffness when placed in an anteroposterior, lateral, or oblique orientation unless the facet joints have been disrupted to allow for placement. This significantly reduces stiffness, predominantly in torsion, and raises a major concern with PLIFs (18).

FUSION RATES

One of the most difficult problems in interpreting the results of anterior interbody fusions has been the large range reported for successful fusion rates. Although the use of threaded cages initially held out hope for improving the fusion rates, in some ways the cages have compounded the already difficult problem of assessing accurately whether a segment is fused. The reported fusion rate for ALIFs has been as low as 18% and has high as 96% (2, 7). This likely reflects differences in technique, patient populations including smokers, and the difficulty in assessing arthrodesis. A recent attempt was made to "average" reported rates of fusion in the literature. Although the validity of such an attempt is questionable, the numbers are interesting. For a single level the fusion rate is approximately 83%. This drops considerably when a second level is included. When three levels are involved, the fusion rate is only approximately 50%. For this reason, multilevel fusions, particularly in heavy smokers, may benefit from the addition of posterior fixation.

COMPLICATIONS

The most worrisome complication in anterior interbody fusion is injury to one of the great vessels, the left iliac vein being the most susceptible. The actual incidence is very low and clearly less than with laparoscopic approaches, particularly above the lumbosacral junction. Retrograde ejaculation varies considerably in frequency, from 0.2 to 17.5%. This potential risk must be explained carefully because it is an unacceptable consequence to some patients or their spouses. Great care should be taken during dissection to minimize the use of cautery and to sweep the soft tissues laterally from the L5–S1 disc to minimize the chance of injury to the presacral plexus. Because of compression and retraction of the iliac veins, venous thrombosis and pulmonary embolus are infrequent but well-known potential complications. Graft extrusion is an infrequent occurrence with most of the new devices. Neurological injury can occur with the approach, including the ilio-inguinal and ilio-hypogastric nerves. The femoral nerve has also been injured (14). Excessive retraction on the psoas can result in injury to the lumbar plexus.

OUTCOMES

Evaluation of outcomes remains unsatisfactory. Two recent studies are cited as examples (15, 19). In both studies, outcome, if based on surveys of patient satisfaction, was reasonably good, with 71% and 72% of patients reporting marked reduction in their painful symptoms. When more objective and detailed assessments of patients' daily function are employed, such as the Low Back Outcome Score (LBOS) or the Japanese Orthopedic Association index, the picture is much different, with only 27% and 34% achieving satisfactory ratings. Interestingly, the outcomes in most of these studies do not correlate with the fusion rate, further complicating analysis.

How does ALIF actually fare when compared with other types of fusions? There are few direct comparison studies in the literature, and it is impossible to compare different surgical series in a valid manor because of the lack of standardized outcome assessment as well as patient selection biases. In a small, nonrandomized series of patients with isthmic spondylolisthesis, with 20 patients in each group, Kim and Lee (10) looked at the fusion rate and successful outcome of ALIF and instrumented posterolateral lumbar fusion. Outcome was judged on subjective changes in symptoms only, but in these groups they could demonstrate no significant difference in fusion rate or outcome.

Greenough et al. (9) compared a much larger group of patients who underwent instrumented posterolateral fusions for intractable low back pain with a second group of patients who underwent ALIF (all patients operated by the senior author). The majority of patients had discogenic low back pain but the group included patients with spondylolisthesis or spondylolysis, failed back surgery, and prior fracture. The results, when expressed by patient satisfaction, were nearly identical, with 65% of posterolateral fusion patients and 68% of ALIF patients reporting marked improvement in their pain. There was a significant difference, however, in the LBOS—the ALIF patients did twice as well as those undergoing posterolateral fusion.

OPEN VERSUS LAPAROSCOPIC

Lastly, should anterior interbody fusion be carried out via an open approach or laparoscopically? Data from the BAK investigational device evaluation clinical trials carried out to satisfy some of the requirements for the United States Food and Drug Administration sheds some light on this (17). Despite the minimally invasive access with laparoscopy, hospital length of stay was reduced minimally. This may be explained in part because patients who underwent a laparoscopic procedure, which was transperitoneal, had a higher incidence of ileus than those who underwent open surgery, although that difference was not statistically significant. There was also a trend for a higher risk of retrograde ejaculation with the laparoscopic approach. Lastly, open ALIF facilitates a more complete removal of the disc if desired. The risk of retropulsed disc herniation was higher in the laparoscopic group, and this did achieve statistical significance.

At the lumbosacral junction, the laparoscopic procedure is relatively easy and safe. It may prove to be the treatment of choice. Above this level, however, the difficulty and risk argue for an open approach. As advances are made in endoscopic retroperitoneal equipment and techniques, this treatment may eventually prove superior.

CONCLUSION

Open ALIF is a safe approach to fuse the lumbar spine, and it has a number of biomechanical advantages compared with posterior approaches. There is limited clinical evidence to suggest better functional outcomes with anterior interbody fusion, but a randomized, prospective study must be carried out to evaluate this accurately. The role of endoscopy will depend on further technical advancements and assessment through valid clinical trials.

REFERENCES

1. Burns BH: An operation for spondylolisthesis. **Lancet** 224:1233, 1933.
2. Calandruccio RA, Benton BF: Anterior lumbar fusion. **Clin Orthop** 35:63–68, 1964.
3. Chen D, Fay L, Lok J, Yuan P, Edwards WT, Yuan HA: Increasing neuroforaminal volume by anterior interbody distraction in degenerative lumbar spine. 20:74–79, 1995.
4. Chow DHK, Luk KDK, Evans JH, Leong JCY: Effects of short anterior lumbar fusion on biomechanics of neighboring unfused segments. **Spine** 21:549–555, 1996.
5. Dennis S, Watkins R, Landaker S, Dillin W, Springer D: Comparison of disc space heights after anterior lumbar interbody fusion. **Spine** 14:876–878, 1989.
6. Esses SI, Doherty BJ, Crawford M, Dreyzin V: Kinematic evaluation of lumbar fusion techniques. **Spine** 21:676–684, 1996.
7. Fujimaki A, Crock HV: The results of 150 anterior lumbar interbody fusion operations performed by two surgeons in Australia. **Clin Orthop** 165:164–167, 1982.

8. Goldner JL, Urbaniak JR, McCollum DE: Anterior disc excision and interbody spinal fusion for chronic low back pain. **Orthop Clin North Am** 2:543–568, 1971.
9. Greenough CG, Peterson MD, Hadlow S, Fraser RD: Instrumented posterolateral lumbar fusion: Results and comparison with anterior interbody fusion. **Spine** 23:479–486, 1998.
10. Kim NH, Lee JW: Anterior interbody fusion versus posterolateral fusion with transpedicular fixation for isthmic spondylolisthesis in adults. **Spine** 24:812–817, 1999.
11. Kumbar A, Kozak JA, Doherty BJ, Dickson JH: Interbody distraction and graft subsidence after anterior lumbar fusion with femoral strut allograft. **Spine** 18:2393–2400, 1993.
12. Lee CK, Langrana NA: Lumbosacral spinal fusion: A biomechanical study. **Spine** 13:357–357, 1984.
13. Luk KDK, Chow DHK, Evans JH, Leons JCY: Lumbar spinal mobility after short anterior interbody fusion. **Spine** 20:813–818, 1995.
14. Papastefanov SL, Stevens K, Mulholland RC: Femoral nerve palsy: An unusual complication of anterior lumbar interbody fusion. **Spine** 19:2842–2847, 1994.
15. Penta M, Fraser RD: Anterior lumbar interbody fusion: A minimum 10 year follow up. **Spine** 22:2429–2434, 1997.
16. Penta M, Sandhu A, Fraser RD: Magnetic resonance imaging assessment of disc degeneration 10 years after anterior lumbar interbody fusion. **Spine** 20:743–747, 1995.
17. Regan JJ, Yuan H, McAfee PC: Laparoscopic fusion of the lumbar spine. Minimally invasive spine surgery. A prospective multicenter study evaluating open and laparoscopic lumbar fusion. **Spine** 24:402–411, 1999.
18. Tencer AF, Hampton D, Eddy S: Biomechanical properties of threaded inserts for lumbar interbody spinal fusion. **Spine** 20:2408–2414, 1995.
19. Tiusanen H, Seitsalo S, Osterman K, Soini J: Anterior interbody lumbar fusion in severe low back pain. **Clin Orthop** 324:153–163, 1996.
20. Weatherley CR, Prickett CF, O'Brien JP: Discogenic pain persisting despite solid posterior fusion. **J Bone Joint Surg Br** 68B:142–143, 1986.
21. Zdeblick TA, Smith GR, Warden KE, McAfee PC: Two point fixation of the lumbar spine: Differential stability in rotation. **Spine** 16[Suppl]:8298–9301, 1991.

CHAPTER

32

Laparoscopic Anterior Lumbar Interbody Fusion

GERALD E. RODTS, JR., M.D., MARK R. MCLAUGHLIN, M.D., JONATHAN ZHANG, M.D., BRIAN R. SUBACH, M.D., REGIS W. HAID, JR., M.D.

The advent of minimally invasive surgery has challenged spine surgeons to refine and to perfect less invasive procedures that have comparable or superior outcomes to standard open techniques. The goals of these procedures are less pain, decreased hospitalization time, and a faster return to functional status. These goals are attained by achieving the same operative result with smaller incisions and reduced tissue dissection. The development and refinement of laparoscopic intraperitoneal surgery has offered spine surgeons new opportunities for anterior approaches to the lumbar spine (26, 30, 33).

Previous reports have documented that anterior lumbar interbody fusions (ALIFs) decrease perioperative blood loss and eliminate nerve root retraction compared with posterior procedures (32). It has also been shown that ALIF procedures have shorter operating times than posterior lumbar interbody fusions with or without pedicle screw instrumentation (24, 25). These advances have led to shorter hospitalization times and comparable fusion rates (23–25).

Currently, the standard approaches for ALIF include transperitoneal or retroperitoneal exposure for interbody fusion at L4–L5 and L5–S1. More cephalad lumbar levels may also be accessible. The development of laparoscopic ALIF has allowed the spine surgeon to place interbody fusion devices with smaller incisions and less bowel irritation and postoperative ileus. Laparoscopic ALIF represents a viable alternative to standard open transperitoneal or retroperitoneal approaches. We review our preliminary experience with laparoscopic ALIF in a series of 32 consecutive patients and describe the lessons learned as this procedure has developed at our institution.

PATIENTS AND METHODS

During a period of 2 years, 32 patients underwent single-level laparoscopic ALIFs at the L4–L5 or L5–S1 interspace. Operative indications included patients with degenerative disc disease characterized by segmental disc degeneration with Modic changes with or without foraminal stenosis demonstrated on magnetic resonance imaging (MRI) with a clinical history of mechanical low back pain with or without leg pain. Other candidates included patients with degenerative lumbar instability, less than grade II spondylolisthesis, postsurgical spinal instability, and pseudoarthrosis after attempted posterior fusions (*Fig. 32.1 and Table 32.1*). All patients had failed conservative therapy, which included any combination of nonsteroidal or narcotic medications, physical therapy, or other local pain procedures. Provocative discography was used only in patients in whom the symptomatic level was in question. In those patients, needles were placed into the disc of interest as well as adjacent disc spaces to serve as a control. Sterile saline solution or contrast material was injected. Discograms were considered positive only if the injection recreated the patient's pain at the appropriate level of interest. Additionally, injection at adjacent levels had to produce either no pain or "discordant" pain. Some patients also underwent diagnostic fact blocks to help confirm the pathological level. Patients with discordant pain dissimilar to the patient's chief complaint in terms of location and intensity were not considered appropriate candidates, did not undergo surgery, and were not included in this analysis. Patients who had evidence of posterior pathology such as a disc fragment within the canal, facet hypertrophy, lateral recess or central spinal stenosis, a history of multiple abdominal procedures, or severe large-vessel atherosclerosis were not considered good candidates for surgery and also were not included in this study (*Table 32.2*).

TECHNIQUE

Positioning

The patient is placed in a supine position on a radiolucent table. Equipment in the room is positioned to allow the surgeon an optimal view of both the C-arm camera and the video monitor (*Fig. 32.2*). Padding is placed under the hips, to ensure normal lumbar lordosis at the lumbosacral junction, and beneath the knees, to prevent hyperextension. Elevating the pelvis also places the patient's arms low enough to prevent interference with the lateral fluoroscopic view (*Fig. 32.3*). Ankle straps are placed on the patient to prevent sliding, because a steep Trendelenburg position is required during the procedure to allow the abdominal viscera to move rostrally out of the pelvis. A nasogastric tube and Foley catheter and are placed to decompress the stomach and bladder respectively. Both catheters are usually removed at the completion of the procedure.

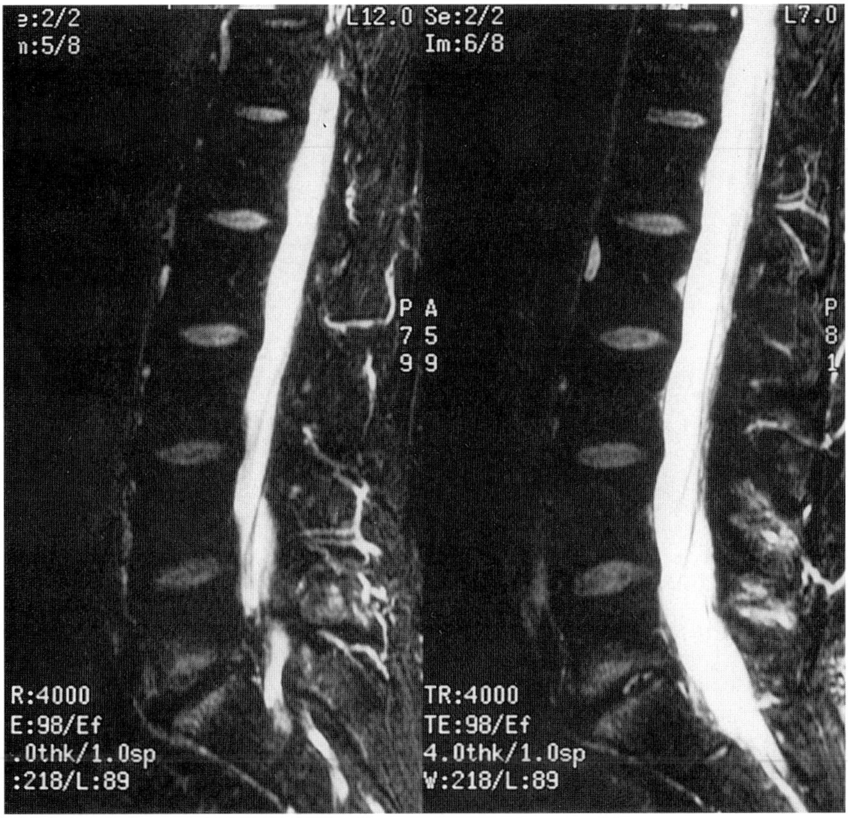

FIG. 32.1 Sagittal MR image with a long repetition time sequence demonstrating a grade I spondylolisthesis with a collapsed disc space in a patient with intractable back pain.

TABLE 32.1
Indications for Laparoscopic ALIF

Degenerative disc disease
Degenerative lumbar instability
Grade 1 or 2 spondylolisthesis
Post surgical spinal instability
Failed posterior fusion

TABLE 32.2
Contraindications for Laparoscopic ALIF

Posterior/Pathology
Multiple abdominal procedures (relative)
Severe atherosclerosis of the aorta and iliac vessels

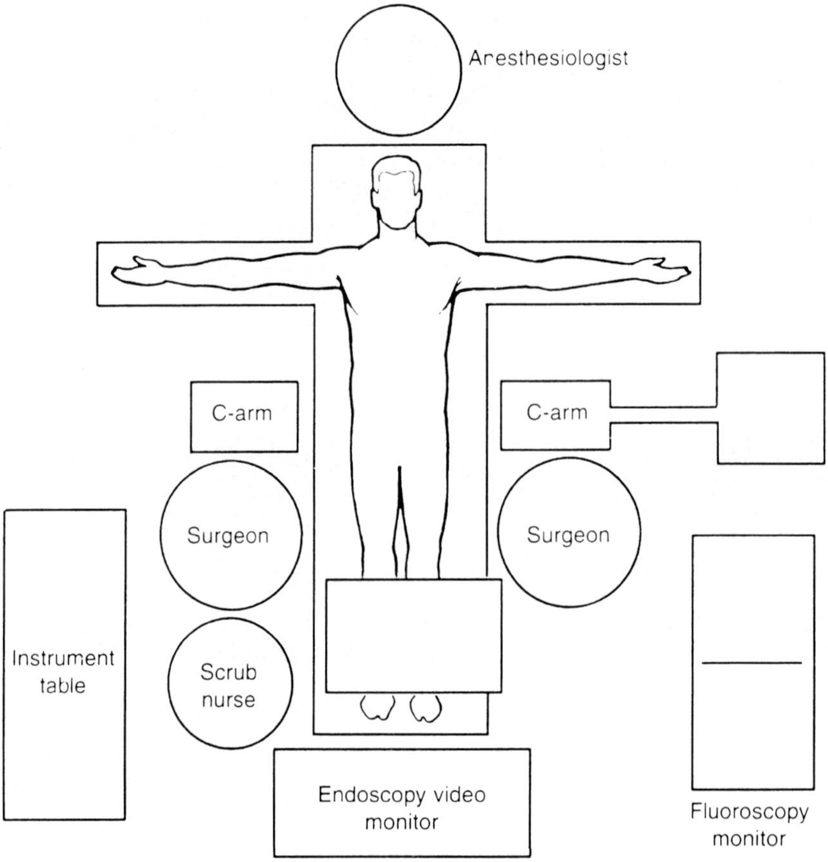

FIG. 32.2 Schematic diagram of the room setup with video-assisted monitors and fluoroscopic equipment with relation to the surgical team.

Technique

Preoperatively, nonsteroidal agents are discontinued at least 1 week before surgery to minimize blood loss and to remove their potential inhibitory effect on bone fusion. The bowel preparation consists of one bottle of magnesium citrate initiated the night before surgery. Consent routinely includes the possibility of an open laparotomy in the event of uncontrolled bleeding or poor visualization, in addition to other potential complications from laparoscopic fusion (*Table 32.3*).

To select implant size, one should examine an adjacent disc space. For most metallic or bone implant systems, a transparent template array is

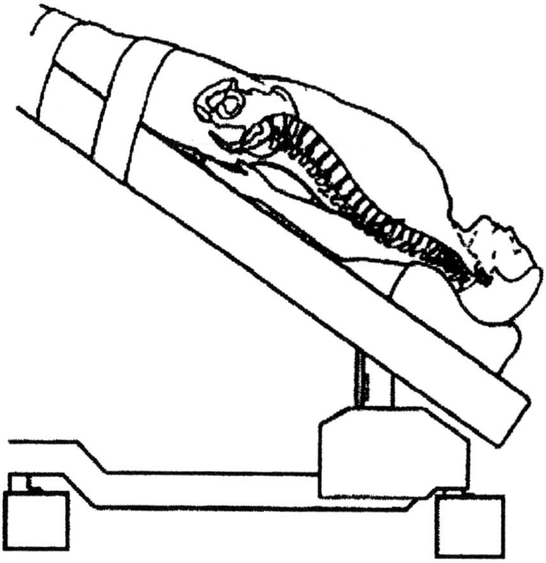

FIG. 32.3 A steep Trendelenburg position causes the abdominal contents to move rostrally out of the pelvis. The arms are tucked under the lumbosacral spine so as not to obscure the fluoroscopic images. A pillow is placed under the knees to prevent hyperextension.

TABLE 32.3
Potential Complications from Laparoscopic ALIF

Major	Minor
Vascular injury	Infection
Deep venous thrombosis	Ileus
Implant migration	Atelectasis
Nerve root contusion	Retrograde ejaculation

available to size the interbody implant. One can anticipate distracting the diseased disc space to approximately the height of an unaffected adjacent segment. A preoperative lateral lumbar radiograph or axial computed tomographic (CT) scan is helpful. MRI is less helpful because this technology subtracts the cortical signal of bone and thus may lead to inaccurate measurements of disc height or the anteroposterior dimensions of the interspace. Selecting the proper size interbody implant is essential. Not only should the implant size approximate the disc height of the adjacent normal interspaces should account for the degree of reaming and tapping into the cortical end plates above and below the disc space.

This allows for the appropriate annular tension to maintain the interbody implant under compression.

The patient is prepped and draped in sterile fashion. Autologous bone is harvested from the anterior iliac crest usually on the right side at the beginning of the procedure. Before insufflation, an incision line is marked that is centered on the midline approximately 1.0 to 3.0 cm wide above the pubis. The fluoroscopic equipment is then brought into place before the incisions are made to verify the midline. It is important to obtain adequate fluoroscopic views for proper intraoperative visualization of the vertebral bodies and to estimate trajectory.

Four incisions are used. The two lower paramedian incisions allow placement of portals for the working forceps (*Fig. 32.4*). The incision for the interbody channel and devices is centered over the midline suprapubic region and measures 2.0 to 4.0 cm in length. The viewing camera

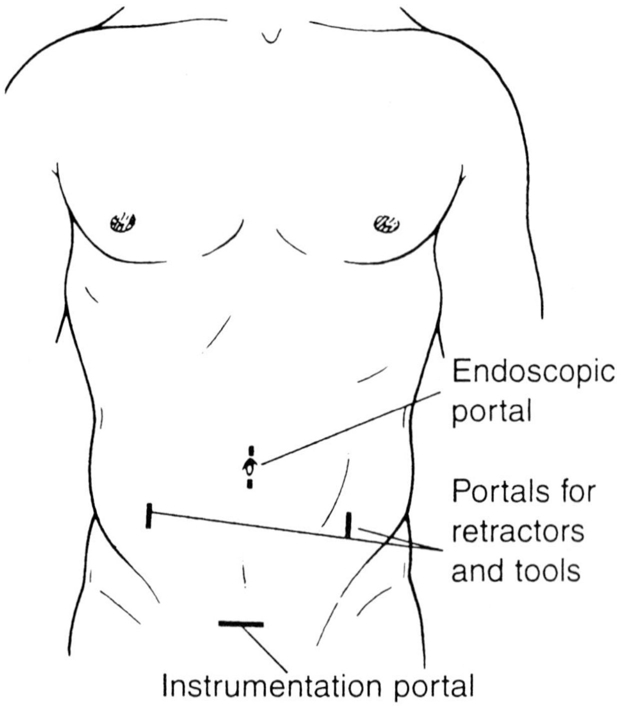

FIG. 32.4 Four incisions are routinely made. Two paramedian incisions provide conduits for the working forceps. The viewing camera is placed through an umbilical incision. The working channel is placed through a midline suprapubic incision measuring 2 to 4 cm in length.

is placed through the curvilinear umbilical incision and is held by a robotic arm (AESOP, Computer Motion, Inc., Goleta, CA). This robotic arm responds to verbal commands from the laparoscopic surgeon and moves the camera to the surgeon's desired position. This allows the surgeon two free hands to place the instrumentation.

As the bone graft is harvested from the iliac crest, the laparoscopic surgeon gains entrance and the abdomen is insufflated. The patient is placed in steep Trendelenburg to mobilize the abdominal contents out of the pelvic inlet. If necessary, the sigmoid colon is tacked to the abdominal wall to gain better exposure.

Adequate disc space exposure is critical. The sacral promontory is identified by palpation and confirmed by fluoroscopy. The peritoneum is then opened sharply. In men, unipolar cautery should be avoided, and a blunt Kittner dissector is used with a gentle sweeping motion to mobilize the presacral sympathetic plexus. This maneuver may decrease the incidence of retrograde ejaculation, a known complication from anterior approaches. In women, monopolar electrocautery can be used to expose the anterior face of the vertebral bodies and disc space.

The first anatomic structure seen is the middle sacral artery and vein (*Fig. 32.5*). Although these vessels do not reliably predict the midline of

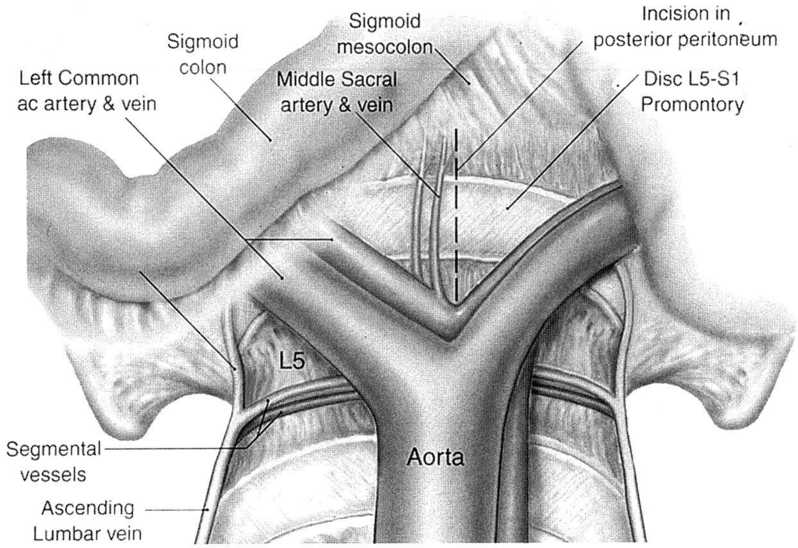

FIG. 32.5 Laparoscopic view of the vascular anatomy of the lower lumbar region. In the artist's depiction the middle sacral artery and vein appear on the midline, however this is not a reliable landmark to determine the midline.

the vertebral body, preoperative MRI may demonstrate their relationship to the midline (10, 16, 27). The preoperative axial images should be reviewed for the presence of eccentric anterior osteophytes, which may give the surgeon a false localization of the lateral convexities. The middle sacral artery and vein are ligated and divided (*Fig. 32.6*). The anterior curvature of the lumbosacral junction is palpated as well as the left and right lateral convexities in conjunction with intermittent fluoroscopy to identify the midline further. The left iliac vein protrudes more anteriorly and may require more retraction. If the midline cannot be identified accurately, the surgeon should consider an open conversion because higher rates of complication are more likely.

After confirmation of the midline, the instrumentation phase can begin (*Fig. 32.7*). Depending on the instrumentation system, the entry sites for the trephines are prepared. Laparoscopic approaches for interbody fusion

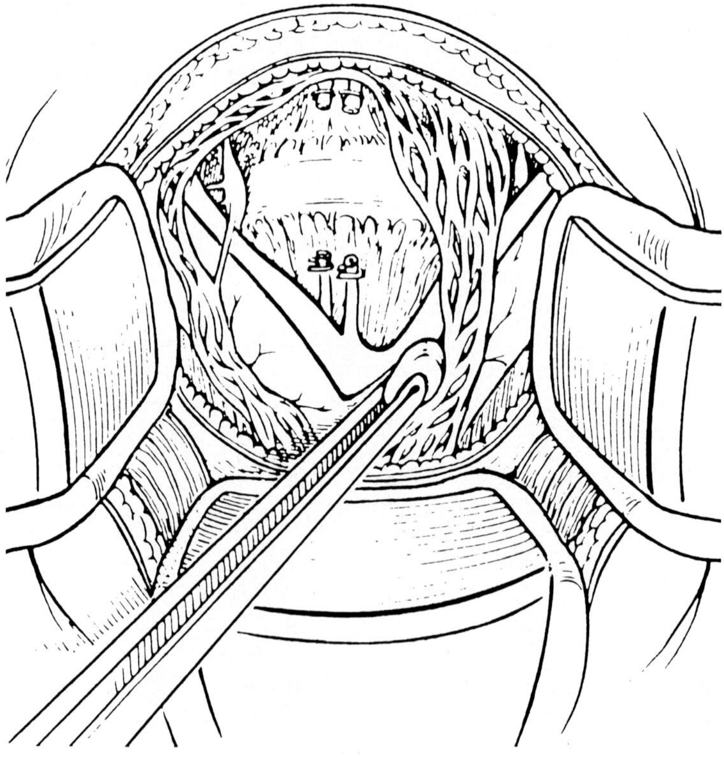

FIG. 32.6 Laparoscopic view of L5–S1 interspace demonstrating clip ligation of middle sacral artery and vein.

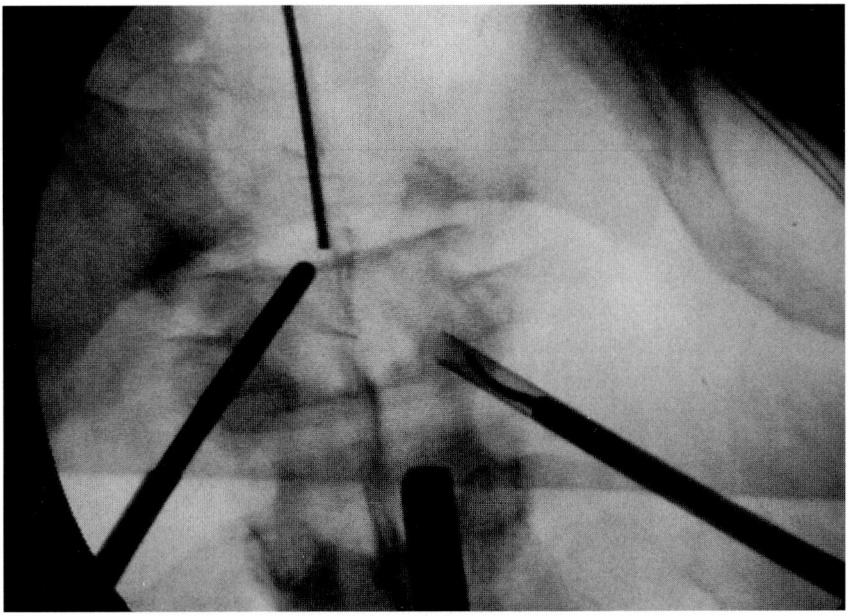

FIG. 32.7 Fluoroscopic view of laparoscopic instruments around the L5–S1 disc space with a K-wire indicating the approximate midline.

may use titanium BAK cages (SpineTech, Minneapolis, MN), allograft bone dowels (Regeneration Technologies, Alachua, FL), or the titanium Interfix cages (Medtronic-Sofamor Danek, Memphis, TN). Lordotic threaded titanium cages (Novus, Medtronic-Sofamor Danek, Memphis, TN) are currently under internal review board evaluation. The trephine is used to core and to remove soft disc material in each paramedian entry site. The trephine should enter the disc space in a trajectory parallel to the end plates to avoid eccentric placement of cages into the vertebral bone. Using the largest trephine possible optimizes maximal disc material removal. Additional disc material is removed with pituitary rongeurs.

Progressively larger distractors are then tamped into the disc space to restore the disc height to the appropriate level and to place tension on the annulus fibrosis (*Fig. 32.8*). When a distractor is in place on one side, the remaining disc material and subjacent cortical bone on the opposite side are removed with a reamer. It is better to ream to a depth longer than the selected interbody implant length to allow placement of additional bone graft anterior to the interbody device and to allow countersinking of the implant if desired. Underreaming may promote

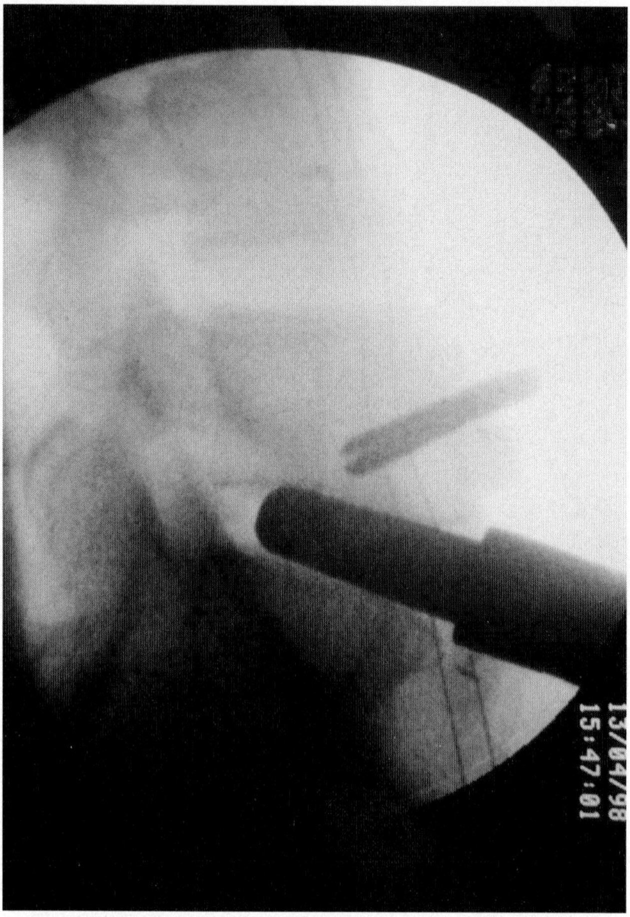

FIG. 32.8 Intraoperative radiograph demonstrating the use of a distractor to increase the disc height and to place tension on the annulus. When the appropriate level of distraction is achieved the graft is placed on the side opposite the distractor.

stripping of the threaded pattern during attempted tapping. This occurs because the tap is prevented from advancing by residual disc material deep in the posterior disc space. The holes are then tapped to the premeasured depth (*Fig. 32.9*). The titanium or bone implant is then inserted in proper alignment (*Fig. 32.10*). Additional bone graft is packed anteriorly and posteriorly to the implant. This promotes additional bone fusion and allows the surgeon to assess better the presence of a solid arthrodesis with anterior bony bridging during postoperative follow-up studies.

The same steps are then repeated on the other side after removing the distractor plug. Ideally, the collapsed disc space should be distracted by the implant to reapproximate its original size.

Anteroposterior and lateral fluoroscopic views are obtained to verify proper positioning of the implants. The peritoneum is closed using clip ligation, and the abdominal wall incisions are closed with interrupted absorbable suture.

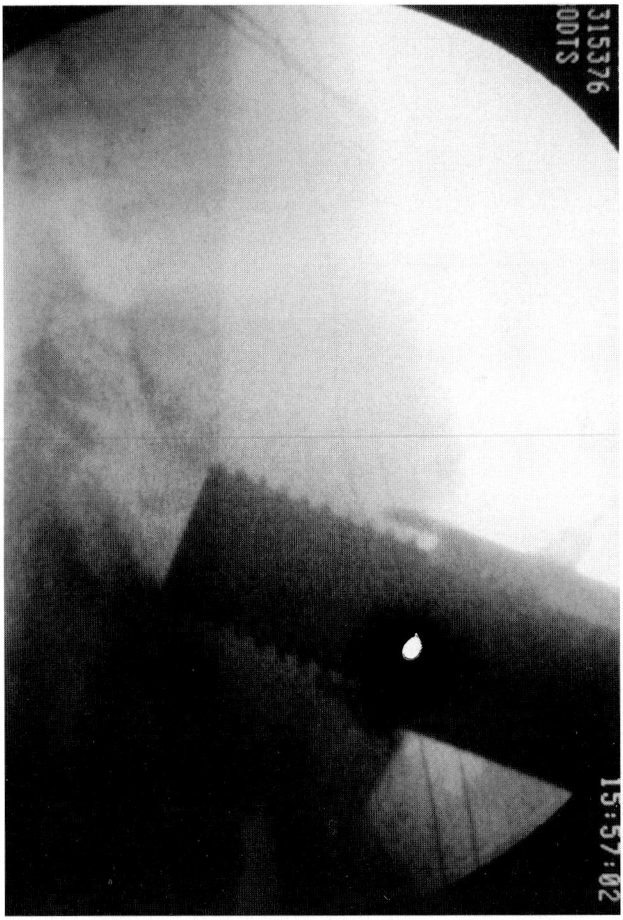

FIG. 32.9 Intraoperative fluoroscopic image showing a tap in the previously reamed trajectory through the disc space. We routinely place additional bone graft anteriorly to promote fusion to allow a better assessment of solid arthrodesis on postoperative studies.

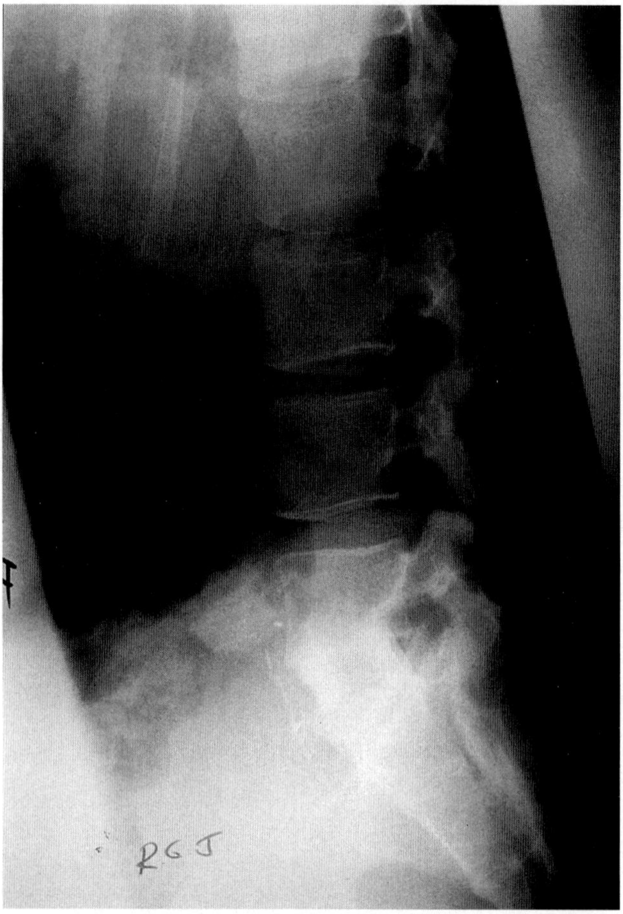

FIG. 32.10 Fluoroscopic image showing threaded allograft cortical bone dowels at the end of the procedure. We routinely place morselized autogenous graft anterior and posterior to the grafts in addition to inside and in between these bone implants.

Postoperative Care

Patients are mobilized early and are allowed to ambulate on postoperative day 1. Diet is advanced as tolerated, provided there are adequate bowel sounds present. A hard or soft lumbar orthosis is used depending on the degree of preoperative instability, the presence of osteoporosis, and the size of the patient. Patients usually are discharged on postoperative day 2. Follow-up radiographs are obtained before discharge, at 6 weeks, at 3 and 9 months, and at 1 and 2 years. Determination of solid arthrodesis can be problematic. A distinction must be made between "stability" versus "arthrodesis." Previously published studies of titanium cages determine "fusion" by absence of lucency around the implant and absence of movement on flexion–extension films (21, 22). Presence of bone within the cage does not necessarily imply sold arthrodesis. Solid bridging bone (between the vertebral end plates) anterior to the cage may signify a solid arthrodesis. We believe evidence of fusion is best demonstrated on reformatted, thin-cut sagittal CT scans, which demonstrate 1) incorporation of cancellous bone within the cage/dowel, 2) a subchondral increase in end plate sclerosis, and 3) a solid arthrodesis in the bone graft placed anterior or posterior to the cage/dowel. With allograft cortical bone dowels, incorporation of the threads can be seen, combined with a progressive diminution in the "halo" seen on the anteroposterior radiographs. An advantage of using bone dowels is a more direct assessment of arthrodesis. Evidence that suggests pseudoarthrosis on plain anteroposterior and lateral radiographs includes lucency around the device, persistent movement at the instrumented level, or lack of a solid bone mass. Movement can be defined by a translational change in position or a change in angulation of the disc space on flexion–extension lateral radiographs.

COMPLICATIONS

In our series of 32 patients there was one disc space infection with a bone dowel that was treated successfully with intravenous antibiotics. Early in the experience we had one nerve root contusion after lateral cut-out of the disc space. This occurred because we had not selected the exact midline properly from the start of the case. Two iliac vein thromboses occurred that required anticoagulation. These thromboses were most likely the result of retraction of the vessels. Three of 15 men reported retrograde ejaculation at their longest follow-up examination. Two other procedures were converted to an open transperitoneal approach for adhesions, and one for better visualization of a spinal deformity. There were no conversions for bleeding.

Other major complications not encountered in our series but that are potential problems in performing this procedure include vascular injury requiring conversion to an open procedure to control bleeding. Minor complications reported in the literature include ileus and retrograde ejaculation. There has been no series reporting problems with impotence or lack of orgasm. We feel it is important to inform the male patient fully preoperatively regarding the risk of retrograde ejaculation.

DISCUSSION

Zucherman et al. (34) were the first to perform the technique of laparoscopic anterior interbody fusion. In their first reported series of 17 patients they had three technical complications, two of which required open conversion to laparotomy secondary to venous bleeding from the middle sacral vein. Subsequently, numerous reports of this technique have been described (1–9, 11–15, 17–20, 28, 29). In a prospective randomized series comparing posterolateral fusion using rigid pedicle screw instrumentation with and without interbody grafting with laparoscopic BAK fusion cages, Zdeblick (31) demonstrated higher fusion rates and shorter hospitalization and return to work. His study confirmed significant cost advantages and outcomes compared with posterior open techniques in patients with L5–S1 disease.

When comparing results relative to interbody fusion it is important to understand the difference between fusion and stability. Fusion is based on the radiographic findings discussed previously, such as increase in subchondral end plate sclerosis, bridging bone incorporating the anterior bone graft, and diminution in the "halo" seen on anteroposterior radiographs. Stability is based on radiographic evidence of nonmovement on flexion–extension roentgenograms. It may be possible to have a stable construct without fusion. Stability rates for threaded interbody cages appear excellent and approach 98% at 3 years in the BAK series. Several large clinical trials have demonstrated marked improvement in pain (10, 21, 22).

CONCLUSIONS

Laparoscopic ALIF is a safe and effective method of placing threaded cylindrical lumbar interbody implants (12, 22, 31, 34). The benefits of this procedure over posterior fusion procedures include the elimination of nerve root retraction and possible dural injury. There is less muscular dissection and thus decreased blood loss and postoperative pain. The drawbacks of the procedure include a steep learning curve and the low but real incidence of retrograde ejaculation. Larger series with long-term follow-up examinations will prove whether one procedure is superior to another or whether they are complementary techniques. Keys to avoiding complications include proper identification of the midline, applying an initial "toe in" force to discourage lateral cut-out, and flexibility to convert to an open approach in the face of inadequate exposure. Laparoscopic fusion with stand-alone interbody devices may have limited success in treating patients with mobile instability and/or high-grade spondylolisthesis. In these cases, supplemental posterior stabilization should be considered.

REFERENCES

1. Arnold W, Gastinger I, Krause W, Schilling HW, Koch A, Grundei H: Endoscopic fusion of the lumbar vertebrae. **Z Chir** 122:1040–1045, 1997.

2. Bhatnagar MK, Mathur SK, Mess CF: Laparoscopic spinal fusion. **Md Med J** 48:161–164, 1999.
3. Boden SD, Martin GJ, Horton WC, Truss TL, Sandhu HS: Laparoscopic anterior spinal arthrodesis with rhBMP-2 in a titanium interbody threaded cage. **J Spinal Disord** 11:95–101, 1998.
4. De Peretti F, Hovorka I, Fabiani P, Argenson C: New possibilities in L2–L5 lumbar arthrodesis using a lateral retroperitoneal approach assisted by laparoscopy: Preliminary results. **Eur Spine J** 5:210–216, 1996.
5. Dickman CA: Internal fixation and fusion of the lumbar spine using threaded interbody cages. **BNI Q** 13:4–25, 1997.
6. Dickman CA, Sonntag VKH, Russell JC: The laparoscopic approach for instrumentation and fusion of the lumbar spine. **BNI Q** 13:26–36, 1997.
7. Heini PF, Krahenbuhl L, Schwarzenbach O, Lottenbach M: Laparoscopic assisted spine surgery. **Dig Surg** 15:185–186, 1998.
8. Henry LG, Cattey RP, Stoll JE, Robbins S: Laparoscopically assisted spinal surgery. **J Soc Laparoendosc Surg** 1:341–344, 1997.
9. Husson JL, Le Huec JC, Trebuchet G, Lesprit E, Bossis JM: Interbody arthrodesis of the lumbar vertebrae using retroperitoneal videoendoscopy. A preliminary study of 38 cases. **Chirurgie** 123:491–499, 1998.
10. Kuslich SD, McAfee PC, Regan JF: Spinal instrumentation, in Regan JF, McAfee PC, Mack MF (eds.): *Atlas of Endoscopic Spine Surgery.* St. Louis, Quality Medical Publishing, 1995, pp 293–331.
11. Lazennec JY, Pouzet B, Ramare S, et al.: Possibilities of anterior approach to the lumbar spine by minimal retroperitoneal access. Anatomical bases. Technical principles and initial results. **Chirurgie** 122:468–477, 1997.
12. Mahvi DM, Zdeblick TA: A prospective study of laparoscopic spinal fusion. Technique and operative complications. **Ann Surg** 224:85–90, 1996.
13. Mathews HH, Evans MT, Molligan HJ, Long BH: Laparoscopic discectomy with anterior lumbar interbody fusion. A preliminary review. **Spine** 20:1797–1802, 1995.
14. McAfee PC, Reagan JJ, Geis WP, Fedder IL: Minimally invasive anterior retroperitoneal approach to the lumbar spine. Emphasis on the lateral BAK. **Spine** 23:1476–1484, 1998.
15. McAfee PC, Regan JR, Zdeblick T, et al.: The incidence of complications in endoscopic anterior thoracolumbar spinal reconstructive surgery. A prospective multicenter study comprising the first 100 consecutive cases. **Spine** 20:1624–1632, 1995.
16. McLaughlin MR, Comey CH, Haid RW, Rodts GE, Erwood SC, Smith CD: Laparoscopic anterior lumbar interbody fusion. **Contemp Neurosurg** 20:1–9, 1998.
17. Nibu K, Panjabi MM, Oxland T, Cholewicki J: Intervertebral disc distraction with a laparoscopic anterior spinal fusion system. **Eur Spine J** 7:142–147, 1998.
18. Ogon M, Maurer H, Wimmer C, Landauer F, Sterzinger W, Krismer M: Minimally invasive approach and surgical procedures in the lumbar spine. **Orthopade** 26:553–561, 1997.
19. Olinger A, Hildebrandt U, Pistorius G, Lindemann W, Menger MD: Laparoscopic 2-level fusion of the lumbar spine with Bagby and Kuslich implants. **Chirurgie** 67:348–350, 1996.
20. Olsen D, McCord D, Law M: Laparoscopic discectomy with anterior interbody fusion of L5–S1. **Surg Endosc** 10:1158–1163, 1996.
21. Ray CD: Threaded fusion cages for lumbar interbody fusions. **Spine** 22:681–685, 1997.
22. Ray CD: Threaded titanium cages for lumbar interbody fusions. **Spine** 22:667–680, 1997.

23. Reagan JJ, McAfee PC, Guyer RD, Aronoff RJ: Laparoscopic fusion of the lumbar spine in a multicenter series of the first 34 consecutive patients. **Surg Laparosc Endosc Percutan Tech** 6:459–468, 1996.
24. Reagan JJ, Yuan H, McAfee PC: Laparoscopic fusion of the lumbar spine: Minimally invasive spine surgery. A prospective multicenter study evaluating open and laparoscopic lumbar fusion. **Spine** 24:402–411, 1999.
25. Regan JJ, Zdeblick T, Zucherman J, et al.: Comparison of open versus laparoscopic fusion of the lumbar spine using the BAK threaded fusion cage. Presented at the 10th annual meeting of the North American Spine Society, Washington, DC, October 18–21, 1995.
26. Riley LH, Eck JC, Yoshida H, et al.: Laparoscopic assisted fusion of the lumbosacral spine. A biomechanical and histologic analysis of the open versus laparoscopic technique in an animal model. **Spine** 22:1407–1412, 1997.
27. Sachs BL, Schwaitzberg SD: Lumbosacral (L5–S1) discectomy and interbody fusion technique, in Regan JF, McAfee PC, Mack MF (eds.): *Atlas of Endoscopic Spine Surgery*. St. Louis, Quality Medical Publishing, 1995, pp 275–291.
28. Scholz–Jager A, Kemen M, Willburger RE, Wittenberg RH, Steffen R, Zumtobel V: Video laparoscopic transperitoneal exposure of the lumbar spine for ventral fusion. **Langenbecks Arch Chir Suppl Kongressbd** 113:956–959, 1996.
29. Silcox DH: Laparoscopic bone dowel fusions of the lumbar spine. **Orthop Clin North Am** 29:655–663, 1998.
30. Weiner BK, Fraser RD: Spine update—lumbar interbody cages. **Spine** 23:634–640, 1998.
31. Zdeblick TA: Laparoscopic spinal fusion. **Orthop Clin North Am** 29:635–645, 1998.
32. Zdeblick TA, Ulschmid S, Dick JC: The surgical treatment of L5–S1 degenerative disc disease. A prospective randomized study. Presented at the 10th annual meeting of the North American Spine Society, Washington, DC, October 18–21, 1995.
33. Zdeblick TA, Warden KE, Zon D, McAfee PC, Abitbol JJ: Anterior spinal fixators: A biomechanical in vitro study. **Spine** 18:513–517, 1993.
34. Zucherman JF, Zdeblick TA, Bailey SA, Mahvi D, Hsu KY, Kohrs D: Instrumented laparoscopic spinal fusion: Preliminary results. **Spine** 20:2029–2035, 1995.

CHAPTER

33

The Biomechanics of Interbody Fusion and the Shortcomings of Lumbar Fusion with Cages and Interbody Bone Dowels

EDWARD C. BENZEL, M.D., F.A.C.S., JORGE J. LASTRA, M.D., IAIN KALFAS, M.D., F.A.C.S., KOANG HUM BAK, M.D., PH.D., LISA A. FERRARA, M.S.

Low back pain is a major cause of disability (17, 42). It is often treated nonoperatively, whereas surgical intervention may provide clinical success in selected patients. The appropriate selection of patients and operative management strategies is critical. Because failed lumbar spinal surgeries are common, the development of effective strategies to minimize the incidence of these failures is clearly needed.

A lumbar interbody fusion is a common treatment alternative for selected cases of low back pain. The use of spinal instrumentation has improved fusion rates, compared with bone graft alone (as low as 46%) (43), but many problems still exist.

Spinal segmental motion is complex. It involves bidirectional motion (axial, rotational, and translational) along or about three axes that represent the displacement of each vertebra relative to its adjacent neighbor in three-dimensional space, as portrayed via the three axes of the Cartesian coordinate system (*Fig. 33.1*) (31, 39). The lumbar spine must bear substantial complex (axial, torsional, and translational) loads that are applied along or about these axes. It is nearly impossible to eliminate segmental micromotion in all three of these planes via dorsal fusion. Lumbar interbody fusion addresses this problem more directly and is, therefore, often the preferred surgical technique to eliminate multidirectional segmental micromotion.

Interbody fusion provides significant theoretical, clinical, and biomechanical advantages over dorsal onlay grafting techniques (10, 12). These include 1) reduced rate of nonunion, 2) an accelerated rate of fusion, 3) increased axial load-bearing capacity, and 4) the provision of an alternative strategy when the dorsal elements have been destroyed (31, 39, 40). It must be remembered, however, that interbody fusion is not without its own set of problems and risks.

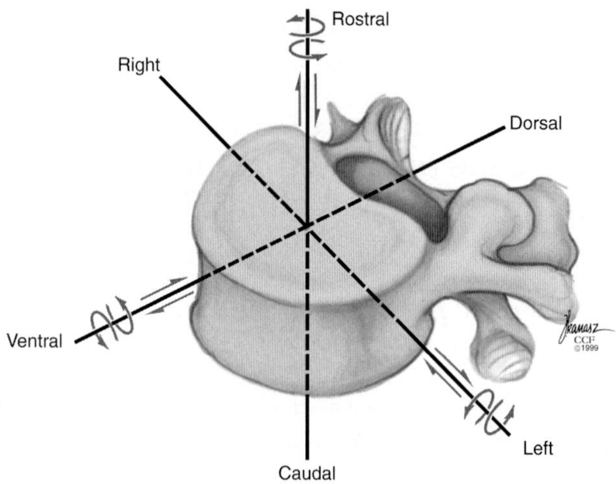

FIG. 33.1 The motion of the lumbar spine as it occurs in a three-dimensional space. The motion is triplanar and rotates along or about the three axes of the spine, as portrayed by the Cartesian coordinate system. The three planes of bidirectional motion are axial, rotational, and translational.

LUMBAR FUSION

Lateral Intertransverse Fusion

Lateral intertransverse fusion is commonly enhanced with pedicle screw fixation. High fusion rates have been achieved with this strategy, often at the expense of an increased risk of complications. Clinically significant lateral soft-tissue injury often results from this approach. In addition, the fusion site is at a significant distance from the instantaneous axis of rotation (IAR) (*Fig. 33.2*). The IAR is the axis about which a vertebral segment rotates. This long moment arm allows for axial loads to cause significant spinal distortion and possibly the failure of spinal fusion. Also, the bone grafts do not "see" significant bone-healing-enhancing stresses (Wolff's Law) (39).

Posterior Lumbar Interbody Fusion (PLIF)

PLIF was popularized as a surgical technique for spinal stabilization in the 1950s by Cloward (15). Although it provides a mechanically favorable fusion with a high rate of arthrodesis, meticulous end plate and graft preparation must be achieved to increase the surface area of contact between the bone graft and the end plate, and to eliminate micromotion across the disc space.

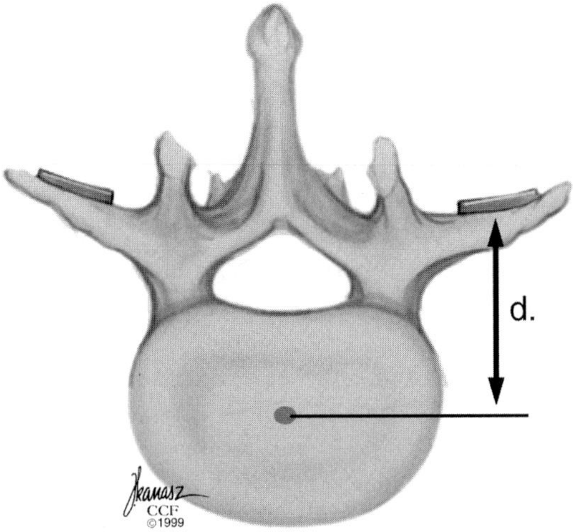

FIG. 33.2 A lateral intertransverse fusion is positioned at a significant distance (*d*) from the IAR (*dot*).

Some researchers have suggested that PLIF, enhanced with dorsal fixation devices such as pedicle screws and plates, adequately reduces spinal deformation and instability while maintaining anatomic alignment of the motion segments (10, 16, 24). Others have raised concerns that combining PLIF with dorsal plate and screw fixation may result in stress-shielding properties that influence fusion rate adversely (6).

The use of pedicle fixation strategies has not eliminated the need for load-bearing support in the anterior column of the spine (10). This underscores the need, in some cases, for interbody fusion. However, the traditional PLIF technique is associated with "complications" that can result in pseudoarthrosis, including excessive epidural bleeding, inadequate graft shaping, graft retropulsion, insufficient donor bone volume, and graft failure resulting from fracture (10).

Anterior Lumbar Interbody Fusion (ALIF)

ALIF has gained in popularity because of the increased interest in minimally invasive surgical approaches to spinal stabilization and the concern associated with PLIF-related morbidity. Decreased surgical morbidity, decreased patient rehabilitation time, and economic factors have heightened interest in minimally invasive approaches to the spine. Although the advantages of ALIF include maximum exposure for visualization of the disc space, resulting in a safe placement of the bone graft without compromising dorsal paraspinous musculature, the disadvantages are as significant as those of the dorsal approach. They include venous and arterial thrombosis, hemorrhage, retrograde ejaculation, impotence, and death (22). Furthermore, ALIFs are commonly augmented with dorsal spinal instrumentation (25, 29), thus incurring the additional risks for stabilization surgery.

INTERBODY STRUTS

An interbody strut is a structure placed between two vertebral bodies for the purpose of functioning as a spacer. It usually becomes an integral part of the fusion mass. A strut may be a bone graft or a cage filled with bone. Cages are of two types, based on the nature of the surface presented to the graft bed—flat and round faced. Flat-faced cages present a flat surface to the graft bed, and round-faced cages present a round surface to the graft bed. The graft bed is composed of either an end plate or vertebral body cancellous bone.

Various interbody strut strategies have been developed and are currently used to support an unstable spinal segment. These include tricortical bone grafts, rectangular and cylindrical bone grafts, bone dowels, threaded bone dowels, carbon fiber implants, and threaded interbody fusion cages (TIFCs) (1, 11, 13, 21, 31, 33).

Once the strut is in place, there are several biomechanical phases of bone healing, remodeling, and revascularization that transpire (39). Autologous cancellous bone is rich in osteogenic substrates, but lacks substantial mechanical strength and exhibits a low resistance to axial loading. Therefore, it is essential that the insertion of this graft type be associated with distraction of the interdiscal space and some means of structural support to counteract high axial loads until it remodels. This may be accomplished by using a hard outer shell (surrounding the cancellous bone), such as cortical bone, a metal shell, or other materials such as carbon fiber that will adequately resist axial loads and, to a lesser extent, the rotational and translational forces impinging on the spinal segment in question.

Tricortical, Rectangular, and Cylindrical Bone Struts

Tricortical struts place cancellous bone in direct contact with the vertebral end plates for revascularization and the incorporation of bone within the interstitial spaces of the trabeculae. This cancellous bone is surrounded by a cortical shell along three sides of the graft for structural support (31, 40). This graft type has several biomechanical advantages if the vertebral end plates remain intact. The graft restores disc height and alleviates foraminal stenosis, while preventing posterior longitudinal ligament invagination (39). Disadvantages of this graft type include graft extrusion if the recipient bed is insufficiently prepared or if a trough is not used to prevent extrusion of the graft (39). A trough increases the risk of subsidence. This type of graft is better suited to end plate geometry than cylindrical spacers. It can be shaped to restore the natural lordosis of the spinal segment.

Rectangular and cylindrical struts, usually allograft cortical bone spacers, are often used in conjunction with morselized autograft. In addition to strut geometry and bone type, these bone struts (tricortical, rectangular, and cylindrical) differ from bone dowels and TIFCs via the lack of a requirement for significant disc distraction to achieve success (see the discussion of restoration and maintenance of disc height).

Bone Dowels

Bone dowels are susceptible to the potential for extrusion and collapse because of the lordotic contoured shape of the intervertebral disc space, and the nonuniform contact between the implant and the vertebral end plates (*Fig. 33.3*) (21, 31). This nonuniformity is amplified with flexion and extension motions. In this regard, they are associated with many of the same problems as metallic TIFCs (see the discussion of TIFCs).

Threaded allograft cortical bone dowels are implanted similarly to metallic TIFCs. Biomechanical studies have demonstrated that dowels can bear an average compressive load of approximately 25 kN under static loading (21). This load exceeds physiological loads considerably,

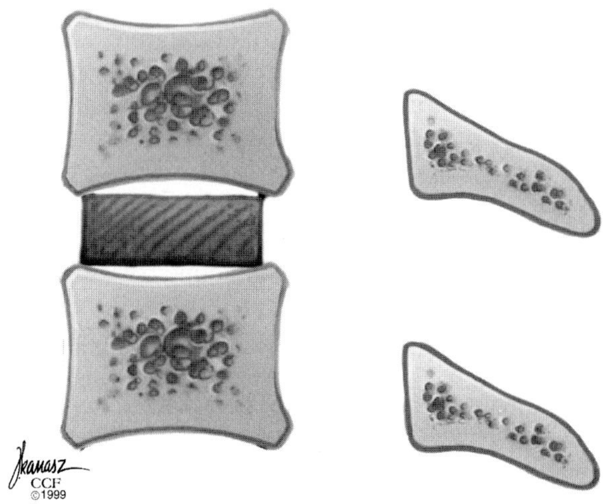

FIG. 33.3 Nonuniform contact between a strut and the elliptical-shaped vertebral end plates.

which range from 1 kN when standing to 10 kN when lifting heavy objects (2, 21). These data indicate that the threaded cortical bone dowels theoretically meet the biomechanical and physiological needs of interbody fusion (21). However, they may not meet the geometrical needs of interbody fusion, as already discussed. On a positive note, the modulus of elasticity of the bone dowels closely matches that of the spine (a physiological need) (35). Bone dowels, however, fail at a greater compressive strength than vertebral bone. Therefore, failure by fracturing through the end plates is possible (6). If failure occurs, bone dowels are easily retrievable. They can be removed in a piecemeal fashion without causing significant local damage. This is unlike the situation associated with TIFCs. With respect to fixation supplementation, this type of interbody fusion, without dorsal instrumentation augmentation, was shown to restore stability except in axial rotation (35).

Carbon Fiber Implants

Alternative biomaterials have been used to construct cages that house autologous or allograft donor bone. One material, a carbon fiber-reinforced polymer, has been used as a cage-like implant with ridges or teeth to resist extrusion (11). Carbon fiber cage implants can withstand physiological loading. Carbon fiber has a modulus of elasticity that approximates that of cortical bone (11). The radiolucency of carbon fiber simplifies the postoperative evaluation of fusion status. Pitfalls associated with this material include 1) the release of the carbon fibers, causing biological reactions in living tissues; 2) fiber brittleness, resulting in breakage; and 3) overt failure (38). To alleviate free fiber release, the fibers are commonly embedded in a composite material such as a polyetherketone. However, minor foreign body reactions have been observed with this modification as well (38). Fortunately, breakage and overt failure is rare.

Threaded Interbody Fusion Cages

Interbody fusion cages have been developed with the aim of overcoming the problems of graft collapse, graft retropulsion, intersegmental micromotion, and eventual pseudarthroses (8, 26, 30, 32, 37, 38). Theoretical advantages of TIFCs are to provide immediate stability, withstand applied axial loads, and reduce segmental motion, translation, and rotation. This should lead to a solid arthrodesis and should correct the existing mechanical deformation (32, 38). Cages are generally constructed from a titanium alloy or surgical-grade stainless steel.

The concept of TIFCs originated in the 1980s (4, 22, 23). They were initially designed for the cervical spine of horses with Wobbler syndrome—a chronic subluxation disorder of the vertebrae. However, they were subsequently applied to lumbar interbody fusion in humans (31, 32, 38). TIFCs are threaded to prevent migration. Holes in the cages allow for bony ingrowth, and theoretically block remnant disc tissue ingrowth. Each cage is packed with morselized autologous bone. Cages have varying pore sizes and alignments. This theoretically affects bone growth into the cage. TIFCs expose intracage bone to the end plate. However, the percentage of surface area of contact of this bone to the end plate ranges from only 4 to 10% of the overall end plate cross sectional surface area. Accurate placement of the holes with respect to the vertebral end plates is crucial for successful bony ingrowth. The high compressive strength of titanium cages shield the bone inside from the mechanical loads (5, 12, 30, 38). However, Bourn et al. (9) demonstrated that cyclical axial loading generates hydrostatic forces within these cages, and hence stimulates bony ingrowth through the cage. The bone generated, however, is woven bone that is not of high quality.

Optimal sizing is important to achieve adequate stabilization (18). If a TIFC is undersize, the segmental stiffness is not increased and the restoration of disc height is not achieved. If the cage is oversize, it will bite into the end plates excessively. An oversize cage inserted dorsally also compromises the posterior spinal structures and may decrease stability because of significant disruption of the facet joints and dorsal ligamentous structures (18). *Figure 33.4* portrays the width of exposure required for TIFC insertion. This is often excessive, necessitating complete facet joint disruption. Excessive distraction of the ligamentous structures may also contribute to postoperative pain.

Placement of a cylindrical device into the disc interspace can alter the trapezoidal relationship of the end plates (e.g., making them parallel), with the loss of lumbar lordosis and sagittal balance. This may be a source of persistent back pain resulting from the loss of sagittal balance (see the discussion of cage geometry and postoperative angular deformation).

Other Techniques

Hybrid devices are rapidly emerging. Hopefully, they will provide advantages over existing techniques.

THE CONSTRUCTION OF AN INTERBODY FUSION: BIOMECHANICAL PRINCIPLES AND CONSIDERATIONS

The modern-day spine surgeon has access to a variety of interbody grafts and devices, including cages. The clinical decision-making process is, therefore, obligatorily complex. It is important to consider multiple variables when designing an interbody fusion construct including 1)

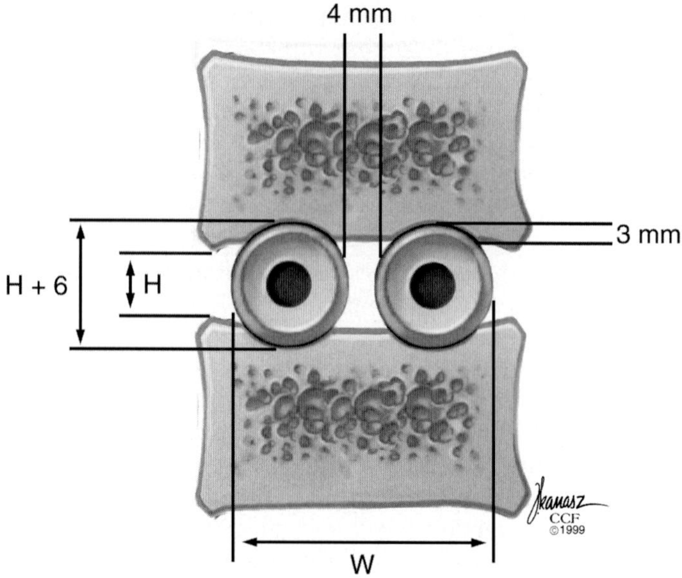

FIG. 33.4 In order for TIFCs to achieve the desired disc interspace height distraction, excessive resection of the dorsal elements is required. The width (*W*) necessary to achieve this interspace distraction is $2(H + 6 \text{ mm}) + 4 \text{ mm} = 2H + 16$ mm. *H* is the desired interspace distraction height. A penetration of 3 mm of the implant in the end plate and a distance of 4 mm between implants is assumed.

shear and axial forces at the disc interspaces; 2) strut location; 3) graft bed preparation; 4) strut preparation, geometry, and surface of contact; 5) strut integrity; 6) load sharing versus load bearing; 7) cage geometry and its relationship with end plate geometry; 8) ligamentous disruption with interbody strut insertion; 9) restoration and maintenance of disc height; 10) subsidence; and 11) postoperative angular deformation. Each variable is considered separately.

Shear and Axial Forces at the Disc Interspaces

The lumbar disc interspaces are not oriented parallel to the floor in the erect human spine. The greatest interspace angle is at the L5–S1 disc interspace. This orientation increases the shear forces imposed at the low lumbar segmental levels because of the resultant force vectors created (*Fig. 33.5*). It is imperative that one remembers that axial loads are desirable (by promoting fusion), whereas nonaxial loads are not desirable with respect to interbody struts and the acquisition of a solid

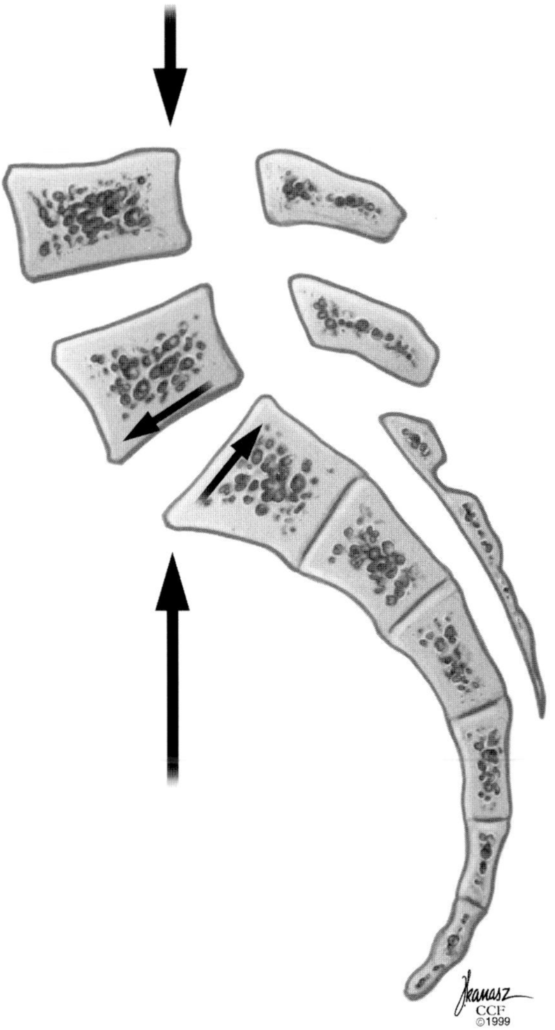

FIG. 33.5 The angular orientation of the lumbosacral disc interspace causes axial loads (*vertical arrows*) to be converted to translational loads (***diagonal arrows***).

arthrodesis. If not respected and controlled, these nonaxial forces contribute pathologically to the high failure rate associated with noninstrumented interbody lumbar and lumbosacral fusions.

TIFCs essentially function as interference screws (*Fig. 33.6A*). In this regard, theoretically they should resist translation (*Fig. 33.6B*). However, they are often ineffective in this regard (*Fig. 33.6C*).

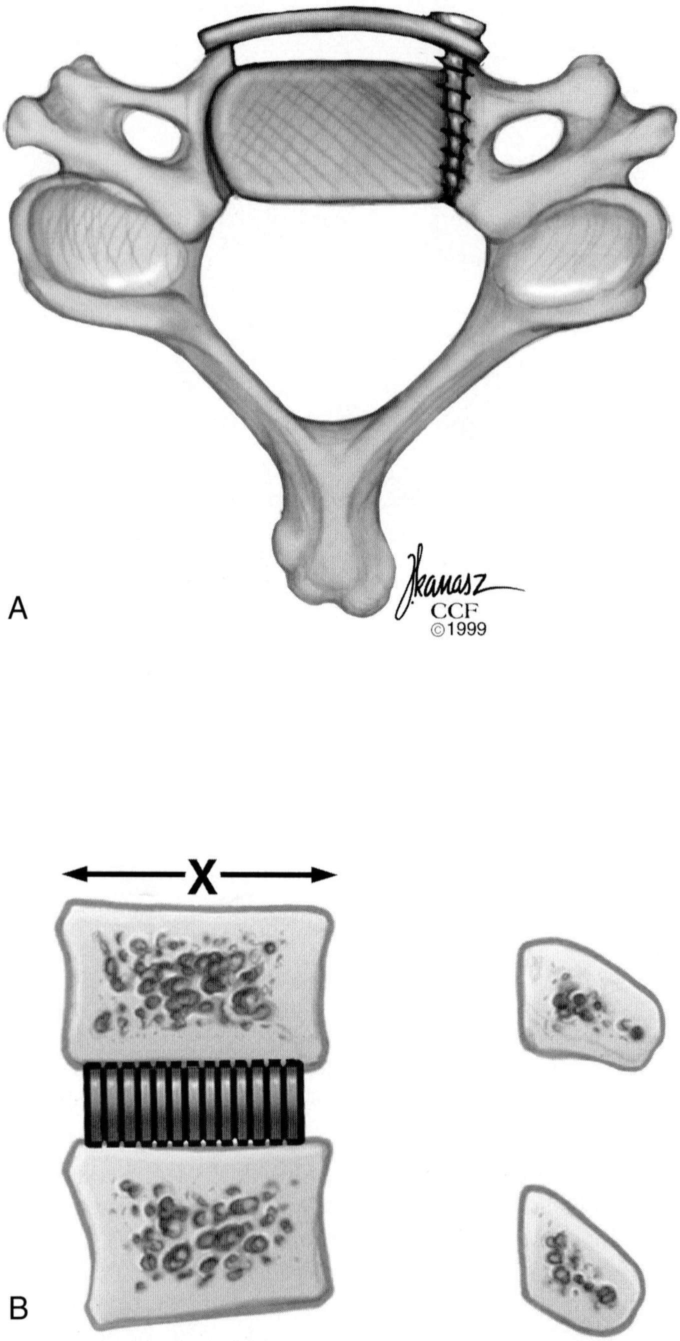
A
CCF
©1999
X
B

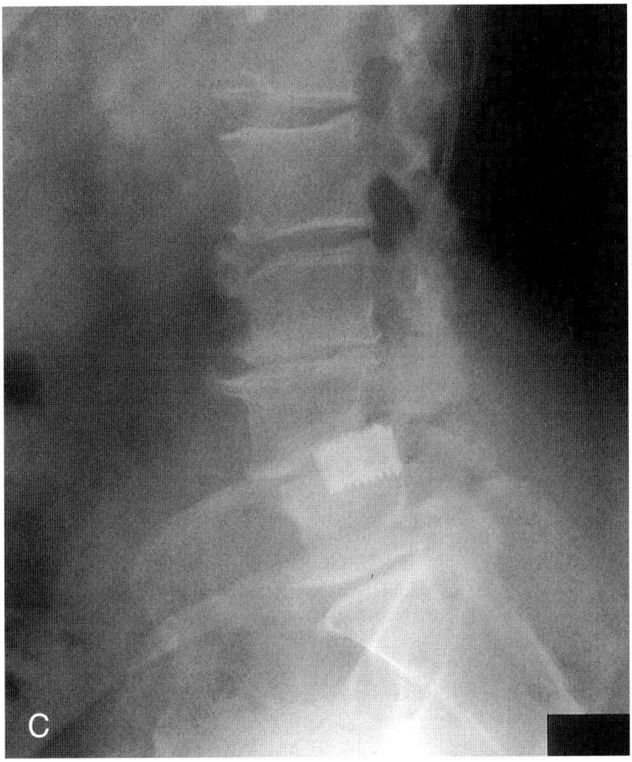

FIG. 33.6 (*A–C*) TIFCs function theoretically as interference screws, as depicted in a cervical spine example (*A*), resisting translation (*B*). (*C*) However, they are often ineffective in this regard, as seen in this lumbar plain radiograph .

Strut Location

The positioning of interbody struts should be accomplished with sagittal, coronal, and axial mechanical loads and while bearing related principles in mind (39). The IAR is a dynamic axis that changes with the mechanical loading of the spine. It describes the axis about which a motion segment rotates. The closer a strut is positioned relative to the IAR, the greater the ability of the strut to resist axial loads. This increases its ability to resist micromotion across the intervertebral segment, decreases sagittal plane motion, and increases spinal column support (*Fig. 33.7*) (6). Conversely, if the fusion site is located at a significant distance from the IAR (a dorsal onlay fusion), the moment arm created by this location will resist angular deformation. In other words, axial load bearing by the fusion mass is poor, but its ability to

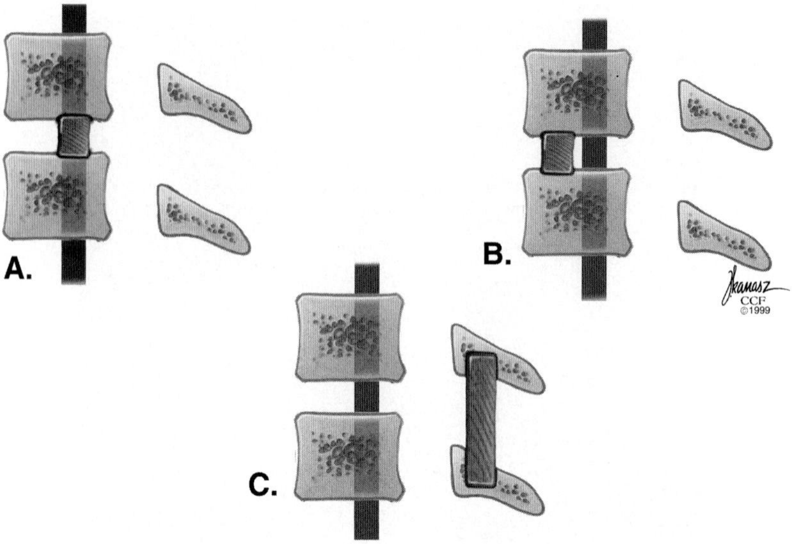

FIG. 33.7 (*A–C*) Bone graft placement close to the original IAR (depicted here by the shaded column that defines the vertical axis, which is the column in the region of the IARs) increases the resistance of applied axial loads (*A*), whereas a graft placed slightly ventral to the IAR resists angular motion (flexion) better (*B*). (*C*) Angular motion resistance is amplified even further with dorsal onlay fusion, when the bone graft is situated at a significant distance from the original IAR. In the lumbar spine, where these axial loads are significant and sagittal plane motion is small, placement of the graft close to the IAR is usually optimal.

resist angular deformation (e.g., flexion) is great. As shown in *Figure 33.8A,* if a force is applied to the lumbar spine along a moment arm, the dynamic nature of the IAR causes it to move, in this case, dorsally. The converse is also true if an interbody fusion mass is placed at a significant distance from the original IAR. The IAR moves toward (or to) the location of the fusion if a solid arthrodesis is achieved (*Fig. 33.8, B and C*). For this reason, it is prudent to place the interbody strut as close as possible to the IAR (*Figs. 33.7 and 33.8*) (6).

An interbody strut should not necessarily be placed ventral to the IAR in the mid to low lumbar spine to resist kyphosis because of the lordotic curvature and the strong intervertebral ligamentous attachments in this region (6, 19). However, this is not true for the cervical spine (despite its lordotic curvature) and the thoracic region. The cervical spine has a greater range of motion than the lumbar spine, whereas the kyphotic curvature of the thoracic spine predisposes it to angular deformation (greater kyphosis). An interbody strut placed slightly ventral to the IAR increases resistance to kyphosis.

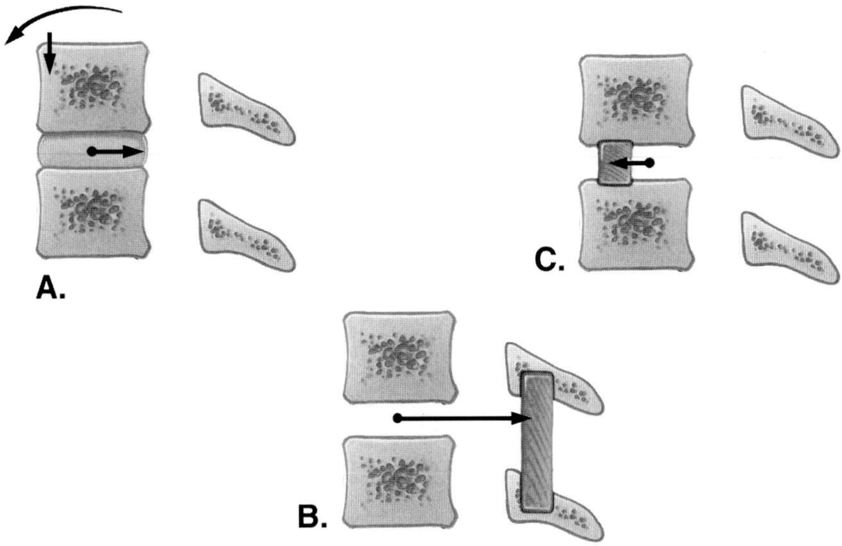

FIG. 33.8 Depiction of the IAR (*dots*). (*A*) Its dynamic nature shows a dorsal shift when the spine is loaded axially and a bending moment is applied. (*B, C*) A solid fusion causes the IAR to move toward the fusion mass.

Graft Bed Preparation

Meticulous preparation of the strut and the graft bed is imperative. Overly aggressive end plate debridement may result in end plate fracture and a loss of load-bearing capacity. Unfortunately, the cancellous bone of the vertebral body functions poorly as a deterrent to subsidence and translation (*Fig. 33.9A*). However, deep mortises created in the vertebral bodies that encompass the strut can help secure the strut to the graft bed, and may also provide some translational resistance (*Fig. 33.9B*). Otherwise, interbody struts by themselves provide little translational resistance (*Fig. 33.9C*). On the other hand, an insufficient debridement of the end plates (inadequate exposure of fresh cancellous bone) may result in inadequate graft bed preparation and pseudoarthrosis.

Strut Preparation, Geometry, and Surface Area of Contact

The capacity to resist axial loads and to minimize micromotion via an interbody fusion is proportional to the surface area of contact between the strut and the graft bed. Thus, the larger the surface area of contact, the more effectively the strut resists axial loads and micromotions in all planes.

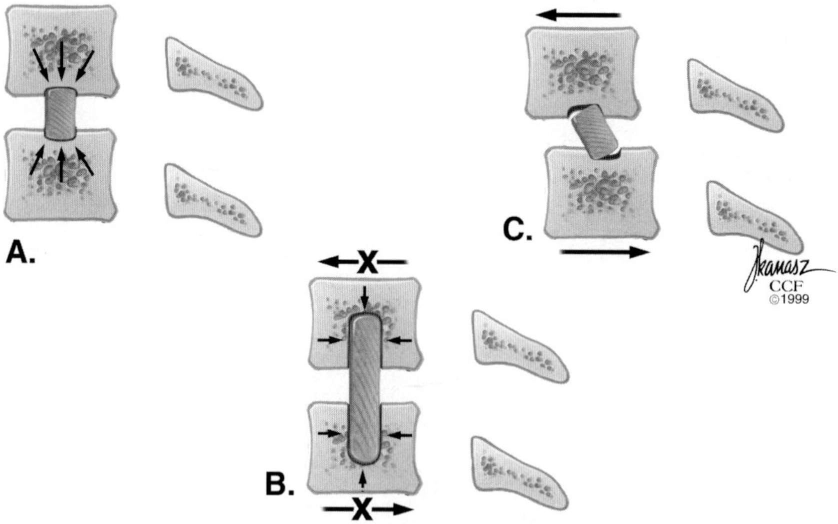

FIG. 33.9 Graft bed preparation. (*A*) Cancellous bone of the vertebral body functions poorly as a deterrent to subsidence. (*B*) Deep mortises encompass a greater bone graft surface area and have a higher ability to oppose graft translation and extrusion. (*C*) Shallow strut placement into the vertebral bodies does not resist translation effectively. The advantages of deep mortises must be compared and contrasted with the disadvantages (e.g., excessive subsidence).

The geometry of an ideal strut should be of appropriate size compared with the graft bed, and should mimic the contour of the two graft beds. Humans have a greater lordosis than quadrupeds and other primates that are only part-time bipeds. This results in a wedge-shaped lumbar intervertebral disc space, particularly in the lumbosacral area (*Fig. 33.10*) (6, 7, 28). This configuration produces a "fish-mouth"-shaped interspace. Keeping this in mind, one should select or prepare a trapezoidal strut that mimics the contour of the lumbar intervertebral disc space, and at the same time increases the surface area of contact between the strut and the graft beds.

Strut Integrity

Strut integrity is essential to minimize "pistoning," collapse, dislodgment, and strut fracture. Strut integrity and the patient's vertebra should be comparable regarding the modulus of elasticity. The modulus of elasticity characterizes the mechanical nature of the material. It is defined as the ratio of stress to strain—the higher the value, the stiffer the material. The elastic modulus is different for each type of strut and

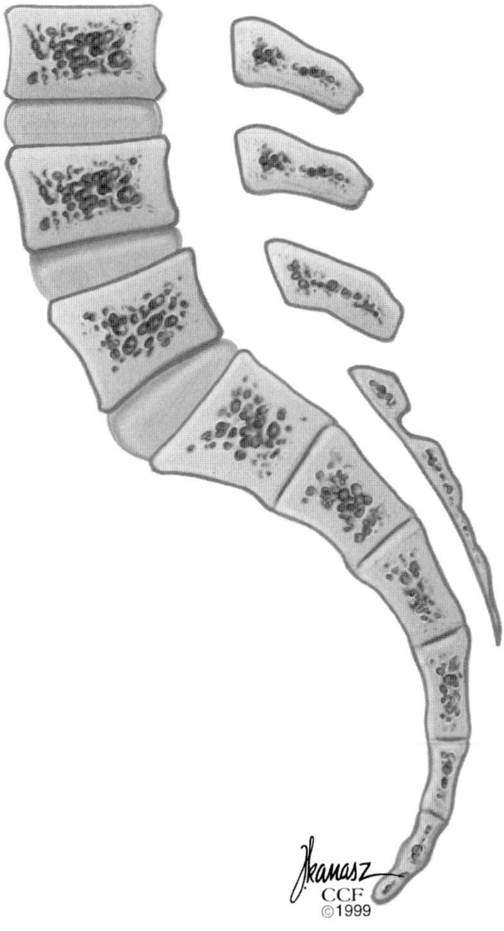

FIG. 33.10 The wedge shape of the intervertebral disc space at L5–S1 dictates the biomechanical behavior of the strut and its ultimate success. If the strut does not conform geometrically, failure is likely.

graft bed (metal cage > carbon fiber cage > cortical bone > cancellous bone > end plate > vertebral body cancellous bone). The quality of the strut and the vertebrae should be assessed before surgery. This can be accomplished in a relatively rudimentary manner by assessing preoperative radiographs of the patient's spine and the mechanical characteristics of the strut, which are usually known.

Pistoning of the strut through the vertebral end plates into the cancellous bone of the vertebrae, or graft collapse is associated with an incompatible modulus of elasticity between the strut and vertebrae, among other variables (*Fig. 33.11, A and B*). In *Figure 33.11,* the strut has a greater stiffness (greater modulus of elasticity) than the vertebral end plates, thereby encouraging the pistoning of the strut through the end plates, and into the cancellous bone of the vertebral body. Furthermore, if a strut has a small surface area of contact, pistoning is also encouraged (*Fig. 33.11C*).

A strut that has a lower modulus of elasticity than the vertebral bodies is at greater risk for fracture and reabsorption. The high axial loads of the intervertebral disc space range from 1000 to 5300 N (40). A weak bone graft will not be able to resist such loads adequately. Eventually, the construct will fail, most often by fracture, collapse, or subsidence.

Load Sharing versus Load Bearing

Load sharing implies that the implant (strut) shares a portion of the construct's load with another implant and/or the spine itself. *Load bearing* implies that the implant (strut) "bears" the entire load.

Per Wolff's Law, bone is formed where stresses are present (for both tensile and compressive forces), and is absorbed where such stresses

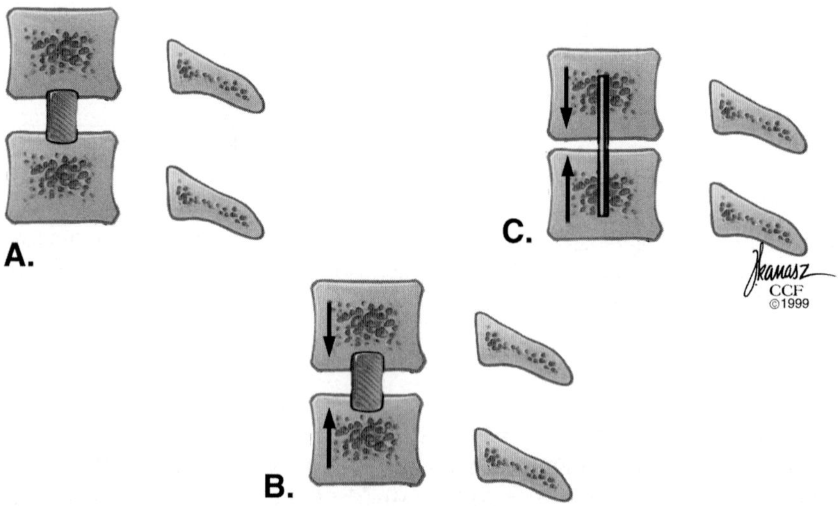

FIG. 33.11 A mismatching of bone integrity between the vertebra and the bone strut. (*A, B*) A denser strut will "piston" through the softer end plate and vertebra. (*C*) If a strut has a small surface area of contact, pistoning is also encouraged.

are not (39). This suggests that pure axial loading promotes bone growth, hence fusion. In this regard, the central region of a healthy, intact intervertebral disc (nucleus pulposus) is exposed to the highest compressive loads. However, in the degenerated state, these stresses are distributed uniformly across the disc space (40). Similarly, an interbody fusion, without dorsal instrumentation, bears the majority of the axial load uniformly across the graft. This enhances the chance of attaining a solid arthrodesis (34). However, if the loading pattern is a combination of axial, shear, and rotational stresses, the fusion process may be impeded. Therefore, strategies that can impede these nonaxial forces may be of benefit.

The addition of dorsal instrumentation is often used to reduce the aforementioned "micromotions." However, a rigid spinal implant "competes" for the axial loads "seen" by the bone graft. Dorsal instrumentation can share axial loads with an interbody strut, thus reducing the stress applied to the interbody strut and strengthening the construct as a whole (39). However, an excessively rigid dorsal fixator may lead to a stress shielding of the bone graft, and ultimately to a pseudoarthrosis (10, 12, 35). In the latter case, the implant only bears loads, whereas the aforementioned strut "sees" less stress (load sharing).

An optimal window of strain (motion) must be maintained for a successful fusion when a combination of spinal implant and bone graft is employed. Too little strain may result in the stress shielding of the bone graft from bone-healing-enhancing forces by the implant. Excessive motion or strain may result in a pseudoarthrosis.

Cage Geometry and Its Relationship to End Plate Geometry

As previously stated, cages can be grouped into two fundamental categories based on the manner in which they interface with the graft bed—flat- or round-faced cages. Flat-faced cages can be square, rectangular, round, or oval. They present a relatively large surface area of contact with the graft bed (*Fig. 33.12A*). They also resist angular motion (e.g., kyphosis) by virtue of their flat surface. Therefore, they function in resisting compressive, angular, and translational deformation (*Fig. 33.12B*). These factors enhance fusion.

Single cages that present a round surface to the graft bed function poorly in resisting angular deformation (*Fig. 33.13A*), but function adequately as paired cages (*Fig. 33.13B*). They usually present a relatively small surface area of bone contact to the graft bed (*Fig. 33.13C*), particularly if not placed appropriately (*Fig. 33.13D*).

The placement of a cylindrical strut (round-faced cage) into an elliptical wedge-shaped space (e.g., a TIFC) results in a nonuniform contact

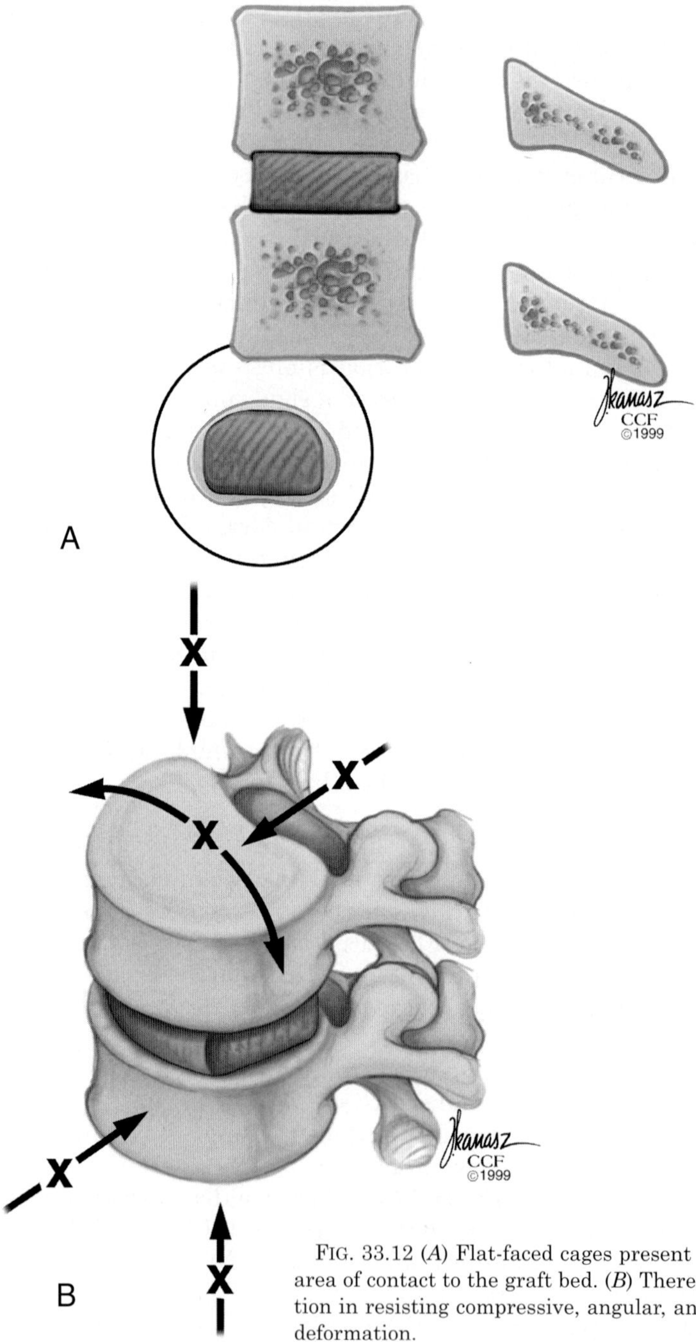

FIG. 33.12 (*A*) Flat-faced cages present a large surface area of contact to the graft bed. (*B*) Therefore, they function in resisting compressive, angular, and translational deformation.

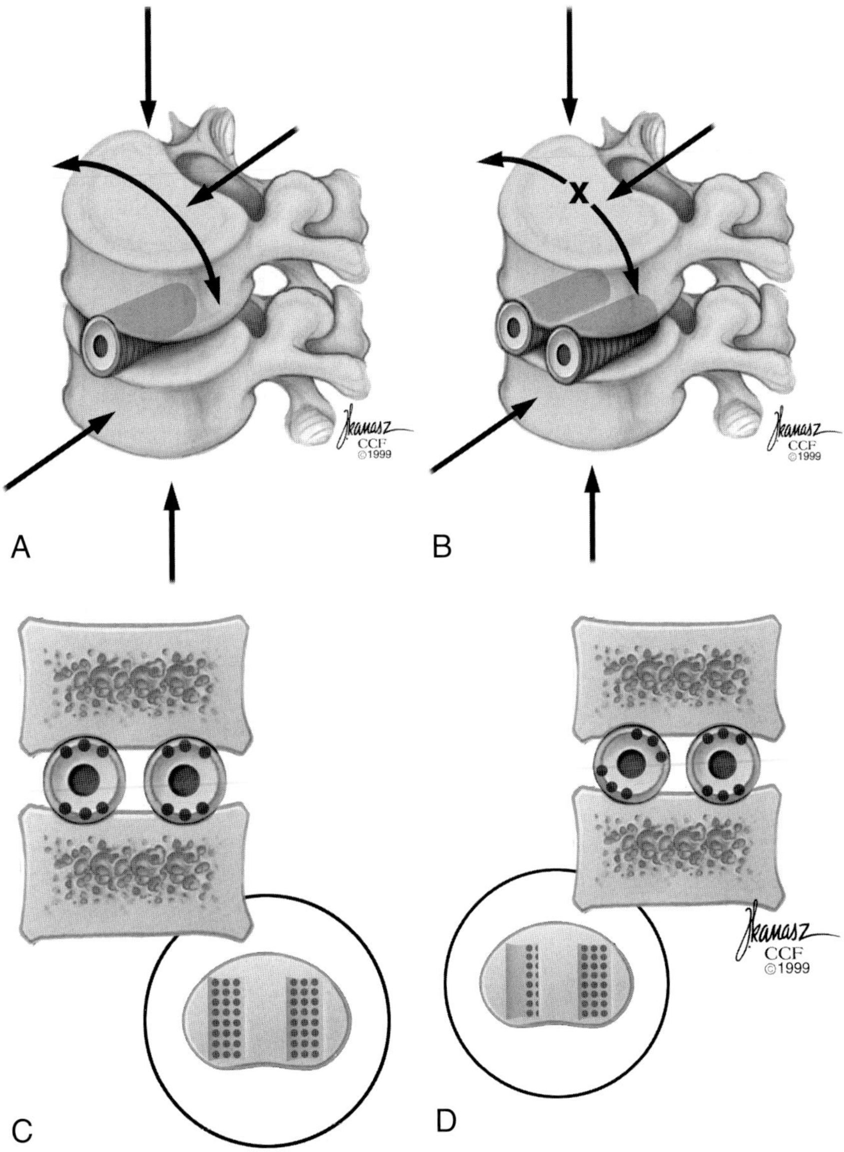

FIG. 33.13 Round-faced cages are so named because of the round surface (face) they present to the graft bed. (*A*) They function poorly in resisting angular deformation as a single cage. (*B*) As paired cages, they function adequately in this regard. They resist compression and translation, but relatively poorly. (*C, D*) They usually present a small surface area of contact for fusion (through holes in the cages) to the bone graft beds (*C*), particularly if not placed appropriately (e.g., inappropriate alignment) (*D*).

between longitudinal regions of the implant with the end plate of the adjacent vertebral bodies (*Fig. 33.14*). Coronal cross sectional views (planes A, B, and C in *Fig. 33.14*) demonstrate the nonuniform nature of the contact between the implant and the end plate. Minimal contact exists in plane A (*Fig. 33.14*) between the implant and the end plate. This may provide a load-bearing capacity resistance in flexion as a result of the tangential relationship between the cage and the end plate, but may increase the micromotion across the interspace. No bone-to-bone contact exists at this location, thus diminishing the arthrodesis rate and degrading the integrity of an acquired fusion. Optimal contact exists between the implant and the end plate in plane B (*Fig. 33.14*). The width of contact of the implant with the end plate is, nevertheless, still very narrow. The implant in plane B (*Fig. 33.14*) has a greater capacity to bear axial loads than the position of the implant in plane C (*Fig. 33.14*). The implant in plane C sits deeper into the end plate bone and invades the vertebral cancellous bone substantially. Because the end plate resists axial loads better than cancellous bone, the implant resists pistoning poorly in this region. The middle portion of the im-

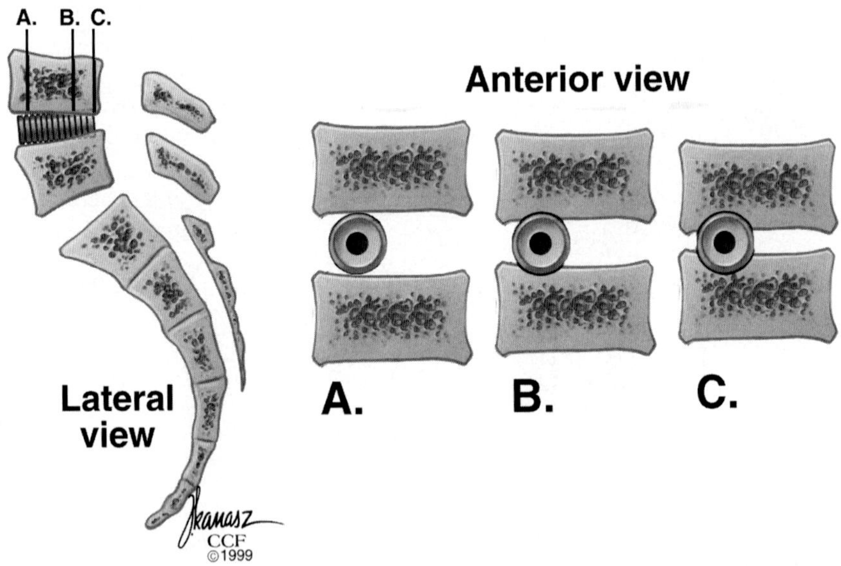

FIG. 33.14 Depiction of three regions of contact of a cylindrical implant in relation to the vertebral body cancellous bone and end plates (*planes A, B, and C*). *Plane A* shows minimal implant–end plate contact, *plane B* shows optimal contact, and *plane C* shows excessive penetration into cancellous bone.

plant can support axial loads relatively well, whereas the dorsal aspect of the implant cannot. The ventral portion only supports axial loads in flexion; however, it presents no intercage bone for contact with the vertebral body. Therefore, this portion of the cage contributes little to the acquisition of a solid arthrodesis.

The elliptical shape of the end plate and its relation to the graft bed was depicted in *Figure 33.3*. In this situation, either penetration of the TIFC into the end plate or gaps between the cage and the end plate exist. Both situations are undesirable.

Lastly, the placement of a cylindrical device into a disc interspace can alter the trapezoidal relationship of the end plates by making them parallel (*Fig. 33.15*). This is more dramatic with multilevel interbody implants (*Fig. 33.16*). Also, this can be accomplished with a Tang distractor (or equivalent). Unfortunately, a loss of lordosis and a disturbance of sagittal balance is the result. This may become a source of prolonged, persistent back pain (e.g., a form of the flat back syndrome). Furthermore, the elliptical shape of the end plate is still not addressed by this strategy (*Fig. 33.3*).

Ligamentous Disruption with Interbody Strut Insertion

Disruption of the ventral annular fibers and the anterior or posterior longitudinal ligaments during an interbody fusion procedure has been postulated to increase the neutral zone and, therefore, the range of motion at the fusion site (28). Although it is true that the anterior longitudinal ligament functions as a tension band in extension, and that the posterior longitudinal ligament functions as a tension band in flexion, the disruption of these ligaments should have an insignificant effect on micromotion and instability across an interspace if the strut

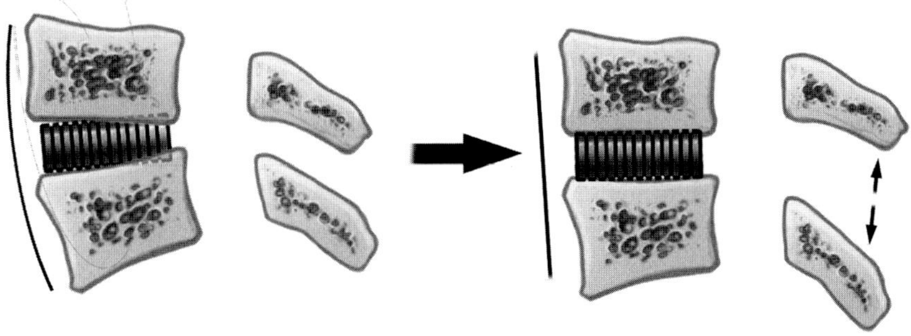

FIG. 33.15 A cylindrical implant, placed into a previously lordotic disc space, may convert the natural lordosis into a nonlordotic, straightened spine configuration.

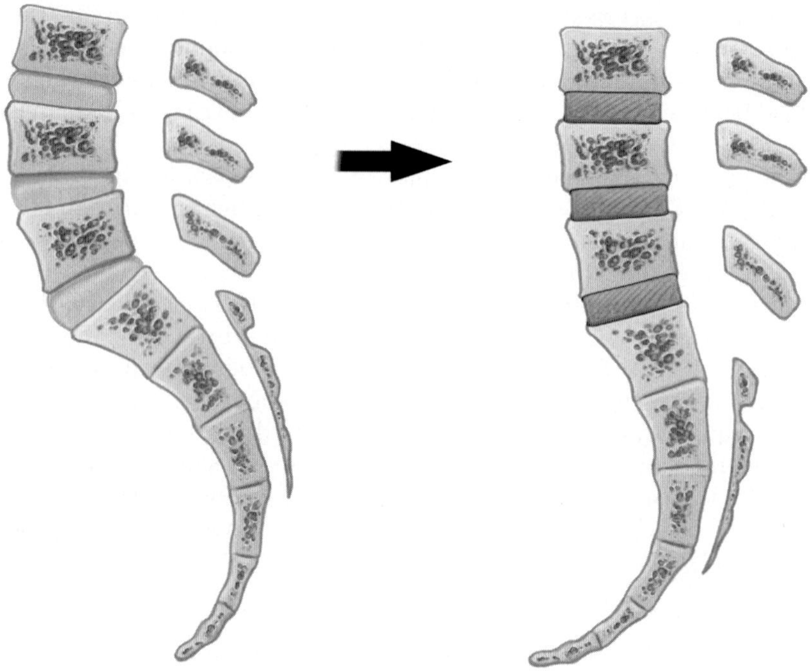

FIG. 33.16 The loss of lordosis of the lumbar spine after the placement of cylindrical devices may alter the normal mechanics, and lead to degenerative changes and chronic pain (e.g., flat back syndrome).

distracts the intervertebral space sufficiently. The restoration of the disc height via strut insertion should place the ligamentous tissues in tension, and should increase the overall stiffness of the interspace (because of the reduced mobility across the segment). If the strut does not conform to the vertebral end plates, an increase in the size of the neutral zone may result, thus increasing the range of motion (28).

In reality, the posterior longitudinal ligament is not the only structure that is disrupted when using the dorsal approach for cage insertion. Significant portions of the facet joints must be removed to attain the benefits associated with disc interspace distraction. In order for the TIFCs to achieve the desired distraction of the interspace height, a cage as large as 17 mm in diameter may be necessary (14, 18, 36). Such an extensive lateral dissection essentially obligates facet joint disruption in most cases, as depicted in *Figure 4.*

Restoration and Maintenance of Disc Height

The lumbar spine has the tendency to lose the normal lordotic posture and the intervertebral disc height with time. One of the major objectives of an interbody fusion via TIFC is the restoration of the intervertebral disc height, which in turn expands the spinal canal and neuroforamina (14, 36). This may alleviate nerve root impingement, which often accompanies degenerative disc disease. It has been shown that TIFCs can adequately increase the size of these anatomic spaces. As previously stated, in order for TIFCs to achieve an adequate disc interspace height, a cage with a diameter as large as 17 mm (or larger) may be necessary (14, 18, 36). This distraction restores the stiffness to the intact spine in flexion and extension, but facet joint efficacy in this regard may be compromised (18). This is not without ramifications. If the cage is undersize, dorsal element disruption is minimized but the distraction is not adequate to achieve stabilization (41). If an oversize cage is used, there is an element of facet joint and end plate disengagement and disruption respectively. The use of an oversize cage may be accompanied by a deeper penetration of the cage into the vertebral end plate, to the point that the cancellous bone is penetrated excessively. This could eventually result in fixation failure via subsidence.

A reconsideration of the tendency of the lumbar spine to lose the intervertebral disc height with time, and the "philosophy" of disc interspace distraction as a goal of surgery, is in order. For this discussion, refer to the collapsed disc interspace depicted in *Figure 33.17.* This disc space is a "victim of entropy." Entropy is a measurement of the degree of disorder in a system (3). The second law of thermodynamics states that "systems will change spontaneously from states of lower probability to states of higher probability" (3). Because states of lower probability are more "ordered" than states of higher probability, the second law of thermodynamics can be restated: "The universe constantly changes so as to become more disordered" (3). Therefore, the greater the disorder, the greater the entropy (3). A decrease of disc interspace height is a manifestation of increased entropy (more disorder). The disc space, in a sense, "sought" (and/or achieved) this state because it is more stable there. One must, therefore, question the wisdom of distracting the interspace to its previous (unstable) height (less entropy; more order). Because the distracted intervertebral space (via a TIFC technique) will indeed have significant axial and nonaxial loads placed on it, it will again seek its state of collapse (greater entropy). Perhaps a strategy that permits this state of high entropy (disc collapse) but encourages fusion as well as spinal alignment and neural element decompression is more prudent.

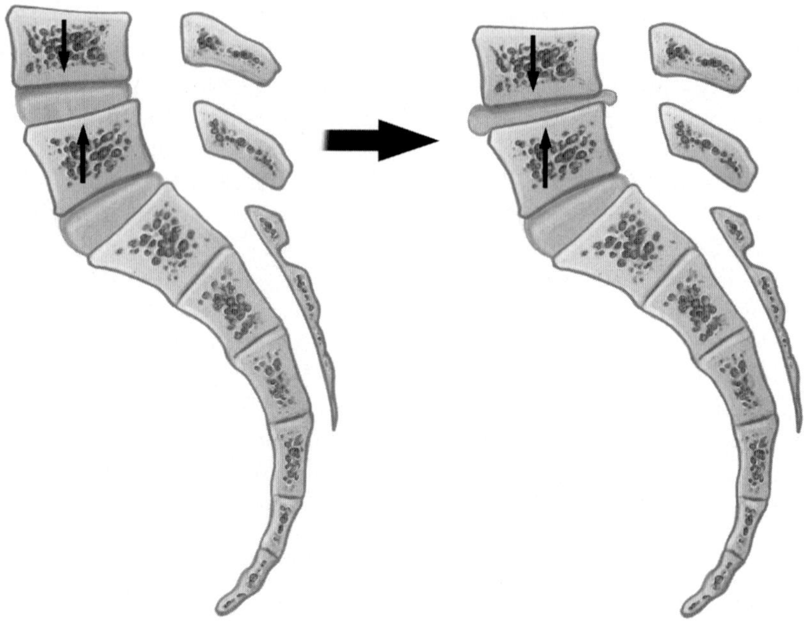

FIG. 33.17 The lumbar spine tends to lose intervertebral disc height with time as a result of repetitive axial loading (*arrows*). The collapsed disc is a "victim of entropy" (*see text*).

Strut Subsidence

Bone can function alone as a spinal instrument by providing support and resisting deformation (6). However, if cortical bone is used, such as a fibular strut graft or bone dowels (all of which fail biomechanically at much higher compressive strengths than cancellous bone), there is an increased risk of postoperative axial deformation (subsidence). This is also true for metallic implants (6, 39). An implant may piston into and through an end plate because of poor vertebral bone quality or because the implant did not encompass an adequate surface area of contact (e.g., adequate or optimal distribution of the axial forces was not achieved). End plate fractures may result in situations in which a strut, with a modulus of elasticity that far exceeds that of the compressive strength of the adjacent vertebrae, subsides excessively.

Postoperative Angular Deformation

The restoration and maintenance of sagittal alignment should be one of the fundamental goals of spinal fusion. A diminished lumbar lordosis after an interbody fusion may result in a progressive kyphosis (20). This process is contributed to by subsidence of the interbody strut. This subsidence process is often accelerated by surgery, but can occur as a manifestation of the degenerative aging process. A loss of lordosis as depicted in *Figures 33.15 and 33.16* creates a moment arm that encourages further kyphotic deformation. This then leads to the creation of longer moment arm, and so forth. In other words, deformity begets deformity (i.e., kyphosis begets kyphosis).

End fusion degenerative changes also have been shown to occur, and to occur at a greater frequency with longer fusions. They occur more frequently if abnormal spinal contours (kyphosis) are created by the fusion. Therefore, the maintenance of a relatively normal spinal alignment is prudent in this regard.

COMPLICATIONS

Complications may arise from an inadequate consideration of the aforementioned principles. Inappropriate strut (cage) placement is a common cause of complications (*Fig. 33.18*). Placement of TIFCs in osteoporotic bone is prone to failure (*Fig. 33.19*). Translational deformation is also common in osteoporotic patients and in patients in whom excessive instability exists (*Fig. 33.20*). Lastly, the determination of pseudoarthrosis is problematic (*Fig. 33.21A*). Close scrutiny is therefore required (*Fig. 33.21B*).

CONCLUSIONS

1. The cross sectional area of contact between the strut and the graft bed (in particular, the end plates) is directly proportional to the construct's capacity to resist axial loads and to minimize micromotion. This distributes the axial forces over a greater area and avoids stress risers (regions of high stress).
2. Placement of the strut close to the IAR (mid-dorsal vertebral body region) minimizes the application of excessive bending moments.
3. Meticulous graft bed preparation and the preservation of the end plate decreases the possibility of pistoning. This will increase the fusion rate and the axial load resistance capacity.
4. Strut type must be selected carefully. The integrity of the strut and the graft beds should be comparable regarding the modulus of elasticity (hardness). If a TIFC is used in poor vertebral bone, subsidence is inevitable. Pistoning, end plate fractures, cage extrusion, and graft nonunion may result.
5. Wedge-shaped intervertebral disc geometry and the trapezoidal design of the strut to match the interspace graft beds closely may minimize

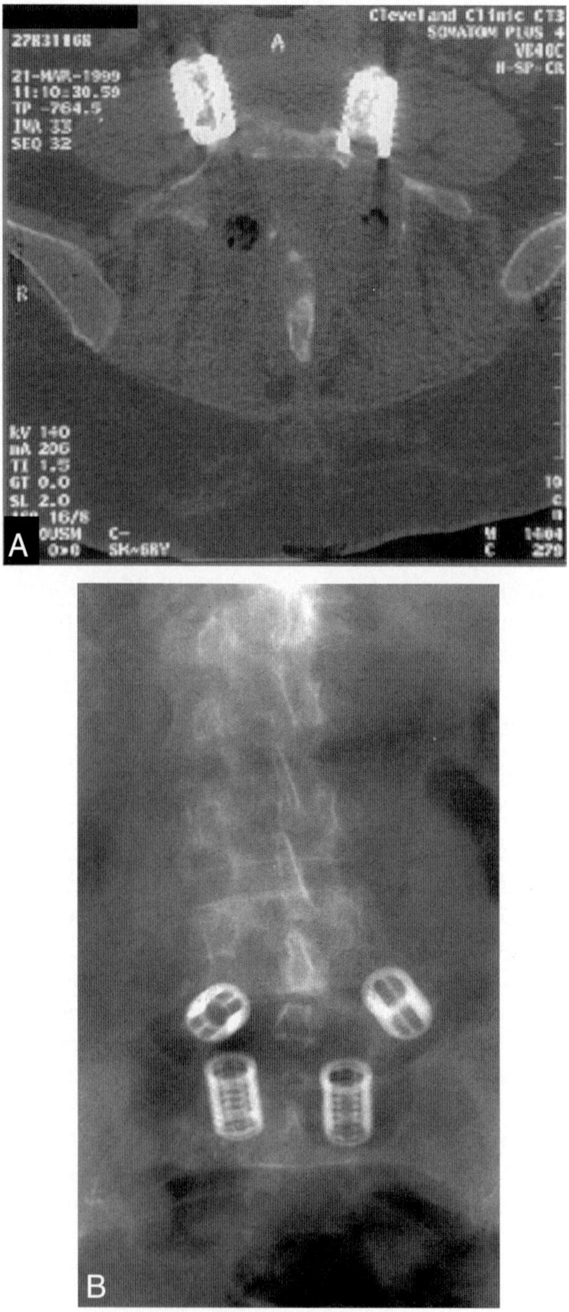

FIG. 33.18 (*A*, *B*) A TIFC placed in a suboptimal position.

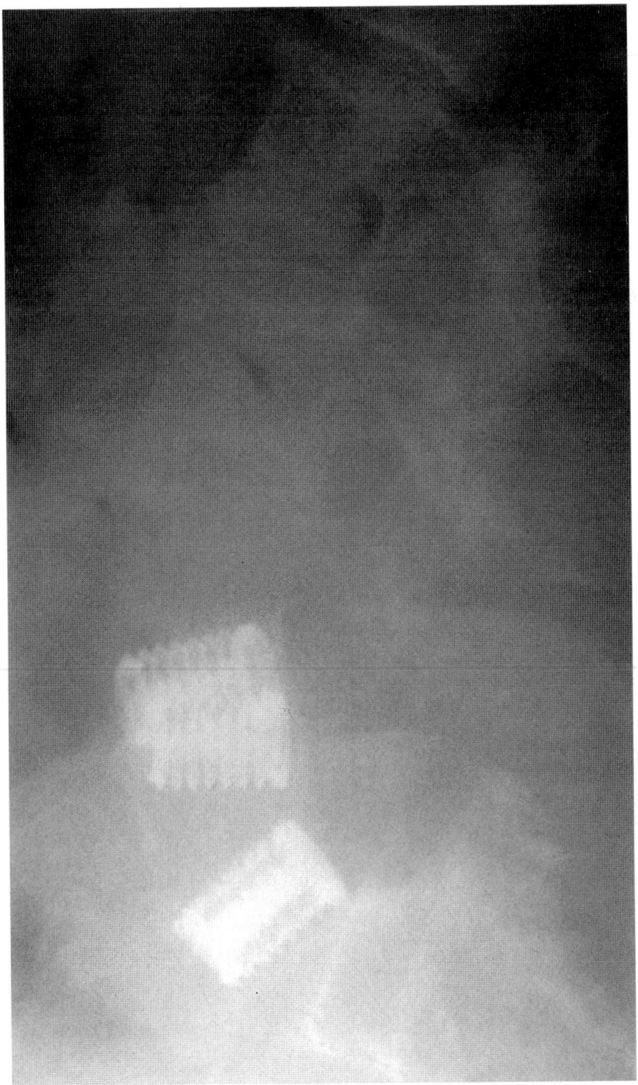

FIG. 33.19 A TIFC placed into osteoporotic bone may be expected to subside excessively, as depicted.

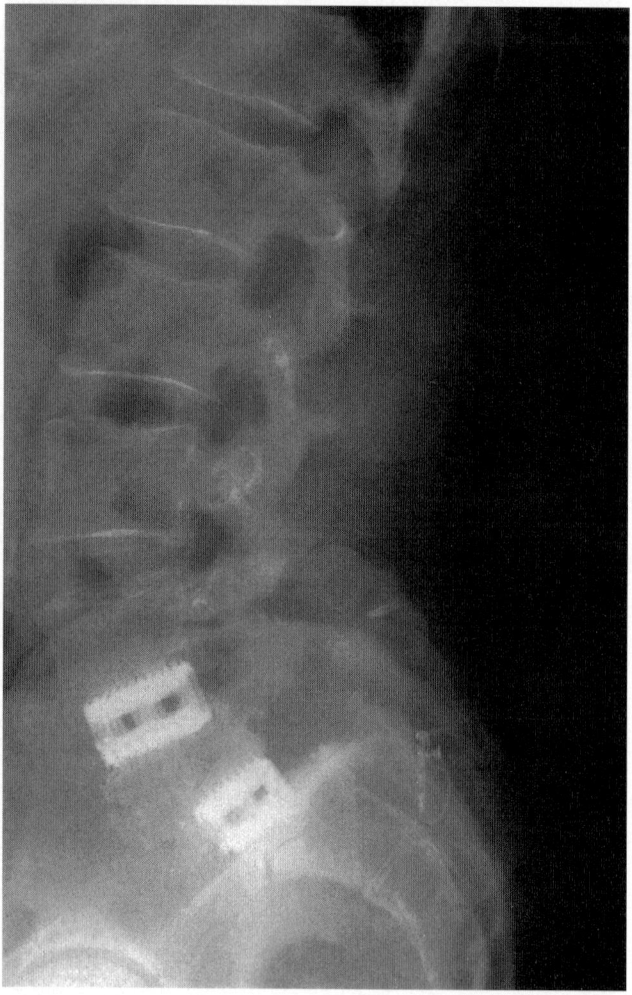

FIG. 33.20 Translational deformation is a common mechanism of failure. TIFCs are poor at preventing such a complication, particularly in osteoporotic patients, as depicted in this lateral plain film.

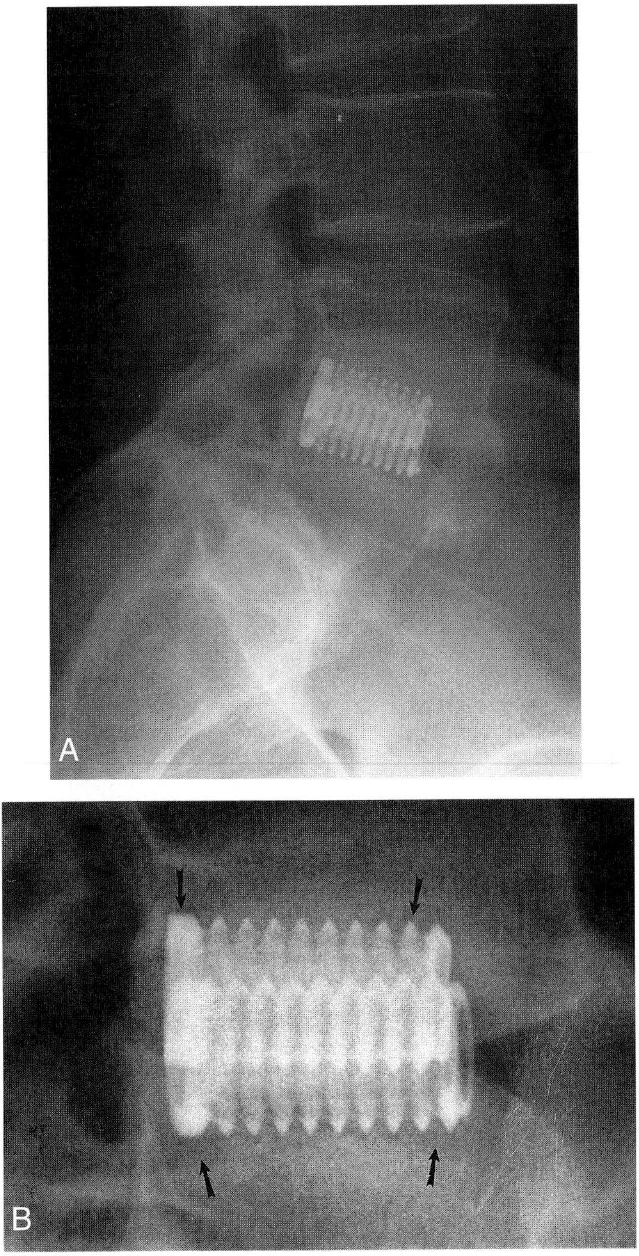

FIG. 33.21 (*A*) The determination of pseudoarthrosis in TIFC patients is often difficult. (*B*) However, close scrutiny may reveal lucency surrounding the cage (*arrows*).

micromotion, loss of stability, and fusion failure. This design and the proper sizing of the strut increase the surface area of contact and maintain (restore) lumbar lordosis.

6. Bone is formed where stresses are present, and it is absorbed where stresses are absent (Wolff's Law). Thus, an adequate understanding of the following concepts is imperative for the planning of a fusion: load bearing, load sharing, and stress shielding.
7. The tendency of the lumbar spine to change from a state of less entropy (healthy disc interspace; less disorder) to a state of higher entropy (collapsed disc interspace; more disorder) with time, should be carefully considered. Perhaps a strategy that permits higher entropy but encourages fusion and spinal alignment, and provides neural element decompression is more prudent than the "philosophy" of the restoration of the intervertebral disc interspace height.

REFERENCES

1. Abitbol JJ, Heim SE: Threaded femoral cortical dowels for the treatment of lumbar degenerative motion segment pain: A radiological analysis and early clinical experience. Presented at the 12th annual meeting of the North American Spine Society, New Orleans, LA, October 22–25, 1997.
2. Adams MA, Hutton WC: Prolapsed intervertebral discs: A hyperflexion injury. **Spine** 7:184–91, 1982.
3. Albers B, et al.: Molecular biology of the cell. 3rd ed. New York, Garland Publishing, 1994, pp. G–9, 668–669.
4. Bagby GW: Arthrodesis by the distraction–compression method using a stainless steel implant. **Orthopedics** 11:931–944, 1988.
5. Bagby GW, Cunningham BW, McAfee PC, Grant BD, Reed SM, Piercy RJ: Bone maturation study within the self-contained implant for spinal arthrodesis. Presented at the 12th annual meeting of the North American Spine Society, New Orleans, LA, October 2–25, 1997.
6. Benzel EC: Biomechanics of spine stabilization: Principles and clinical practice. New York, McGraw-Hill, 1995, pp 89–107.
7. Benzel EC, Ferrara LA, Baldwin NG: Multidirectional stabilizing potential of BAK interbody spinal fusion system for anterior surgery. **J Spinal Disord** 11(5):454–455, 1998.
8. Boden SD, Horton WC, Martin G, Truss T, Sandhu H: Laparoscopic anterior spinal arthrodesis with rhBMP-2 in a titanium interbody threaded cage. Presented at the 12th annual meeting of the North American Spine Society, New Orleans, LA, October 22–25, 1997.
9. Bourn SM, Ghanayem AJ, Havey R, Patwardhan A: Hydrostatic forces within intervertebral fusion cages. Presented at the 12th annual meeting of the North American Spine Society, New Orleans, LA, October 22–25, 1997.
10. Brantigan JW: Pseudarthrosis rate after allograft posterior lumbar interbody fusion with pedicle screw and plate fixation. **Spine** 19:1271–1280, 1994.
11. Brantigan JW, Steffee AD, Geiger JM: A carbon fiber implant to aid interbody lumbar fusion: Mechanical testing. **Spine** 16[6 Suppl]:277–282, 1991.

12. Brodke DS, Dick JC, Kunz DN, McCabe R, Zbedlick TA: Posterior lumbar interbody fusion: A biomechanical comparison, including a new threaded cage. **Spine** 22:26–31, 1997.
13. Brooke NSR, Rorke AW, King AT, Gullan RW: Preliminary experience of carbon fibre prostheses for treatment of cervical spine disorders. **Br J Neurosurg** 11:221–227, 1997.
14. Chen D, Fay LA, Lok J, Yuan P, Edwards WT, Yuan HA: Increasing neuroforaminal volume by interbody fusion in the reduction of foraminal stenosis. **Spine** 20:74–79, 1995.
15. Cloward R: Bone as a spinal instrument, in Benzel EC (ed.): *Spinal Instrumentation.* Park Ridge, IL, American Association of Neurological Surgeons, 1994, pp 185–210.
16. Coric D, Branch CL, Jenkins JD: Postlaminectomy spondylolisthesis treated with allograft PLIF and transpedicular screw fixation. Presented at the 12th annual meeting of the North American Spine Society, New Orleans, LA, October 22–25, 1997.
17. Frymoyer JW: Magnitude of the problem, in Wiesel SW, Weinstein JN, Herkowitz H, Dvorak J, Bell G (eds.): *The Lumbar Spine.* 2nd ed. Philadelphia, WB Saunders, 8–16, 1996.
18. Goh JCH, Yu CS, Thambyah A, Wong HK, Bose K: Influence of PLIF cage size on lumbar spine stability. Presented at the 12th annual meeting of the North American Spine Society, New Orleans, LA, October 22–25, 1997.
19. Goldstein JA, Griffith SL, McAfee PC: Effect of anterior lumbar interbody fusion cages on segmental lordosis: Two year follow-up. Presented at the 12th annual meeting of the North American Spine Society, New Orleans, LA, October 22–25, 1997.
20. Kitchel SH: Improvement in sagittal plane alignment following anterior lumbar interbody fusion with threaded titanium cages. Presented at the 12th annual meeting of the North American Spine Society, New Orleans, LA, October 22–25, 1997.
21. Kitchel SH: Threaded cortical bone dowels: Biomechanical properties and early clinical results. Presented at the 12th annual meeting of the North American Spine Society, New Orleans, LA, October 22–25, 1997.
22. Kuslich SD, Ahern JW: Analysis of complications in large personal series of lumbar interbody fusions using the BAK instrumentation. Presented at the 12th annual meeting of the North American Spine Society, New Orleans, LA, October 22–25, 1997.
23. Kuslich SD, Oxland TR, Jansen RC, Ulstrom CL: The BAK interbody fusion system: Early clinical results of treatment for chronic low back pain. Presented at the 8th annual meeting of the North American Spine Society, San Diego, CA, October 14–16, 1993.
24. Lin PM: Posterior lumbar interbody fusion. **Clin Orthop** 180:154–165, 1983.
25. Mathews HH, Evans MT, Molligan HJ, Long BH: Laparoscopic discectomy with anterior lumbar interbody fusion. **Spine** 20:1797–1802, 1995.
26. McCulloch JA: Point of view. **Spine** 20:2034–2035, 1995.
27. Moore DK, Cheng B, Tribus CB, Zdeblick TA: Radiographic analysis of laparoscopic BAK anterior spinal fusion. Presented at the 12th annual meeting of the North American Spine Society, New Orleans, LA, October 22–25, 1997.
28. Nibu K, Panjabi MM, Oxland T, Cholewicki J: Multidirectional stabilization potential of BAK interbody spinal fusion system for anterior surgery. **J Spinal Disord** 10:357–362, 1997.
29. Penta M, Sandhu A, Fraser RD: Magnetic resonance imaging assessment of disc degeneration 10 years after anterior lumbar interbody fusion. **Spine** 20:743–747, 1995.

30. Rapoff AJ, Ghanayem AJ, Zdeblick TA: Biomechanical comparison of posterior lumbar interbody fusion cages. **Spine** 22:2375–2379, 1996.
31. Ray CD: Spinal interbody fusions: A review, featuring new generation techniques. Neurosurg Q 7:135–156, 1997.
32. Ray CD: Threaded fusion cages for lumbar interbody fusions: An economic comparison with 360 degree fusions. **Spine** 22:681–685, 1997.
33. Ray CD: Threaded titanium cages for lumbar interbody fusions. **Spine** 22:667–680, 1997.
34. Shirazi–Adl SA, Shrivastava SC, Ahmed AM: Stress analysis of the lumbar disc–body unit in compression: A three-dimensional nonlinear finite element study. **Spine** 9:120–134, 1984.
35. Spiegel DA, Cunningham BW, Kanayama M, Haggerty CJ, McAfee PC, Drummond, DS: Augmentation of anterior instrumentation with threaded bone dowels. A biomechanical study. Presented at the 12th annual meeting of the North American Spine Society, New Orleans, LA, October 22–25, 1997.
36. Vamvanij V, Fay LA, Hai Y, Zhao J, Kolata R, Yuan HA: Changes in spinal canal dimensions using interbody distraction for spondylolisthesis. Presented at the 12th annual meeting of the North American Spine Society, New Orleans, LA, October 22–25, 1997.
37. van Erp AJ, de Gruijter AJ, Zeegers WS: A multi-center study of anterior lumbar interbody fusion using the anterior lumbar I/F cage. Presented at the 12th annual meeting of the North American Spine Society, New Orleans, LA, October 22–25, 1997.
38. Weiner BK, Fraser RD: Spine update—lumbar interbody cages. **Spine** 23:634–640, 1998.
39. White AA, Panjabi MM: Clinical biomechanics of the spine. 2nd ed. Philadelphia, JB Lippincott, 1990, pp 547–560, 649.
40. White AA, Panjabi MM: Clinical biomechanics of the spine. 2nd ed. Philadelphia, JB Lippincott, 1990, p 42.
41. Wong HK, Goh JCH, Chen J, Goh PS, Tan L, Bose K: Cylindrical interbody fusion cage fit and facetectomy in PLIF. Presented at the 12th annual meeting of the North American Spine Society, New Orleans, LA, October 22–25, 1997.
42. Yuan HA, Kuslich SD, Dowdle JA, Ulstrom CL, Griffith SL: Prospective multi-center clinical trial of the BAK interbody fusion system. 1–8. www.spine-tech.com/productsClinicalResults.html
43. Zdeblick TA: A prospective, randomized study of lumbar fusion: Preliminary results. **Spine** 18:983–999, 1993.

CHAPTER

34

Resident Curriculum Guidelines for Neurosurgery

Congress of Neurological Surgeons Education Committee

VINCENT C. TRAYNELIS, MD, CHAIR, BRIAN T. ANDREWS, MD, ISSAM A. AWAD, MD, H. H. BATJER, MD, ALLAN BELZBERG, MD, LYAL LEIBROCK, MD, WILLIAM COULDWELL, MD, KENNETH FOLLETT, MD, ALLAN FRIEDMAN, MD, CHRISTOPHER M. LOFTUS, MD, ALLEN MANIKER, MD, TIMOTHY MAPSTONE, MD, BRUCE E. POLLOCK, MD, SYDNEY S. SCHOCHET, JR., MD, ALEX VALADKA, MD, AND CHRIS WOLFLA, MD

CONTENTS

Spinal Surgery
Stereotactic and Functional Neurosurgery

INTRODUCTION

This curriculum was created to detail the body of knowledge that should be attained by an individual completing residency training in neurological surgery. The specific structure of resident education in neurological surgery is defined by the American Board of Neurological Surgery, and each program is examined periodically by the Residency Review Committee. It is not the intent of this curriculum to direct or influence these two entities in any way. The curriculum is meant to serve as a template to be used by individual neurosurgery residency program directors and residents as they see fit. In many respects, this comprehensive and specific curriculum delineates the "ideal," and therefore complete compliance to the curriculum will be difficult or impossible to achieve for most if not all programs. Nevertheless, it represents a goal toward which to strive.

This document will assist program directors, faculty, and residents in structuring an adequate postgraduate experience in neurological surgery. It should serve to create an organizational structure of academic, clinical, and technical criteria for the training of residents in neurological surgery. The curriculum should prompt members of established training programs to examine their educational experience and to assist new program developers in designing a comprehensive educational experience. The goal is to improve patient care by ensuring that residents completing training have achieved the highest possible level of competency in neurological surgery.

Although each portion of the curriculum has been examined by a number of recognized experts and leading educators in neurological surgery, it is recognized that an absolute consensus concerning the definition of essential knowledge for the practice of neurological surgery has not and will not be achieved. Despite this inevitable shortcoming, wide distribution of this resource to program directors, faculty, and residents will allow for each program to maximize its strengths, to address its weaknesses, and to promote constructive dialog among all involved parties.

It is noted that there is redundancy in the curriculum. This has arisen because many areas of neurosurgery overlap. The curriculum structure is based on performance. Hopefully, this will facilitate self-directed resident study and will impart some objectivity to periodic resident evaluations. The curriculum is constructed in such a manner that the educational experience is divided into three levels—junior, middle, and senior. The resident should display competency in each level before progressing to the next. Those individuals who do not stay on track will be promptly identified in an objective manner, thereby enabling more timely remedial attention or dismissal. Furthermore, it will force each program to examine its faculty and the structure of the basic and clinical training programs to ensure an optimal educational experience. The curriculum does not define how information is imparted, only the body of knowledge that must be mastered. It is up to the program developers to determine whether achievement of the goals will be accomplished through conferences, required readings, scheduled lectures or workshops, and so forth.

Adequate supervision of resident performance is critical to ensure proper care of the patient and learning of the resident. It is recognized, however, that a great deal of learning also takes place without supervision. Programs should be structured to allow residents to act independently at various tasks commensurate with their skills and the specific medical situation.

Although the assessment of resident, faculty, and program performance is extremely important, the curriculum does not include specific outcomes measures. Currently, a resident evaluation is performed in a nonuniform manner by the faculty and directors of each individual program. Hopefully there will be homogeneous evaluation of the knowledge and performance for each level of residency in the future.

Lastly, it should be recognized that a great number individuals have provided input and reviewed this work. Many of these persons are not listed as authors, but without their assistance the completion of this curriculum would not be possible.

NEUROANATOMY

Unit Objective

Demonstrate knowledge of anatomy that is pertinent to the diagnosis of diseases of the nervous system and the practice of neurological surgery.

Competency-Based Knowledge Objectives

JUNIOR LEVEL

General

1. Review the embryological development of the brain, cerebellum, brainstem, glial elements, spinal cord, conus medullaris, cauda equina, sympathetic and parasympathetic systems, and the peripheral nervous system.
2. Discuss the embryological development of the skull, craniovertebral junction, and spine.

3. Describe and differentiate the different types of neurons.
4. Discuss the microanatomy of the neuron including the
   a. cell body
   b. dendritic process
   c. axonal process
5. Diagram and describe the microanatomy of the synapse.
6. List the microglial elements and review their microanatomy.
   a. astrocytes
   b. oligodendrocytes
   c. microglia
   d. ependyma
   e. choroid epithelium
7. Diagram and describe in detail the carotid and vertebral arteries and their branches that provide blood supply to the face, scalp, skull, meninges, brain, brainstem, cerebellum, and rostral spinal cord.
8. Discuss in detail the arterial blood supply to the spinal cord. Include in the discussion the spinal and radicular arteries and the concept of watershed ischemia.
9. Identify and review the venous drainage of the central nervous system (CNS).
10. List and identify the bones of the skull.
11. Describe each of the sutures of the skull.
12. Identify each named foramen of the skull and list its contents.
13. Describe the anatomy of the meninges including the
    a. dura mater
    b. arachnoid mater
    c. pia mater
14. Describe the anatomy of the dura including the falx cerebri and tentorium.
15. Review the layers of the scalp and discuss its innervation.
16. Diagram the cerebral ventricles.
17. Discuss the major arachnoid cisterns.
18. Review the anatomy of the arachnoid villi.
19. Discuss the anatomic correlates pertinent to the production, flow, and reabsorption of cerebrospinal fluid (CSF).
20. Identify and describe the gross anatomy of the spine including
    a. atlas
    b. axis
    c. subaxial cervical vertebrae
    d. thoracic vertebrae
    e. lumbar vertebrae

   f. sacrum
   g. coccyx
   h. intervertebral disc complex
   i. supporting ligaments of the spine
21. List the muscles related to the skull and spine.
22. Describe the gross anatomy of the neck.
23. Discuss the anatomic basis for the blood–brain barrier in detail.

Central Nervous System

1. Describe the gross anatomy of the brain, brainstem, cerebellum, cranial nerves, and spinal cord in detail.
2. Describe the anatomy of the cerebral cortex in detail including
   a. cortical layers
   b. sensory areas
   c. motor areas
   d. prefrontal cortex
   e. fiber tracts
   f. calcarine cortex
3. Describe the anatomy of the olfactory pathways, hippocampal formation, and amygdala in detail including
   a. rhinencephalon
   b. olfactory pathways
   c. anterior commissure
   d. hippocampal formation (including cytoarchitecture)
   e. amygdala
   f. limbic system
4. Describe the anatomy of the corpus striatum in detail including
   a. striatum
   b. globus pallidus
   c. claustrum
   d. subthalamic region
   e. striatal afferent and efferent connections
   f. pallidal afferent and efferent connections
   g. pallidofugal fiber systems
5. Describe the anatomy of the hypothalamus and pituitary in detail including
   a. cytoarchitecture of the hypothalamus
   b. afferent and efferent connections of the hypothalamus
   c. supraoptic nuclei and tracts
   d. hypophysial portal system
   e. anatomy of the pituitary stalk
   f. anterior and posterior pituitary

   g. cellular organization of the anterior pituitary
   h. hormonally active cells of the hypothalamus and pituitary
6. Describe the anatomy of the diencephalon in detail including
   a. midbrain–diencephalon junction
   b. caudal diencephalon
   c. epithalamus
   d. thalamus (including nuclei)
   e. thalamic radiations
   f. internal capsule
   g. visual pathways
7. Describe the anatomy of the cerebellum in detail including
   a. cerebellar cortex including organization
   b. deep cerebellar nuclei
   c. cerebellar connections
   d. cerebellar peduncles
8. Describe the anatomy of the mesencephalon in detail including
   a. superior colliculus
   b. inferior colliculus
   c. pretectal region
   d. posterior commissure
   e. mesencephalic nuclei
   f. oculomotor nerve
   g. tegmentum
   h. mesencephalic reticular formation
   i. substantia nigra
   j. crus cerebri
   k. ascending and descending tracts
9. Describe the anatomy of the pons in detail including
   a. vestibulocochlear nerve
   b. facial nerve
   c. abducens nerve
   d. trigeminal nerve
   e. ascending and descending tracts
10. Describe the anatomy of the medulla in detail including
   a. olivary nucleus
   b. medullary reticular formation
   c. cranial nerves of the medulla
   d. ascending and descending tracts
11. Review the location and connections of each cranial nerve nuclei. Trace the course of each cranial nerve from nucleus to end organ termination.

12. Describe the external topography and landmarks of the fourth ventricle.
13. Describe the anatomy of the spinal cord in detail including
    a. nuclei and cell groups
    b. cytoarchitectural lamination (Rexed laminae)
    c. somatic and visceral efferent neurons
    d. posterior horn neurons
    e. descending tracts
    f. ascending tracts
    g. upper and lower motor neurons
    h. somatotopic organization

Autonomic Nervous System

1. Distinguish pre- and postganglionic neurons.
2. Describe the sympathetic nervous system.
3. Describe the parasympathetic nervous system.
4. Review the visceral afferent fibers.
5. Describe the structure of the autonomic ganglia.
6. Discuss the central autonomic pathways.

Peripheral Nervous System

1. Differentiate between segmental and peripheral innervation.
2. Diagram the anatomy of the spinal nerve root.
3. Diagram and discuss the cervical, brachial, and lumbosacralplexi.
4. Outline the anatomy of the major peripheral nerves of the upper and lower extremities including
    a. axillary
    b. suprascapular
    c. median
    d. ulnar
    e. radial
    f. long thoracic
    g. musculocutaneous
    h. lateral femoral cutaneous
    i. femoral
    j. obturator
    k. sciatic
    l. saphenous
    m. peroneal
    n. tibial
5. Describe the microanatomy of the peripheral nerves in detail.
6. Explain the difference between myelinated and unmyelinated nerves.

7. Review the anatomy of the Schwann cell.
8. List the peripheral afferent receptors and describe the anatom of each.
9. Segregate peripheral neurons by size and explain the rationale for such a classification scheme.

Muscle

1. Explain the concept of the motor unit.
2. Describe the anatomy of the motor end plate.
3. Describe the microscopic anatomy of striated and smooth muscle.
4. Discuss the subcellular components of muscle.

MIDDLE LEVEL

1. Discuss the clinical presentation in anatomic terms of syndromes of the brain and its coverings including
   a. epidural hematoma
   b. acute subdural hematoma
   c. chronic subdural hematoma
   d. subgaleal hematoma
   e. injury to innervation of the scalp
2. Discuss the syndromes produced by mass lesions affecting the cranial nerves including
   a. suprasellar lesions
   b. lesion of the jugular foramen
   c. lesion of the internal auditory canal
   d. lesions or distortion at the incisura
3. Review the expected effects of stroke or mass lesion at different locations within the brainstem and cerebellum.
4. List the expected effects of destructive lesions in the basal ganglia and cerebellum.
5. Describe the expected effects of ischemic or destructive lesions of the white matter tracts of the cerebrum.
6. Discuss the expected effect of destructive lesions of specific regions of the cerebral cortex.
7. Review the clinical presentation of stroke in the distribution of the supratentorial cerebral blood vessels.
8. Discuss the relationship of the spinal nerves to the vertebral level of exit.
9. Diagram the structures comprising the boundaries of the spinal neural foramina.
10. Discuss the clinical manifestation of injury for each of the major peripheral nerves.

11. Describe the anatomy and presentation of common entrapment syndromes of peripheral nerves including
    a. thoracic outlet syndrome
    b. carpal tunnel syndrome
    c. ulnar nerve entrapment syndrome at the wrist and elbow
    d. anterior interosseous syndrome
    e. posterior interosseous syndrome
    f. meralgia paresthetica
    g. peroneal nerve palsy
    h. tarsal tunnel syndrome
12. Describe the surgical exposure of common peripheral nerve entrapments including
    a. carpal tunnel
    b. ulnar nerve at the elbow
    c. ulnar nerve at the wrist
    d. lateral femoral cutaneous nerve
    e. peroneal nerve
13. Discuss the clinical presentation and neurological deficits associated with common lesions of and injuries to the spinal cord and nerve roots.

Competency-Based Performance Objectives

MIDDLE LEVEL

1. Identify at the time of surgery
    a. occipital artery
    b. superficial temporal artery
    c. frontalis muscle
    d. pterion
    e. inion
    f. asterion
    g. coronal suture
    h. sagittal suture
    i. middle meningeal artery
    j. sagittal sinus
    k. transverse sinus
    l. foramen rotundum
    m. foramen ovale
    n. foramen spinosum
    o. superior orbital fissure
    p. jugular foramen
    q. internal auditory canal

r. superior sagittal sinus
s. sigmoid sinus
t. incisura
u. each cranial nerve
v. each named cerebral artery and vein
w. components of the brainstem
x. named structures on the floor of the fourth ventricle
y. foramina of Magendie and Luschka
z. cerebral peduncles
aa. components of the cerebellum
bb. cerebellar tonsils
cc. brachium cerebelli
dd. vermis
ee. major supratentorial gyri
ff. supratentorial lobes
gg. Sylvian fissure
hh. central sulcus

2. Identify at the time of surgery structures visible in the lateral ventricles including
   a. foramen of Monro
   b. fornix
   c. caudate
   d. thalamus
   e. choroidal fissure
   f. named veins
   g. glomus of the choroid plexus
   h. hippocampus
3. Identify the parts of the vertebral column, spinal cord, and nerve roots at the time of surgery including
   a. spinous process
   b. lamina
   c. superior facet
   d. inferior facet
   e. pedicle
   f. pars interarticularis
   g. uncovertebral joint
   h. neural foramen and nerve root
   i. nerve root ganglion
   j. disc space
   k. vertebral artery
   l. dorsal column and lateral column of the spinal cord
   m. intradural afferent and efferent rootlets

NEUROPHYSIOLOGY

Unit Objective

Demonstrate knowledge of physiology that is pertinent to the understanding of neurological disease.

Competency-Based Knowledge Objectives

JUNIOR AND MIDDLE LEVELS

1. Review the basic biology of the nerves including
   a. synthesis and movement of proteins in the nerve
   b. membrane potential and membrane properties
   c. ion channels
   d. generation and conduction of an action potential
2. Discuss synaptic transmission including
   a. types of synaptic transmission
   b. transmitter release
   c. nerve–muscle transmission
   d. chemical messengers
   e. direct gated receptors
   f. second messenger linked receptors
3. Describe the physiology of the sensory systems including
   a. sensory receptor physiology
   b. anatomy of the somatic sensory system
   c. coding of modality-specific sensory information
   d. pain and analgesia
   e. cortical integration of sensory perception
   f. visual system
      i. processing of information in the retina
      ii. processing of vision in the central visual pathways
      iii. columnar units of the visual cortex
      iv. processing in the geniculate nucleus
      v. visual perception of motion and form
   g. auditory system. Within this description, review the processing of hearing in the cochlea and the central auditory pathways.
   h. olfaction and taste
4. Discuss the physiology of the motor system including
   a. mechanisms of muscle contraction
   b. muscle receptors and spinal reflexes
   c. spinal reflexes concerned with position
   d. brainstem reflexes controlling motion
   e. vestibular nuclei control of movement and posture
   f. red nucleus control of movement

g. cortical control of movement
h. cerebellar control of movement
    i. regional and cellular organization of the cerebellum
    ii. functional divisions of the cerebellum
    iii. the role of the cerebellum in planning movement
i. basal ganglia
    i. the anatomy of basal ganglia pathways
    ii. neural transmitters in the circuits within the basal ganglia
j. thalamus

5. Describe the attributes of the autonomic nervous system including both the sympathetic and parasympathetic systems.
6. Review the physiological basis of arousal and emotion. Include within this review the
    a. noradrenergic systems
    b. limbic system. Include within this review the physiological basis for emotion and memory.
    c. sleeping and sleep states
    d. reticular activating system
7. Describe the higher cortical functions including
    a. anatomy of language
    b. function of association cortex
8. Describe the physiological basis for CSF production and reabsorption.
9. Review the physiological control of the cerebral vasculature.
10. Discuss in detail the physiology of the hypothalamus and pituitary, particularly as they relate to endocrinology.

NEUROPATHOLOGY

Unit Objective

Demonstrate knowledge of neuropathology that is pertinent to the diagnosis of diseases of the nervous system and practice of neurological surgery.

Competency-Based Knowledge Objectives

MIDDLE LEVEL

General Neuropathology

1. Describe the techniques available for examination of surgical specimens from the CNS, peripheral nervous system, skeletal muscle, pineal, and pituitary.
2. Review the use of standard chromatic, histochemical, and selected immunohistochemical stains used to evaluate surgical

specimens from the CNS, peripheral nervous system, skeletal muscle, pineal, and pituitary.
3. List the techniques available for morphological examination of CSF and the abnormalities observed in CSF from patients with meningeal carcinomatosis, meningeal lymphomatosis, pyogenic meningitis, and aseptic meningitis.

Central Nervous System

1. Describe the gross and histopathological features and, when applicable, the genetic basis of the following congenital and perinatal disorders
   a. encephaloceles and cranial meningoceles
   b. myelomeningoceles and meningoceles
   c. hydromyelia
   d. diastematomyelia and diplomyelia
   e. syringomyelia and syringobulbia
   f. Chiari I malformation
   g. Chiari II malformation
   h. Dandy–Walker malformation
   i. arachnoid cysts
   j. porencephaly
   k. aqueductal stenosis
   l. subependymal germinal matrix hemorrhages
   m. posthemorrhagic hydrocephalus
   n. periventricular leukomalacia (white matter infarcts)
2. Describe the gross and histopathological features and characteristics of the causative agents of the following infectious diseases
   a. cranial and spinal epidural abscesses
   b. cranial and spinal subdural abscesses
   c. pyogenic bacterial meningitis and ventriculitis
   d. brain abscesses
   e. tuberculous meningitis and tuberculomas
   f. CNS sarcoidosis
   g. CNS cryptococcosis
   h. CNS mucormycosis
   i. CNS toxoplasmosis
   j. CNS cysticercosis
   k. herpes simplex encephalitis
   l. CNS human immunodeficiency virus infections
   m. CNS cytomegalovirus infection

3. Describe the gross and histopathological features of the following vascular lesions
   a. acute, subacute, and remote infarcts
   b. border zone and watershed infarcts
   c. manifestations of embolic infarcts including those secondary to atheromatous embolization and embolization from extracorporeal pumps
   d. vasculitis including temporal arteritis, primary CNS vasculitis, granulomatous angiitis, and Wegener's granulomatosis
   e. moyamoya
   f. hypertensive intracerebral hemorrhages
   g. lobar intracerebral hemorrhages
   h. amyloid angiopathy
   i. malformations including arteriovenous malformations, cavernous angiomas, venous angiomas, and capillary telangiectases
   j. vein of Galen "aneurysms"
   k. saccular aneurysms
   l. infectious ("mycotic") aneurysms
   m. giant aneurysms
   n. traumatic and dissecting aneurysms
   o. venous and dural sinus occlusive disease
   p. vascular malformations of the spinal cord
   q. spinal cord infarcts
4. Describe the gross and histopathological features of the following traumatic lesions.
   a. skull fractures
   b. entrance and exit gunshot wounds of the skull
   c. gunshot wounds of the brain including internal ricochet
   d. epidural hematomas
   e. acute subdural hematomas
   f. chronic subdural hematomas
   g. recent and remote cerebral contusions
   h. traumatic intraparenchymal hemorrhages
   i. diffuse axonal injury
   j. traumatic cranial nerve injuries
   k. spinal cord injuries
   l. cerebral herniation syndromes
   m. fat embolization
   n. CNS trauma in infancy
   o. CNS radiation injuries
   p. manifestations of prior surgical intervention

5. Describe the gross and histopathological features and, when applicable, the metabolic basis for the following intoxications and deficiency states.
   a. hypoxic–anoxic encephalopathy
   b. carbon monoxide intoxication
   c. ethanol intoxication
   d. alcoholic cerebellar degeneration
   e. central pontine myelinolysis
   f. CNS complications of diagnostic agents including contrast material
   g. CNS complications of antimicrobial therapy
   h. CNS complications of antineoplastic therapy
   i. CNS complications of "street drugs"
   j. Wernicke's encephalopathy and thiamine deficiency
   k. subacute combined degeneration and B12 deficiency
6. Describe the gross and histopathological features of the following demyelinating diseases.
   a. multiple sclerosis
   b. progressive multifocal leukoencephalopathy
   c. human immunodeficiency virus vacuolar myelopathy
   d. postinfectious encephalomyelitis
7. Describe the gross and histopathological features and the metabolic basis for the following leukodystrophies.
   a. adrenoleukodystrophy and adrenomyeloneuropathy
   b. Krabbe's disease
   c. metachromatic leukodystrophy
8. Describe the gross and histopathological features and, when applicable, the genetic basis for the following dementias and degenerations.
   a. Alzheimer's disease including familial forms
   b. vascular dementia including Binswanger's disease and cerebral autosomal dominant arteriopathy
   c. Pick's disease
   d. other frontotemporal dementias
   e. Creutzfeldt–Jacob's disease and other prion diseases
   f. Parkinson's disease
   g. diffuse Lewy body disease
   h. Huntington's disease
   i. amyotrophic lateral sclerosis
   j. paraneoplastic degenerative diseases
9. Describe the gross and histopathological features and, when applicable, the biochemical and genetic basis for the following metabolic diseases.

a. Wilson's disease
b. Tay Sachs disease and other GM-2 gangliosidoses
c. neuronal ceroid lipofuscinoses
d. hepatic encephalopathy
e. Reye's syndrome

10. Describe the gross and histopathological features and, when applicable, the grading criteria for the following CNS neoplasms.
    a. diffuse fibrillary astrocytomas
    b. gemistocytic astrocytomas
    c. anaplastic astrocytomas
    d. glioblastoma multiforme including giant cell glioblastoma and gliosarcomas
    e. pilocytic astrocytomas including cerebellar, diencephalic, dorsal exophytic pontine, and cerebral pilocytic astrocytomas
    f. subependymal giant cell astrocytomas
    g. pleomorphic xanthoastrocytoma
    h. oligodendrogliomas including anaplastic oligodendrogliomas and mixed oligoastrocytomas
    i. ependymomas including myxopapillary ependymomas
    j. subependymomas
    k. choroid plexus tumors
    l. colloid cysts
    m. gliomatosis cerebri
    n. gangliocytomas and gangliogliomas
    o. dysembryoplastic neuroepithelial neoplasms
    p. central neurocytomas
    q. medulloblastomas
    r. atypical teratoid/rhabdoid tumors
    s. primitive neuroectodermal tumors and cerebral neuroblastomas
    t. olfactory neuroblastoma
    u. spinal paragangliomas
    v. meningiomas including meningothelial (syncytial) fibrous, transitional, psammomatous, angiomatous, and papillary meningiomas
    w. anaplastic and malignant meningiomas
    x. meningeal hemangiopericytomas
    y. other meningeal mesenchymal tumors
    z. meningeal melanomatosis and melanomas
    aa. hemangioblastomas

- bb. lipomas
- cc. primary CNS lymphomas
- dd. metastatic carcinomas including leptomeningeal carcinomatosis
- ee. teratomas
- ff. dermoids and epidermoids
- gg. schwannomas including acoustic neurinomas or vestibular schwannomas, schwannomas of other cranial nerves, and spinal root schwannomas

11. Describe the gross and histopathological features and the genetic basis for the following tumor syndromes.
    - a. neurofibromatosis type 1
    - b. neurofibromatosis type 2
    - c. von Hippel–Lindau syndrome
    - d. tuberous sclerosis
    - e. Cowden syndrome
    - f. Turcot syndrome

Peripheral Nervous System

1. Describe the gross and histopathological features and, when applicable, the genetic and biochemical basis for the following disorders of peripheral nerves.
    - a. compressive and traumatic neuropathies
    - b. leprosy
    - c. diabetic and uremic neuropathy
    - d. Charcot–Marie–Tooth disease
    - e. Guillain–Barré syndrome
    - f. sympathetic dystrophy
2. Describe the gross and histopathological features of the following neoplastic and tumorous disorders of peripheral nerves.
    - a. peripheral schwannoma
    - b. neurofibromas
    - c. malignant peripheral nerve sheath tumors
    - d. spinal root and peripheral nerve root cysts

Pituitary and Pineal

1. Describe the gross and histopathological features of the following pituitary conditions.
    - a. pituitary adenomas including null cell adenomas, growth hormone-secreting adenomas, prolactin-secreting adenomas, ACTH-secreting adenomas, and oncocytomas

   b. craniopharyngiomas including adamantinomatous and squamopapillary craniopharyngiomas
   c. Rathke pouch (cleft) cysts
   d. pituitary involvement by metastatic neoplasms
   e. lymphocytic hypophysitis
   f. pituitary infarcts including pituitary “apoplexy”
   g. pituitary lesions resulting from closed head trauma
   h. empty sella syndromes
2. Describe the gross and histopathological features of the following lesions of the pineal.
   a. germinomas
   b. teratomas and embryonal carcinomas
   c. pineoblastomas and pineocytomas
   d. metastatic carcinoma

Skull and Spine (Including Intervertebral Discs)

1. Describe the gross and histopathological features of the following disorders of the skull.
   a. dermoids and epidermoids
   b. hemangiomas
   c. osteomas
   d. chordomas
   e. solitary and multifocal eosinophilic granulomas
   f. Paget’s disease including secondary osteosarcomas
   g. metastatic carcinomas
   h. plasmacytoma including myeloma
2. Describe the gross and histopathological features of the following disorders of the spine and intervertebral discs.
   a. herniated intervertebral discs
   b. pyrophosphate disease including involvement of the ligamentum flavum
   c. tumorous calcinosis
   d. hemangiomas
   e. chordomas
   f. eosinophilic granulomas
   g. metastatic carcinomas including epidural metastases
   h. plasmacytoma including myeloma
   i. lymphomas
   j. primary bone tumors
   k. spinal osteomyelitis including tuberculous and fungal spinal osteomyelitis

Eye and Orbit

1. Describe the gross and histopathological features of the following ocular lesions.
   a. retinoblastomas
   b. ocular melanomas
2. Describe the gross and histopathological features of the following orbital lesions.
   a. optic nerve gliomas
   b. optic nerve meningiomas
   c. orbital lymphomas and pseudotumors
   d. orbital metastases

Miscellaneous

1. List the gross and histopathological features found in temporal lobectomy and cerebral hemispherectomy specimens removed during epilepsy surgery.
2. Review the gross, histopathological, and cytopathological features that can be observed in shunt revision specimens.
3. Describe the gross, histopathological, and cytopathological features that can be observed with indwelling pump and intrathecal catheter specimens.
4. Cite the techniques for the examination of foreign objects removed from the nervous system and the need for documentation of chain of custody when of potential legal significance.
5. Describe the histopathological features of myotonic dystrophy and central core myopathy and list the potential implications of these diseases with regard to adverse anesthetic reactions including development of malignant hyperthermia.

NEUROPHARMACOLOGY

Unit Objective

Demonstrate knowledge of pharmacology that is pertinent to the treatment of neurological disorders and diseases that affect the nervous system.

Competency-Based Knowledge Objectives

JUNIOR LEVEL

1. Review basic cellular neurotransmission. During the course of this review discuss
   a. the synapse
   b. membrane potentials

   c. ion pumps
   d. ion channels
   e. transmitter secretion
   f. transmitter identification
2. Define and discuss receptors and receptor pharmacodynamics including
   a. receptor classification
   b. receptor identification
   c. dose–response curves
   d. agonists and antagonists
   e. receptor modulation
3. Discuss the neurotransmitter acetylcholine in detail. Include within the context of the discussion
   a. cholinergic receptor classification
   b. functional aspects of cholinergic receptors
   c. synthesis, storage, and release of acetylcholine
4. Discuss the catecholamine neurotransmitters (norepinephrine and dopamine) in detail. Include within the context of the discussion
   a. biosynthesis of catecholamines
   b. storage and release of catecholamines
   c. anatomy of catecholamine receptors
   d. α and β adrenergic receptors
   e. dopaminergic receptors
5. Discuss the neurotransmitter serotonin in detail. Include within the context of the discussion
   a. anatomy of serotonin receptors
   b. biosynthesis, storage, and release of serotonin
   c. subtypes of serotonin receptors
6. Discuss the neurotransmitter glutamate in detail. Include within the context of the discussion
   a. biosynthesis, storage, and release of glutamate
   b. inotropic glutamate receptors
      i. NMDA receptors and subunits
      ii. non-NMDA receptors and subunits
   c. metabotropic glutamate receptors
      i. group I metabotropic receptors and subunits
      ii. group II metabotropic receptors and subunits
      iii. group III metabotropic receptors and subunits
   d. role in neurological disorders
7. Discuss the neurotransmitters gamma aminobutyric acid and glycine in detail. Include within the context of the discussion
   a. synthesis, uptake, and release

   b. physiology and pharmacology
   c. clinically relevant agonists and antagonists of gamma aminobutyric acid and glycine receptors
8. Discuss the peptide neurotransmitters.
9. Describe the pharmacology of each of the drugs used to treat neurological disorders.

NEUROLOGY

Unit Objective

Demonstrate an understanding of the neurological examination, diagnostic neurological testing, and neurological diseases and their treatment.

Competency-Based Knowledge Objectives

JUNIOR AND MIDDLE LEVELS

1. Discuss electroencephalography (EEG). Recognize normal and abnormal EEG patterns. Identify specific epileptic conditions by EEG findings.
2. Describe the principles of sensory evoked potential (SEP) testing. Discuss how SEPs may be useful diagnostically.
3. List the indications for using intraoperative SEP monitoring and describe in detail how the procedure may be performed.
4. Describe the principles of visual evoked potential (VEP) testing. Discuss how VEPs may be useful diagnostically.
5. Describe the principles of motor evoked potential (MEP) testing. Discuss how MEPs may be useful diagnostically.
6. List the indications for using intraoperative MEP monitoring and describe in detail how the procedure may be performed.
7. Discuss electromyographic (EMG) testing in detail. Describe how the testing is performed and review the diagnostic capabilities of EMG testing. Describe the EMG changes associated with neuromuscular pathology.
8. List the indications for using intraoperative EMG testing and describe in detail how the procedure may be performed.
9. Discuss nerve conduction velocity (NCV) testing in detail. Describe how the testing is performed and review its diagnostic capabilities. List the transmission velocities of the major nerves. Describe NCV changes observed in neuropathy.
10. Define delirium and dementia. List the differential diagnoses for each.
11. Define and discuss coma and altered states of consciousness.

12. Describe the evaluation of a patient with syncope.
13. Describe the etiology and pathogenesis of cerebrovascular disease.
14. Review the clinical presentation and discuss the radiographic evaluation, clinical evaluation, and management of the following.
    a. transient ischemic attacks
    b. cerebral infarction
    c. cerebral and cerebellar hemorrhage
    d. subarachnoid hemorrhage
    e. venous infarction
15. Identify the primary causes of stroke in the pediatric population.
16. Discuss comprehensively the etiology, clinical presentation, diagnostic evaluation, and management of cerebral vasculitis.
17. Differentiate between basal occlusive disease with and without telangiectasia. Review the prognosis and treatment options for each.
18. Describe the acute and chronic effects of ionizing radiation on the CNS.
19. Review the diagnosis and management of pseudotumor cerebri.
20. Discuss the diagnosis and management of normal pressure hydrocephalus.
21. Discuss the management of hyperosmolar hyperglycemic nonketotic diabetic coma.
22. Review the neurological manifestations of altitude sickness.
23. List the neurological manifestations of decompression sickness.
24. Describe autism.
25. Review the general topic of chromosomal abnormalities as they may relate to the CNS, including etiology, inheritance patterns, penetrance, and laboratory diagnosis.
26. List the major syndromes characterized by obesity and hypogonadism, including Prader–Willi syndrome.
27. Discuss agenesis of the corpus callosum.
28. Discuss anencephaly, microencephaly, and megalencephaly.
29. List the major disorders of amino acid and purine metabolism. Discuss the neurological manifestations of each.
30. Review each of the major storage diseases including
    a. GM1 gangliosidoses
    b. GM2 gangliosidoses
    c. Fabry disease
    d. Gaucher disease
    e. Niemann–Pick disease
    f. Farber disease

   g. Wolman disease
   h. Refsum disease
   i. cerebrotendinous xanthomatosis
   j. neuronal ceroid lipofuscinoses
31. Review each of the major leukodystrophies including
   a. Krabbe leukodystrophy
   b. metachromatic leukodystrophy
   c. X-linked leukodystrophies with and without adrenal involvement
32. Review each of the major mucopolysaccharidoses including
   a. Hurler syndrome (MPS IH)
   b. Hunter syndrome (MPS II)
   c. Sanfilippo syndrome (MPS III)
   d. Morquio syndrome (MPS IV)
   e. Maroteaux–Lamy syndrome (MPS VI)
33. Review the disorders of carbohydrate metabolism including
   a. glycogen storage diseases
   b. Lafora disease and other polyglucose storage diseases
34. Discuss hyperammonemia as it relates to neurological dysfunction.
35. Discuss adrenoleukodystrophy as it relates to neurological dysfunction including Reye's syndrome.
36. Review the major syndromes of dysfunctional copper metabolism including
   a. hepatolenticular degeneration (Wilson disease)
   b. trichopoliodystrophy (Menkes' syndrome)
37. Review the pathogenesis, clinical presentation, diagnosis, and treatment of acute intermittent porphyria. List drugs to avoid in patients with porphyria (e.g., sulfa drugs).
38. Review the pathogenesis, clinical presentation, diagnosis, and treatment of abetalipoproteinemia.
39. List the neurological disorders associated with xeroderma pigmentosum.
40. List the major cerebral degenerative disorders of childhood including
   a. progressive sclerosing poliodystrophy
   b. spongy degeneration
   c. infantile neuraxonal dystrophy
   d. Hallervorden–Spatz disease
   e. Pelizaeus–Merzbacher disease
   f. Alexander disease
   g. Cockayne syndrome

    h. peroxisomal diseases
    i. Leigh disease
41. Review in detail the major neurocutaneous disorders including
    a. neurofibromatosis, types 1 and 2
    b. encephalotrigeminal angiomatosis
    c. incontinentia pigmenti
    d. tuberous sclerosis
42. Discuss Leber hereditary optic atrophy.
43. Review the salient features of progressive external ophthalmoplegia.
44. Define peripheral neuropathy, polyneuropathy, mononeuropathy, mononeuropathy multiplex, and neuritis.
45. Review the major inherited neuropathies including
    a. peroneal muscle atrophy
    b. Dejerine–Sottas disease
    c. Refsum disease
    d. hereditary sensory neuropathy
    e. porphyric neuropathy
46. Discuss the etiology, clinical presentation, diagnosis, treatment, and prognosis of Guillain–Barré syndrome.
47. List the major acquired neuropathies other than Guillain–Barré syndrome including
    a. chronic demyelinating polyneuritis
    b. acute and chronic idiopathic sensory neuropathy
    c. acute pandysautonomia
    d. tick paralysis
    e. brachial neuropathy (neuralgic amyotrophy)
    f. radiation neuropathy
    g. cold neuropathy
    h. cryoglobulin neuropathy
    i. diabetic neuropathy
    j. hypothyroid neuropathy
    k. acromegalic neuropathy
    l. vasculitic neuropathy
    m. uremic neuropathy
    n. hepatic neuropathy
    o. infectious neuropathies
        i. leprosy
        ii. acquired immunodeficiency syndrome
        iii. Lyme
        iv. herpes zoster
    p. sarcoid neuropathy

q. paraneoplastic neuropathy
r. amyloid neuropathy
s. polyneuropathy associated with plasma cell dyscrasia
t. polyneuropathy associated with dietary deficiencies
u. neuropathy induced by metals
  i. arsenic
  ii. lead
  iii. mercury
  iv. thallium
v. drug-induced neuropathy
w. neuropathy produced by aliphatic chemicals

48. Discuss the major hereditary ataxias including
  a. Friedreich ataxia
  b. Levy–Roussy syndrome
  c. hereditary cerebellar ataxia
49. Review the major noninherited forms of cerebellar ataxia including
  a. acute cerebellar ataxia in children
  b. ataxia telangiectasia
  c. Marinesco–Sjögren syndrome
  d. Ramsay–Hunt syndrome
  e. Joseph disease
50. Discuss the pathophysiology, clinical presentation, treatment, and prognosis of Alzheimer's disease, Pick's disease, and diffuse Lewy body disease.
51. Define hemichorea and hemiballismus.
52. Review the pathophysiology, clinical presentation, treatment, and prognosis of Sydenham chorea, Huntington's disease, and senile chorea.
53. Define myoclonus.
54. Review Tourette's syndrome.
55. Review the major general and focal dystonic conditions.
56. Define benign essential tremor.
57. Discuss the pathophysiology, clinical presentation, diagnosis, treatments, and prognosis of parkinsonism in detail.
58. Define progressive supranuclear palsy.
59. Review the pathophysiology, clinical presentation, diagnosis, and treatment of tardive dyskinesia.
60. Discuss hereditary spastic paraplegia.
61. List the major generalized and focal forms of spinal muscular atrophy including
  a. Wernig–Hoffmann disease

   b. Kugelberg–Welander syndrome
   c. benign focal amyotrophy
62. Describe the pathophysiology and neurological manifestations of poliomyelitis.
63. Review the pathophysiology, clinical presentation, diagnosis, treatment, and prognosis of amyotrophic lateral sclerosis.
64. Review the pathophysiology, clinical presentation, diagnosis, treatment, and prognosis of subacute combined degeneration of the spinal cord.
65. Review the pathophysiology, clinical presentation, diagnosis, treatment, and prognosis of juvenile and adult myasthenia gravis.
66. Review the pathophysiology, clinical presentation, diagnosis, treatment, and prognosis of botulism.
67. Review the common muscular dystrophies including
   a. Duchenne muscular dystrophy
   b. fascioscapulohumeral muscular dystrophy
   c. myotonic muscular dystrophy
   d. myotonia congenita
   e. congenital muscular dystrophy
68. Review the major periodic paralysis syndromes including
   a. familial periodic paralysis
   b. hypokalemic periodic paralysis
   c. hyperkalemic periodic paralysis
   d. paramyotonia congenita
69. Discuss polymyositis.
70. Review the epidemiology, pathophysiology, clinical presentation, diagnosis, treatment, and prognosis of multiple sclerosis.
71. Define Marchiafava–Bignami disease.
72. Review central pontine myelinolysis in detail.
73. Discuss multiple-system atrophy.
74. Review the pathophysiology, clinical presentation, diagnosis, treatment, and prognosis of migraine headaches.
75. Discuss the diagnosis and management of nonmigrainous headache syndromes.
76. Review the pathophysiology, clinical presentation, diagnosis, treatment, and prognosis of the common epileptic disorders in detail.
77. Define status epilepticus and discuss its medical treatment.
78. Describe the neurological implications of the common collagen–vascular diseases.
79. Describe the neurological implications of alcoholism.

80. Discuss the neurological aspects of pregnancy.
81. Review malignant hyperthermia.

NEURORADIOLOGY

Unit Objective

Demonstrate an understanding of neuroradiological imaging and interventions as they relate specifically to neurosurgical patients.

Competency-Based Knowledge Objectives

JUNIOR LEVEL

1. Describe the precautions that should be taken when performing radiological examinations.
2. Identify the normal anatomic structures of the skull on anteroposterior, lateral, Towne, and submental vertex radiographs.
3. List the indications for carotid and cerebral angiography.
4. Review the potential complications to intravenous contrast agents and discuss their management.
5. Identify the major arteries and veins of the neck and brain on angiograms.
6. Describe the concepts of computed tomographic (CT) scanning.
7. Identify the normal anatomic structures of the scalp, skull, dura, brain, and cranial vasculature on CT scans.
8. Describe the concepts of magnetic resonance imaging (MRI). Review the various imaging sequences that may be obtained.
9. Identify the normal anatomic structures of the scalp, skull, dura, brain, and cranial vasculature on MR images.
10. Recognize common traumatic injuries that may be detected by skull radiographs including
    a. linear skull fractures
    b. depressed skull fractures
    c. pneumocephalus
    d. foreign bodies
11. Recognize common pathological conditions that may be detected by skull radiographs including
    a. neoplasms
    b. fibrous dysplasia
    c. congenital bone diseases
    d. metabolic bone disorders
    e. infections

12. Recognize common traumatic injuries that may be detected by CT head scans including
    a. skull fractures
    b. pneumocephalus
    c. intracranial hematomas
        i. epidural
        ii. acute subdural
        iii. chronic subdural
        iv. intraparenchymal
        v. intraventricular
    d. cerebral contusions
    e. subarachnoid hemorrhage
    f. foreign bodies
13. Recognize common pathological conditions that may be detected by CT head scans including
    a. ischemic infarction
    b. venous infarction
    c. hydrocephalus
    d. cysts
    e. tumors
    f. cerebral edema
    g. infections
    h. congenital abnormalities
    i. infections
14. Recognize common traumatic injuries that may be detected by MR head images including
    a. pneumocephalus
    b. intracranial hematomas
        i. epidural
        ii. acute subdural
        iii. chronic subdural
        iv. intraparenchymal
        v. intraventricular
    c. cerebral contusions
    d. diffuse axonal injury
15. Recognize common pathological conditions that may be detected by MR head images including
    a. ischemic infarction
    b. venous infarction
    c. hydrocephalus
    d. cysts
    e. tumors

   f. cerebral edema
   g. vascular occlusions
   h. infections
   i. congenital abnormalities
16. Identify the normal anatomic structures of the craniovertebral junction on plain radiographs.
17. Review the radiographic diagnoses of platybasia and cranial settling.
18. Describe the plain radiographic findings of common traumatic injuries to the craniovertebral junction including
   a. occipital condyle fractures
   b. atlanto-occipital dislocation
   c. Jefferson fractures
   d. posterior atlas fractures
   e. dens fractures
   f. axis body fractures
   g. hangman's fracture
   h. atlas and axis facet fractures
   i. atlantoaxial rotatory dislocation
19. Distinguish between orthotropic and dystropic os odontoideum.
20. Describe the common congenital abnormalities of the craniovertebral junction.
21. Recognize common spinal congenital abnormalities on plain radiographs.
22. Recognize common spinal traumatic injuries that may be detected by plain radiographs including
   a. vertebral body fractures
   b. facet fractures and dislocations
   c. posterior element fractures
   d. transverse process fractures
   e. vertebral subluxation/dislocation
23. Recognize common spinal degenerative conditions that may be detected by plain radiographs.
24. Discuss the indications for CT scanning and MRI of the spine in the setting of trauma.
25. Describe the appearance of the CT scan for each of the traumatic spinal lesions listed previously.
26. Describe the appearance of the MR image of
   a. spinal ligament injury
   b. traumatic disc herniation
   c. spinal cord contusion
   d. spinal epidural hematoma

27. Recognize common spinal degenerative conditions that that may be detected by MRI including
    a. disc degeneration
    b. disc herniation
    c. degenerative spinal stenosis
    d. facet hypertrophy
    e. osteophyte formation
    f. foraminal stenosis
    g. degenerative spondylolisthesis
    h. degenerative scoliosis
    i. ossification of the posterior longitudinal ligament
28. Identify spinal and spinal cord tumors on CT scans and MR images.
29. Discuss the indications for spinal myelography.
30. Review the indications for spinal angiography.
31. Discuss the use of both the radiographic contrast and radionuclide shuntogram in evaluating neurosurgical patients.

MIDDLE LEVEL

1. Identify the common carotid and vertebral circulation congenital variants on angiograms.
2. Recognize intracranial aneurysms on angiograms.
3. Identify and characterize intracranial vascular malformations on angiograms. Recognize
    a. arteriovenous malformations
    b. venous angiomas
    c. arteriovenous fistulas
    d. feeding vessels
    e. draining veins
    f. associated aneurysms
    g. degree of shunting
4. Discuss the angiographic evaluation of carotid and vertebral disease.
5. Review the role of MR angiography and venography in the evaluation of cerebrovascular disease, neoplasms, and trauma.
6. Describe the radiological evaluation of CNS vasculitis.
7. Describe the radiological evaluation of spinal vascular malformations.
8. Discuss the role of myelography in the evaluation of neurosurgical patients.
9. Discuss the radiological evaluation of suspected CNS and spinal infection.

10. Review MR neurography.
11. Describe the appearance of peripheral nerve tumors on MR images.
12. Review the role of radionuclide scans in the evaluation of patients with suspected cranial and spinal disease.
13. Discuss the use of intraoperative radiographs and fluoroscopy.
14. List the indications for CT- and MR-guided biopsies.
15. Describe the concepts of ultrasonography.
16. Review the findings of normal and abnormal neonatal cranial ultrasonic images.
17. Review the findings of normal and abnormal carotid ultrasonic images.
18. Discuss the use of transcranial Doppler ultrasonography in the management of patients with subarachnoid hemorrhage, trauma, and occlusive vascular disease.

SENIOR LEVEL

1. Review the indications for interventional endovascular therapies for
   a. aneurysms
   b. vasospasm
   c. cranial vascular malformations
   d. spinal vascular malformations
   e. tumor embolization
   f. carotid and vertebral stenosis
   g. carotid and vertebral dissection
2. Describe the indications and techniques of endovascular trial occlusions.
3. Review the role of quantitative cerebral blood flow studies in the management of neurosurgical patients.
4. Describe the concepts of positron emission tomography. Review the indications for obtaining these scans.
5. Describe the concepts of functional MRI. Review the indications for obtaining these images.
6. Describe the concepts of MR spectroscopy. Review the indications for obtaining such evaluations in neurosurgical patients.
7. Discuss the indications and technique of discography. Describe the procedure.
8. Discuss the indications for percutaneous vertebroplasty. Describe the procedure.

Competency-Based Performance Objectives

JUNIOR LEVEL

1. Order appropriate radiological evaluations in a timely fashion.
2. Complete radiological requisitions properly.
3. Demonstrate the ability to interpret accurately the radiographic studies of trauma patients.

MIDDLE LEVEL

1. Demonstrate the ability to interpret accurately carotid and vertebral angiograms.
2. Demonstrate the ability to interpret accurately spinal angiograms.
3. Demonstrate the ability to interpret accurately spinal myelograms and postmyelogram CT scans.
4. Demonstrate the ability to interpret accurately cranial and spinal CT scans and MR images of nontraumatic lesions.

SENIOR LEVEL

1. Demonstrate the ability to interpret accurately radiological examinations of neurosurgical patients.
2. Demonstrate the ability to use intraoperative ultrasonography.

FLUIDS, ELECTROLYTES, AND NUTRITION

Unit Objectives

Demonstrate an understanding of normal and pathological fluid and electrolyte homeostasis. Demonstrate an ability to maintain normal electrolyte balance. Demonstrate an understanding of the basics of nutritional management in neurosurgical patients.

Competency-Based Knowledge Objectives

JUNIOR AND MIDDLE LEVELS

1. Discuss the normal distribution of intracellular and extracellular fluid and electrolytes including
   a. sodium and water distribution and metabolism
   b. clinical assessment of water and sodium balance and the concept of osmolality
   c. normal maintenance requirements
   d. management of pathological conditions such as diabetes insipidus and the syndrome of inappropriate antidiuretic hormone secretion
   e. cerebral salt wasting

2. Review the potential implications of diuresis and fluid restriction on water and electrolyte balance.
3. Review briefly the potential clinical implications of calcium, phosphorous, and magnesium excesses and deficiencies, and the treatment of same.
4. Review the criteria for nutritional assessment including
   a. history of significant weight loss
   b. hypoalbuminemia
   c. impaired immune response including diminished total lymphocyte count and anergy
   d. physical signs of malnutrition
5. Describe briefly the metabolic responses to starvation and stress.
6. Describe and contrast the indications, contraindications, complications, and benefits of enteral and parenteral nutrition.
7. Analyze the implications of specific nutritional deficiencies as they relate to neurological and neurosurgical diseases.
8. Review briefly swallowing disorders.
9. Describe the common changes of metabolism and nutritional requirements of trauma patients and their evaluation.

Competency-Based Performance Objectives

JUNIOR AND MIDDLE LEVELS

1. Demonstrate an ability to manage the fluid and electrolyte requirements of neonatal, pediatric, and adult neurosurgical patients.
2. Demonstrate the ability to place central venous catheters.
3. Demonstrate the ability to place enteral feeding tubes.
4. Demonstrate the ability to prescribe appropriate parenteral and enteral nutrition.
5. Recognize and treat the complications of parenteral and enteral feeding including
   a. line sepsis
   b. glucose intolerance
   c. diarrhea
   d. dehydration
6. Recognize swallowing disorders and manage them.

GENERAL CRITICAL CARE

Unit Objectives

Demonstrate an ability to perform triage for neurosurgical patients in and out of a critical care setting. Demonstrate a knowledge of and the ability to manage neurosurgical patients in the critical care setting.

Competency-Based Knowledge Objectives

JUNIOR LEVEL

1. Define the adult and pediatric patient who would be best served in a critical care setting. Include both medical and neurosurgical issues within the context of this discussion.
2. Review general medical issues pertinent to the management of neurosurgical patients in a critical care setting including
   a. prophylaxis of gastrointestinal hemorrhage
   b. prophylaxis of pulmonary morbidity
   c. prophylaxis, diagnosis, and treatment of venous thrombosis and pulmonary embolism
   d. skin care
   e. eye care
   f. physical therapy to maintain strength and joint range of motion
   g. universal precautions
   h. workup and treatment of sepsis
3. Describe the indications and pharmacokinetics for medications commonly used in the management of critically ill neurosurgical patients including
   a. vasoactive drugs
   b. inotropic drugs
   c. bronchodilators
   d. diuretics
   e. antiarrhythmics
   f. antihypertensives
   g. antimicrobials
   h. anticonvulsants
4. Describe the clinical presentation, evaluation, and treatment of infections that commonly occur in critical care neurosurgical patients.
5. Review the indications for intubation including
   a. loss of patient airway
   b. respiratory insufficiency
   c. inability to protect airway
6. Discuss commonly used pulmonary values including
   a. measured pulmonary functions
      i. rate
      ii. minute ventilation
      iii. spontaneous tidal volume
      iv. forced vital capacity
      v. functional residual capacity
      vi. maximum ventilatory volume

b. ventilator modes and settings
   i. pressure versus volume ventilation
   ii. continuous positive airway pressure
   iii. intermittent positive airway pressure
   iv. pressure support
   v. assist control
   vi. intermittent mandatory ventilation
   vii. positive end expiratory pressure
   viii. rate
   ix. tidal volume

7. Review the indications for weaning patients from ventilatory support. Describe the methods by which this is accomplished and the general pulmonary parameters a patient must demonstrate before extubation.
8. Discuss the medications used to improve pulmonary function.
9. Review briefly the following cardiac function parameters.
   a. preload
   b. afterload
   c. contractility
10. Review the indications for implementing the following monitoring devices. Describe briefly how the information obtained is used to optimize patient management.
    a. arterial catheters
    b. central venous catheters
    c. Swan–Ganz catheters
    d. pulse oximetry
    e. electrocardiographic monitoring
    f. end-tidal carbon dioxide monitors
11. List the signs of acute myocardial ischemia and briefly discuss the emergent treatment of this condition.
12. Review the impact of renal insufficiency as it pertains to the management of neurosurgical patients.
13. Discuss briefly the diagnosis and management of acute renal insufficiency.
14. Describe the diagnosis and management of an ileus. List the differential diagnosis for an ileus.
15. Review the diagnosis and management principles of the following endocrine disorders.
    a. hypo- and hyperthyroidism
    b. hypo- and hyperparathyroidism
    c. adrenal cortical excess and deficiency
    d. diabetes mellitus
    e. diabetes insipidus

16. Review the medical and legal definitions of brain death.
17. Discuss moral and ethical issues pertaining to critically ill neurosurgical patients including
    a. patient or family requests to withhold or withdraw treatment
    b. organ donation
18. Summarize the physiology of hydrogen ion production and excretion.
19. Discuss briefly the acute and chronic buffering systems.
20. Discuss metabolic acidosis and alkalosis.
21. Discuss respiratory acidosis and alkalosis.
22. Review the effects of acid–base disturbances on the CNS and intracranial pressure (ICP).

Competency-Based Performance Objectives

JUNIOR AND MIDDLE LEVELS

1. Obtain ACLS and ATLS certification.
2. Demonstrate the ability to perform an initial evaluation and management of critically ill neurosurgical patients.
3. Perform the following procedures.
    a. orotracheal intubation
    b. nasogastric intubation
    c. bladder intubation
4. Serve on a trauma team.
5. Demonstrate an ability to manage neurosurgical patients in a critical care setting.
6. Diagnose and treat acid–base abnormalities in neurosurgical patients.
7. Demonstrate an understanding of the management of complex acid–base disturbances in the critical care setting.

SENIOR LEVEL

1. Oversee and direct the junior- and middle-level resident management of critically ill neurosurgical patients.

INFECTION

Unit Objectives

Demonstrate an understanding of the factors related to the acquisition, diagnosis, and treatment of infections as they pertain to neurosurgical patients. Describe the typical presentation and treatment of common neurosurgical infections. Review the methods used to minimize infectious complications in neurosurgical patients. Demonstrate an understanding of the techniques to minimize the risk of spread of viral infections, including hepatitis and human immunodeficiency virus.

Competency-Based Knowledge Objectives

JUNIOR AND MIDDLE LEVELS

1. List the common organisms responsible for meningitis in an age-related fashion.
2. List the common CNS infections and describe the populations that are most at risk for each.
3. List the common opportunistic CNS infections and describe the populations that are most at risk for each.
4. Describe in detail the clinical and pathological symptoms and findings associated with CNS infections.
5. Discuss the radiological evaluation of patients with suspected and known CNS infections.
6. Review the indications for alerting individuals at risk for infections based on exposure to a patient with a known CNS infectious process.
7. Review each major class of antimicrobial drugs.
   a. Describe the potential of resistance to each drug.
   b. List the potential complications of each agent.
   c. Review the serological monitoring of each antimicrobial agent including the need for monitoring renal, hepatic, and hemopoietic function.
   d. Indicate those drugs that will traverse the blood–brain barrier and those that will not.
   e. Demonstrate a knowledge of the pharmacokinetics of each antimicrobial agent.
   f. Describe the potential complications of each antimicrobial drug and explain how to monitor for and detect them.
   g. Review the rationale for monitoring drug levels and list the therapeutic levels of antimicrobials commonly used to treat neurosurgical infections.
8. Discuss the advantages and disadvantages of treatment of CNS infections with corticosteroids.
9. Review the role of anticonvulsant therapy in the management of CNS infections.
10. List the universal precautions for prevention of infection as they pertain to health care workers in general and neurosurgeons in particular.
11. Discuss the role of hand washing as the most important method of preventing infection.
12. Describe the role of the clinical epidemiologist in tracking infectious disease incidence and potential sources of infection within the hospital and community settings.

13. Review the mode of transmission, diagnosis, and treatment of non-CNS infections that may commonly arise in neurosurgical patients, such as
    a. respiratory infections
    b. urinary tract infections
    c. wound infections
14. Review the prevention, diagnosis, and management of sepsis.
15. List the common sources of a postoperative fever.
16. Describe the workup for a febrile patient.
17. Discuss the use of prophylactic antibiotics.
18. Review the symptoms, clinical evaluation, and management of patients with shunt infections.
19. Discuss prion disease and precautions to be taken when it is suspected.

Competency-Based Performance Objectives

JUNIOR AND MIDDLE LEVELS

1. Demonstrate the ability to use universal precautions.
2. Demonstrate the ability to use sterile technique.
3. Diagnose and treat appropriately non-CNS infections in neurosurgical patients.
4. Diagnose and treat appropriately CNS infections in neurosurgical patients.

PRACTICE LEGAL, AND SOCIOECONOMIC ISSUES

Unit Objective

Demonstrate an understanding of the principles of practice management and the business aspects associated with the delivery of health care.

Competency-Based Knowledge Objectives

JUNIOR AND MIDDLE LEVELS

1. Discuss the ethical and moral factors associated with the practice of neurosurgery.
2. Review the role of the neurosurgical leadership in the community and hospital settings.
3. Explain the neurosurgeon's responsibilities in terms of health care cost containment.
4. Review the features and relationships of the health care system including

   a. treatment facilities
   b. third-party payment systems
      i. Medicare
      ii. Medicaid
      iii. employer-provided insurance
      iv. private insurance
   c. physician practice organizations
   d. medical equipment manufacturers
   e. pharmaceutical companies
5. Recite the rules and regulations of the training hospitals as they pertain to the practice of neurosurgery in which the residency is performed.
6. Name the institutional and social service agencies in your community and review their roles in the overall management of neurosurgical patients.
7. Demonstrate a knowledge of the rules and regulations of your state medical board.
8. Discuss the concept of informed consent.
9. Discuss mandatory reporting laws.
10. Discuss issues pertinent to the topic of the impaired physician.
11. Name and describe the local, regional, and national neurosurgical organizations including their purposes, roles, activities, and interactions.
12. Discuss the importance of tracking morbidity, mortality, and patient outcomes.
13. Review the career options available at the completion of neurosurgical residency in detail including
   a. private practice
   b. academic practice
   c. subspecialty fellowship
   d. research
   e. administration
   f. military
14. Discuss postresidency fellowship training program availability, application process, and career usefulness.
15. Describe the types and characteristics of surgical practice organizations including
   a. solo practice
   b. group practice
      i. partnership
      ii. professional association
      iii. corporation

   c. academic practice
   d. health maintenance organizations (HMOs)
      i. preferred provider organizations (PPOs)
      ii. individual practice associations
      iii. staff model (Kaiser–Permanente type)
   e. federal
      i. Department of Veterans Affairs
      ii. military
      iii. Public Health Service
16. Discuss hospital payment systems (e.g., DRGs per diem rates), and describe their incentives and how they affect hospital profitability.
17. Discuss the role and influence of national quality oversight and review organizations for hospitals and health plans (Joint Commission on Accreditation of Healthcare Organizations, NCQA).
18. Discuss the history, changes, eligibility, funding, and problems associated with the Medicare program.
19. Describe the Medicare program features, such as eligibility, funding, administration, federal–state relationship, benefits, and payment methods.
20. Discuss federal funding of graduate medical education and how current federal budget allocations and proposals for changes in funding affect or will affect neurosurgical training programs.
21. Discuss the significance of the following issues as they relate to the practice of neurosurgery.
   a. legislative/regulatory requirements
      Americans with Disabilities Act
      Clinical Laboratory Improvement Amendments
   b. federal/professional regulatory institutions
      i. Health Care Financing Administration
      ii. Joint Commission on Accreditation of Healthcare Organizations
      iii. Occupational Safety and Health Administration
   c. miscellaneous
      i. affirmative action
      ii. equal opportunity
      iii. sexual harassment
22. Discuss the common causes of malpractice actions and effective measures to reduce the risk of malpractice complaints.
23. Describe the ways, means, and reasons physicians influence the political process at the national, state, and local levels.

24. Discuss the demographics of neurosurgeon distribution, numbers, workload studies, and workforce needs.
25. Outline the requirements for certification by the American Board of Neurological Surgery.
26. Formulate a strategy to evaluate personal and professional considerations in making a career choice.
27. Appraise the importance of family involvement in making career choices, including geographic location.

SENIOR LEVEL

1. Review the requirements to obtain certification from the American Board of Neurological Surgery.
2. Discuss the available opportunities to obtain continuing medical education credits.
3. Describe the political, economic, and social factors that impact the practice of medicine generally and neurosurgery specifically.
4. Demonstrate a working knowledge of the International Classification of Diseases and current procedural terminology (CPT) coding and analysis.
5. Discuss the concept of relative values units.
6. Summarize the process of impairment determination as it relates to the neurosurgical patient population.
7. Review the availability, requirements, and application procedures for postresidency fellowship if appropriate.
8. Discuss the following issues as they relate to planned neurosurgical practice.
   a. health care delivery systems, including managed care
   b. health care economics
   c. political and legislative processes in health care
9. Obtain a demographic profile of potential practice locations including population and medical demographics.
10. Outline the essential business characteristics of neurosurgical practice including
    a. content and interpretation of financial reports
    b. management of human resources
    c. facility design and maintenance
    d. billing and collection processes
11. Discuss the key elements of a provider professional services agreement, such as a PPO or HMO contract, and identify provisions that require particular attention.
12. Describe the typical provisions and considerations in a physician employment contract including what to look for and what to avoid.

13. Describe, compare, and contrast partnership versus corporate practice structures, including the tax and liability advantages and disadvantages of each.
14. Describe the advantages and disadvantages of solo, single-specialty group, and multispecialty group practices.
15. Review the financial issues associated with the neurosurgical career options under consideration.
16. Describe the administrative structures and processes required for managing an office practice including
    a. billing and collection for medical services
    b. financial accounting and reporting
    c. scheduling
    d. transcription
    e. medical record management
    f. appointment scheduling
    g. information systems
    h. facility selection and maintenance
    i. secretarial services
17. Describe the content, interpretation, and use of the following financial documents.
    a. balance sheet
    b. income and expense statement
    c. accounts payable and receivable
    d. collection analysis
18. Discuss the insurance requirements associated with neurosurgical practice including
    a. personal and professional liability
    b. personal health and disability
    c. casualty, fire, and theft
    d. personal life
19. Discuss the issues of quality assurance as related to neurosurgical practice including
    a. maintenance of the clinical record
    b. review and documentation of morbidity and mortality
    c. risk management
20. Discuss the theory and organization of CPT coding, along with examples of complex procedural coding.
21. Describe the considerations in evaluation and management coding, including documentation requirements.
22. Describe the work, practice expense, and malpractice expense components of Medicare's Resource-Based Relative Value Scale (RBRVS) and how they are derived.
23. Explain how Medicare and commercial payer conversion factors are derived and used to create a fee schedule from the RBRVS.

24. Describe commonly used methods of physician risk contracting, such as capitation payment, and explain the considerations in negotiating such a contract.
25. Describe the practice information necessary to manage a neurosurgical risk contract safely and profitably.
26. Review the features, similarities, and differences in various third-party payment systems including
    a. Medicare
    b. Medicaid
    c. commercial insurance
    d. worker's compensation
27. Contrast HMO and PPO health plans.
28. Describe the meaning of "managed care" and its typical components including
    a. contractual discounts
    b. provider risk arrangements
    c. use management
    d. provider report cards
    e. practice guidelines
    f. restricted access models
        i. primary gatekeeper
        ii. point of service
        iii. open access
29. List and discuss the ethical issues and conflicts of interest involved in managed care treatment decisions such as
    a. capitation reimbursement
    b. risk pools
    c. cost-saving incentive bonuses
30. Discuss antitrust considerations faced by physicians in payer contract negotiations including the concepts of collective bargaining, price fixing, and group boycott.
31. Describe the types of retirement plans, and funding considerations and limitations.
32. Explain the differences between occurrence and claims-made professional liability insurance and considerations made in selecting insurer and coverage levels.

Competency-Based Performance Objectives

JUNIOR AND MIDDLE LEVELS

1. Demonstrate an ability to interact effectively, professionally, and respectfully with
    a. patients and their families
    b. fellow residents

   c. allied health care personnel
   d. hospital staff
   e. medical students
   f. faculty physicians
   g. referring physicians
2. Demonstrate the ability to maintain accurate and current medical records.
3. Discuss neurosurgical career options with
   a. faculty
   b. peers
   c. family
   d. nonfaculty neurosurgeons and other mentors
4. Accumulate information about postresidency career options.
5. Create and keep current a resume/curriculum vitae.
6. Record CPT codes for office visits and procedures performed on service.
7. Document accurately H&P and consultations according to the American Medical Association CPT evaluation and management documentation guidelines.

SENIOR LEVEL

1. Demonstrate the ability to code neurosurgical activities properly.
2. Assign accurately and justify medical impairment ratings for neurosurgical patients.
3. Outline a postresidency career track.
4. Apply for postresidency fellowship if appropriate.
5. Obtain information about specific practice, research, or administrative career opportunities as appropriate.
6. Compose a list of questions to ask and things to see when interviewing for a neurosurgical position.
7. Read and interpret a financial report.
8. Design a structure for an office practice including a listing of the generic office processes and how to arrange staffing.
9. Prepare lists of neurosurgical instruments/equipment needed for specific operative procedures.
10. Select a proper practice, research, or administrative opportunity if appropriate.
11. Complete license and registration requirements for your chosen location.
12. Complete applications for hospital staff membership and clinical privileges.

13. Complete a resident case data sheet for the American Board of Neurological Surgery and have it signed by the program chair.

CEREBROVASCULAR SURGERY

Unit Objectives

Demonstrate an understanding of the anatomy, physiology, pathophysiology, and presentation of cerebrovascular diseases, including ischemic and hemorrhagic stroke, and other diseases and malformations of intracranial, extracranial, and spinal vasculature. Demonstrate the ability to formulate and implement a diagnostic and treatment plan for cerebrovascular diseases, including medical and surgical management.

Competency-Based Knowledge Objectives

JUNIOR LEVEL

1. Describe the anatomy of the extracranial and intracranial vessels, including the carotid, vertebral, and spinal arteries.
2. Describe the location of key perforating arteries involving the anterior and posterior circulation, their target distribution, and the consequence of occlusion or injury.
3. Review the anatomy of the venous circulation as it pertains to the CNS.
4. Identify the classic syndromes of vessel occlusion of the following.
   a. internal carotid artery
   b. middle cerebral artery
   c. anterior cerebral artery
   d. recurrent artery of Heubner
   e. anterior choroidal artery
   f. vertebral artery
   g. posterior inferior cerebellar artery
   h. lower and upper basilar trunk
5. Identify the classic brainstem ischemic syndromes.
6. Explain the concepts of cerebral blood flow, cerebral autoregulation (hemodynamic and metabolic), ischemic thresholds, ICP, and cerebral perfusion pressure. Describe the impact on cerebral blood flow of intracranial hypertension with and without mass lesion.
7. Recognize the common causes of brain ischemic states including
   a. cardiac embolism
   b. embolism from proximal vasculature
   c. large-vessel occlusion
   d. intracranial conducting vessel occlusion

   e. small-vessel disease
8. Associate CT and MR evidence of ischemic injury with likely anatomic substrates.
9. Describe the epidemiology, physiology, and underlying pathophysiology of ischemic brain injury, including concepts of the critical therapeutic window.
10. Recognize the common causes of intracranial and intraspinal hemorrhage including
    a. aneurysmal disease
    b. vascular malformations
    c. hypertension
    d. vasculopathies
    e. degenerative diseases
    f. hemorrhagic arterial infarction
    g. venous infarction.
11. Relate typical imaging characteristics of CNS hemorrhagic lesions to probable causes.
12. Categorize common causes of intracranial hemorrhage, subarachnoid hemorrhage, and ischemic stroke.
13. Explain the principles of fluid and electrolyte resuscitation and maintenance, respiratory physiology, cardiac physiology, and nutritional physiology, as applied to the neurological patient following ischemic or hemorrhagic stroke. Integrate this knowledge with the specific issues of the perioperative period.
14. Recognize the need for laboratory evaluation for systemic illness.
15. List the appropriate diagnostic neuroimaging studies used to evaluate ischemic and hemorrhagic stroke.
16. Recognize the typical clinical course of patients with ischemic and hemorrhagic stroke, including peak risk intervals for edema, vasospasm, rebleeding, and so forth.
17. Identify the periods of high vulnerability to systemic complications of cerebrovascular illness, including deep venous thrombosis, pulmonary embolism, bacterial pneumonia, aspiration, congestive heart failure, and so on.
18. Explain the principles of augmentation of cerebral blood flow during cerebral vasospasm.
19. Discuss the principles and indications for medical, endovascular, and surgical interventions for ischemic and hemorrhagic stroke.
20. Relate the principles of timing of medical, endovascular, and surgical intervention in these same disease states.
21. Explain the principles, indications for, and complications of barbiturate coma.

22. Recognize the principles and interpretation of normal and common abnormal findings on skull, chest, and abdominal radiographs in the critical care unit.
23. Describe the fundamentals of CT scanning, including the typical appearance of acute, subacute, and chronic blood, calcification, ventricular anatomy, and mass effect.
24. Describe the typical CT appearance of hemorrhagic and ischemic stroke. Provide a detailed explanation for the typical delay between the onset of stroke and appearance of confirmatory CT findings.
25. Explain the fundamentals of MRI. Distinguish between normal and abnormal findings within the realm of cerebrovascular disease. Recognize the classic MR appearance of
    a. arteriovenous malformations
    b. venous angiomas
    c. cavernous malformations
    d. aneurysms
26. List the indications for noninvasive vascular imaging, including ultrasound, MR angiography, and CT angiography. Recite the limitations of noninvasive studies.
27. Describe the practical application of commonly employed noninvasive studies, such as transcranial Doppler, in the setting of cerebral vasospasm.
28. List the indications for catheter angiography. Interpret the findings of angiography in ischemic and hemorrhagic cerebrovascular conditions. Identify the key segments of the internal carotid artery including the upper cervical, petrous, cavernous, and supraclinoid components.
29. Recite the principles of localizing focal intracranial and spinal vascular pathology by the use of traditional topographic measurements and the application of stereotactic guidance.
30. Describe the surgical anatomy and the principles of exposure of the cervical carotid artery.
31. Describe the principles of pterional craniotomy, including scalp and bony anatomy, as well as the anatomy of the sphenoid ridge.
32. Explain the principles of cerebrovascular surgery detailed in the previous objectives to medical students and allied health personnel during conferences.

MIDDLE LEVEL

1. Recognize controversies regarding the basic neuroscience knowledge concepts mastered during junior residency.

2. Explain the principles of ischemic neuronal protection and salvage.
3. Review the principles of guideline development and outcome assessment related to the basic knowledge objectives achieved during junior residency.
4. Display an understanding of the principles of hypothesis development and testing, and statistical analysis as applied to clinical research trials, as well as the critique of scientific manuscripts.
5. Recognize areas of controversy related to management protocols in cerebrovascular patients achieved during junior residency.

SENIOR LEVEL

1. Demonstrate a sophisticated understanding of current literature related to basic neuroscience knowledge objectives acquired as a junior and middle resident. Define scientific hypotheses in relation to controversies and evolving knowledge regarding these same objectives, and demonstrate the ability to interpret and adapt new knowledge to evolving patient care paradigms.
2. Demonstrate a mature fundamental knowledge in clinical and teaching conferences, specialty conferences, and in publications and scientific presentations.
3. Understand the guidelines, protocols, and literature controversies regarding the diagnostic imaging modalities available in cerebrovascular disease.

Competency-Based Performance Objectives

JUNIOR LEVEL

1. Perform a comprehensive neurological history and clinical examination.
2. Perform a comprehensive systemic evaluation.
3. Adapt comprehensive evaluations to specific, pertinent positives and negatives with regard to ischemic and hemorrhagic stroke.
4. Demonstrate an understanding of urgency and the ability to prioritize during emergent aspects of hemorrhagic and ischemic disease states.
5. Demonstrate the ability to manage cardiac and pulmonary complications following cerebrovascular illness and therapy, and review the need for specialty and subspecialty consultations.
6. Apply the principles of perioperative care after common endovascular and surgical procedures directed at cerebrovascular disease.
7. Demonstrate the ability to be vigilant in the clinical detection of subtle neurological change during the acute and subacute phases of illness.

8. Demonstrate the ability to place an arterial catheter, central venous catheter, and pulmonary artery catheter. Perform placement of a ventricular catheter via a burr-hole or twist-drill craniotomy.
9. Perform lumbar puncture and CSF reservoir tapping.
10. Define the proper placement of a craniotomy flap in the planned surgical evacuation of hematoma. This should be performed using both topographical as well as stereotactic-assisted navigation techniques.
11. Assist in the opening, exposure, and closure of cervical carotid procedures.
12. Assist during pterional craniotomy for vascular disease.
13. Assist in the performance of intracranial hematoma evacuation.
14. Demonstrate the ability to keep accurate and timely records.

MIDDLE LEVEL

1. Perform pterional craniotomy for vascular disease.
2. Demonstrate the ability to make independent management decisions regarding ischemic and hemorrhagic stroke states.
3. Supervise care delivered by PGY1 and junior resident physicians for cerebrovascular patients.
4. Demonstrate efficient prioritization skills for clinical assessment of multiple simultaneous problems in the same or different patients. Display a clear sense of prioritization regarding timing and urgency of medical and surgical intervention for ischemic and hemorrhagic stroke states. Recognize the impact of systemic conditions on prioritization and timing issues.
5. Interpret and respond correctly to changes in patient status related to systemic and neurological parameters.
6. Implement patient care protocols regarding perioperative management.
7. Display independence in making decisions regarding the critical care of cerebrovascular patients. Recognize the need for reporting such decisions to the senior resident and attending staff.
8. Demonstrate the ability to obtain appropriate medical and surgical consultation.
9. Display skills in prioritization of diagnostic interventions, including the choice and sequence of studies in the setting of ischemic and hemorrhagic states.
10. Interpret invasive and noninvasive diagnostic imaging studies in relation to cerebrovascular disease.
11. Formulate preliminary and surgical planning.
12. Perform frameless navigation procedures.

13. Perform routine and complicated twist-drill or burr-hole procedures for the drainage of the ventricular system or intracranial hematomas.
14. Perform exposure of the cervical carotid artery for endarterectomy or proximal arterial control.
15. Observe and assist in the performance of plaque removal and arterial closure during carotid endarterectomy.
16. Practice microsurgical techniques in the laboratory setting.
17. Demonstrate a mature understanding of the planning and performance of pterional craniotomy for intracranial vascular pathology. Perform pterional craniotomy with initiation of microsurgical clinical skills. Observe the microsurgical dissection of the Sylvian fissure and basal cisterns for vascular pathology.
18. Perform the surgical approach to vascular structures via a craniotomy other than pterional.
19. Supervise and assist junior residents in burr-hole and twist-drill procedures for ventricular access or ICP monitoring.
20. Realize an increasingly progressive teaching responsibility to medical students, interns, and junior residents in the various educational objectives of the cerebrovascular curriculum.
21. Supervise the junior residents in the technical performance of cerebrovascular procedures, as well as critical care catheter procedures commensurate with their level of expertise.
22. Organize clinical and teaching rounds and conferences, as well as the presentation of cases.
23. Prepare topic reviews in lecture and manuscript formats, including literature summaries and reference compilations.

SENIOR LEVEL

1. Review fundamental concepts of cerebrovascular disease during conferences and clinical rounds with the house staff and medical students.
2. Demonstrate mature clinical judgment related to the spectrum of problems encountered in hemorrhagic and ischemic stroke states.
3. Formulate independent plans for patient assessment and management, including prioritization in cerebrovascular disease, while maintaining a clear reporting relationship with the faculty.
4. Supervise house staff and medical student teams in daily patient assessment and care.
5. Identify the indications and controversies of endovascular catheter procedures, perioperative management, and follow-up. Implement and supervise patient care protocols related to these procedures.

6. Display a mature and detailed understanding of indications, principles, and interpretation of the full spectrum of the neurodiagnostic armamentarium. Formulate independent management plans based on sophisticated interpretation of diagnostic studies for concise presentation to faculty.
7. Apply evolving technology and new methods to patient protocols and to the education of house staff and medical students.
8. Demonstrate a mature understanding of surgical strategies and approaches to common and unusual vascular disease.
9. Apply the principles of intraoperative anesthetic management, proximal and distal control, temporary arterial occlusion, brain protective strategies, and intraoperative localization as applied to vascular disease.
10. Complete the planning, positioning, and execution of pterional craniotomy for common vascular disease.
11. Perform microsurgical dissection of the Sylvian fissure and exposure of the basal cisterns for vascular disease.
12. Perform microsurgical exposure and clipping of an intracranial aneurysm.
13. Complete the planning, positioning, and execution of nonpterional craniotomy for intracranial vascular disease.
14. Assist in the microsurgical management of highly complex cerebrovascular disease.
15. Plan and execute a craniotomy for the evacuation of intracranial hematomas.
16. Supervise other house staff in meeting their surgical objectives.
17. Describe the exposure and treatment of intraspinal vascular lesions. Assist in such operations.
18. Oversee all aspects of patient care and identify appropriate cases for database analysis, morbidity, mortality, conferences, and discussions. Supervise medical students and house staff in every aspect of patient care.
19. Report appropriate patient care issues to responsible faculty members in a timely fashion.
20. Organize and administer teaching conferences.
21. Display mature participation in specialty conferences.
22. Assign responsibilities to junior residents and residents, with the aim of fulfilling their respective educational objectives.

NEUROSURGICAL ONCOLOGY

Unit Objectives

Demonstrate an understanding of the anatomy, physiology, pathophysiology, and presentation of tumor-related diseases of the cranium.

Demonstrate the ability to formulate and implement a diagnostic and treatment plan for tumor-related diseases of the cranium that are amenable to surgical intervention.

Competency-Based Knowledge Objectives

JUNIOR LEVEL

1. Summarize the epidemiology, incidence, and risk factors for intracranial neoplasms.
2. Summarize the tenets of tumor biology including genetic factors and biochemical processes associated with invasion. Describe the natural history of intracranial neoplasms.
3. List a differential diagnosis of lesions requiring biopsy and describe their pathophysiology.
4. List the various types of bone tumors involving the calvarium.
5. Describe and differentiate
   a. astrocytomas, including the accepted World Health Organization grading scheme
   b. gliomas other than astrocytomas
   c. metastatic tumors, including location and common origins
   d. infectious, granulomatous, and cystic lesions that may present in a tumor-like manner
6. Define the cell or origin of meningioma, its common intracranial locations, and the expected presentation for each location.
7. Define the embryological origin of arachnoid cysts and their natural history. List the etiologies of other cystic lesions of the brain, including tumorous and infectious lesions.
8. Describe the anatomic location, cell of origin, clinical presentation, age at presentation, and natural history of common intrinsic posterior fossa neoplasms, including cerebellar astrocytoma, medulloblastoma, and ependymoma.
9. Describe the anatomy of the posterior fossa and the relation of the cranial nerves to the brainstem and skull.
10. Illustrate the relationship of the facial, vestibular, and cochlear components of the acoustic nerve at the internal auditory meatus.
11. Describe the various tumors that may arise in the cerebellopontine angle.
12. Describe the management of a patient with a brain abscess, including the role of stereotactic drainage or open drainage.
13. Explain the medical workup of a patient with a diagnosed brain abscess.
14. Specify the follow-up and evaluation of the patient with a brain abscess after surgical treatment.

15. Describe the embryological origin of craniopharyngioma. List the common locations of the tumor.
16. Describe the common presentations of pituitary tumors, the cell of origin, and endocrinopathies associated with
    a. null cell adenomas
    b. somatotrophic adenomas
    c. prolactinomas
    d. corticotrophic secreting adenomas
    e. thyrotrophic secreting adenomas
17. Define the medical management of the secreting pituitary tumors. Explain the role of surgery in each of the tumors just listed.
18. Describe the etiology of fibrous dysplasia, its presentation, and general management. List the indications for surgery for benign tumors of bone at the base of the skull, and potential adjuvant therapy.
19. List the tumors that may be approached routinely through a transtemporal route.
20. Describe the indications for use of lumbar spinal drainage in skull base surgery, and its implementation. List all complications associated with continuous lumbar spinal drainage.
21. Illustrate the general principles of stereotaxis and the underlying localization techniques used in the currently used frame-based and frameless systems.

MIDDLE LEVEL

1. Describe appropriate postoperative management with drainage of brain abscess or cyst.
2. Describe the appropriate surgical management and postoperative treatment of bony skull lesions.
3. Describe the role of surgery in arachnoid cysts, infectious cysts, and tumor-related cystic lesions. Describe the adjuvant treatment of parasitic cysts.
4. Explain the rationale and indications for various skull base approaches to the anterior, middle, and posterior cranial fossae. Identify the important anatomic landmarks for each approach. Illustrate the general principles used in prophylaxis of CSF leaks employed in skull base surgery.
5. Describe the neurosurgical management for the following tumors involving the anterior cranial fossa.
    a. meningioma
    b. fibrous dysplasia

   c. esthesioneuroblastoma
   d. osteoma of the frontal sinus
   e. chondroma, chordoma
   f. mucocele
   g. bony metastasis
6. Explain the use of the balloon occlusion test of the carotid artery, its indication for use in skull base tumor surgery, how it is performed, and how the information gained influences surgical management.
7. Explain the surgical advantage of transposing the facial nerve during a transtemporal skull base approach.
8. Describe the transcondylar approach, the relationship of the lower cranial nerves, and the exposure gained over a routine suboccipital craniectomy.
9. Illustrate the transpetrosal approach and the relationship of the transverse and sigmoid sinuses with skull bony landmarks such as the asterion, mastoid, and inion.
10. Describe the intradural course of the trochlear nerve, trigeminal nerve through Meckel's cave, and the abducens nerve and Dorello's canal.
11. Describe the surgical management of the frontal sinus that has been exposed during craniotomy for anterior skull base surgery. Illustrate the development and use of a frontal vascularized pericranial flap and explain its indication. Similarly, illustrate the use of a musculocutaneous flap of the temporalis muscle and list the locations for application.
12. Describe the general methods used for embolization of tumors of the head and neck, and the indications for such procedures.
13. Compare and contrast the methods for stereotactic radiation, including particle beam, gamma ray, or linear accelerator, and the indications for each technique.

SENIOR LEVEL

1. Describe the indications for transcranial orbitotomy and list the lesions that require this approach.
2. Discuss the surgical management and postoperative treatment of astrocytomas, gliomas other than astrocytomas, metastatic brain tumors, infectious granulomas, and cystic lesions presenting in a tumor-like manner. Review the role of radiotherapy, chemotherapy, and other adjunctive treatments of these neoplasms.
3. Describe the role of surgery for intracranial meningioma, and the relation between the surgical option and the location of the

tumor. Discuss adjuvant treatments of meningioma and their efficacy.

4. Discuss the surgical treatment of common, intrinsic posterior fossa neoplasms, including cerebellar astrocytoma, medulloblastoma, and ependymoma, including the roles of ventricular drainage and surveillance imaging. Present adjuvant treatment options and outcomes for the various posterior fossa intrinsic tumors.
5. Address the surgical goals of treatment, complications of surgical treatment, and adjuvant therapy for posterior fossa meningioma.
6. List and illustrate the various approaches for removal of a vestibular schwannoma, and the rationale and indication for each approach.
7. Describe the role of stereotactic radiosurgery and microsurgery in the management of vestibular schwannoma.
8. List the various approaches to the midline clivus and review the indications for each approach. Outline the surgical and medical management of tumors of the clivus and midline skull base.
9. Explain the management goal for a patient with craniopharyngioma, and the risks of surgical treatment and conservative treatment. Describe the various surgical approaches used to resect craniopharyngiomas and the options for adjuvant treatment, including radiotherapy and chemotherapy (systemic and local).
10. Illustrate the transnasal–transsphenoidal approach and its indications. Define the options for treatment of recurrent pituitary tumors of all types (including medical management). Describe the risks of the approach and the management of the complication of CSF leak.
11. Illustrate the various skull base approaches to the anterior, middle, and posterior cranial fossae in detail, explaining the key anatomic landmarks and strict indications for the approach. List the complications relevant to each approach and the management of each complication.
12. List a differential diagnosis of orbital tumors, their usual location within the orbit, medical and surgical management of the tumor, and the approach used to remove the tumor if indicated.
13. List the various tumors and their locations in which an orbitocranial approach may be indicated for their removal.
14. Compare and contrast the exposure offered by the pre- and postauricular infratemporal approach, and the indications for each approach.

15. Illustrate transposition of the facial nerve during a transtemporal skull base approach.
16. Describe the location of meningiomas intracranially that are amenable to preoperative embolization.

Competency-Based Performance Objectives

JUNIOR LEVEL

1. Perform a complete history and physical examination on patients with intracranial neoplasms.
2. Review appropriate radiographic studies with a radiologist and formulate a differential diagnosis for patients with intracranial neoplasms.
3. Prepare patients for cranial tumor surgery.
4. Understand the positioning of patients for craniotomy and craniectomy.
5. Assist in the opening and closing of craniotomies and craniectomies for neoplasms.
6. Place lumbar drains.
7. Demonstrate the ability to open and close scalp incisions.
8. Perform ventriculostomies.
9. Demonstrate proper postoperative wound care.

MIDDLE LEVEL

1. Determine independently a differential diagnosis based on the patient's history, physical examination, and radiographic studies.
2. Position patients for craniotomy and craniectomy.
3. Perform the opening and closing of craniotomies and craniectomies.
4. Assist in the resection of intracranial neoplasms.
5. Resect skull lesions.
6. Treat supra- and infratentorial brain abscesses surgically.
7. Demonstrate the ability to manage postoperative complications including
   a. brain edema
   b. meningitis
   c. cranial flap infection
   d. postoperative seizures
8. Assess the need for appropriate pre-, intra-, and postoperative monitoring.
9. Obtain proper non-neurosurgical consultation in tumor patients.
10. Identify patients requiring rehabilitation services.
11. Use appropriate support agencies and groups for patients with intracranial neoplasms.

SENIOR LEVEL

1. Demonstrate the capability to function independently in all phases of management of patients with intracranial neoplasms.
2. Perform resection of supra- and infratentorial intra-axial and extra-axial neoplasms.
3. Perform resection of pituitary lesions.
4. Perform or serve as first assistant for skull base procedures.
5. Oversee the pre- and postoperative management of patients with intracranial neoplasms.
6. Assume teaching responsibilities for junior residents as assigned.
7. Assume responsibility for managing the psychosocial aspects of intracranial neoplasms.

NEUROTRAUMA AND NEUROSURGICAL CRITICAL CARE

Unit Objectives

Demonstrate an understanding of the anatomy, physiology, pathophysiology, and presentation of traumatic injuries of the brain, spinal cord, and peripheral nervous system, including their supporting structures. Demonstrate the ability to formulate and implement appropriate diagnostic and treatment plans for traumatic injuries to the nervous system, including both surgical and nonsurgical management.

Competency-Based Knowledge Objectives

JUNIOR LEVEL

1. Describe the systematic assessment of polytrauma patients.
2. Rank management priorities in polytrauma patients appropriately.
3. Discuss principles of resuscitation of polytrauma patients, including appropriate fluid resuscitation, and explain the anticipated effects of shock and resuscitation on fluid shifts and on electrolyte balance.
4. Name an initial choice for intravenous fluids for newly admitted intensive care unit (ICU) patients with the following diagnoses and explain changes in that choice based on specific changes in the patient's diagnosis, clinical condition, and electrolyte and volume status.
   a. head injury
   b. stroke
   c. tumor
   d. infection
   e. hydrocephalus
5. Propose appropriate initial ventilator settings for patients with different types of common neurosurgical conditions and explain

changes in that choice based on specific changes in the patient's metabolic or pulmonary status.

6. List the mechanisms of action and potential complications of commonly used pressors and hypotensive agents.
7. Discuss indications, pharmacological mechanism, duration of action, and effect on the neurological examination for sedative, paralytic, and analgesic agents commonly used in the ICU.
8. Explain the indications, advantages, and risks for various hemodynamic monitoring tools (e.g., pulmonary artery catheters, indwelling arterial lines) used in critically ill patients.
9. Discuss the pathophysiology and management of coagulopathy after head injury.
10. Describe basic principles of nutritional management in neurosurgical critical care.
11. Explain the treatment of post-traumatic seizures.
12. Outline basic principles of ICU management of patients with spinal cord injury.
13. Name the major structures supplied by the major vessels of the brain and spinal cord.
14. Discuss the evaluation, treatment, and prognosis of subarachnoid hemorrhage, both traumatic and spontaneous.
15. Explain the pathophysiology and treatment of cerebral vasospasm.
16. Formulate a diagnostic and treatment plan for patients with cerebral ischemia.
17. Explain the evaluation and management of birth-related intracranial hemorrhage, spinal cord injury, and brachial plexus injury.
18. Describe a systematic approach to the examination of the peripheral nervous system.
19. Describe the basic principles of management of peripheral nerve injuries.
20. List the principles of rehabilitation of different types of neurosurgical patients.
21. Define brain death and discuss methods of making such a diagnosis.
22. Describe the pathophysiology of electrical injuries to the nervous system and review their treatment.

MIDDLE LEVEL

1. Describe the pathophysiology of intracranial hypertension and explain a plan for its management, including arguments for and against various treatments.

SENIOR LEVEL

1. Discuss management priorities in polytrauma patients with severe neurological and systemic trauma.

Competency-Based Performance Objectives

JUNIOR LEVEL

1. Perform and document pertinent history, physical findings, and radiological findings in a polytrauma patient.
2. Differentiate central from peripheral nervous system injuries.
3. Insert intravascular monitoring devices for use in the hemodynamic management of critically ill patients, including central venous lines, pulmonary artery catheters, and arterial catheters.
4. Insert ICP monitoring devices, including ventriculostomy catheters and electronic (fiberoptic or miniaturized strain gauge) devices.
5. Perform twist-drill or burr-hole drainage of subdural fluid collections.
6. Decide appropriately which patients require emergency craniotomy and other procedures.
7. Position patients appropriately for procedures/surgery and begin emergency procedures if more experienced neurosurgeons have not yet arrived.
8. Assist with opening and closure of craniotomies.
9. Perform elective tracheotomies and be able to perform emergency tracheotomies.
10. Be able to intubate patients in both emergency and elective situations.

MIDDLE LEVEL

1. Perform the following surgical procedures in uncomplicated cases.
   a. craniotomy for subdural and/or epidural hematoma
   b. craniotomy for penetrating head injury
   c. craniotomy for intracerebral hematoma or contusion
   d. craniotomy for depressed skull fracture
   e. decompressive craniectomy
   f. repair/cranialization of frontal sinus fracture
   g. craniotomy/craniectomy for posterior fossa epidural, subdural, or intracerebral hematoma
   h. simple cranioplasty

2. Manage traumatic skull base fractures with a CSF leak.
3. Manage infections associated with open CNS injuries.

SENIOR LEVEL

1. Perform the procedures for middle level, item 1, in complicated cases.
2. Reconstruct complex cranial defects with assistance from other specialties as indicated.
3. Reconstruct traumatic skull base defects with assistance from other specialties as indicated.
4. Explore and repair peripheral nerve injuries.
5. Supervise and teach junior- and middle-level residents with patients appropriate for their level.
6. Lead the critical care team in the treatment of patients with neurological injuries, either in isolation or in polytrauma patients.

PAIN MANAGEMENT

Unit Objectives

Demonstrate an understanding of the anatomic and physiological substrates of pain and pain disorders. Demonstrate an ability to formulate and execute diagnostic and therapeutic plans for management of pain and disorders giving rise to pain.

Competency-Based Knowledge Objectives

JUNIOR LEVEL

1. Describe the anatomy and physiology of nociception within the peripheral and central nervous systems.
2. Differentiate the basic categories of pain syndromes.
   a. acute
   b. chronic
   c. nociceptive
   d. neuropathic (including complex regional pain syndromes)
   e. musculofascial
   f. cancer related
   g. postoperative
3. Explain the concept of pain as a biopsychosocial disorder.
4. Discuss the role of rehabilitation in pain management.
5. Describe methods for assessing pain in pediatric patients.
6. Discuss ethical standards in pain management and research.
7. Discuss methods of assessing outcomes of pain treatment and describe common assessment tools.

8. Describe a typical history of a patient with trigeminal neuralgia, trigeminal neuropathic pain, and atypical facial pain.
9. Diagram the anatomy of the trigeminal nerve divisions (ophthalmic, maxillary, and mandibular nerves), foramen ovale, Meckel's cave, trigeminal (gasserian) ganglion, cistern of Meckel's cave, retrogasserian root, descending tract and nuclei, nervus intermedius, and glossopharyngeal nerve.
10. Illustrate the appropriate medical management of patients with trigeminal neuralgia, trigeminal neuropathic pain, and atypical facial pain.
11. Discuss the potential complications of percutaneous procedures for trigeminal neuralgia.
12. Describe the brainstem anatomy and physiology of the spinothalamic and trigeminothalamic systems.
13. Describe the anatomy of the primary sensory cortex (S1), Rolandic fissure, and the relationship of S1 to the primary motor cortex.
14. Describe the functional anatomy of the following thalamic nuclei: ventral posterolateral, ventralis caudalis externus, ventral posteromedial, and ventralis caudalis internus. Review the functional anatomy of the medial thalamic nuclei (e.g., nervus parafascicularis).
15. Identify the primary indications for spinal cord stimulation (SCS), peripheral nerve stimulation, and intraspinal (epidural, intrathecal) drug infusion therapy.
16. Diagram the spinal anatomy pertinent to SCS and intraspinal drug administration, including the spinous process–interspinal ligament–spinous process complex, ligamentum flavum, and dorsal epidural space. Review the different degrees of angulation of the spinous processes at various spine levels in the cervical and thoracic areas.
17. Diagram the spinal cord anatomy pertinent to spinal ablative procedures for pain management.
18. Recognize complications arising from implantation of pulse generators/receivers and infusion pumps.
19. Describe the anatomy of the major peripheral nerves, brachial plexus, and lumbosacral plexus.
20. Describe the anatomy of the sympathetic nervous system and explain its role in pain.
21. List the common mechanisms of peripheral nerve injury and describe the changes that occur in an injured nerve at both the microscopic and macroscopic levels. Explain the theories of pain generation in peripheral nerve injury.

22. Describe the pharmacology of local anesthetic agents (e.g., lidocaine, procaine, tetracaine, bupivacaine) and the use of epinephrine with local anesthetic agents.
23. Discuss the indications for a peripheral neural blockade. Explain the principles of blocking procedures including the techniques and expected outcomes. Cite the complications of a peripheral neural blockade (including anaphylaxis, neural injury, and intravascular or intrathecal administration). List the alternatives to a temporary blockade including neurolytic blocks, ablative neurosurgical procedures, augmentative neurosurgical procedures, alternative traditional pain management procedures, and alternative medicine approaches.
24. Review the indications for radiofrequency facet rhizolysis.
25. Discuss the anatomy and biomechanics of the facet complex with emphasis on bone, cartilage, fibrous capsule, synovial fluid, and innervation of this structure.

MIDDLE LEVEL

1. Name and differentiate the major classes of medications that are used commonly for pain treatment (opioids, nonsteroidals and acetaminophen, antidepressants, anticonvulsants).
2. Review the psychosocial issues that may influence a pain disorder and describe the role of behavioral interventions in pain management.
3. Explain the rationale for multidisciplinary management of pain disorders.
4. Contrast impairment and disability.
5. Explain the basis of chemical, balloon compression, and radiofrequency neurolysis in the treatment of trigeminal neuralgia.
6. Relate subcortical and brainstem sites that appear to be involved in the modulation of nociception to targets for deep brain stimulation for pain control.
7. Explain how central neurostimulation (cortical, subcortical) is thought to produce analgesia.
8. Explain the role of ablative brain and brainstem procedures (e.g., cingulotomy, mesencephalic tractotomy, trigeminal tractotomy) in the management of chronic benign pain and cancer pain.
9. Discuss the possible complications of subcortical and brainstem ablative procedures for deafferention pain.
10. List the primary indications for the following spinal ablative lesions.
    a. dorsal root entry zone (DREZ) lesion

   b. open and percutaneous anterolateral cordotomy
   c. myelotomy
11. Discuss SCS, including types of stimulation systems and electrodes available, basic techniques of insertion of percutaneous and plate electrodes, the rationale and goals of intraoperative SCS testing (paresthesia coverage of painful area, avoidance of undesirable stimulation), the rationale and techniques for testing SCS, and the advantages and disadvantages of different sites of implantation of a SCS pulse generator/receiver.
12. Explain the key aspects of intraspinal drug administration, including the pharmacology of intraspinal drugs, the various types of infusion systems available, the rationale for testing intraspinal drug infusions, basic techniques for insertion of intrathecal and epidural catheters, and the proper location for infusion pump implantation.
13. Discuss the role of neurectomy and neurolysis for pain control in nerve injury and compare alternative techniques for pain control.
14. Describe the anatomy of the dorsal root ganglion, the bony anatomy of the nerve root foramen, and the location of the ganglion within that foramen. Discuss indications for ganglionectomy and describe long-term outcome from ganglionectomy with emphasis on pain recurrence and deafferentation.
15. Describe the indications for peripheral nerve stimulation and contrast them with SCS.
16. Describe indications for ablative peripheral neurolysis. Review the pharmacology and histopathological effects of neurolytical agents (e.g., phenol, glycerine/glycerol, chlorocresol, absolute alcohol, ammonium chloride/sulfate).
17. Discuss basic principles of ablative neurolytic procedures in terms of technique, expected outcomes, and complications including neural injury, injury to surrounding soft tissue, and inadvertent intravascular or intrathecal administration. Describe the alternatives to neurolysis, including temporary anesthetic blocks, ablative neurosurgical procedures, augmentative procedures, alternative traditional pain management procedures, and alternative medicine approaches.
18. Describe the principles of radiofrequency lesioning. Include in the discussion the following topics.
   a. probe
   b. thermocouple and thermistor
   c. time

   d. intensity of heat
   e. isotherm fields
19. Discuss basic principles of radiofrequency facet rhizolysis and list the equipment used, technique employed, expected outcomes, and complications (including damage to other nerve root branches, potential for spinal instability, inadvertent damage to the radicular artery, CSF leak, and spinal cord injury).
20. Compare the alternatives to radiofrequency lesioning.
   a. local anesthetic facet blocks
   b. epidural injections
   c. neurolytical facet blocks
   d. ablative neurosurgical procedures
   e. augmentative neurosurgical procedures
   f. alternative traditional pain management procedures
   g. alternative medicine approaches
   h. surgical intervention such as instrumentation and fusion

SENIOR LEVEL

1. Distinguish the indications for surgical and nonsurgical treatment of pain.
2. Construct a management strategy relating to the application of percutaneous trigeminal neurolytical procedures, retrogasserian rhizotomy, and microvascular decompression in the care of patients with trigeminal neuralgia.
3. Describe and contrast the approaches to the cerebellopontine angle for microvascular decompression or rhizotomy of the trigeminal and glossopharyngeal nerves.
4. Identify the various target spine levels for SCS according to the pain topography (simple and complex).
5. Identify the various intraspinal structures based on their responses to mechanical and electrical stimulation (dura mater, lateral canal wall, dorsal columns, dorsal roots, ventral roots, motor neurons).
6. Compare the different methods of intraspinal drug administration (epidural, intrathecal, tunneled catheter, implanted infusion system).
7. Describe the techniques for testing intraspinal drugs.
8. Compare the pharmacodynamics of different drugs delivered intrathecally (e.g., hydrophilic versus lipophilic).
9. Describe the possible complications of SCS electrode or spinal catheter insertion and their evaluation and treatment.
   a. paralysis

   b. nerve root damage
   c. electrode or catheter migration
   d. electrode or catheter breakage
   e. epidural hematoma
   f. CSF leak
10. Describe the common drug side effects associated with intraspinal analgesic administration.
11. Describe the correct placement of lesions for DREZ, cordotomy, and myelotomy, including lesion depth and structures affected.
12. Discuss the possible neurological sequelae of spinal ablative procedures with both correct and incorrect lesion placement, with anatomic correlates.
13. Describe the role of DREZ lesioning in the overall management of the patient with deafferented pain.
14. Describe the techniques for exposure of the major peripheral nerves.
15. Demonstrate knowledge of the basic principles of nerve grafting, including regeneration, graft length considerations, and use of allograft donor nerves.
16. Describe the role and outcomes of ganglionectomy in the management of various pain syndromes, contrasting it with augmentative techniques.
17. Discuss in detail the surgical technique of ganglionectomy.
18. Describe percutaneous methods of gangliolysis.
19. Explain the effects of blocking agents at the membrane and synaptic cleft, and the biochemistry and histology of neurotoxicity.
20. Explain the histological effects of neurolytic agents at the membrane level and display a comprehensive level of understanding with regard to toxicity.
21. Describe the histological effects of radiofrequency lesioning.
22. Discuss in detail the evaluation and management of a patient selected for radiofrequency lesioning of the facets.
23. Discuss the alternatives to radiofrequency lesioning, with particular emphasis on the potential surgical remedies including decompression, instrumentation, and fusion.

Competency-Based Performance Objectives

JUNIOR LEVEL

1. Obtain a pertinent history and perform an appropriate physical examination for a patient with a primary complaint of pain.
2. Formulate and implement treatment plans for simple pain syndromes (e.g., acute postoperative pain, acute low back pain).

3. Evaluate and diagnose a patient with trigeminal neuralgia, trigeminal neuropathic pain, and atypical facial pain.
4. Assist with radiofrequency, glycerol, or balloon compression neurolysis of the trigeminal nerve in patients with trigeminal neuralgia.
5. Assist with surgical exploration of the trigeminal nerve, nervus intermedius, or glossopharyngeal nerve for MVD or rhizotomy.
6. Illustrate appropriate patient selection for spinal ablative or augmentative procedures for pain management.
7. Locate the spinal epidural space and place a percutaneous SCS electrode with supervision.
8. Assist with the implantation of a plate electrode for SCS.
9. Insert with supervision a spinal catheter for drug administration.
10. Implant with supervision an SCS system pulse generator/receiver and extension wire.
11. Implant with supervision an intraspinal drug infusion pump.
12. Assist with a spinal ablative procedure for pain management (cordotomy, myelotomy, DREZ).
13. Perform, record, and report complete patient evaluation and assessment for peripheral nerve repair, neurectomy, and neurolysis, including a comprehensive neuromuscular examination of affected nerve distributions.
14. Evaluate electrodiagnostic studies pertaining to peripheral nerve injury.
15. Recognize and treat the potential complications of peripheral nerve repair, neurectomy, and neurolysis, including hematoma formation, infection, and local wound problems.
16. Assist in the surgical treatment of peripheral nerves.
17. Assist with the implantation of a peripheral nerve stimulation system.
18. Perform, record, and report a complete patient evaluation and assessment for dorsal root ganglionectomy.
19. Recognize and treat the potential complications of dorsal root ganglionectomy including CSF leak, infection, and local wound problems.
20. Assist in foraminotomy and exposure of dorsal root ganglion.
21. Assess patients for appropriateness of local anesthetic blocks.
22. Perform simple superficial blocks with supervision and assist in complicated procedures. After these procedures
    a. Assess the outcome of the nerve block.
    b. Recognize and treat complications.
    c. Record and monitor the effects of the block over a specified time interval.

   d. Assess the need for repeat blocks.
23. Assess the patient for appropriateness of ablative neurolysis. Perform simple superficial neurolysis with supervision and assist in complicated procedures. After ablative neurolysis
   a. Assess the outcome of the procedure.
   b. Recognize and treat complications.
   c. Record and monitor the effects of neurolysis over a specified time interval.
   d. Assess the need for repeat procedures.

MIDDLE LEVEL

1. Formulate and implement an appropriate treatment program for complicated pain syndromes (e.g., chronic back pain, "failed back surgery syndrome").
2. Assess the need for multidisciplinary management of pain disorders.
3. Demonstrate appropriate management of psychosocial factors complicating a pain disorder.
4. Employ the Hartel technique to perform radiofrequency, glycerol, or balloon compression neurolysis of the trigeminal nerve in patients with trigeminal neuralgia.
5. Implant a plate electrode.
6. Demonstrate appropriate methods for testing SCS and intraspinal drug administration systems.
7. Implant a peripheral nerve stimulation system.
8. Assess the patient for appropriateness of radiofrequency facet blocks. Perform radiofrequency facet blocks with supervision. After performing these procedures
   a. Assess the outcome of the facet blocks.
   b. Recognize and treat complications.
   c. Record and monitor the effects of the facet blocks over a specified time interval.
   d. Assess the need for repeat facet blocks.
9. Diagnose and formulate appropriate treatment plans for sympathetically maintained pain.
10. Diagnose and formulate an appropriate treatment plan for a patient with occipital neuralgia.

SENIOR LEVEL

1. Recognize and execute intelligent treatment choices for different pain syndromes including nociceptive, neuropathic, and cancer pain.

2. Demonstrate the appropriate use of each of the major classes of medications in common use for treating pain.
3. Demonstrate the appropriate selection of patients for surgical treatment of pain disorders.
4. Perform microvascular decompression and rhizotomy of the trigeminal nerve and glossopharyngeal nerves.
5. Assist a junior resident in performing a percutaneous ablative procedure for trigeminal neuralgia.
6. Formulate and implement an appropriate treatment plan for management of pain using spinal ablative and augmentative techniques according to pain etiology, pain topography, and status of spinal column (e.g., previous surgery at implant level, scoliosis, stenosis, etc.).
7. Select and implant an appropriate SCS system, recognizing how to modify the electrode insertion technique and location based on intraoperative responses.
8. Implant a plate electrode in a patient with previous spinal surgery at the same level.
9. Demonstrate proficiency with maintenance and programming of spinal drug administration systems and SCS systems.
10. Recognize and evaluate malfunctions of SCS and intraspinal drug administration systems.
11. Perform surgical revision of SCS and intraspinal drug administration systems.
12. Demonstrate proficiency in identification and lesioning of the DREZ, even in cases of nerve root avulsion.
13. Demonstrate proficiency in performing myelotomy and cordotomy.
14. Expose major peripheral nerves and perform closure of extremity incision for peripheral neurectomy/neurolysis.
15. Demonstrate proficiency in neurolysis and nerve grafting techniques.
16. Plan and execute surgical approaches to injuries of the major peripheral nerves.
17. Plan a peripheral nerve reconstruction including exposure, preparation of donor site, and nerve graft.
18. Demonstrate proficiency in the technique of ganglion resection.
19. Incorporate ganglionectomy as one part of an integrated approach to the patient with intractable pain.
20. Display appropriate patient selection for local anesthetic blocks.
21. Perform simple superficial blocks with minimal supervision. Relative to these blocks perform the following.
    a. Assess the outcome of the block.

   b. Recognize and treat complications.
   c. Maintain detailed records of the effects of the block and follow-up.
   d. Assess the need for repeat blocks.
22. Provide information regarding alternatives for a failed nerve block.
23. Perform complicated nerve block procedures with direct supervision. Recognize and treat the complications of these procedures.
24. Display appropriate patient selection for ablative peripheral neurolysis.
25. Perform simple neurolytic procedures with minimal supervision. Relative to these procedures perform the following.
   a. Assess the outcome of the procedure.
   b. Recognize and treat complications.
   c. Maintain detailed records of the effects of neurolysis and follow-up.
   d. Assess the need for repeat neurolysis.
26. Provide information regarding alternatives for failed neurolysis.
27. Perform complicated neurolytic procedures with direct supervision.
28. Display appropriate patient selection for radiofrequency facet rhizolysis.
29. Perform simple facet blocks with minimal supervision. Relative to these procedures perform the following.
   a. Assess the outcome of the procedure.
   b. Recognize and treat complications.
   c. Maintain detailed records of the effects of the facet blocks and follow-up.
   d. Assess the need for repeat facet blocks.
30. Provide information regarding alternatives for failed facet blocks.
31. Perform complicated facet blocks with direct supervision.
32. Perform sympathectomy.

PEDIATRIC NEUROSURGERY

Unit Objectives

Demonstrate an understanding of the anatomy, physiology, pathophysiology, and presentation of diseases in children that a neurosurgeon may be called on to diagnose and treat. Demonstrate the ability to formulate and implement a diagnostic and treatment plan for these diseases.

Competency-Based Knowledge Objectives

JUNIOR LEVEL

Myelomeningocele and Its Variants, Meningocele, Encephalocele, Chiari Malformations, Occult Spinal Dysraphism, Split Cord Anomalies, Segmentation Anomalies, Craniofacial Syndromes, and Phakomatosis

1. Review the embryology of the CNS and its supporting structures.
2. List the abnormalities a neurosurgeon may treat that are congenital/developmental in nature and classify them with respect to their embryological defect.
3. Describe the incidence, epidemiology, and inheritance patterns.
4. State other disorders associated with this set of diseases.
5. Describe the anatomic and pathophysiological parameters that distinguish among these diseases.
6. Develop a diagnostic treatment plan along with a prognostication of the outcome with optimal management.
7. List disorders that may be referred for neurosurgical care but do not require surgery.
8. Display current knowledge of the molecular basis for these diseases when known.
9. Describe the expected outcome if treatment is not undertaken.

Hydrocephalus and Other Disorders of CSF Circulation

1. Describe the normal physiology of CSF.
2. Delineate the different etiologies of hydrocephalus and their relative incidence.
3. Explain how to differentiate between CSF collections that require treatment and those that do not.
4. Indicate the various treatment options for the management of hydrocephalus.
5. Distinguish between treatment options for hydrocephalus with normal CSF and contaminated CSF (e.g., infection, blood).
6. List the complications associated with each treatment option for hydrocephalus and the diagnosis and their treatment.
7. Differentiate between low-pressure and high-pressure hydrocephalus.
8. Describe the presentation and diagnostic approach to a patient with suspected shunt malfunction.
9. Define how the diagnosis of hydrocephalus is made.
10. List nonsurgical diseases that may be mistaken for hydrocephalus but require treatment different than surgery.

11. Review the causes of cerebral atrophy.

Neoplasia

1. Delineate the differences between pediatric and adult tumors.
2. List the common tumor types occurring in children and their typical location.
3. Describe the changing tumor type and location based on age.
4. Identify lesions that require biopsy as part of the treatment and diagnostic plan.
5. Describe the typical presentations of tumors.
6. Describe the appropriate evaluation for patients suspected of having a tumor.
7. Classify tumor types regarding degree of malignancy, role of surgical versus nonsurgical therapy, and outcomes of optimal treatment.
8. Discuss the possible complications associated with specific tumor types.
9. Describe the pertinent anatomy for surgical treatment of midline or hemispheric cerebellar tumors and hemispheric cerebral tumors.
10. Discuss the appropriate preoperative management of patients with tumors.
11. Compare the role of biopsy, subtotal resection, and total resection in the management of tumors.
12. List the possible complications of the treatment options, their diagnostic evaluation, and treatment.

Infection

1. Describe the presentations of a shunt infection.
2. List the indications for ventricular lumbar and subarachnoid CSF sampling.
3. List the common organisms seen in shunt infections.
4. Describe treatment plans for shunt infection.
5. List risk factors, risks of shunt infection, and the proper diagnostic protocol to establish the presence of a shunt infection.
6. Describe the common presentations of intracranial and intraspinal suppuration.
7. List the host risk factors that are associated with CNS infections.
8. Describe the appropriate diagnostic protocol to establish the presence of CNS infection.
9. Discuss the timeliness and usefulness of surgical therapy for the treatment of CNS infection both shunt related and nonshunt related.

Other

1. Delineate the various types of spasticity and movement disorders seen in children.
2. List seizure types.
3. Describe surgical lesions that may be related to seizures.
4. Describe surgical and nonsurgical treatment options regarding the alleviation of spasticity in children.
5. Discuss the pathophysiology of craniosynostosis.

Cerebrovascular

1. Delineate the possible causes of an atraumatic intracerebral or subarachnoid hemorrhage.
2. Delineate the possible causes of cerebral infarction/ischemia.
3. Discuss the common locations of arteriovenous shunts and their presentation, evaluation, and treatment (includes dural arteriovenous malformations).
4. Discuss the embryology of the cerebral and spinal vasculature and its possible role in vascular anomalies in children.
5. Describe the common locations and types of aneurysms seen in children and how they differ from those seen in adults.
6. List the possible presentations of vein of Galen aneurysms, their diagnosis, and management.
7. List the possible causes of aneurysms in children that are not congenital in nature.
8. Describe the pathophysiology, treatment, and outcome of intraventricular hemorrhage in the neonate.

Trauma

1. List the appropriate diagnostic tests to evaluate a child who has sustained multisystem trauma.
2. Describe the Glasgow Coma Scale and its use.
3. List the salient historical and examination features that lead one to the diagnosis of nonaccidental trauma.
4. Discuss the management of the cervical spine in a child who is comatose.
5. Describe the anatomy of the child's spine that causes the epidemiology of spinal cord injury to differ from adults.
6. Describe the common injuries seen as a result of birth trauma and discuss their diagnosis and management.
7. Describe the use of antibiotics and anticonvulsants in CNS trauma.
8. Review the evaluation and management of a child who has

sustained a head injury with loss of consciousness but is now awake.

9. Discuss the management of depressed skull fractures, both open and closed.
10. Describe the diagnosis and management of spinal column injury.
11. Discuss the diagnosis and management of spinal cord injury without radiological abnormality.
12. Describe the ICP compliance curve and discuss its usefulness in the management of head injury.
13. List the parameters needed to decide on letting an athlete who has sustained a CNS injury return to activity.
14. Discuss the concept of brain death, its diagnosis, and its role in organ donation.
15. Discuss the importance and interplay between ICP and cerebral perfusion pressure in the management of head and spinal cord injury.
16. Define the concept of "secondary injury."
17. Discuss the role of invasive monitoring in all its forms in closed head injury.

MIDDLE LEVEL

Myelomeningocele and Its Variants, Meningocele, Encephalocele, Chiari Malformations, Occult Spinal Dysraphism, Split Cord Anomalies, Segmentation Anomalies, Craniofacial Syndromes, and Phakomatosis

1. Enumerate the indications for surgery, surgical options, and expected outcomes for each disease entity.
2. Explain the indications for and the usefulness of intraoperative monitoring.
3. Describe the appropriate timing of intervention and its rationale.
4. Describe the pathophysiology and presentation of the tethered cord syndrome.

Hydrocephalus and Other Disorders of CSF Circulation

1. Describe normal ICP dynamics and their relation to establishing a differential diagnosis of CSF flow disturbance.
2. Define "slit ventricle system" and how it is diagnosed and treated.
3. Define "brain compliance" and relate how it can affect ventricular size.
4. List indications for and describe the technique of accessing a shunt for CSF samples.

5. List disease states that are commonly associated with hydrocephalus.

Neoplasia

1. Discuss the differential diagnosis and evaluation of tumors located in the following areas.
   a. suprasellar
   b. pineal
   c. intraventricular
2. Discuss the treatment and diagnostic options for tumors in each location listed in item 1 including surgical approaches.
3. Describe the appropriate evaluation and treatment of patients with neoplastic processes associated with
   a. neurofibromatosis
   b. tuberous sclerosis
   c. von Hippel Lindau
4. Discuss the appropriate use of skull base approaches for specific tumor locations.
5. List tumors that will require adjunctive therapy and describe those therapies and their potential complications.
6. Discuss the global management of tumorous hydrocephalus.
7. Cite the long-term outcome and complications for treatment of the common cerebellar and supratentorial hemispheric tumors.

Infection

1. Compare the differing patterns of infection as seen in immune-compromised patients with those with a functioning immune system.
2. Discuss the sequelae of CNS infection, both shunt related and nonshunt related.
3. List all acceptable treatment options for CNS infection with the pros and cons of each plan.
4. Demonstrate an understanding of the different etiologies for subdural and epidural empyema and brain abscess and their different treatments.
5. Provide a complete differential diagnosis with regard to infectious disease for ring-enhancing brain lesions.
6. Discuss the role of osteomyelitis in CNS infection.
7. Differentiate radiographically between infection and tumor of bone.

Other

1. Discuss variance in the surgical management of tumorous versus nontumorous seizure foci.

2. Discuss surgical options, indications, and outcome for nonlesional approaches (e.g., callosotomy).
3. Discuss various surgical options for the management of spasticity.
4. Discuss preoperative evaluation and planning for seizure treatment.
5. Discuss preoperative evaluation and planning for treatment of spasticity and postoperative management.

Cerebrovascular

1. Describe the nomenclature for congenital vascular anomalies and what role, if any, inheritance plays.
2. Describe the pathology, risk factors, diagnosis, and treatment of moyamoya in children.
3. List the phakomatoses that have vascular anomalies associated with them and their treatment.

Trauma

1. Discuss the role of apoptosis in brain and spinal cord injury.
2. Compare the usefulness of epidural, subdural, parenchymal, and intraventricular ICP monitoring.
3. Differentiate between retinal hemorrhages and Terson's syndrome.
4. Describe the role of electrophysiological monitoring in the management and prognostication of the CNS-injured patient.
5. Discuss the evidence for and role of steroid therapy in CNS injury.
6. Discuss the prognosis and management of penetrating injuries to the brain and spine.
7. Discuss the management of CSF leaks after head injury.
8. Describe the diagnosis and treatment of a traumatic leptomeningeal cyst.

SENIOR LEVEL

Myelomeningocele and Its Variants, Meningocele, Encephalocele, Chiari Malformations, Occult Spinal Dysraphism, Split Cord Anomalies, Segmentation Anomalies, Craniofacial Syndromes, and Phakomatosis

1. Differentiate between the use of rigid and nonrigid skeletal fixation in the appropriate surgical setting for this group of disorders.

2. Explain the rationale for surgical treatment of a symptomatic disease.

Hydrocephalus and Other Disorders of CSF Circulation

1. Discuss the usefulness of expansion craniotomy in the treatment of hydrocephalus.
2. Differentiate between ventriculomegaly, compensated hydrocephalus, and pseudotumor cerebri.
3. Describe the pertinent anatomy of the ventricular system and prepontine cisterns.
4. Describe the role of venous outflow obstruction in hydrocephalus.

Neoplasia

1. Describe the pertinent surgical anatomy for approaches to tumors in the following locations.
   a. suprasellar
   b. pineal
   c. intraventricular
2. Discuss the role of endoscopic third ventriculostomy in the management of tumorous hydrocephalus.
3. Cite the long-term outcome and complications of all treatment options for tumors arising in the following locations.
   a. suprasellar
   b. pineal
   c. intraventricular
4. Discuss the usefulness of preoperative embolization and/or chemotherapy in the surgical management of specific tumors.
5. Discuss the role of stereotactic radiosurgery in the management of selected tumors.
6. Describe the presentations of hypothalamic hamartomas and the role of surgery in management.
7. Describe options for CNS monitoring during surgical therapy and their efficacy.
8. Discuss options for treatment and expected outcomes for recurrent tumors.

Infection

1. Describe in detail the differential diagnosis, evolution, and treatment options of an immune-compromised patient with a ring-enhancing brain lesion.
2. List the important aspects of the patient's history that may lead one to entertain the diagnosis of CNS infection, both shunt related and nonshunt related.

3. List diagnostic tools, other than CSF culture, that are used to diagnose a shunt infection.

Cerebrovascular

1. List the locations for traumatic vascular lesions and their risk factors, diagnosis, and treatment.
2. Discuss the management options and controversies in the treatment of vascular disease in children.

Trauma

1. Discuss the potential complications and evaluation of comatose patients with skull base fractures.
2. Discuss the usefulness of lumbar drains and expansion craniectomy and the removal of the frontal or temporal lobes in the management of refractory, elevated ICP.
3. Describe the approaches to the management of traumatic intracranial hemorrhage and its supporting data, both surgical and nonsurgical.
4. List the vascular and endocrine complications seen after head injury.
5. Discuss the long-term management of a child who has sustained CNS trauma including rehabilitation and neurocognitive issues.
6. Discuss the management of peripheral nerve injuries in a child.

Competency-Based Performance Objectives

JUNIOR LEVEL

1. Perform a complete history, physical examination, and assessment on newborns, infants, and children.
2. Interpret the results of the physical examination, and laboratory and radiological studies to arrive at a differential diagnosis.
3. Perform subdural, intraventricular, and lumbar punctures in children.
4. Perform a shunt tap.
5. Perform a twist drill or burr hole for subdural, parenchymal, or ventricular access or as part of a craniotomy.
6. Perform a craniotomy or craniectomy for evacuation of a subdural or epidural lesion.
7. Perform a craniectomy as part of a skull biopsy.
8. Perform craniotomy for elevation of a depressed skull fracture.
9. Place a ventriculoperitoneal, jugular, or pleural shunt.
10. Revise a ventriculoperitoneal, jugular, or pleural shunt.
11. Perform a cranioplasty with artificial material or homologous material.
12. Perform a laminectomy in a patient with normal spinal anatomy.

13. Position a patient for intracranial or intraspinal surgery.
14. Demonstrate an ability to open and close cranial and spinal wounds including dural opening and repair.
15. Complete a sagittal synostectomy.

MIDDLE LEVEL

1. Close an open spinal or cranial neural tube defect.
2. Repair an intracranial encephalocele.
3. Make the opening for a complex craniofacial repair.
4. Perform the exposure for supratentorial and infratentorial lesions (excluding pineal, suprasellar, and intraventricular locations).
5. Perform the exposure for spinal exploration in a patient with abnormal spinal anatomy or reoperation.
6. Evacuate an intraparenchymal hematoma.
7. Accomplish an endoscopic third ventriculostomy in uncomplicated settings.
8. Apply and use frameless or framed stereotactic modalities for lesion location and shunt placement.
9. Accomplish repair of a Chiari malformation.
10. Accomplish an uncomplicated detethering procedure.
11. Perform a cranial vault expansion.
12. Perform placement of baclofen-type pumps.
13. Perform spinal fusion without instrumentation.
14. Apply a vagal nerve stimulator.

SENIOR LEVEL

1. Perform exposure for a suprasellar, pineal, and intraventricular lesion (including orbitofrontal, transcallosal, and supracerebellar).
2. Remove uncomplicated posterior fossa and supratentorial lesions.
3. Repair complex tethered cords (e.g., lipomyelomeningocele, retethering, and diastematomyelia).
4. Accomplish exposure for intradural spinal neoplasms.
5. Use an endoscope to communicate trapped CSF spaces.
6. Remove an intracranial vascular malformation less than 3 cm in size and in noneloquent brain.
7. Perform the placement of grids for seizure monitoring.
8. Perform a rhizotomy for spasticity.
9. Perform a temporal lobectomy in an uncomplicated patient.
10. Perform a stereotactic biopsy of a supratentorial lesion.
11. Perform a spinal fusion using instrumentation.

12. Accomplish endoscopic third ventriculostomy in uncomplicated settings.
13. Assist with complex craniofacial surgery.
14. Assist with a vascular procedure for moyamoya disease.

SURGERY OF THE PERIPHERAL NERVOUS SYSTEM

Unit Objectives

Demonstrate an understanding of the anatomy, physiology, pathophysiology, and presentation of peripheral nerve diseases. Demonstrate the ability to formulate and implement a diagnostic and treatment plan for diseases of the peripheral nerves that are amenable to surgical intervention.

Competency-Based Knowledge Objectives

JUNIOR LEVEL

1. Define the peripheral nervous system versus the CNS.
2. Discuss the major structural elements of a peripheral nerve.
   a. epineurium
   b. perineurium
   c. endoneurium
   d. axon
   e. fascicle
   f. Schwann cell
   g. connective tissue
   h. motor end plate
   i. sensory receptor
3. Discuss the blood supply of the peripheral nerves.
4. Discuss the blood–nerve barrier.
5. Define axonal transport and differentiate fast from slow.
6. Describe an action potential including the flow of ions.
7. Describe the various nerve fibers in terms of size.
8. Discuss the significance of fiber size in terms of function (e.g., c-fiber, nociceptive).
9. Discuss the various forms of action potential propagation.
10. Discuss the pathophysiological response to various injuries by a nerve.
    a. compression
    b. ischemia
    c. metabolic
    d. concussive
    e. stretch

11. Define and discuss apoptosis.
12. Define Wallerian degeneration.
13. Discuss nerve regeneration.
    a. sprouting
    b. nerve growth factors
    c. rate of growth
    d. remyelination
14. Define neuroma.
    a. axonal tangle
    b. mechanosensitivity
    c. neuroma-in-continuity
15. Define and discuss the pathophysiology and clinical significance of Tinel's sign.
16. Describe the symptoms and signs of typical nerve injuries.
    a. entrapment syndromes
    b. stretch injuries
    c. laceration injuries
    d. concussive injuries
    e. injection injuries
17. Distinguish upper versus lower motor neuron symptoms and signs in nerve injury.
    a. anatomic definition
    b. degree of atrophy
    c. distribution of weakness
    d. reflex changes
    e. potential for recovery
18. Describe the classification of nerve injury.
    a. Seddon classification
    b. Sunderland classification
19. List the major peripheral nerves of the body. Describe the motor and sensory innervation of each.
20. Draw the major components of the brachial plexus.
21. Describe the rating scales for motor power.
22. Describe the various sensory modalities and how to examine each.
23. Describe the symptoms and signs of common nerve entrapments.
    a. carpal tunnel
    b. ulnar entrapment at the elbow
    c. lateral femoral cutaneous nerve
    d. peroneal at the fibular head
24. Define EMG and NCV.
25. Describe the changes in EMG and NCV in nerve entrapment.

26. Describe the nonoperative and operative treatment of entrapment syndromes.
27. Define
    a. coaptation
    b. neurorrhaphy
    c. neurotization
    d. nerve transfer

MIDDLE LEVEL

1. Define the autonomic nervous system.
    a. Differentiate between sympathetic and parasympathetic.
    b. Discuss anatomic distribution.
    c. Identify the various neurotransmitters.
    d. Discuss Horner's syndrome.
2. Compare and contrast a peripheral nerve to a cranial nerve.
    a. histology
    b. response to injury
    c. root entry zone
3. Describe nerve regeneration in terms of
    a. specificity
    b. pruning of sprouts
    c. end-to-side sprouting
4. Draw the complete brachial plexus.
5. Discuss the lumbar plexus.
6. Discuss stretch injury, missile injury, and avulsion injury.
    a. definition
    b. typical etiology
    c. physical findings
    d. electrical findings
    e. nonoperative management
    f. indications for surgery
    g. intraoperative findings
    h. potential for recovery
7. Describe the anatomic location of the common entrapment sites. List the various bands and arcades that produce entrapment.
8. Provide a differential diagnosis for common entrapment syndromes.
    a. Differentiate radiculopathies from entrapments.
    b. Discuss repetitive strain disorder.
9. Discuss uncommon entrapment neuropathies.
    a. Guyon's canal
    b. suprascapular entrapment

   c. radial tunnel/PIN
   d. median nerve in the forearm/AIN
   e. tarsal tunnel (anterior and posterior)
   f. pyriformis syndrome
10. Explain the use of EMG and NCV in the management of peripheral nerve disorders.
   a. physiology
   b. typical findings in neuropathy
   c. typical findings in nerve injury
   d. typical findings in nerve regeneration
11. Discuss the common metabolic/inherited neuropathies.
12. Discuss burn and electrical injury effects on nerves.
13. Classify peripheral nerve tumors.
14. Discuss the pathophysiology of neurofibromatosis types 1 and 2.
15. Discuss the timing of peripheral nerve surgery.
   a. laceration injury
   b. blunt injury
   c. missile injury
   d. iatrogenic injury
   e. surgical injury
   f. injection injury
16. Discuss outcome priorities in brachial plexus surgery.
   a. motor versus sensory
   b. functional outcome (e.g., elbow flexion, shoulder abduction, etc.)
17. Discuss tension at the nerve repair site.
18. Discuss nerve repair techniques.
   a. direct coaptation
   b. nerve graft
   c. nerve transfer
   d. donor (graft) nerves
   e. epineurial repair
   f. fascicular repair
19. Describe intraoperative nerve evaluation.
   a. visual
   b. palpation
   c. internal neurolysis
   d. nerve conduction
   e. biopsy

SENIOR LEVEL

1. Discuss with the aid of diagrams the anatomy of the peripheral nervous system.
   a. common sites of entrapments

   b. the brachial and lumbar plexus
   c. innervation of the bladder
2. Discuss the use of nerve grafting.
   a. types of fixation (suture/glue)
   b. types of grafts (nerve, vein, artificial)
   c. end to side
3. Discuss entrapment syndromes.
   a. thoracic outlet
   b. double-crush syndrome
   c. repetitive strain
4. Discuss ulnar nerve decompression.
   a. in situ decompression
   b. transposition (subcutaneous, intramuscular, submuscular)
   c. medial epicondylectomy
5. Differentiate brachial plexus injury from brachial plexitis.
6. Formulate a management plan for
   a. birth brachial plexus injury
   b. acute nerve injury (stretch, compression, laceration, injection)
   c. chronic nerve injury
   d. failed nerve decompression
   e. painful nerve/neuroma
7. Describe the management of nerve tumors.
   a. imaging techniques, including MR neurography
   b. indications for surgery in neurofibromatosis type 1
   c. operative and adjuvant treatment for malignant peripheral nerve sheath tumors
   d. use of monitoring during tumor surgery
   e. fascicular dissection
8. Describe adjuvant therapies in nerve injury.
   a. muscle and tendon transfers
   b. prosthesis
   c. joint fusion

Competency-Based Performance Objectives

JUNIOR LEVEL

1. Obtain a history and perform a motor and sensory examination of the peripheral nervous system.
2. Based on the history and physical examination, localize the lesion anatomically.
3. Obtain appropriate ancillary tests.
   a. EMG and NCV
   b. metabolic screens
   c. imaging studies

4. Formulate a differential diagnosis for common entrapments.
5. Position and prepare for common entrapment releases.
6. Perform a diagnostic nerve and muscle biopsy.
7. Obtain the sural nerve for grafting.

MIDDLE LEVEL

1. Provide pre- and postoperative care of the patient with a peripheral nerve injury.
2. Evaluate a child with birth palsy.
3. Position a patient for nerve surgery.
   a. all entrapment sites
   b. brachial plexus surgery
4. Perform a neurolysis/decompression.
5. Expose the brachial plexus.
6. Manage the pain associated with nerve injury.
   a. use of medications
   b. use of rehabilitation
   c. use of stimulation

SENIOR LEVEL

1. Perform a consultation concerning a nerve injury.
2. Discuss the risks versus benefits of a surgical repair of a given nerve injury.
3. Determine the parameters confirming anticipated nerve regeneration.
   a. anticipated advancing Tinel's sign
   b. order of muscle reinnervation
4. Perform a nerve decompression.
   a. carpal tunnel
   b. ulnar nerve at the elbow
   c. peroneal nerve
5. Perform a nerve repair.
   a. neurolysis
   b. internal neurolysis
   c. intraoperative nerve conductions
   d. neuroma excision
   e. placement and suture of nerve graft
6. Excise a nerve sheath tumor.
7. Expose a brachial plexus injury.
   a. Determine possible repairs including nerve transfers.
   b. Expose the spinal accessory nerve.
   c. Expose the intercostal nerves.

SPINAL SURGERY

Unit Objectives

Demonstrate an understanding of the anatomy, physiology, pathophysiology, and presentation of disorders of the spine, its connecting ligaments, the spinal cord, the cauda equina, and the spinal roots. Demonstrate the ability to formulate and implement a diagnostic and treatment plan for diseases of the spine, its connecting ligaments, the spinal cord, the cauda equina, and the spinal roots that are amenable to surgical intervention.

Competency-Based Knowledge Objectives

JUNIOR LEVEL

1. Review the anatomy of the craniocervical junction; cervical, thoracic, and lumbar spine; sacrum; and pelvis.
2. Interpret plain and dynamic radiographs, bone scans, myelograms, CT scans, and MR images of patients with spinal disorders.
3. Review the signs, symptoms, and pathophysiology of common syndromes of degenerative spinal disorders: radiculopathy, myelopathy, instability, and neurogenic claudication.
4. Identify the common syndromes of spinal cord injury, including complete transverse injury, anterior cord injury, Brown–Sequard injury, central cord injury, cruciate paralysis, syringomyelia, conus syndrome, and sacral sparing. Describe the pathophysiology of spinal cord injury.
5. Describe the cauda equina syndrome.
6. Recite the differential diagnosis of cervical, thoracic, and lumbar pain.
7. Discuss the indications for cervical, thoracic, and lumbar discectomy.
8. Identify nonsurgical spinal cord syndromes including amyotrophic lateral sclerosis, demyelinating conditions, and combined systems disease.
9. Review the initial management of spine- and spinal cord-injured patients including immobilization, traction, reduction, appropriate radiographic studies, and medical management.
10. Classify fractures, dislocations, and ligament injuries of the craniocervical region; subaxial cervical spine; thoracic and thoracolumbar junction; and lumbar and sacral spine. Describe the mechanism of injury and classify the injuries as stable or unstable. Review the indications for surgical management.

11. Discuss briefly the concept of grading schemes for spinal cord injury and myelopathy.

MIDDLE LEVEL

1. Review the biomechanics of the craniocervical junction, cervical spine, and thoracolumbar and lumbar spine.
2. Review the biomechanics of common internal spinal fixators.
3. Review the definition of spinal instability based on the principles of Punjabi and White and other authors.
4. Recognize the radiographic signs of degenerative neoplastic, traumatic, and congenital spinal instability.
5. Review the indications for, uses, and relative effectiveness of common spinal orthoses. Discuss the degree of segmental and regional immobilization these orthoses provide.
6. Review the indications for and physiology of intraoperative spinal cord monitoring. Describe the technical aspects of intraoperative spinal cord monitoring.
7. Compare and contrast indications for anterior and posterior approaches to the cervical spine for the treatment of herniated cervical discs, spondylosis, and instability.
8. Discuss the role of corpectomy in the management of cervical disorders.
9. Compare and contrast the indications for anterior cervical discectomy with and without anterior interbody fusion.
10. Discuss the indications and techniques for anterior and posterior cervical spinal internal fixators.
11. Explain the biology of bone healing and options for bone grafting in spinal surgery.
12. Review the diagnosis and management of primary spinal tumors, spinal cord tumors, and spinal metastatic disease including indications for dorsal decompression, ventral decompression, and radiotherapy.
13. Discuss the management principles for gunshot and other penetrating wounds to the spine.
14. Review the signs, symptoms, and management options in the treatment of the adult tethered cord syndrome and syringomyelia.
15. Review management principles for spontaneous and postoperative spinal infections.
16. Review the management principles for intraoperative and postoperative CSF leaks.
17. Discuss the surgical management of intradural congenital, neoplastic, and vascular lesions.

SENIOR LEVEL

1. Describe indications for the use of angiography and endovascular procedures in the management of spinal disorders.
2. Discuss the management of cervical degenerative disease secondary to rheumatoid arthritis. Describe factors that make it different from the management of nonrheumatoid disease.
3. Compare and contrast the treatment options for cervical spondylotic myelopathy and ossification of the posterior longitudinal ligament, including multilevel anterior cervical corpectomy and fusion, laminectomy, laminectomy and fusion, laminoplasty, and nonoperative therapies.
4. Discuss the indications for posterior cervical spinal internal fixators.
5. Compare and contrast the transthoracic, transpedicular, costotransverse, and lateral extracavitary approaches to a herniated thoracic disc, thoracic tumor, or thoracic spinal injury.
6. Discuss the indications for lumbar fusion for congenital disorders, iatrogenic disease, and degenerative disease, ranking indications from least to most controversial.
7. Compare and contrast the indications for anterior or posterior lumbar interbody fusion and intertransverse fusion for lumbar disease.
8. Discuss internal fixation options for posterior lumbar interbody fusion and intertransverse fusion.
9. Summarize the most common types of spinal tumors in the following categories.
   a. intradural/intramedullary
   b. intradural/extramedullary
   c. extradural/extramedullary
10. Discuss nonoperative and operative treatment options for fractures and dislocations affecting the atlas and axis.
11. Compare and contrast the indications for nonoperative treatment, anterior approaches, and posterior operative approaches for the treatment of fractures and dislocations of the subaxial cervical spine.
12. Describe the indications for anterior, posterior, and posterolateral procedures in the management of thoracolumbar tumor, trauma, or infection.
13. Compare and contrast the indications for anterior and posterior spinal fixators in the management of thoracolumbar tumor, trauma, or infection.
14. Discuss reconstruction options for vertebral body defects after corpectomy for tumor, trauma, or infection.

Competency-Based Performance Objectives

JUNIOR LEVEL

1. Perform a complete history and physical examination on patients with spinal disorders.
2. Interpret plain radiographs, dynamic radiographs, myelograms, CT scans, and MR images of patients with spinal disorders.
3. Prepare patients for spinal surgery, including proper positioning, protection of pressure points, and placement of indicated arterial and central venous catheters, indwelling urinary catheters, and antiembolism devices.
4. Perform lumbar punctures and placement of lumbar drains.
5. Demonstrate the ability to place and manage cranial traction devices for reduction and immobilization of the unstable cervical spine.
6. Demonstrate the ability to place and manage a halo vest, including indications for placement and criteria for removal.
7. Demonstrate the ability to place properly the Mayfield head holder and other headrests.
8. Demonstrate the ability to harvest autologous bone graft from the calvarium, rib, fibula, and anterior or posterior iliac crest.
9. Perform dorsal exposure of the spinous processes, laminae, and facets of the cervical, thoracic, and lumbar spine.
10. Demonstrate the ability to close dorsal, ventral, and lateral spinal incisions.
11. Demonstrate proper postoperative wound care.
12. Demonstrate appropriate postoperative management of patients who have undergone spinal procedures.
13. Demonstrate the ability to perform, with supervision, a lumbar decompressive laminectomy for spinal stenosis.
14. Demonstrate the ability to excise, with supervision, a herniated lumbar disc.
15. Demonstrate the appropriate use of the operating microscope.

MIDDLE LEVEL

1. Demonstrate the ability to prepare structural allografts for use in spinal surgery.
2. Determine the need for postoperative inpatient or outpatient rehabilitation in patients with spinal disorders.
3. Demonstrate the ability to perform a ventral exposure of the cervical spine followed by anterior cervical discectomy.
4. Demonstrate the ability to perform an anterior cervical interbody arthrodesis.

5. Demonstrate the ability to place anterior cervical instrumentation.
6. Demonstrate the ability to perform posterior cervical decompressive laminectomy.
7. Demonstrate the ability to perform posterior cervical foraminotomy with or without discectomy.
8. Demonstrate the ability to perform medial and lateral approaches to a far lateral lumbar disc herniation.
9. Demonstrate appropriate surgical technique in the management of recurrent lumbar disc herniations and recurrent lumbar stenosis.
10. Demonstrate the ability to perform posterior lumbar arthrodesis with or without the use of interbody instrumentation.
11. Demonstrate exposure of the cervical lateral masses, thoracic and lumbar transverse processes, and the sacral ala.
12. Demonstrate the ability to perform posterior/intertransverse arthrodesis in the cervical, thoracic, and lumbar regions.
13. Demonstrate the ability to perform a laminectomy with or without transpedicular decompression for tumor, infection, or trauma.
14. Demonstrate techniques for spinous process arthrodesis of the subaxial cervical spine for fracture or dislocation.
15. Demonstrate the ability to manage postoperative complications of spinal surgery including
    a. hematoma
    b. infection
    c. spinal fluid leak
    d. new neurological deficit
16. Demonstrate the ability to perform a tethered cord release.

SENIOR LEVEL

1. Demonstrate the ability to function independently in all phases of management of patients with spinal disorders.
2. Demonstrate the ability to perform occipital–cervical arthrodesis.
3. Demonstrate the ability to place properly sublaminar wires, lateral mass screws, lower cervical/upper thoracic pedicle screws, C2 pars interarticularis screws, and C1–C2 transarticular screws for the management of cervical spine disorders.
4. Demonstrate the ability to perform, with assistance if necessary, transoral odontoidectomy.
5. Demonstrate common techniques for performing C1–C2 arthrodesis.

6. Demonstrate the ability to perform anterior cervical corpectomy followed by arthrodesis.
7. Demonstrate the ability to perform, with assistance if necessary, transthoracic, thoracoabdominal, retroperitoneal, and transabdominal approaches to the thoracic and lumbar spine.
8. Demonstrate the ability to perform costotransverse and lateral extracavitary approaches to the thoracolumbar spine.
9. Demonstrate the ability to excise a herniated thoracic disc by use of the previously mentioned approaches.
10. Demonstrate the ability to perform vertebral corpectomy of the thoracolumbar spine for tumor, infection, or trauma using the previously mentioned approaches.
11. Demonstrate the ability to perform anterior arthrodesis of the thoracolumbar spine.
12. Demonstrate the proper placement of transpedicular screws in the thoracic and lumbar spine.
13. Demonstrate the proper placement of laminar, transverse process, and pedicle hooks in the thoracic and lumbar spine.
14. Demonstrate the ability to resect intradural spinal neoplasms.
15. Demonstrate the ability to perform methylmethacrylate vertebroplasty.
16. Demonstrate techniques of open reduction of fractures and dislocations of the cervical, thoracic, and lumbar spine.
17. Demonstrate the ability to manage arachnoid cysts and spinal cord syrinx surgically.
18. Demonstrate the ability to perform intradural procedures for congenital, neoplastic, and vascular lesions.

STEREOTACTIC AND FUNCTIONAL NEUROSURGERY

Unit Objectives

Define neurosurgical stereotactic procedures and recognize their proper application. Describe the appropriate anatomy, physiology, and presentation of patients who are candidates for stereotactic procedures.

Competency-Based Knowledge Objectives

JUNIOR LEVEL

1. Discuss the considerations of stereotactic frame placement with regard to target localization and purpose of procedure (biopsy, craniotomy, functional, radiosurgery).
2. Describe the direct and indirect basal ganglion–thalamocortical motor pathways.

3. Define and distinguish each of the following entities.
   a. tremor
   b. rigidity
   c. dystonia
   d. chorea
   e. athetosis
4. Describe the pathophysiology of Parkinson's disease and cerebellar tremor.
5. Explain the primary symptoms treated by ventrolateral (VL) thalamotomy pallidotomy.
6. Discuss the advantages and disadvantages of stereotactic biopsy compared with open biopsy procedures.
7. Discuss the differential diagnosis of a newly discovered ring-enhancing intracranial mass.
8. Discuss the differential diagnosis of a newly discovered nonenhancing intracranial mass.
9. Define different seizure types (partial, partial–complex, generalized, etc.).
10. Define medically intractable epilepsy.
11. Describe the anatomy of the mesial temporal lobe.
12. Define brachytherapy.
13. Define conventional care for patients with high-grade gliomas.
14. Review the limitations of conventional care for patients with high-grade gliomas.
15. Describe the anatomy of the trigeminal nuclei, root, ganglion, and divisions.
16. Define typical trigeminal neuralgia, atypical trigeminal neuralgia, and trigeminal neuropathy.
17. Explain the potential causes for trigeminal neuralgia.
18. Define stereotactic radiosurgery.
19. Explain the differences between radiosurgery and radiation therapy.
20. List the potential indications for radiosurgery.
21. List the reported complications of radiosurgery.
22. Compare advantages and disadvantages of frame-based or frameless stereotactic craniotomies to nonstereotactic craniotomies.

MIDDLE LEVEL

1. Describe factors guiding the choice of neuroimaging (CT, MRI, MR angiography) for stereotactic procedures.

2. Explain the rationale for various MRI sequences used for tumor localization and functional procedures.
3. Discuss the benefits and limitations of frame-based stereotactic procedures.
4. Discuss patient selection for VL thalamotomy and pallidotomy.
5. Discuss the advantages and disadvantages of ablative procedures.
6. List the potential complications of VL thalamotomy, pallidotomy, and bilateral thalamotomies or pallidotomies.
7. Discuss technical considerations to minimize the potential for an intracranial hemorrhage after a stereotactic biopsy.
8. Discuss technical considerations to minimize the potential for a nondiagnostic stereotactic biopsy.
9. Describe the appropriate trajectories to acquire a biopsy specimen of a lesion in the pineal region, midbrain, pons, and medulla.
10. Compare the advantages and disadvantages of radiosurgery and surgical resection for tumors and vascular malformations.

SENIOR LEVEL

1. Identify the microelectrode recordings of the thalamus and globus pallidus.
2. Identify the primary indications for medial thalamotomy and cingulotomy.
3. Describe the evaluation of a patient with medically intractable epilepsy.
4. Discuss the indications for placement of depth electrodes.
5. Describe the surgical treatment of epilepsy in detail.
6. Discuss the theoretical advantages of brachytherapy over external beam radiation therapy.
7. Describe the most common complications of brachytherapy and their treatment.
8. Explain the effect of patient selection on the reported results of brachytherapy for high-grade gliomas.
9. Describe the methods used to localize and penetrate percutaneously the foramen ovale.
10. List the potential advantages and disadvantages for the following trigeminal rhizotomy procedures.
    a. glycerol
    b. radiofrequency
    c. balloon compression

11. Discuss the dose–volume relationships for radiation-related complications after radiosurgery.
12. Discuss potential sources of inaccuracy for stereotactic procedures.
13. Discuss the advantages and disadvantages of deep brain stimulation compared with ablative techniques.

Competency-Based Performance Objectives

MIDDLE LEVEL

1. Perform simple radiosurgery dose planning.

SENIOR LEVEL

1. Perform complex radiosurgery dose planning.
2. Perform stereotactic craniotomies.

Author Index

Subject Index